Keratoconus

Sujata Das
Editor

Keratoconus

Diagnosis and Treatment

Springer

Editor
Sujata Das
L V Prasad Eye Institute
Bhubaneswar, Odisha, India

ISBN 978-981-19-4264-8 ISBN 978-981-19-4262-4 (eBook)
https://doi.org/10.1007/978-981-19-4262-4

This Springer imprint is published by the registered company Springer Nature Singapore Pte Ltd.
The registered company address is: 152 Beach Road, #21-01/04 Gateway East, Singapore 189721, Singapore

Foreword

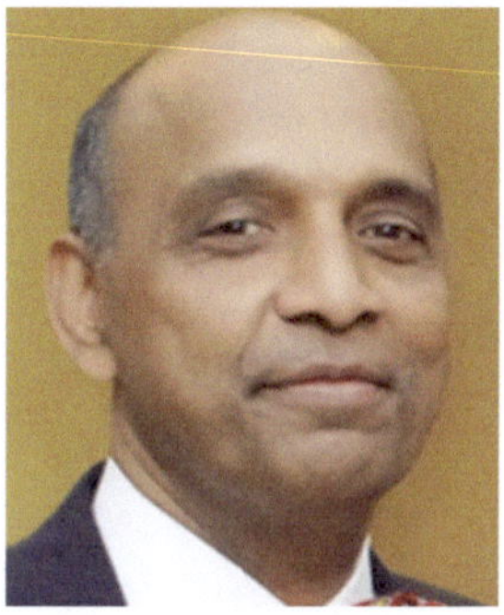

The problem of keratoconus is gaining increasing attention all over the world as the newer diagnostic approaches made it possible to recognize this entity earlier and better. This is now considered the most common ectatic disorder of the cornea. Multiple factors contribute to the causation of keratoconus—genetic, mechanical, and other factors.

The management of this problem has several options ranging from simple optical correction in the early stages to a variety of surgical procedures in the later stages, usually with high degree of success.

Dr Sujata Das is a very experienced and accomplished clinician with special interest in keratoconus. Other contributing authors are all very well-known corneal specialists with excellent record of publishing. This book has benefitted immensely from this pool of talent and hence provided a comprehensive coverage of this topic.

I congratulate the authors on this effort and recommend this volume to all those who wish to get more information on keratoconus from a single source.

L V Prasad Eye Institute,
L V Prasad Marg, Banjara Hills
Hyderabad, Telangana, India

Gullapalli N. Rao

Foreword

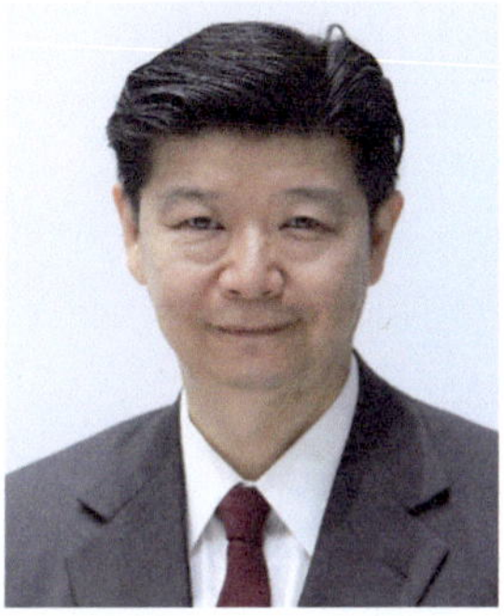

It is a great honor that I have been given the privilege to write the foreword for the book *Keratoconus* edited by Sujata Das.

Dr Das is actively involved in cornea and anterior segment disorders, including keratoconus, corneal infections, and eye banking. She is one of the leaders in the field, who has received numerous awards such as the Developing Country Eye Researcher Award from the Association for Research in Vision and Ophthalmology Foundation and the Achievement Award from the American Academy of Ophthalmology.

Keratoconus is a classic disease that has been known for a long time, and it is relatively common among corneal diseases. However, the cause of keratoconus has not yet been determined, and the diagnosis and treatment of keratoconus have changed with time. In the past, keratoconus was a non-inflammatory corneal thinning disorder and the only way to control its progression was to let it grow naturally, but now keratoconus is considered to be a chronic inflammatory disease whose progression can be suppressed. The paradigm shift in keratoconus care requires eye care specialists to be up to date.

The book comprises 23 chapters, with the topics ranging from public health and epidemiology to the newer paradigms in diagnosis and management. So, undoubtedly this textbook fulfils the needs of practitioners. My hearty congratulations to the authors for taking this great initiative.

Department of Ophthalmology
Osaka University Graduate School of Medicine,
Suita City, Osaka, Japan

Naoyuki Maeda

Preface

Keratoconus is an eye problem that affects young individuals. It is associated with significantly impaired vision-related quality of life (VRQoL). Many times, patients with keratoconus have associated allergy, which additionally impacts their daily activities. While early cases can be managed by glasses, there are various options for moderate to advanced disease. Whenever I examine these patients, especially children, I feel the challenges are many despite newer diagnostic techniques and treatment modalities.

Coming across the increasing number of patients with keratoconus in my clinical practice drove me to editing a comprehensive book on keratoconus to help cornea specialists and general ophthalmologists to better manage keratoconus cases. The authors are experts in their field and from various parts of the world.

Technology is emerging fast for the diagnosis of keratoconus. Similarly, the armamentarium of its visual rehabilitation procedures has expanded. Collagen crosslinking is a boon for these patients. Research is underway to understand the pathogenesis of the disease and its progression. I hope this book will be a useful guide and a ready reference for ophthalmologists in managing cases of keratoconus.

Bhubaneswar, Odisha, India — Sujata Das

Contents

About the Editor

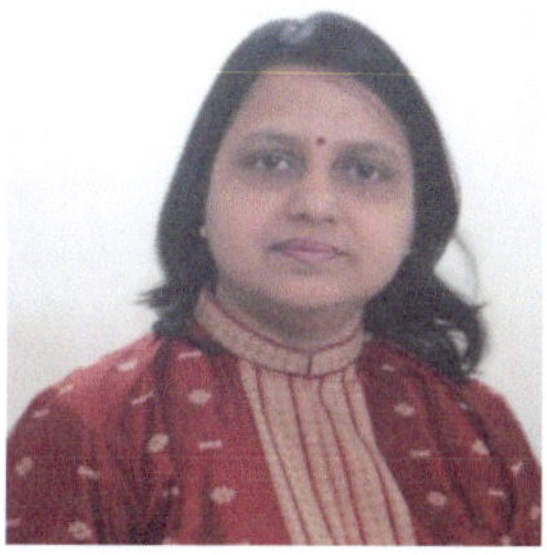

Sujata Das, MS, FRCS, AMPH, D.Sc.(h.c.) is a faculty member at the L V Prasad Eye Institute (LVPEI), Bhubaneswar, India. She received her postgraduate training in ophthalmology from MKCG Medical College and Hospital, Odisha, India, and FRCS (Glasgow) in ophthalmology. She completed her subspecialty training in cornea and anterior segment from LVPEI, Hyderabad, India. Further, she completed her ICO fellowship in cornea at the University of Erlangen-Nuremberg, Germany, and clinical fellowship in cornea at the Royal Victorian Eye and Ear Hospital and CERA, Melbourne University, Australia. She has pursued an advanced management program for health care from the Indian School of Business, Hyderabad, India, and received a DSc. (honoris causa) from the Ravenshaw University, Odisha, India. She is a recipient of several national and international awards.

Dr Das is presently involved in research encompassing corneal infections, eye banking, keratoconus, and genetic analysis of Fuchs' endothelial corneal dystrophy. She has authored over 140 peer-reviewed papers and book chapters to her credit. She has published a book entitled *Infections of the Cornea and Conjunctiva.*

1 Epidemiology of Keratoconus

Smruti Rekha Priyadarshini and Sujata Das

1.1 Introduction

Keratoconus (KC) is a bilateral, noninflammatory, progressive disorder characterized by thinning, ectasia resulting in conical protrusion of the cornea, irregular astigmatism, and myopia resulting in mild to marked impairment of vision. There lies a lack of understanding and clarity related to the etiology, inheritance, and pathophysiology of keratoconus. Epidemiology data has been largely collected and compiled based on hospital-based studies across the world.

1.2 Epidemiology

1.2.1 Incidence and Prevalence

The prevalence of keratoconus has been reported to vary widely across the world geographically between 0.0003% in Russia [1] and as high as 2.3% in Central India [2]. One of the earliest studies by Hofstetter has reported an incidence of 600 per 100,000 population where Placido disc was used for diagnosis [3]. Another study from the United States has reported a prevalence of 0.54% where scissors reflex and keratometry were used for diagnosis [4]. In this clinical and epidemiological study spanning over 48 years (1935–1982), it was observed that there was no significant trend noted in the incident rate. The prevalence figures from various epidemiological studies varied from 0.0003% [1] to 0.054% [4], 0.086% [5], 2.3% [2], and 2.34% [6]. Increased awareness among ophthalmologists and the emergence of better diagnostic modalities like topography and tomography have improved the sensitivity and early detection of this disorder as compared to the past. The annual incidence of keratoconus also varies geographically ranging from 50 to 230 per 100,000 population [7].

1.2.2 Age of Onset

A study by Lass et al. observed that almost two-thirds of patients present between 21 and 40 years of age, with only 10% presenting beyond 50 years [8]. Similar incidence and prevalence in the older population have been seen in other studies [9]. Ertan and coworkers have studied the distribution pattern in younger, middle, and older age groups to be 17.2%, 75.3%, and 7.5%, respectively [10]. Studies across the globe have observed that the mean age of presentation in Asians is early (21.5 years) as compared to the white population (26.4 years) [11]. A study from Saudi Arabia has shown the mean age of presentation as 15.5 ± 3.8 years [12], whereas in the United States, the mean age is 31.7 ± 10.9 (median 25 years) [4]. The disease is likely to progress to any stage till the age of 30 years and rarely

S. R. Priyadarshini · S. Das (✉)
L V Prasad Eye Institute, Bhubaneswar, Odisha, India
e-mail: drsmruti@lvpei.org; sujatadas@lvpei.org

S. Das (ed.), *Keratoconus*, https://doi.org/10.1007/978-981-19-4262-4_1

beyond 40 [13]. Factors such as genetic inheritance, availability of experienced ophthalmologists, diagnostic instruments, and lack of awareness may influence the age of the first presentation and hence diagnosis. With age, the interfibrillar spacing decreases, and collagen bundles become thicker. Such changes affect the rigidity and elasticity of the cornea which may be the possible hypothesis for the decrease in incidence of keratoconus with increase in age [14]. The onset is usually at puberty and progresses till the third to fourth decade of life, after which it usually stabilizes [15]. The average age of presentation in various studies is 29 years [4], 25 years [16], 28 years [9], and 22.9 years [17]. Saini et al. have reported that eyes with severe disease present early (18.8 ± 5.35 years) as compared to moderate disease (23.69 ± 8.07 years) [18]. Few studies have also reported a low percentage of patients beyond the fifth decade, ranging from 7.4% to 15% [19–21]. The disease is usually asymptomatic in the initial years; hence, the age of diagnosis may not be the age of onset in most cases.

1.2.3 Gender

A female preponderance has been reported in various ratios ranging from 57% to 66.7% [2, 7, 22]. However, Palimeris et al. had a different observation and reported male preponderance (69.8%) [23]. Other studies also found a male predominance, such as 57% [24], 62% [25], 62% [19], 59% [17], 53% [26], and 62% [10]. Another study based on gender differences (CLEK study) showed that women were much older, were more likely to report a family history of keratoconus, and were mostly non-whites. The mean age of female subjects was 40 years versus male subjects which was 38.3 years [27].

1.2.4 Laterality

Keratoconus is usually a bilateral disease, often asymmetric. Clinically, it may manifest unilaterally in one eye first, but careful examination like the presence of scissors reflex, keratometry readings, topography, and tomography will help to pick up early stages of keratoconus especially the forme fruste variant. In many cases, this disorder affects one eye first and eventually the fellow eye. Such observations have been reported by Li and coworkers where 50% of the fellow eye which were normal at presentation progressed to Keratoconus within 16 years of follow-up [28]. Krachmer in his case series has reported unilaterality in 14.3% [7]. Kennedy in his 48-year-long epidemiology study mentioned the disease to be unilateral (41%) and bilateral (59%) at the time of diagnosis [4]. This may be due to the initial asymmetric presentation and lack of investigational modalities in those early days. Also, 6 out of 26 patients were found to have the other eye involvement later during follow-up.

1.3 Risk Factors

Keratoconus is a multifactorial disorder. It is a biomechanical and biochemical disorder resulting from a complex interplay of genetic and environmental risk factors.

1.3.1 Genetic

Keratoconus most commonly presents as a sporadic disorder. A very small subset may exhibit an autosomal dominant mode of inheritance. Further investigations point toward the complete penetrance of predisposing factors with various phenotypic expressions as underlying etiology. In a few patients, heterozygous mutation of the VSX1 gene has also been detected [29, 30]. There have also been anecdotal reports of keratoconus in identical twins across the world. Females are more predisposed to develop this clinical condition which points toward the possibility of an X-linked transmission. A review of 304 cases by Hallerman and Wilson concluded that the frequency of inheritance was 7% with a multifactorial mode of transmission [31]. Autosomal mode of inheritance has been reported in 20 cases [32]. Rabinowitz had reported that the two important factors responsible were positive family history and habit of eye rubbing. A family history of keratoconus has been reported to be 0.05–0.23% [15] and 13.5% [33]. First-degree relatives have been found to have more prevalence (3.34%) [34].

Both genetic and environmental factors have been studied (twin studies) in 21 monozygotic twins and have been found to have a 54% concordance rate [35, 36]. There have been studies where discordance among monozygotic twins was also seen [17, 37, 38]. In such cases, a possible role of environmental factors such as eye rubbing and hormonal effects may be responsible. Further genetic studies by Li et al. was also done where fine mapping of keratoconus patients along with ethnically matched controls suggested that SNPrs4954218 near the RAB3GAP1 gene may be a possible locus [39]. Recent study by Burdon and coworkers have found genetic variation at hepatocyte growth factor (HGF) locus to be responsible [40].

Varying rates of prevalence among different ethnic groups from the same geographical area point toward the genetic basis of the entity, which has been observed in a UK-based study where higher prevalence was observed in Indians and Pakistanis as compared to British natives [41]. Consanguinity also contributes to the genetic basis of the disease [42].

Family history plays a very significant role affecting 10% versus 0.05% of an age-matched control group [43]. Other studies suggesting such familial contribution is the CLEK study (13.5%) [9]. A study from New Zealand also reported a very high rate in families of twins (23.5%) with several families reporting multiple cases of keratoconus [17]. Among them, 11 pairs of twins were detected with at least 1 keratoconic sibling.

1.3.2 Ethnic Groups

Keratoconus affects people across the whole world. The prevalence may range widely among different ethnic groups residing in the same geographical location. Both ethnic preponderances along with environmental factors together contribute to the etiology of the disorder.

Surveys from the United Kingdom have observed a higher prevalence in the Asian population (4.4 and 7.5 times) respectively in two different studies as compared to white Caucasians [11, 41]. It was also observed that Asian patients (predominantly Indian origin) had a fourfold increase in incidence, present early, and require keratoplasty earlier in life as compared to white patients [41]. In a study at a UK-based hospital, it was found that the incidence of keratoconus was more in Asians of north Pakistani origin (25 per 100,000) as compared to whites (3.3 per 100,000) [11]. A possibility of consanguineous marriage especially with the first cousin may be a strong genetic factor for such high incidence. A study by Millodot et al. has shown a higher prevalence in Middle East countries, Israeli Arabs (3.0%) and Israeli Jews (2.0%) [6]. Similarly, Maori and Pacific ethnicity were also found to have a larger prevalence [17]. Studies from Iran have reported an annual incidence rate of 22.3 (excluding suspected cases) and 24.9 (including suspected cases) per 100,000 population [44].

1.3.3 Eye Rubbing

Chronic habits of abnormal rubbing (CHAR) are considered a major environmental stress factor in the development of keratoconus. It may be incorporated into their daily activity as a repetitive habitual ritualistic behavior without being self-aware. This association has been much earlier reported to be an important etiological factor with a prevalence between 66% and 73% [7]. Eye rubbing is frequently seen in patients with vernal keratoconjunctivitis (VKC) and atopy [45]. Chronic eye rubbing is commonly associated among keratoconus patients with Leber congenital amaurosis, Down syndrome, atopic disease, contact lens wear, floppy eyelid syndrome, and nervous habitual eye rubbing [46]. A study by Bawazeer et al. involved assessment of potential risk factors, including atopy, family history, eye rubbing, and contact lens wear in 120 keratoconus subjects [47]. In the univariate analysis, there were associations between KC and atopy, family history, and eye rubbing. However, in the multivariate analysis, only eye rubbing was found to be a significant predictor of KC. Various other studies have reported approximately rigorous eye rubbing of at least 1 eye in 50% of keratoconus subjects [9, 48]. The mechanism in response to eye rubbing sequentially involves increased corneal temperature, epithelial thinning, increased levels of inflammatory mediators, anomalous enzyme activity, raised intraocular pressure, and hydrostatic tissue pressure. As a result, decreased viscosity and temporary displacement from the corneal apex lead to buckling, flexure of fibrils, and corneal indentation. Furthermore, this biomechanically coupled curvature may transfer to the cone apex resulting in the slippage between collagen fibrils due to mechanical trauma and/or high hydrostatic pressure, in addition to scar formation [49]. A case series by Jafri et al. reported patients with very asymmetric KC and found a clear history of mechanical trauma to the more affected eye within 1 month [50]. The possible underlying mechanism was microtrauma due to eye rubbing which injures the epithelium, leading to cytokine release, myofibroblast differentiation, a change in biomechanical forces, and thinning of corneal tissue and thereby ectasia. A case report of bilateral recurrent keratoconus following keratoplasty in a patient with self-induced keratoconus secondary to compulsive eye rubbing has also been reported [51].

Another correlation between disease asymmetry and sleeping on the worse side, often with the hand under the pillow, may over time lead to abnormalities such as a floppy eyelid and unilateral eyelash misdirection which points toward chronic nocturnal eyelid pressure [52]. Keratoconus patients usually rub with either a middle knuckle or a fingertip in a circular motion over the cornea often with significant posterior pressure. The intensity and duration (10–180 s or even up to 300 s) are much severe and repetitive.

1.3.4 Atopy

Atopy is associated with keratoconus and has been reported in the literature in the past [4, 53, 54]. Rahi et al. in their study of 182 cases of keratoconus found a definite history of atopy in 35% as compared to 12% in the matched control group. The serum IgE was also significantly raised ($p < 0001$) in these patients especially those with associated atopic disease [45]. The atopic individuals in the keratoconus series showed a female preponderance, and the commonest allergic disorder was hay fever, asthma, and eczema. The CLEK study reported a history of asthma (14.9%) and eczema (8.4%), with a higher percentage of hay fever (52.9%) and atopic history (53%) [9]. The DUSKS study reported a history of atopic diseases including asthma (23%), eczema (14%), and hay fever (30%) [48]. A recent study by Shajari et al. found a notable difference in the mean age between the control group (36.1 ± 11.7) and the atopic group, 32.8 ± 9.6 ($p = 0.002$) with 1 atopic trait, and 30.4 ± 7.5 with 2 or more atopic traits ($p = 0.002$) [55]. This finding may point that atopic syndrome can trigger the earlier manifestation of keratoconus, thereby suggesting frequent examination and early intervention.

1.3.5 Ultraviolet and Sun Exposure

Ultraviolet light (UV) is a source of reactive oxygen species (ROS). In keratoconus eyes, there is a reduced amount of the enzymes including aldehyde dehydrogenase class 3 (ALDH3) and superoxide dismutase which are necessary to remove the ROS. So, it has been observed that excessive exposure to sunlight results in oxidative damage to these keratoconic corneas [56, 57]. Therefore, a higher prevalence of KC is found in hot, sunny countries like Saudi Arabia, Iran, New Zealand, India, and some Pacific Islands.

Animal experiments further suggest that mice when exposed to UV light demonstrated degeneration of stromal collagen and stromal thinning resulting in apoptotic cell death and marked loss of keratocytes [58, 59]. Thus, sun exposure, especially in genetically susceptible individuals, poses a risk factor for the development of keratoconus.

However, it must also be kept in mind that UV radiations have a beneficial role by inducing cross-linking of corneal collagen, thus a useful surgical technique for halting the progression of keratoconus.

1.3.6 Hormonal

Hormones play a critical role in regulating tissue function by promoting cell survival, proliferation, and differentiation. Because keratoconus usually starts by puberty, hormones have been presumed as a possible cause. Also, there have been reports of sudden progression during pregnancy and after hormone replacement therapy. A study by McKay et al. has shown that both male and female KC patients had increased dehydroepiandrosterone sulfate (DHEA-S) levels (1.8-fold, $P = 0.047$) compared to the healthy controls supporting a role for elevated DHEA-S and reduced estrone in KC pathogenesis [60]. There have been case reports where keratoconus progression has been observed following pregnancy [61, 62], in vitro fertilization (IVF) [63], and the postmenopausal patient treated with hormone replacement therapy (HRT) [64].

1.3.7 Associated Systemic and Ocular Disorders

Keratoconus often occur as an isolated disorder. However, keratoconus has also been associated with other ocular, syndromic, and systemic disorders [7, 15, 65], which include Marfan syndrome, mitral valve prolapse, collagen vascular disease, pigmentary retinopathy, Leber congenital amaurosis, and Down syndrome. Previous studies have reported that approximately 0.5–15% of patients with Down syndrome can manifest keratoconus [65] or even a 10–300-fold higher prevalence [66]. Elder et al. have reported keratoconus in approximately 35% of patients with Leber congenital amaurosis, a clinically heterogeneous group of childhood retinal degenerations inherited in an autosomal recessive manner [67]. There seems to be a possibility of gene mutations in aryl hydrocarbon-interacting protein-like 1 (AIPL1) and crumbs homolog 1 (CRB1) in patients with Leber congenital amaurosis contributing toward keratoconus susceptibility [68–72]. Other connective tissue disorders which have been reported to be associated are osteogenesis imperfecta, GAPO syndrome, type IV Ehlers-Danlos syndrome, and mitral valve prolapse [73–76]. Also, a prevalence of keratoconus in immune-mediated disorders such as rheumatoid arthritis, ulcerative colitis, autoimmune chronic hepatitis, Hashimoto thyroiditis, arthropathy, irritable bowel syndrome, and asthma has been observed [77]. Case reports of Tourette syndrome associated with compulsive eye rubbing, a causative factor of keratoconus, have been reported [78, 79].

1.4 Conclusion

Keratoconus is the most common ectatic disorder of the cornea. It usually develops in the second decade of life around puberty time and progresses in the next two decades. It can affect either gender or all ethnic groups. Keratoconus is certainly multifactorial, and genetics plays an important role in pathogenesis as proved through twin studies, family-based linkage studies, and genetic association studies. A "two-hit" hypothesis in the pathogenesis is increasingly accepted suggesting that keratoconus patients need a genetic predisposition and an environmental factor for clinical manifestation of the disease (Table 1.1).

Table 1.1 Summary of previous epidemiologic studies in keratoconus patients

Study	Year	Method of diagnosis	Prevalence	Incidence	Gender	Laterality	Associated factors	Place of study	Age	Eye rubbing
Hofstetter et al. [3]	1959	Placido disc keratoscopy	0.6%	–	Female	–	–	Indianapolis, USA	–	–
Kennedy et al. [4]	1986	Scissors reflex, keratometry	0.54%	0.02%	Male	Bilateral (59%)	Asthma, eczema, hay fever (36%), mitral valve prolapse (5%)	Mayo Clinic, Rochester	25 (median)	25%
Ihalainen et al. [20]	1986	Clinically	0.03%	0.0015%	Male (67.5%)	–	Familial (19% North Finland, 9% South Finland), connective tissue disorders (67%)	Finland	Male, 26.5 ± 8.24; female, 30.6 ± 13.7	–
Owens et al. [17]	2003	Questionnaire based—optometrists, ophthalmologists	–	–	Male (59%)	Bilateral	Familial (23.5%), ethnicity (M/P descent), twins, atopy	New Zealand	22.9 years	63%
Saini et al. [18]	2004	Clinical findings, topography	–	–	Female	–	VKC (36%), eye rubbing (44%)	India	20.2 ± 6.4 years	44.3%
Georgiou et al. [11]	2004	Myopic astigmatism, clinical signs	–	Asian (25 per 100,000), whites (3.3 per 100,000)	Male (72%)	–	Ethnic (Asian of North Pakistan), atopy (whites)	U.K.	Asian (21.5 years), white (26.4 years)	50%
Assiri et al. [12]	2005	Keratometry, retinoscopy	–	Asir province 20 per 100,000	Female	–	Asir province (ethnic), atopy (56%), family h/o (16%), atopic dermatitis (16%)	Saudi Arabia	18.5 years	44.8%
Jonas et al. [2]	2009	Keratometry, pachymetry, biometry	2.3 ± 0.2 (>30 years)	–	Female	–	Low height, poor education, myopia, thin cornea	Central India	49.4 ± 13.4 (median: 46 years)	–
Sharma et al. [80]	2009	Keratometry, pachymetry, videokeratography			Males	Bilateral (88%)	VKC, atopy, eye rubbing	India	20.07 ± 6.4	55.8%
Millodot et al. [6]	2011	Videokeratography	2.34%	–	Male	–	Family history (21.7%), male, atopy (40.9)	Israel	24.4 ± 5.7	36.4%
Ziaei et al. [44]	2012	Topography	–	22.3–24.9 per 100,000	Male (54.4%)	–	–	Iran	28.5 ± 8.9	–

References

1. Gorskova EN, Sevost'ianov EN. Epidemiologiia keratokonusa na Urale [Epidemiology of keratoconus in the Urals]. Vestn oftalmol. 1998;114(4):38–40.
2. Jonas JB, Nangia V, Matin A, Kulkarni M, Bhojwani K. Prevalence and associations of keratoconus in rural Maharashtra in central India: the Central India eye and medical study. Am J Ophthalmol. 2009;148(5):760–5.
3. Hofstetter HW. A keratoscopic survey of 13,395 eyes. Am J Optom Arch Am Acad Optom. 1959;36(1):3–11.
4. Kennedy RH, Bourne WM, Dyer JA. A 48-year clinical and epidemiologic study of keratoconus. Am J Ophthalmol. 1986;101(3):267–73.
5. Nielsen K, Hjortdal J, Aagaard Nohr E, Ehlers N. Incidence and prevalence of keratoconus in Denmark. Acta Ophthalmol Scand. 2007;85(8):890–2.
6. Millodot M, Shneor E, Albou S, Atlani E, Gordon-Shaag A. Prevalence and associated factors of keratoconus in Jerusalem: a cross-sectional study. Ophthalmic Epidemiol. 2011;18(2):91–7.
7. Krachmer JH, Feder RS, Belin MW. Keratoconus and related noninflammatory corneal thinning disorders. Surv Ophthalmol. 1984;28(4):293–322.
8. Lass JH, Lembach RG, Park SB, Hom DL, Fritz ME, Svilar GM, Nuamah IF, Reinhart WJ, Stocker EG, Keates RH, et al. Clinical management of keratoconus. A multicenter analysis. Ophthalmology. 1990;97(4):433–45.
9. Zadnik K, Barr JT, Edrington TB, Everett DF, Jameson M, McMahon TT, Shin JA, Sterling JL, Wagner H, Gordon MO. Baseline findings in the Collaborative Longitudinal Evaluation of Keratoconus (CLEK) Study. Invest Ophthalmol Vis Sci. 1998;39(13):2537–46.
10. Ertan A, Muftuoglu O. Keratoconus clinical findings according to different age and gender groups. Cornea. 2008;27(10):1109–13.
11. Georgiou T, Funnell CL, Cassels-Brown A, O'Conor R. Influence of ethnic origin on the incidence of keratoconus and associated atopic disease in Asians and white patients. Eye (Lond). 2004;18(4):379–83.
12. Assiri AA, Yousuf BI, Quantock AJ, Murphy PJ. Incidence and severity of keratoconus in Asir province, Saudi Arabia. Br J Ophthalmol. 2005;89(11):1403–6.
13. Jacobs DS, Dohlman CH. Is keratoconus genetic? Int Ophthalmol Clin. 1993;33(2):249–60.
14. Francois M, Ancele E, Butterworth J. Epidemiology of keratoconus. In: Barbera A, editor. Textbook on keratoconus: new insights. New Delhi: Jaypee Digital; 2012. p. 1–11.
15. Rabinowitz YS. Keratoconus. Surv Ophthalmol. 1998;42(4):297–319.
16. Tuft SJ, Fitzke FW, Buckley RJ. Myopia following penetrating keratoplasty for keratoconus. Br J Ophthalmol. 1992;76(11):642–5.
17. Owens H, Gamble G. A profile of keratoconus in New Zealand. Cornea. 2003;22(2):122–5.
18. Saini JS, Saroha V, Singh P, Sukhija JS, Jain AK. Keratoconus in Asian eyes at a tertiary eye care facility. Clin Exp Optom. 2004;87(2):97–101.
19. Pobelle-Frasson C, Velou S, Huslin V, Massicault B, Colin J. Kératocône: que deviennent les patients âgés? [Keratoconus: what happens with older patients?]. J Fr Ophtalmol. 2004;27(7):779–82.
20. Ihalainen A. Clinical and epidemiological features of keratoconus genetic and external factors in the pathogenesis of the disease. Acta Ophthalmol Suppl. 1986;178:1–64.
21. Romagnani S. The increased prevalence of allergy and the hygiene hypothesis: missing immune deviation, reduced immune suppression, or both? Immunology. 2004;112(3):352–63.
22. Hammerstein W. Zur Genetik des Keratoconus [Genetics of conical cornea (author's transl)]. Albrecht Von Graefes Arch Klin Exp Ophthalmol. 1974;190(4):293–308.
23. Palimeris G. Some observations on the pathogenesis and management of keratoconus. In: Trevor-Roper PD, editor. Sixth congress of the European Society of Ophthalmology: the cornea in health and disease. Published jointly by the Royal Society of Medicine [and] Academic Press; 1981. p. 927–931.
24. Pouliquen Y, Forman MR, Giraud JP. Vitesse d'évolution du kératocone. Etude des relations entre l'âge de découverte t l'âge auquel il est opéré [Evaluation of the rapidity of progression of keratoconus by a study of the relationship between age when first detected and age at operation (author's transl)]. J Fr Ophtalmol. 1981;4(3):219–21.
25. Street DA, Vinokur ET, Waring GO 3rd, Pollak SJ, Clements SD, Perkins JV. Lack of association between keratoconus, mitral valve prolapse, and joint hypermobility. Ophthalmology. 1991;98(2):170–6.
26. Fatima T, Acharya MC, Mathur U, Barua P. Demographic profile and visual rehabilitation of patients with keratoconus attending contact lens clinic at a tertiary eye care centre. Cont Lens Anterior Eye. 2010;33(1):19–22.
27. Fink BA, Wagner H, Steger-May K, Rosenstiel C, Roediger T, McMahon TT, Gordon MO, Zadnik K. Differences in keratoconus as a function of gender. Am J Ophthalmol. 2005;140(3):459–68.
28. Li X, Rabinowitz YS, Rasheed K, Yang H. Longitudinal study of the normal eyes in unilateral keratoconus patients. Ophthalmology. 2004;111(3):440–6.
29. Dash DP, George S, O'Prey D, Burns D, Nabili S, Donnelly U, Hughes AE, Silvestri G, Jackson J, Frazer D, Héon E, Willoughby CE. Mutational screening of VSX1 in keratoconus patients from the European population. Eye (Lond). 2010;24(6):1085–92.
30. Héon E, Greenberg A, Kopp KK, Rootman D, Vincent AL, Billingsley G, Priston M, Dorval KM, Chow RL, McInnes RR, Heathcote G, Westall C, Sutphin JE,

Semina E, Bremner R, Stone EM. VSX1: a gene for posterior polymorphous dystrophy and keratoconus. Hum Mol Genet. 2002;11(9):1029–36.
31. Hallermann W, Wilson EJ. Genetische Betrachtungen über den Keratokonus [Genetic aspects of keratoconus (author's transl)]. Klin Monatsbl Augenheilkd. 1977;170(6):906–8.
32. Falls HF, Allen AW. Dominantly inherited keratoconus. J Genet Hum. 1969;17(3):317–24.
33. Wagner H, Barr JT, Zadnik K. Collaborative Longitudinal Evaluation of Keratoconus (CLEK) Study: methods and findings to date. Cont Lens Anterior Eye. 2007;30(4):223–32.
34. Wang Y, Rabinowitz YS, Rotter JI, Yang H. Genetic epidemiological study of keratoconus: evidence for major gene determination. Am J Med Genet. 2000;93(5):403–9.
35. Bechara SJ, Waring GO 3rd, Insler MS. Keratoconus in two pairs of identical twins. Cornea. 1996;15(1):90–3.
36. McMahon TT, Shin JA, Newlin A, Edrington TB, Sugar J, Zadnik K. Discordance for keratoconus in two pairs of monozygotic twins. Cornea. 1999;18(4):444–51.
37. Harrison RJ, Klouda PT, Easty DL, Manku M, Charles J, Stewart CM. Association between keratoconus and atopy. Br J Ophthalmol. 1989;73(10):816–22.
38. Parker J, Ko WW, Pavlopoulos G, Wolfe PJ, Rabinowitz YS, Feldman ST. Videokeratography of keratoconus in monozygotic twins. J Refract Surg. 1996;12(1):180–3.
39. Li X, Bykhovskaya Y, Haritunians T, Siscovick D, Aldave A, Szczotka-Flynn L, Iyengar SK, Rotter JI, Taylor KD, Rabinowitz YS. A genome-wide association study identifies a potential novel gene locus for keratoconus, one of the commonest causes for corneal transplantation in developed countries. Hum Mol Genet. 2012;21(2):421–9.
40. Burdon KP, Macgregor S, Bykhovskaya Y, Javadiyan S, Li X, Laurie KJ, Muszynska D, Lindsay R, Lechner J, Haritunians T, Henders AK, Dash D, Siscovick D, Anand S, Aldave A, Coster DJ, Szczotka-Flynn L, Mills RA, Iyengar SK, Taylor KD, Phillips T, Montgomery GW, Rotter JI, Hewitt AW, Sharma S, Rabinowitz YS, Willoughby C, Craig JE. Association of polymorphisms in the hepatocyte growth factor gene promoter with keratoconus. Invest Ophthalmol Vis Sci. 2011;52(11):8514–9.
41. Pearson AR, Soneji B, Sarvananthan N, Sandford-Smith JH. Does ethnic origin influence the incidence or severity of keratoconus? Eye (Lond). 2000;Pt 4:625–8.
42. Gordon-Shaag A, Millodot M, Essa M, Garth J, Ghara M, Shneor E. Is consanguinity a risk factor for keratoconus? Optom Vis Sci. 2013;90(5):448–54.
43. Rabinowitz YS. The genetics of keratoconus. Ophthalmol Clin N Am. 2003;16(4):607–20.
44. Ziaei H, Jafarinasab MR, Javadi MA, Karimian F, Poorsalman H, Mahdavi M, Shoja MR, Katibeh M. Epidemiology of keratoconus in an Iranian population. Cornea. 2012;31(9):1044–7.
45. Rahi A, Davies P, Ruben M, Lobascher D, Menon J. Keratoconus and coexisting atopic disease. Br J Ophthalmol. 1977;61(12):761–4.
46. Krachmer JH. Eye rubbing can cause keratoconus. Cornea. 2004;23(6):539–40.
47. Bawazeer AM, Hodge WG, Lorimer B. Atopy and keratoconus: a multivariate analysis. Br J Ophthalmol. 2000;84(8):834–6.
48. Weed KH, MacEwen CJ, Giles T, Low J, McGhee CN. The Dundee University Scottish Keratoconus study: demographics, corneal signs, associated diseases, and eye rubbing. Eye (Lond). 2008;22(4):534–41.
49. McMonnies CW. Mechanisms of rubbing-related corneal trauma in keratoconus. Cornea. 2009;28(6):607–15.
50. Jafri B, Lichter H, Stulting RD. Asymmetric keratoconus attributed to eye rubbing. Cornea. 2004;23(6):560–4.
51. Koenig SB. Bilateral recurrent self-induced keratoconus. Eye Contact Lens. 2008;34(6):343–4.
52. Carlson AN. Expanding our understanding of eye rubbing and keratoconus. Cornea. 2010;29(2):245.
53. Galin MA, Berger R. Atopy and keratoconus. Am J Ophthalmol. 1958;45(6):904–6.
54. Spencer WH, Fisher JJ. The association of keratoconus with atopic dermatitis. Am J Ophthalmol. 1959;47(3):332–44.
55. Shajari M, Eberhardt E, Müller M, Al Khateeb G, Friderich S, Remy M, Kohnen T. Effects of atopic syndrome on keratoconus. Cornea. 2016;35(11):1416–20.
56. Cristina Kenney M, Brown DJ. The cascade hypothesis of keratoconus. Cont Lens Anterior Eye. 2003;26(3):139–46.
57. Gondhowiardjo TD, van Haeringen NJ, Völker-Dieben HJ, Beekhuis HW, Kok JH, van Rij G, Pels L, Kijlstra A. Analysis of corneal aldehyde dehydrogenase patterns in pathologic corneas. Cornea. 1993;12(2):146–54.
58. Newkirk KM, Chandler HL, Parent AE, Young DC, Colitz CM, Wilkie DA, Kusewitt DF. Ultraviolet radiation-induced corneal degeneration in 129 mice. Toxicol Pathol. 2007;35(6):819–26.
59. Podskochy A, Gan L, Fagerholm P. Apoptosis in UV-exposed rabbit corneas. Cornea. 2000;19(1):99–103.
60. McKay TB, Hjortdal J, Sejersen H, Asara JM, Wu J, Karamichos D. Endocrine and metabolic pathways linked to keratoconus: implications for the role of hormones in the stromal microenvironment. Sci Rep. 2016;6:25534.
61. Bilgihan K, Hondur A, Sul S, Ozturk S. Pregnancy-induced progression of keratoconus. Cornea. 2011;30(9):991–4.
62. Soeters N, Tahzib NG, Bakker L, Van der Lelij A. Two cases of keratoconus diagnosed after pregnancy. Optom Vis Sci. 2012;89(1):112–6.
63. Yuksel E, Yalinbas D, Aydin B, Bilgihan K. Keratoconus progression induced by in vitro fertilization treatment. J Refract Surg. 2016;32(1):60–3.

64. Coco G, Kheirkhah A, Foulsham W, Dana R, Ciolino JB. Keratoconus progression associated with hormone replacement therapy. Am J Ophthalmol Case Rep. 2019;15:100519.
65. Romero-Jiménez M, Santodomingo-Rubido J, Wolffsohn JS. Keratoconus: a review. Cont Lens Anterior Eye. 2010;33(4):157–66.
66. Shapiro MB, France TD. The ocular features of Down's syndrome. Am J Ophthalmol. 1985;99(6):659–63.
67. Elder MJ. Leber congenital amaurosis and its association with keratoconus and keratoglobus. J Pediatr Ophthalmol Strabismus. 1994;31(1):38–40.
68. McMahon TT, Kim LS, Fishman GA, Stone EM, Zhao XC, Yee RW, Malicki J. CRB1 gene mutations are associated with keratoconus in patients with Leber congenital amaurosis. Invest Ophthalmol Vis Sci. 2009;50(7):3185–7.
69. Dharmaraj S, Leroy BP, Sohocki MM, Koenekoop RK, Perrault I, Anwar K, Khaliq S, Devi RS, Birch DG, De Pool E, Izquierdo N, Van Maldergem L, Ismail M, Payne AM, Holder GE, Bhattacharya SS, Bird AC, Kaplan J, Maumenee IH. The phenotype of Leber congenital amaurosis in patients with AIPL1 mutations. Arch Ophthalmol. 2004;122(7):1029–37.
70. McKibbin M, Ali M, Mohamed MD, Booth AP, Bishop F, Pal B, Springell K, Raashid Y, Jafri H, Inglehearn CF. Genotype-phenotype correlation for Leber congenital amaurosis in northern Pakistan. Arch Ophthalmol. 2010;128(1):107–13.
71. Damji KF, Sohocki MM, Khan R, Gupta SK, Rahim M, Loyer M, Hussein N, Karim N, Ladak SS, Jamal A, Bulman D, Koenekoop RK. Leber's congenital amaurosis with anterior keratoconus in Pakistani families is caused by the Trp278X mutation in the AIPL1 gene on 17p. Can J Ophthalmol. 2001;36(5):252–9.
72. Stoiber J, Muss WH, Ruckhofer J, Thaller-Antlanger H, Alzner E, Grabner G. Recurrent keratoconus in a patient with Leber congenital amaurosis. Cornea. 2000;19(3):395–8.
73. Balasubramanian SA, Pye DC, Willcox MD. Are proteinases the reason for keratoconus? Curr Eye Res. 2010;35(3):185–91.
74. Beckh U, Schönherr U, Naumann GO. Autosomal dominanter Keratokonus als okuläres Leitsymptom bei Osteogenesis imperfecta tarda Lobstein [Autosomal dominant keratoconus as the chief ocular symptom in Lobstein osteogenesis imperfecta tarda]. Klin Monatsbl Augenheilkd. 1995;206(4):268–72.
75. Wajntal A, Koiffmann CP, Mendonça BB, Epps-Quaglia D, Sotto MN, Rati PB, Opitz JM. GAPO syndrome (McKusick 23074)—a connective tissue disorder: report on two affected sibs and on the pathologic findings in the older. Am J Med Genet. 1990;37(2):213–23.
76. Robertson I. Keratoconus and the Ehlers-Danlos syndrome: a new aspect of keratoconus. Med J Aust. 1975;1(18):571–3.
77. Nemet AY, Vinker S, Bahar I, Kaiserman I. The association of keratoconus with immune disorders. Cornea. 2010;29(11):1261–4.
78. Mashor RS, Kumar NL, Ritenour RJ, Rootman DS. Keratoconus caused by eye rubbing in patients with Tourette syndrome. Can J Ophthalmol. 2011;46(1):83–6.
79. Kandarakis A, Karampelas M, Soumplis V, Panos C, Makris N, Kandarakis S, Karagiannis D. A case of bilateral self-induced keratoconus in a patient with Tourette syndrome associated with compulsive eye rubbing: case report. BMC Ophthalmol. 2011;11:28.
80. Sharma R, Titiyal JS, Prakash G, Sharma N, Tandon R, Vajpayee RB. Clinical profile and risk factors for keratoplasty and development of hydrops in north Indian patients with keratoconus. Cornea. 2009;28(4):367–70.

2 Etiology and Risk Factors of Keratoconus

Mark Daniell and Srujana Sahebjada

2.1 Introduction

Keratoconus (KC) is a complex degenerative disorder characterized by progressive corneal ectasia and thinning [1]. The occurrence of the disease is bilateral, ultimately affecting both eyes, but asymmetric in progression [2, 3]. Disease progression is manifested with vision distortion and potential blindness, primarily due to irregular astigmatism and myopia and secondarily due to corneal deformation and scarring. Treatment and management vary depending on disease severity. Early stages of treatment begin with glasses or soft contact lenses to correct vision problems or corneal cross-linking (CXL) to arrest and regress the progression of the disease [4]. Treatment for later stages of the disease requires hard contact lenses, and when intolerance to contact lens develops, corneal transplantation is required to restore vision [5]. Thus, early or asymptomatic diagnosis is crucial for the most effective treatment outcome, but early signs and symptoms are nonspecific for diagnosing KC. The characteristic histopathologic findings of KC are thinning of the corneal stroma, breakage of Bowman's layer, and iron deposition in the basal layers of the corneal epithelium [6]. Although several studies have provided strong indications for genetic and environmental risk factors to play a major role in the etiology of KC, there are currently no known direct causes that allow for onset prediction and reliable symptomatic detection [7].

2.2 The Genetics of Keratoconus

Genetic studies are providing insights into KC pathogenesis. It is a feature of many genetic syndromes, and twin studies also demonstrate genetic inheritance [8]. Depending on the study, 6–23% of patients have a positive family history, and the disorder is almost always bilateral [8]. The advent of computerized corneal topography to detect subtle or early cases of KC (usually called forme fruste) has led to an increased ability to detect familial KC and to study the segregation in large pedigrees. The subclinical indices derived from corneal topography are themselves heritable, and several studies have supported a major gene effect with variable phenotypic expression [9, 10]. A comprehensive study of a large series of KC cases and their nuclear families showed at least a 15-fold increase in KC in the first-degree relatives compared to the general population [10]. Together, these studies indicate a clear genetic component to KC (Table 2.1).

M. Daniell (✉) · S. Sahebjada
Centre for Eye Research Australia, Royal Victorian Eye and Ear Hospital,
East Melbourne, VIC, Australia
e-mail: daniellm@unimelb.edu.au; srujana.sahebjada@unimelb.edu.au

S. Das (ed.), *Keratoconus*, https://doi.org/10.1007/978-981-19-4262-4_2

Table 2.1 List of keratoconus genes and identified variants [Adapted from Bykhovskaya and Rabinowitz [11], updated May 2021]

Method (reference)	Gene name	Position	Variant(s)	Location	Gene function/phenotype
GWAS, TG [12]	PNPLA2	11p15.5	rs61876744	Intron	Catalyzes the initial step in triglyceride hydrolysis
GWAS, TG [12]	MAML2	11a21	rs10831500	Intron	Transcriptional factor
S [13]	TGFBI	5q31.1	Multiple rare variants	Extron	Transforming growth factor beta induced, involved in corneal dystrophies
GWLS/LD/FM/S/ NA/TG [13]	LOX	5q23.2	rs10519694	Intron	Lysyl oxidase, participates in collagen cross-linking
			rs2956540	Missense	
			rs1800449	Missense	
			rs2288393		
			rs41407546		
GWLS/FM/GWAS/MA/ WES [14–16]	COL5A1	9q34.2.3	rs1536482	5′ near gene	Collagen type V, alpha 1 chain; variants are associated with population in CCT
			rs7044529	Intron	
			IVS50-4C > G	Splice site	
GWAS, TG [17, 18]	RAB3GAP1	2q21.3	rs4954218	5′ near gene	Regulates exocytosis; mutations are associated with ocular diseases
			rs6730157	Intron	
GWAS, TG [19]	HGF	7q21.1	rs3735520	Promoter	Involved in corneal wound healing, decreased serum levels in KC patients carrying minor allele
GWAS, MA [14, 20]	FNDC3B	3q26.31	rs4894535	Intron	Fibronectin extracellular matrix protein; variants are associated with population variation in CCT, CH, CRF
GWAS, MA, TG [14, 18, 20]	FOXO1	13q14.1	rs2721051	3′ near gene	Transcription factor; variants are associated with population variation in CCT, CH, CRF
GWLS/GWAS/S [21]	DOCK9	13q32.2	c.2262A > C	Missense	Guanine nucleotide exchange factor
			p.Gln754His		
GWAS/TG [14, 18, 20, 22]	MPDZ/NF1B	9p23	rs1324183	Intergenic	Intergenic region involved in genetic regulation of CCT, CH, CRF
S	TSC1	9q34	rs751398082	Missense	Hamartin, regulates cell growth and proliferation
			rs550526986		
GWAS/TG/S/TA [20, 23, 24]	ZNF469	16q24.2	rs9938149	3′ near gene	Transcription factor, regulates corneal collagen structure and synthesis, involved in genetic regulation of CCT, CH, CRF
			Multiple rare variants	Exons	
GWLS, LD, FM, S [25]	PPIP5K2	5q21.2	c.1255 T > G S419A	Missense	Kinase/phosphatase involved in normal corneal function; defects lead to pathological corneal thinning in mouse model of KC
			c.2528 A > G N843S		

GWLS genome-wide linkage study, *S* sequencing, *GWAS* genome-wide association study, *TG* targeted genotyping, *LD* linkage disequilibrium, *MA* meta-analysis, *FM* fine mapping

2.2.1 Genome-Wide Association Studies (GWAS)

GWAS study findings provide valuable insights into the possible pathogenesis of KC. The number of identified susceptibility genes implicated in the genetic evidence of KC has increased a dozen since the first GWAS using pooled DNA of KC patients (identifying HGF gene variant) published in 2011 [19] and the first GWAS of individual KC patients (identifying RAB3-GAP1 gene variant) published in 2012 [17]. Even though majority of the gene variants identified by GWAS came from European populations, a large number have been replicated in one or more patient populations of different ethnic origins [18, 22]. The recent KC GWAS led to the identification and subsequently confirmation of two more genomic loci (PNPLA2 and MAML2) [12]. With more powerful GWAS studies and larger sample sizes, the number of KC-related loci will increase. A multiethnic large-scale recent GWAS reported common variants associated with KC to explain 12.5% of the genetic variance, which shows potential for the future development of a diagnostic test to detect susceptibility to disease [26]. These results provide attractive targets to investigate in terms of their gene expression patterns as well as their effect on clinical phenotype.

2.2.2 GWAS of Central Corneal Thickness (CCT) and Corneal Biomechanical Properties

Using endophenotypes (a heritable quantitative trait that is associated with the disease of and is measurable in both healthy and affected individuals and is genetically correlated to the disease) has been a successful strategy for identifying genetic basis for KC. Central corneal thickness (CCT) and corneal biomechanical properties are the commonly investigated endophenotypes for the KC.

Central corneal thickness (CCT) is one of the most heritable human traits with a broad-sense heritability estimate ranging from 0.68 to 0.95 [27]. The high heritability of this trait has led to successful identification of genetic network behind CCT variation in several association studies. The most recent published CCT meta-analysis identified 98 genomic loci (41 novel) and explained 14.2% of CCT variance [27]. Variation exists between different ethnic groups, with some genes identified in multiethnic panels and some novel genes specific to certain populations like LOC100506532 in Hispanics [28] and STON2 gene in Japanese [29].

Corneal biomechanical properties are reliably assessed by corneal hysteresis (CH) and corneal resistance factor (CRF) using Ocular Response Analyzer (ORA) [30]. The most recent GWAS of 10,000 individuals with significantly increased power identified and replicated over 200 genome-wide loci associated with CH or CRF [20] with multiple novel candidate loci identified for corneal diseases that lead to severe visual impairment.

The number of KC-associated loci increased as CCT GWAS became more powerful, with 20 out of 98 CCT-associated genomic loci to be associated with KC [27]; STON2 gene identified is also thought to be associated with KC in Japanese population [29]. The main pathway between CCT regulation and KC susceptibility is identified to be collagen and extracellular matrix regulation in all CCT studies. CCT studies also consistently found genetic overlap with corneal dystrophies and Mendelian connective tissue disorders [27].

Several studies have reported that identified CH- and CRF-associated genomic-wide loci do not contribute greatly to the susceptibility of KC [31]. Out of the 200+ loci identified in CH and CRF GWAS, only 4 loci (FNDC3B, ZNF469, MPDZ, and FOXO1) have showed significance in association with KC and CCT variation [20].

In summary, while there is suggestive association of KC with these endophenotypes, larger studies are needed to confirm the genetic links between these measures and the condition.

2.3 KC and Family History

The most significant risk factor for developing KC remains being a first-degree relative of a subject with KC [32]. Even in the absence of clinically manifest KC, abnormal corneal topography

(KC suspect) is frequently diagnosed [33] and showed significantly increased risk of progression from subclinical to clinical KC [34].

Prior to the advent and use of high-throughput next-generation sequencing of familiar samples, multiple linkage studies in individual families and family sets were undertaken and led to the identification of genomic positions but not specific genes or variants [13]. However, the nature of a genetically complex disorder presents major complications and challenges even with the use of modern highly powerful technologies [35]. In recent successes, evidence for specific genes and variants have been identified: ZNF469 gene and multiple variants in multiple KC families [23], a functional variant in DOCK9 responsible for exon skipping in KC family [21], a functional splice variant in COL5A1 gene in KC family [16], and two familial variants in PPIP5K2 gene in a four-generation KC family [36].

In summary, as discussed above, research to date has not identified a single major gene, although in some families the inheritance pattern does suggest such a model.

2.4 Functional Studies of Candidate Genes

Genetic linkage studies have reported at least 17 gene loci, indicating the likely presence of multiple genes involved in KC [37]. However, the identification of true disease-causing genes has been scarce. For the many candidate genes reported to be associated with KC, few of the early detected genes have been replicated.

2.4.1 DOCK9 and PPIP5K2

Expression constructs using wild-type and mutant alleles of DOCK9 showed that c.2262A > C in exon 20 of DOCK9 led to aberrant splicing [21]. This resulted in different ratios of normal and truncated transcripts.

The expression of either wild-type PPIP5K2 protein or each of the two familial variants (S419A and N843S) was determined using HEK cells as a host. A significant reduction in PPIP5K2 phosphatase activity was seen in N843S variant, while elevated kinase activities in vitro were seen in both variants, albeit at various levels [25]. The biochemical effects of PPIP5K2 (elevated kinase and reduced phosphatase activity) were studied using a PPIP5K2 gene trap mouse model [25], followed by histological staining and slit lamp biomicroscopy for visualization of the anterior segment of the eye including the cornea. Abnormalities on the anterior corneal surface, decreased anterior chamber depth, and corneal opacity were demonstrated in both heterozygous and homozygous affected allele mice starting at 3 months of age. These irregularities demonstrated the critical role PPIP5K2 play in maintaining physiological function of the mouse cornea. Thus, the potentially critical role that PPIP5K2 gene defects play in the pathogenesis of KC may be concluded.

2.5 Genetic Determinants of Syndromic and Non-syndromic KC

Non-syndromic form of KC is a type of KC with absence of other tissue involvements; this is commonly seen in about 97% of cases. The other 3% of KC cases have been reported to be linked with systemic genetic disorders, including Down syndrome, Ehlers-Danlos syndrome (EDS), Bardet-Biedl syndrome, nail-patella syndrome, and others in a syndromic form [7].

EDS is a group of connective tissue disorders affecting the joints, skin, and blood vessel walls. Symptoms include hyperflexible joints, hyperextensible skin, and abnormal scar formation. Generalized corneal thinning and KC have also been frequently described in patients with EDS. Studies of clinically diagnosed patients with classic EDS have indicated that 50% of patients have mutations in COL5A1 and COL5A2 gene, encoding the alpha1 and alpha2 chain of type V collagen, respectively [38]. Multiple genome-wide scans in multiple populations have identified other variants of COL5A1 gene (rs1536482 and 7044529) that are consistently involved in the regulation of CCT [14]. Targeted analysis that was subsequently done revealed that both SNPs, rs1536482 and rs7044529, were consistently associated with KC in case-control panels and in a familial panel [15]. However, even though variants of COL5A1 are involved in the regulation of CCT, patients who carry minor alleles of COL5A1 SNPs revealed only diffuse corneal thinning with no evidence of focal ectasia.

On isolated occasions, patients with tuberous sclerosis complex (TSC) have shown KC phenotype. TSC is a rare multisystem genetic disorder that causes growth of benign tumors in the brain and on other vital organs such as the kidneys, heart, liver, eyes, lungs, and skin. Mutations in two genes, TSC1 (9q34) and TSC2 (16p13), were found to play a critical role in TSC patients, as the genes are important in coding for tumor suppressors hamartin and tuberin, which are critical regulators of cell growth and proliferation [39]. Coincidentally, TSC patients carrying both TSC1 and TSC2 mutations have shown KC phenotype [40]. Additionally, pathogenic mutations in TSC1 gene were recently identified, with Q765X in TSC patients with KC (syndromic KC) and D1136E/R1093Q in patients with non-syndromic KC [41]. This shows that TSC1 protein function in different tissues including the eye and therefore the different clinical manifestations can be influenced by different variants of TSC1 gene. Our developing understanding of phenotypic spectrum and molecular diversity of germline mutations has furthered since the identification of TSC1 as a potential novel gene for syndromic and non-syndromic KC and has since led to further exploration of complex genetic disorders with overlapping clinical features.

2.6 Transcriptomic and Expression Studies

The extensive use of gene expression studies has resulted in significant advances in the understanding of functional genes and pathways important for KC pathogenesis. This has recently been complemented with newly developed and now widely used high-throughput RNA sequencing (RNA-seq), which has shown multiple genes involved in KC cornea abnormalities, especially those that affect biomechanical properties of the corneal tissue.

Expression analysis and targeted expression analysis have been undertaken to reveal the differential expression patterns of the identified candidate genes (including LOX, SPARC, ZNF469, and TGFBI), between the human KC and non-KC corneal tissues [13, 24]. Analysis of the pathways has indicated the enrichment of extracellular matrix genes, genes involved in protein binding, glycosaminoglycan binding, and cell migration [42]. Thus, it proves useful that analysis of transcriptomic data from different populations and patient groups may help develop biomarkers for KC [43].

2.6.1 Noncoding RNA (lncRNAs and miRNAs) Involved in KC

Noncoding RNA plays a critical role in the regulation and modulation of gene expression affecting multiple biological processes. Recent studies aimed to explore the potential role of noncoding RNAs in the pathogenesis of KC [44]. Two studies that focused on analyzing long noncoding RNA (transcripts exceeding 200 nucleotides that do not translate into proteins) found several lncRNAs possibly regulating gene expression and biological pathways with known or plausible links to the susceptibility of KC [45, 46]. miRNA and histological analyses of keratoconic corneal epithelia revealed downregulation of 12 miRNAs which participated in cell junction, cell division, and motor activity. Further high-throughput bioinformatic analysis of KC-associated genomic regions found nonrandom distribution of miRNA genes and single-nucleotide variants in regions containing KC loci [47]. Further investigation may lead to new discovery of miRNAs and its role as a potential therapeutic target and diagnostic marker for KC.

2.7 Environmental Risk Factors

Along with genetic factors, there are various environmental factors that influence the development and progression of KC. There have been numerous studies to explore the effect of the environmental risks (Table 2.2); however, the exact triggers for keratoconus remain largely elusive.

2.7.1 Eye Rubbing

Eye rubbing has been established as an environmental risk factor with the strongest association to the etiology of KC. It has been studied since the 1960s when the association between KC and atopic disease was first identified as patients reported intense eye rubbing due to the allergy [48]. Numerous studies have been performed ever since. In 2009, McMonnies described numerous mechanisms of eye rubbing and corneal trauma leading to KC, such as increased corneal temperature due to friction increasing the activity of collagenases, scar formation, increased inflammatory mediators (IL6, TNFa, MMP9) in tears, cellular changes of keratocytes and epithelial cells, and increased intraocular pressure that causes much movement of aqueous humor over the cornea leading to tissue remodeling [49]. A case-control study performed in France demonstrated a strong correlation with OR 8.29 when rubbed using knuckles and OR 5.34 when using fingertips [50]. Rabinowitz stated that, currently, the predominant model is that corneal trauma, including eye rubbing, provides the "second hit" required in the development of KC in a genetically susceptible individual [51]. Recent meta-analysis conducted by Sahebjada et al. also suggested eye rubbing to be consistently associ-

Table 2.2 Strongly associated risk factors with keratoconus

Authors	Year	Country	Study design	Total study participants (n)	Risk factor(s) analyzed
Macsai et al. [63]	1990	USA	Retrospective cohort	199	Contact lens
Donnenfeld et al. [55]	1991	USA	Case report	5	Floppy eyelid syndrome
Bawazeer et al. [71]	2000	Canada	Case-control study	120	Atopy, eye rubbing
Owens et al. [67]	2003	New Zealand	Survey questionnaire	673	Age, gender, consanguinity, allergy, and asthma
Moon et al. [64]	2006	South Korea	Cross-sectional study	42	Contact lens wear
Millodot et al. [70]	2011	Jerusalem	Cross-sectional study	981	Atopy
Merdler et al. [66]	2015	Israel	Cross-sectional study	807	Allergic diseases
Gordon-Shaag et al. [68]	2015	Israel	Case-control study	219	Asthma, UV exposure, and parental education
Naderan et al. [69]	2017	Iran	Case-control study	2411	Allergy
Moran et al. [50]	2020	France	Case-control study	557	Eye rubbing, pattern of eye rubbing, dominant hand, allergies, history of dry eye, screen time, sleep position, and night-time work
Sorbara et al. [65]	2021	Canada	Cross-sectional study	56	Contact lens wear
Sahebjada et al. [62]	2021	Australia	Cross-sectional study	260	All known environmental risk factors including asthma, BMI, smoking, diabetes, rheumatoid arthritis, eczema

ated with KC; however, the results limited to only a small number of case-control studies [52]. Taken together, the current evidence suggests that KC is heterogeneous in nature and more studies are needed to investigate the detailed relationship of eye rubbing and its initiation, ongoing progression, and severity of keratoconus.

2.7.2 Comorbidities

KC has been reported be associated with many systemic and ocular comorbidities including connective tissue diseases, with particularly strong associations with mitral valve prolapse and Ehlers-Danlos syndrome [53, 54]. Ocular conditions including floppy eyelid syndrome [50, 55] and vernal keratoconjunctivitis are strongly associated [56], while cataract, granular dystrophy type II and Fuchs dystrophy, and others have also been reported in concomitance with KC [57]. Tourette syndrome with obsessive-compulsive eye rubbing is also linked [58]. Obesity and obstructive sleep apnea are more frequently found in the keratoconic population than the general population [59, 60]. Diabetes may be protective for KC possibly because it accelerates age-induced cross-linking in the cornea [61, 62]. Metabolic diseases and complex genetic syndromes, congenital hip dysplasia, mitral valve prolapse, and Marfan and Down syndromes have also been associated with KC [57].

In summary, it should be noted that it is not clear whether these associations with KC are true comorbidity or occur by chance due to limited number of cases. Thus, it is currently difficult to dissect specific contributions.

2.7.3 Contact Lens Wear

The relationship between contact lens wear and KC has been controversial. This association is of high significance since many KC patients wear contact lenses as part of their management. In 1990, a retrospective review of 199 KC patients noted that those who had been wearing contact lens were younger at the time of diagnosis but also commented on the inability to prove the influence of contacts on the disease development [63]. More recently, contact lens wear has been reported to produce ocular changes that are also seen in KC—central corneal thinning, decreased keratocyte density, and squamous metaplasia—but a clear association still warrants further research [64]. A study in South Korea evaluated ocular surface changes with tear film breakup times and conjunctival impression cytology and stated that these ocular changes may be due to contact lens wear, rather than the disease. Tear film breakup times and goblet cell densities were significantly lower in KC patients who had been wearing RGP contact lenses for an average of 5.54 ± 2.11 years compared to patients who did not wear them and controls [64]. On the other hand, Sorbara et al.'s study displayed no relationship of central corneal epithelial changes on histology with length of contact lens wear, but rather the duration of the disease [65]. The difference in results may be because Sorbara et al.'s study comprised only of patients of advanced KC who were currently wearing RGP lenses or had worn them in the past.

To summarize, the current literature leaves the conundrum that KC is a typically progressive disease that is often managed with contact lenses but progresses with or without contact lens wear; thus, the contribution of possible pathogenic contact lens-related phenomena remains speculative.

2.7.4 Asthma

Asthma has also been reported to increase not only the risk but also the severity of KC. There have been multiple studies that have noted the positive relationship between asthma and KC. A study of 662,644 Israeli adolescents demonstrated increased odds ratio of 2.0 for asthma in 807 KC patients [66], and a New Zealand study showed an association of $p = 0.0002$ [67]. The Australian Study of keratoconus states asthma to be significantly associated with the severity of the disease as KC patients with asthma had a steeper corneal curvature than those without asthma by 2.2 diopters [62]. A possible shared genetic path involving the interleukin-6 receptor (IL6R) gene with common environmental factors is a proposed mechanism for linking the two diseases [62]. However, a study performed on Israeli population denied a significant association with OR of 0.92 among 73 KC patients and 145 controls [68].

2.7.5 Allergy

Association of KC and other allergic conditions has also been studied, with a consensus on the positive relationship. A cross-sectional study conducted to estimate the epidemiologic relationship between KC and allergic diseases in Israel found a significant association between allergic rhinitis and KC [odds ratio (OR) 1.6], and the combination of allergic conjunctivitis, chronic blepharitis, and vernal keratoconjunctivitis demonstrated OR of 6.0. Furthermore, after stratification of the combined allergic diseases according to severity, the association became stronger with OR of 36.5 [66]. Another case-control study added to these findings, illuminating that only VKC and allergic conjunctivitis had substantial correlation to KC severity [69]. Hence, the severity of the allergic status is without doubt established with a greater risk of having KC, while the mechanism causing this association is still unclear.

2.7.6 Atopy

Atopy refers to a genetic predisposition to develop an allergic reaction, such as allergic rhinitis or atopic dermatitis. Results from various studies on the effect of atopy on KC are unable to clearly outline a relationship. A study in Jerusalem showed a positive relationship between atopy and KC (OR = 3.0) [70]. However, a case-control study presented association only in the univariate model and not multivariate regardless of how the term "atopy" was defined [71], and another study did not find association between the two conditions with OR of 1.0 [66]. In addition, atopy is strongly associated with eye rubbing [71], and taking these risk factors into consideration, it is therefore precise to presume a multifactorial causal pathway for KC.

2.7.7 UV Exposure

Although the effect of UV exposure on development of KC has not been well established, prevalence rates of KC reveal marked differences related to geographical locations. Countries of hotter climates, such as India, Lebanon, Israel, Iran, and Saudi Arabia, tend to have higher rates than countries of cooler climates, including Northern USA, Europe, and Russia [68]. The differences can be explained by UV light being a source of oxidative stress. However, a study in New Zealand exhibited no significance ($p = 0.12$), albeit acknowledging that calculations of UV exposure throughout patients' childhood and adolescent years are limited [67]. Gordon-Shaag et al. reported that wearing a hat outdoors was protective of the disease (OR = 3.13), spending time in the shade was a risk (OR = 0.45), and limiting time in the sun was not associated with KC ($p = 0.51$). The variation in results was explained by how UV radiations may provide a beneficial effect to the cornea by inducing collagen cross-linking. Furthermore, the complexity is compounded by ethnic differences in people living in the same geographic location. In summary, the causal relationship between UV and KC needs to be further explored before considering it as a risk factor.

2.8 Conclusion

Keratoconus is a complex disease with the exact etiology remaining unclear. It appears to be a heterogeneous disorder caused by both genetic and environmental factors. While some families present with obvious Mendelian inheritance, other individuals display multiple contributory factors.

As with most complex diseases, candidate gene and linkage studies of multiple small families have failed to explain the overall genetic contribution to the disease. In addition, many studies were conducted on very small cohorts and without replication or subsequent follow-up. One of the main limitations of existing studies on keratoconus has been the relatively small number of patients who have been studied and reported, leading to underpowered analyses and false-positive findings that limit generalizability of the results. Recent advances in genomic methodologies such as well-powered GWASs for keratoconus and CCT have highlighted multiple risk loci and high-throughput RNA-seq to identify the disease pathways have helped improve the understanding of KC pathogenesis. The challenge now lies in identifying the full spectrum of genetic risk in various ethnic groups and determining how specific environmental risk factors contribute to disease development. A global initiative, where researchers from across the world collect, share, and combine clinical data with genetic and proteomic testing, will further improve our understanding of the relative contributions of genetic and environmental factors in the etiology and progression of the disease. This in turn will result in developing precision medicine treatments focused on the molecular cause of the disease.

References

1. Loukovitis E, Kozeis N, Gatzioufas Z, Kozei A, Tsotridou E, Stoila M, Koronis S, Sfakianakis K, Tranos P, Balidis M, Zachariadis Z, Mikropoulos DG, Anogeianakis G, Katsanos A, Konstas AG. The proteins of keratoconus: a literature review exploring their contribution to the pathophysiology of the disease. Adv Ther. 2019;36(9):2205–22.
2. Dienes L, Kránitz K, Juhász E, Gyenes A, Takács A, Miháltz K, Nagy ZZ, Kovács I. Evaluation of intereye corneal asymmetry in patients with keratoconus. A scheimpflug imaging study. PLoS One. 2014;9(10):e108882.
3. Wang YM, Pang CC. Molecular genetics of keratoconus: clinical implications. In: Ocular surface diseases: some current date on tear film problem and keratoconic diagnosis. London: IntechOpen; 2019.
4. Tan P, Mehta JS. Collagen crosslinking for keratoconus. J Ophthalmic Vis Res. 2011;6(3):153–4.
5. Fournié P, Touboul D, Arné JL, Colin J, Malecaze F. Kératocône [Keratoconus]. J Fr Ophtalmol. 2013;36(7):618–26.
6. Naderan M, Jahanrad A, Balali S. Histopathologic findings of keratoconus corneas underwent penetrating keratoplasty according to topographic measurements and keratoconus severity. Int J Ophthalmol. 2017;10(11):1640–6.
7. Rabinowitz YS. Keratoconus. Surv Ophthalmol. 1998;42(4):297–319.
8. Rabinowitz YS. The genetics of keratoconus. Ophthalmol Clin N Am. 2003;16(4):607–20.
9. Rabinowitz YS, Garbus J, McDonnell PJ. Computer-assisted corneal topography in family members of patients with keratoconus. Arch Ophthalmol. 1990;108(3):365–71.
10. Wang Y, Rabinowitz YS, Rotter JI, Yang H. Genetic epidemiological study of keratoconus: evidence for major gene determination. Am J Med Genet. 2000;93(5):403–9.
11. Bykhovskaya Y, Rabinowitz YS. Update on the genetics of keratoconus. Exp Eye Res. 2021;202:108398.
12. McComish BJ, Sahebjada S, Bykhovskaya Y, Willoughby CE, Richardson AJ, Tenen A, Charlesworth JC, MacGregor S, Mitchell P, Lucas SEM, Mills RA, Mackey DA, Li X, Wang JJ, Jensen RA, Rotter JI, Taylor KD, Hewitt AW, Rabinowitz YS, Baird PN, Craig JE, Burdon KP. Association of genetic variation with keratoconus. JAMA Ophthalmol. 2020;138(2):174–81.
13. Bykhovskaya Y, Gromova A, Makarenkova HP, Rabinowitz YS. Abnormal regulation of extracellular matrix and adhesion molecules in corneas of patients with keratoconus. Int J Keratoconus Ectatic Corneal Dis. 2016;5(2):63–70.
14. Lu Y, Vitart V, Burdon KP, Khor CC, Bykhovskaya Y, Mirshahi A, Hewitt AW, Koehn D, Hysi PG, Ramdas WD, Zeller T, Vithana EN, Cornes BK, Tay WT, Tai ES, Cheng CY, Liu J, Foo JN, Saw SM, Thorleifsson G, Stefansson K, Dimasi DP, Mills RA, Mountain J, Ang W, Hoehn R, Verhoeven VJ, Grus F, Wolfs R, Castagne R, Lackner KJ, Springelkamp H, Yang J, Jonasson F, Leung DY, Chen LJ, Tham CC, Rudan I, Vatavuk Z, Hayward C, Gibson J, Cree AJ, MacLeod A, Ennis S, Polasek O, Campbell H, Wilson JF, Viswanathan AC, Fleck B, Li X, Siscovick D, Taylor KD, Rotter JI, Yazar S, Ulmer M, Li J, Yaspan BL, Ozel AB, Richards JE, Moroi SE, Haines JL, Kang JH, Pasquale LR, Allingham RR, Ashley-Koch A, NEIGHBOR Consortium, Mitchell P, Wang JJ, Wright AF, Pennell C, Spector TD, Young TL, Klaver CC, Martin NG, Montgomery GW, Anderson MG, Aung T, Willoughby CE, Wiggs JL, Pang CP, Thorsteinsdottir U, Lotery AJ, Hammond CJ, van Duijn CM, Hauser MA, Rabinowitz YS, Pfeiffer N, Mackey DA, Craig JE, Macgregor S, Wong TY. Genome-wide association analyses identify multiple loci associated with central corneal thickness and keratoconus. Nat Genet. 2013;45(2):155–63.
15. Li X, Bykhovskaya Y, Canedo AL, Haritunians T, Siscovick D, Aldave AJ, Szczotka-Flynn L, Iyengar SK, Rotter JI, Taylor KD, Rabinowitz YS. Genetic association of COL5A1 variants in keratoconus

patients suggests a complex connection between corneal thinning and keratoconus. Invest Ophthalmol Vis Sci. 2013;54(4):2696–704.
16. Lin Q, Zheng L, Shen Z, Jie L. A novel splice-site variation in COL5A1 causes keratoconus in an Indian family. J Ophthalmol. 2019;2019:2851380.
17. Li X, Bykhovskaya Y, Haritunians T, Siscovick D, Aldave A, Szczotka-Flynn L, Iyengar SK, Rotter JI, Taylor KD, Rabinowitz YS. A genome-wide association study identifies a potential novel gene locus for keratoconus, one of the commonest causes for corneal transplantation in developed countries. Hum Mol Genet. 2012;21(2):421–9.
18. Liskova P, Dudakova L, Krepelova A, Klema J, Hysi PG. Replication of SNP associations with keratoconus in a Czech cohort. PLoS One. 2017;12(2):e0172365.
19. Burdon KP, Macgregor S, Bykhovskaya Y, Javadiyan S, Li X, Laurie KJ, Muszynska D, Lindsay R, Lechner J, Haritunians T, Henders AK, Dash D, Siscovick D, Anand S, Aldave A, Coster DJ, Szczotka-Flynn L, Mills RA, Iyengar SK, Taylor KD, Phillips T, Montgomery GW, Rotter JI, Hewitt AW, Sharma S, Rabinowitz YS, Willoughby C, Craig JE. Association of polymorphisms in the hepatocyte growth factor gene promoter with keratoconus. Invest Ophthalmol Vis Sci. 2011;52(11):8514–9.
20. Simcoe MJ, Khawaja AP, Hysi PG, Hammond CJ, UK Biobank Eye and Vision Consortium. Genome-wide association study of corneal biomechanical properties identifies over 200 loci providing insight into the genetic etiology of ocular diseases. Hum Mol Genet. 2020;29(18):3154–64.
21. Karolak JA, Rydzanicz M, Ginter-Matuszewska B, Pitarque JA, Molinari A, Bejjani BA, Gajecka M. Variant c.2262A>C in DOCK9 leads to exon skipping in keratoconus family. Invest Ophthalmol Vis Sci. 2015;56(13):7687–90.
22. Hao XD, Chen P, Chen ZL, Li SX, Wang Y. Evaluating the association between keratoconus and reported genetic loci in a Han Chinese population. Ophthalmic Genet. 2015;36(2):132–6.
23. Davidson AE, Borasio E, Liskova P, Khan AO, Hassan H, Cheetham ME, Plagnol V, Alkuraya FS, Tuft SJ, Hardcastle AJ. Brittle cornea syndrome ZNF469 mutation carrier phenotype and segregation analysis of rare ZNF469 variants in familial keratoconus. Invest Ophthalmol Vis Sci. 2015;56(1):578–86.
24. Karolak JA, Ginter-Matuszewska B, Tomela K, Kabza M, Nowak-Malczewska DM, Rydzanicz M, Polakowski P, Szaflik JP, Gajecka M. Further evaluation of differential expression of keratoconus candidate genes in human corneas. PeerJ. 2020;8:e9793.
25. Khaled ML, Bykhovskaya Y, Gu C, Liu A, Drewry MD, Chen Z, Mysona BA, Parker E, McNabb RP, Yu H, Lu X, Wang J, Li X, Al-Muammar A, Rotter JI, Porter LF, Estes A, Watsky MA, Smith SB, Xu H, Abu-Amero KK, Kuo A, Shears SB, Rabinowitz YS, Liu Y. PPIP5K2 and PCSK1 are candidate genetic contributors to familial keratoconus. Sci Rep. 2019;9(1):19406.
26. Hardcastle AJ, Liskova P, Bykhovskaya Y, McComish BJ, Davidson AE, Inglehearn CF, Li X, Choquet H, Habeeb M, Lucas SEM, Sahebjada S, Pontikos N, Lopez KER, Khawaja AP, Ali M, Dudakova L, Skalicka P, Van Dooren BTH, Geerards AJM, Haudum CW, Faro VL, Tenen A, Simcoe MJ, Patasova K, Yarrand D, Yin J, Siddiqui S, Rice A, Farraj LA, Chen YI, Rahi JS, Krauss RM, Theusch E, Charlesworth JC, Szczotka-Flynn L, Toomes C, Meester-Smoor MA, Richardson AJ, Mitchell PA, Taylor KD, Melles RB, Aldave AJ, Mills RA, Cao K, Chan E, Daniell MD, Wang JJ, Rotter JI, Hewitt AW, MacGregor S, Klaver CCW, Ramdas WD, Craig JE, Iyengar SK, O'Brart D, Jorgenson E, Baird PN, Rabinowitz YS, Burdon KP, Hammond CJ, Tuft SJ, Hysi PG. A multi-ethnic genome-wide association study implicates collagen matrix integrity and cell differentiation pathways in keratoconus. Commun Biol. 2021;4(1):266.
27. Choquet H, Melles RB, Yin J, Hoffmann TJ, Thai KK, Kvale MN, Banda Y, Hardcastle AJ, Tuft SJ, Glymour MM, Schaefer C, Risch N, Nair KS, Hysi PG, Jorgenson E. A multiethnic genome-wide analysis of 44,039 individuals identifies 41 new loci associated with central corneal thickness. Commun Biol. 2020;3(1):301.
28. Gao X, Gauderman WJ, Liu Y, Marjoram P, Torres M, Haritunians T, Kuo JZ, Chen YD, Allingham RR, Hauser MA, Taylor KD, Rotter JI, Varma R. A genome-wide association study of central corneal thickness in Latinos. Invest Ophthalmol Vis Sci. 2013;54(4):2435–43.
29. Hosoda Y, Miyake M, Meguro A, Tabara Y, Iwai S, Ueda-Arakawa N, Nakano E, Mori Y, Yoshikawa M, Nakanishi H, Khor CC, Saw SM, Yamada R, Matsuda F, Cheng CY, Mizuki N, Tsujikawa A, Yamashiro K, Nagahama Study Group. Keratoconus-susceptibility gene identification by corneal thickness genome-wide association study and artificial intelligence IBM Watson. Commun Biol. 2020;3(1):410.
30. Luce DA. Determining in vivo biomechanical properties of the cornea with an ocular response analyzer. J Cataract Refract Surg. 2005;31(1):156–62.
31. Khawaja AP, Rojas Lopez KE, Hardcastle AJ, Hammond CJ, Liskova P, Davidson AE, Gore DM, Hafford Tear NJ, Pontikos N, Hayat S, Wareham N, Khaw KT, Tuft SJ, Foster PJ, Hysi PG. Genetic variants associated with corneal biomechanical properties and potentially conferring susceptibility to keratoconus in a genome-wide association study. JAMA Ophthalmol. 2019;137(9):1005–12.
32. Lapeyre G, Fournie P, Vernet R, Roseng S, Malecaze F, Bouzigon E, Touboul D. Keratoconus prevalence in families: a French study. Cornea. 2020;39(12):1473–9.
33. Shneor E, Frucht-Pery J, Granit E, Gordon-Shaag A. The prevalence of corneal abnormalities in first-degree relatives of patients with keratoconus: a prospective case-control study. Ophthalmic Physiol Opt. 2020;40(4):442–51.

34. Li X, Yang H, Rabinowitz YS. Longitudinal study of keratoconus progression. Exp Eye Res. 2007;85(4):502–7.
35. Magalhães OA, Kowalski TW, Wachholz GE, Schuler-Faccini L. Whole-exome sequencing in familial keratoconus: the challenges of a genetically complex disorder. Arq Bras Oftalmol. 2019;82(6):453–9.
36. Bykhovskaya Y, Li X, Taylor KD, Haritunians T, Rotter JI, Rabinowitz YS. Linkage analysis of high-density SNPs confirms keratoconus locus at 5q chromosomal region. Ophthalmic Genet. 2016;37(1):109–10.
37. Lucas SEM, Burdon KP. Genetic and environmental risk factors for keratoconus. Annu Rev Vis Sci. 2020;6:25–46.
38. Malfait F, De Paepe A. Molecular genetics in classic Ehlers-Danlos syndrome. Am J Med Genet C Semin Med Genet. 2005;139C(1):17–23.
39. Caban C, Khan N, Hasbani DM, Crino PB. Genetics of tuberous sclerosis complex: implications for clinical practice. Appl Clin Genet. 2016;10:1–8.
40. Lyall DA, Tobias ES, Srinivasan S, Willoughby C. Bilateral keratoconus in tuberous sclerosis: is there a molecular link? Can J Ophthalmol. 2012;47(6):e41–2.
41. Bykhovskaya Y, Fardaei M, Khaled ML, Nejabat M, Salouti R, Dastsooz H, Liu Y, Inaloo S, Rabinowitz YS. TSC1 mutations in keratoconus patients with or without tuberous sclerosis. Invest Ophthalmol Vis Sci. 2017;58(14):6462–9.
42. Sharif R, Khaled ML, McKay TB, Liu Y, Karamichos D. Transcriptional profiling of corneal stromal cells derived from patients with keratoconus. Sci Rep. 2019;9(1):12567.
43. Shinde V, Hu N, Mahale A, Maiti G, Daoud Y, Eberhart CG, Maktabi A, Jun AS, Al-Swailem SA, Chakravarti S. RNA sequencing of corneas from two keratoconus patient groups identifies potential biomarkers and decreased NRF2-antioxidant responses. Sci Rep. 2020;10(1):9907.
44. Beermann J, Piccoli MT, Viereck J, Thum T. Non-coding RNAs in development and disease: background, mechanisms, and therapeutic approaches. Physiol Rev. 2016;96(4):1297–325.
45. Szczesniak MW, Kabza M, Karolak JA, Rydzanicz M, Nowak DM, Ginter-Matuszewska B, Polakowski P, Ploski R, Szaflik JP, Gajecka M. KTCNlncDB—a first platform to investigate lncRNAs expressed in human keratoconus and non-keratoconus corneas. Database (Oxford). 2017;2017:baw168.
46. Khaled ML, Bykhovskaya Y, Yablonski SER, Li H, Drewry MD, Aboobakar IF, Estes A, Gao XR, Stamer WD, Xu H, Allingham RR, Hauser MA, Rabinowitz YS, Liu Y. Differential expression of coding and long noncoding RNAs in keratoconus-affected corneas. Invest Ophthalmol Vis Sci. 2018;59(7):2717–28.
47. Nowak DM, Gajecka M. Nonrandom distribution of miRNAs genes and single nucleotide variants in keratoconus loci. PLoS One. 2015;10(7):e0132143.
48. Ridley F. Eye-rubbing and contact lenses. Br J Ophthalmol. 1961;45(9):631.
49. McMonnies CW. Mechanisms of rubbing-related corneal trauma in keratoconus. Cornea. 2009;28(6):607–15.
50. Moran S, Gomez L, Zuber K, Gatinel D. A case-control study of keratoconus risk factors. Cornea. 2020;39(6):697–701.
51. Rabinowitz YS, Galvis V, Tello A, Rueda D, García JD. Genetics vs chronic corneal mechanical trauma in the etiology of keratoconus. Exp Eye Res. 2021;202:108328.
52. Sahebjada S, Al-Mahrouqi HH, Moshegov S, Panchatcharam SM, Chan E, Daniell M, Baird PN. Eye rubbing in the aetiology of keratoconus: a systematic review and meta-analysis. Graefes Arch Clin Exp Ophthalmol. 2021;259(8):2057–67.
53. Robertson I. Keratoconus and the Ehlers-Danlos syndrome: a new aspect of keratoconus. Med J Aust. 1975;1(18):571–3.
54. Siordia JA, Franco JC. The association between keratoconus and mitral valve prolapse: a meta-analysis. Curr Cardiol Rev. 2020;16(2):147–52.
55. Donnenfeld ED, Perry HD, Gibralter RP, Ingraham HJ, Udell IJ. Keratoconus associated with floppy eyelid syndrome. Ophthalmology. 1991;98(11):1674–8.
56. Singhal D, Sahay P, Maharana PK, Raj N, Sharma N, Titiyal JS. Vernal keratoconjunctivitis. Surv Ophthalmol. 2019;64(3):289–311.
57. Ferrari G, Rama P. The keratoconus enigma: a review with emphasis on pathogenesis. Ocul Surf. 2020;18(3):363–73.
58. Mashor RS, Kumar NL, Ritenour RJ, Rootman DS. Keratoconus caused by eye rubbing in patients with Tourette syndrome. Can J Ophthalmol. 2011;46(1):83–6.
59. Pellegrini M, Bernabei F, Friehmann A, Giannaccare G. Obstructive sleep apnea and keratoconus: a systematic review and meta-analysis. Optom Vis Sci. 2020;97(1):9–14.
60. Slater JA, Misra SL, Braatvedt G, McGhee CN. Keratoconus and obesity: can high body mass alter the shape of the cornea? Clin Exp Ophthalmol. 2018;46(9):1091–3.
61. Naderan M, Naderan M, Rezagholizadeh F, Zolfaghari M, Pahlevani R, Rajabi MT. Association between diabetes and keratoconus: a case-control study. Cornea. 2014;33(12):1271–3.
62. Sahebjada S, Chan E, Xie J, Snibson GR, Daniell M, Baird PN. Risk factors and association with severity of keratoconus: the Australian study of keratoconus. Int Ophthalmol. 2021;41(3):891–9.
63. Macsai MS, Varley GA, Krachmer JH. Development of keratoconus after contact lens wear. Patient characteristics. Arch Ophthalmol. 1990;108(4):534–8.
64. Moon JW, Shin KC, Lee HJ, Wee WR, Lee JH, Kim MK. The effect of contact lens wear on the ocular surface changes in keratoconus. Eye Contact Lens. 2006;32(2):96–101.
65. Sorbara L, Lopez JCL, Gorbet M, Bizheva K, Lamarca JM, Pastor JC, Maldonado López MJ, Hileeto

D. Impact of contact lens wear on epithelial alterations in keratoconus. J Optom. 2021;14(1):37–43.
66. Merdler I, Hassidim A, Sorkin N, Shapira S, Gronovich Y, Korach Z. Keratoconus and allergic diseases among Israeli adolescents between 2005 and 2013. Cornea. 2015;34(5):525–9.
67. Owens H, Gamble G. A profile of keratoconus in New Zealand. Cornea. 2003;22(2):122–5.
68. Gordon-Shaag A, Millodot M, Kaiserman I, Sela T, Barnett Itzhaki G, Zerbib Y, Matityahu E, Shkedi S, Miroshnichenko S, Shneor E. Risk factors for keratoconus in Israel: a case-control study. Ophthalmic Physiol Opt. 2015;35(6):673–81.
69. Naderan M, Rajabi MT, Zarrinbakhsh P, Bakhshi A. Effect of allergic diseases on keratoconus severity. Ocul Immunol Inflamm. 2017;25(3):418–23.
70. Millodot M, Shneor E, Albou S, Atlani E, Gordon-Shaag A. Prevalence and associated factors of keratoconus in Jerusalem: a cross-sectional study. Ophthalmic Epidemiol. 2011;18(2):91–7.
71. Bawazeer AM, Hodge WG, Lorimer B. Atopy and keratoconus: a multivariate analysis. Br J Ophthalmol. 2000;84(8):834–6.

3 Biomechanics of Keratoconus

Kanwal Singh Matharu, Jiaonan Ma, Yan Wang, and Vishal Jhanji

3.1 Introduction

The optimal cornea is an optically transparent prolate-positive lens that focuses light on the retina. To achieve this function, corneal microstructure and macrostructure are highly regular and regulated. Pathological changes to the density and cross-linking between collagens and microfibrils at the microscopic level result in structural instability or ectasia, producing visual disturbance via multiple orders of aberration. Keratoconus (KCN) is a progressive corneal ectasia, frequently bilateral and asymmetric, characterized by thinning and protrusion at the apex and its surrounding areas. The disease likely has multiple etiologies including genetic, environmental, and mechanical [1], with the final pathway yielding a weakened Bowman's layer, stromal instability, and decreased corneal stiffness [2]. Increasing astigmatism, often irregular, can cause intractable vision loss. Meanwhile, corneal thinning causes structural and biomechanical instability, resulting in breaks in Descemet's and ultimately scarring. Thus, end-stage KCN may necessitate partial- or full-thickness corneal transplantation. Interventions earlier in the course of the disease, including intracorneal inlay procedures such as Intacs and the ultraviolet procedure cross-linking (CXL), stabilize the cornea and prevent progression of disease.

There has been a recent surge of interest in assessing corneal biomechanics due to the potential correlation between keratoconus and corneal biomechanics. Identifying patients with structurally and biomechanically unstable corneas susceptible to ectasia is important to prevent vision loss in patients with KCN and those considering refractive surgery. To date, ophthalmologists have used topography [3] and more recently tomography of the anterior and posterior surfaces of the cornea to screen for ectasia and forme fruste KCN (ffKCN). Specifically, the Belin-Ambrosio enhanced ectasia display criteria available in the Pentacam (Oculus Optikgerate GmbH, Wetzlar, Germany) has become almost universally adopted [4]. Greater than six diopters of corneal astigmatism, irregular astigmatism with skewed axis, against-the-rule astigmatism in a young patient [5], corneal thinning on pachymetry maps, and increased epithelial thickness are other topographical signs of brewing disease [6].

K. S. Matharu · V. Jhanji (✉)
UPMC Eye Center, University of Pittsburgh School of Medicine, Pittsburgh, PA, USA
e-mail: matharuks@upmc.edu; jhanjiv@upmc.edu

J. Ma
Clinical College of Ophthalmology, Tianjin Medical University, Tianjin, China

Y. Wang
Clinical College of Ophthalmology, Tianjin Medical University, Tianjin, China

Tianjin Eye Hospital, Tianjin Eye Institute, Tianjin Key Laboratory of Ophthalmology and Visual Science, Nankai University Affiliated Eye Hospital, Tianjin, China

S. Das (ed.), *Keratoconus*, https://doi.org/10.1007/978-981-19-4262-4_3

Posterior corneal elevation is one tomographic change [7]. Algorithms evaluating topographies have been developed and refined to screen for ectasia [4]. However, this method still does not allow for a definitive diagnosis. Biomechanical properties independently [8] and as additional parameters in these models are increasing sensitivity and specificity for KCN and ffKCN [9].

The first widely used in vivo biomechanical biometer introduced in 2005 was the Ocular Response Analyzer (ORA®, Reichert Ophthalmic Instruments, Inc., Buffalo, NY, USA). This non-contact tonometer uses an infrared beam to measure the deformation of the eye caused by a pressurized column of air indenting the central 3–6 mm of the apical cornea. In 2010, the Corneal Visualization Scheimpflug Technology (Corvis ST, Oculus Optikgerate GmbH, Wetzlar, Germany) was introduced [10]. This in vivo biometer captures the effects of a standardized air puff with a Scheimpflug camera and generates upward of 12 biomechanical parameters [7, 11]. Currently, other devices utilize ultrasound, applanation, interferometry, and Brillouin optical microscopy among other technologies to detail the biomechanical properties of the cornea with a variety of spatial and temporal regimes and at various depths [7]. Studies have shown that biomechanical changes are one of the characteristics of the KCN, even before the morphological changes of the cornea; therefore, identifying the biomechanical properties is important in the diagnosis of KCN and suspected KCNs. However, validation of these technologies in human eyes will be essential before using them to improve the accuracy of KCN diagnosis. Leveraging this wealth of data with artificial intelligence may provide the next step change in diagnostic capability.

3.2 Background

The cornea is composed of multiple layers of which the stroma constitutes approximately 90% of its thickness. The compact, mostly acellular, stroma is composed of primarily type I collagen fibrils and fibronectin organized into lamellae by proteoglycans [12]. The stroma also has elastins, which give the tissue plasticity. The polar, water-absorbent glycosaminoglycans attached to proteoglycans provide viscosity [12]. This microstructure results in a viscoelastic stroma that provides the bulk of the resistance to shear and tensile forces of the cornea. The inclination angle, azimuthal angle, and diameter of fibrils vary precisely in an anterior to posterior direction, with the anterior 40% of lamellae more interwoven [7, 12] and therefore the strongest [7]. The cornea also has a specific lateral arrangement of its fibrils [12] resulting in higher corneal stiffness following the direction of the collagen fibrils in the longitudinal *x*- and *y*-axes compared to the perpendicular *z*-axis [7]. To further complicate matters, spatial heterogeneity results in anisotropy or different values measured along a single radial meridian [12]. These properties of the cornea introduce many variables and boundaries into measuring the biomechanics of a single patient and are important for interpreting the output from current biometers. The variation in structure and function at different depths has ramifications for refractive and disease-modifying interventions.

Almost every layer of the cornea in KCN has microstructural changes [12]. Alterations in lysyl oxidase and matrix metalloproteins correspond to disease severity in KCN [13], along with other inflammatory signals [1], distort the stromal collagen interlamellar and intralamellar network [14]. The subsequent changes to the cornea result in myriad eponymous clinical findings and topographic and tomographic changes, which are briefly summarized above. The next step change in our understanding of the keratoconic and ectatic corneas in general involves biomechanics; and in fact, biomechanics are already being used for diagnosis, staging, progression, and prognosis of disease [7].

The biomechanical properties of a sample describe how the sample changes in response to an applied force. Shearing forces are applied in opposite directions, often parallel to the surface, while compression forces are collinear. The elasticity of a sample refers to its ability to resist distortion from a loading force and return to its original shape after unloading. Viscosity quantifies a fluid's resistance to flow. Important mechanical properties of the viscoelastic cornea include the elastic modulus, shear modulus, and loss modulus. The loss modulus is related to viscosity, creep, and hysteresis. Hysteresis describes the effect on a delayed output in a dynamically changing system for a given input. The hysteresis of the sample is proportional to the amount of energy dissipated as heat during a single loading and unloading cycle. For example, a rubber ball will have a larger absolute value for its hysteresis than a steel bar for a given force. Each layer of the cornea has specific biomechanical properties, which have been described in multiple studies [12]. Specific structural changes occurring in the corneal stroma as part of the disease process can be linked to alterations in the viscous and elastic properties of the cornea in keratoconus.

There is extensive ex vivo studies using techniques such as tensile test and inflation test to analyze the biomechanical properties of the normal cornea, such as viscosity, elasticity, and anisotropy; few have investigated the keratoconus using above classical biomechanical experiments. Recent research has focused on measuring corneal deformation parameters in vivo using two commercially available instruments to reflect its biomechanical properties since those can be used clinically.

The ORA calculates corneal hysteresis (CH) and corneal resistance factor (CRF) using an infrared-based optical system to measure the bidirectional movement of the cornea in response to an air pulse. The inward motion of the cornea during the ingoing phase is marked by the first applanation moment, *A*1. Based on this data, the air pump then modulates its stream to create a pulse with a Gaussian configuration. The outgoing phase is marked by the second applanation, *A*2. CH is the difference between *A*1 and *A*2; CRF equals $a[A1 - 0.7A2] + d$. The two constants maximize correlation with central corneal thickness (CCT) [7]. Additional parameters that measure the waveform have been derived.

The Corvis ST (and brand name with FDA is STL) also analyzes the dynamic behavior of the cornea, when temporarily deformed by an air puff; however, the output parameters of these two instruments are not directly comparable due to differences in the characteristics of the air puff and output parameters. First, the Scheimpflug technology captures 140 horizontal 8-mm frames in 33 ms. Compared to the ORA, the Corvis ST outputs at least 11 primary corneal deformation parameters (Fig. 3.1). The Corvis ST utilizes different aspects of the electromagnetic spectrum, rendering it less susceptible to tear film and sur-

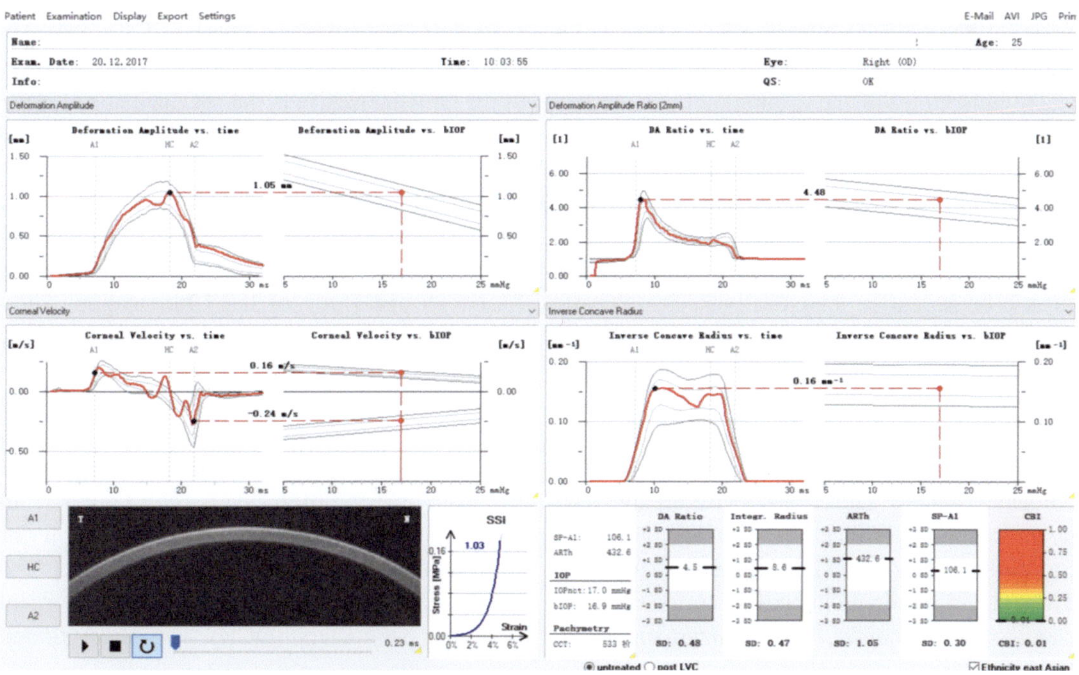

Fig. 3.1 Corneal deformation parameters measured by the Corvis ST

face irregularities [2]. Second, the Corvis ST has a fixed peak pressure per air puff [7]. The primary measured values—*A*1 length, *A*2 length, and *A*1 velocity—are repeatable in healthy and KCN corneas. The output biomarker describing corneal stiffness is the SP-*A*1. SP-*A*1 equals the loading forces (air pressure minus biomechanically measured intraocular pressure) divided by the displacement of the corneal apex at the first applanation moment [7].

In addition to detailed analysis of the ectasia spectrum, the Corvis ST has also been used to compare the biomechanics after laser-assisted subepithelial keratectomy (LASEK, also laser epithelial keratomileusis) [15], laser-assisted in situ keratomileusis (LASIK), and small incision lenticule extraction (SMILE) refractive surgery [16].

3.3 Biomechanical Changes

Before examining the biomechanics of the keratoconic cornea, here, we review the biomechanical properties and natural history in the healthy cornea. Each layer, including the tear film, contributes to the cornea's viscoelastic properties, with Bowman's layer, stroma, and Descemet's membrane having higher elastic moduli. Each layer also has spatiotemporal pattern. In addition to the anisotropy of the stroma, animal models have demonstrated biomechanical variability along the nasal-temporal and superior-inferior axes. Finally, the stroma has a depth-dependent gradient function that follows logically from its collagen lamellar structure, with the anterior stroma being stiffer than the posterior stroma. Notably, the degree of lamellar interweaving does not fully account for the empirical strength of the depth-dependent gradient; so, other forces are also at play.

Many supraocular and ocular variables affect corneal hysteresis. The cornea's viscous and elastic properties vary linearly with age [17, 18]. Stiffness increases while viscosity decreases. These age-dependent changes in corneal biomechanics occur secondary to nonenzymatic cross-links in the stroma. Similarly, hyperglycemia induces corneal cross-linking [12]. Thyroid hormone concentrations and the menstrual cycle also affect corneal biomechanics, but differences at the population level between men and women have not been described [12, 19]. Ethnicity affects corneal biomechanics [19].

Given this multitude of variables affecting corneal biomechanics, the first step in developing a KCN screening test is collecting population-level data on corneal parameters in healthy subjects, which is currently underway [17–23]. Data from patients with common diseases such as ocular hypertension and glaucoma [22] is key for developing generalizable and applicable algorithms. Normative data in multiple populations have shown that intraocular pressure (IOP) [18, 24] and CCT [18, 19] are major determinants of biomechanical properties, especially when measured by the Corvis ST.

3.3.1 Biomechanical Changes in KCN

Studies using these two instruments have reported significant differences between KCN and healthy corneas. Eyes with KCN have a significant lower CCT, CH, and CRF compared with normal eyes [25]. This may be the consequence of distortion of the lamellar matrix in the stroma that no longer follows an orthogonal pattern, with regions of highly aligned collagen intermixed with regions of little aligned collagen [14].

The deformation amplitude has been the best predictive parameter of KCN with a sensitivity of 81.7% in one study of the Chinese population [23]. After controlling for age, CCT, and IOP, deformation amplitude and radius of corneal curvature were significantly different in a study based in Hong Kong [26]. The sagittal Scheimpflug image of the cornea provides data for pachymetry profiles and progression from apex to periphery, enabling calculation of Ambrosio's relational thickness (ARTh) [7]. The ARTh, along with other dynamic corneal response parameters (DCR), was incorporated into the Corvis biomechanical index (CBI) [9]. Using the CBI, researchers correctly classified healthy and keratoconic corneas with 98.4% specificity and 100% sensitivity [9]. The Corvis ST now also has the tomographic/biomechanical index (TBI) that incorporates tomography which improves its discriminative ability with a sensitivity and specificity of 100% in one study [8]. This same study showed no statistical difference in the area under the curve between the parameters of the ORA and Corvis ST [8]. The next frontier for this line of research involves developing optimized artificial intelligence functions with these data sets [7].

*A*2 velocity, *A*2 length, and the difference between the first and second applanation lengths are parameters sensitive enough to discriminate between keratonic and healthy corneas. These parameters also change significantly after CXL [7].

Interestingly, in a pediatric population seen at a tertiary hospital in north India, both CH and CRF as measured by the ORA had a statistically significant, negative correlation with severity of KCN, as graded on the scale of I–IV as described previously [27].

3.3.2 Biomechanical Changes in ffKCN

Reliably differentiating KCN from ffKCN (subclinical KCN) is arguably the most important next step in KCN diagnostics. One study differentiated ffKCN from normal eyes in terms of CCT, CH, and CRF: in the low CCT group (<500 mm), CH achieves 87% sensitivity, whereas CRF achieves 91% sensitivity [28]. Another study found statistically significant differences between KCN and normal eyes in the following parameters after matching patients for IOP and CCT: maximum deformation amplitude, curvature radius at the highest concavity, *A*2 length, and *A*2 corneal velocity. These parameters did not generate a receiver operating characteristic curve with a high enough area under the curve. Velocity at *A*2 was the best single parameter to diagnose ffKCN [2].

3.3.3 Biomechanical Changes After Intrastromal Corneal Ring Segments

Intrastromal corneal ring segments are a well-established part of ophthalmologist's armamentarium to stabilize keratoconus [29]. However, in a study based in France, the biomechanical parameters of CH and CRF did not change at postoperative month 6 despite changing of the corneal curvature [30]. Statistically significant postoperative changes included a decrease in the mean maximum height of *A*2 and the width of the peak during *A*1 [30].

3.3.4 Biomechanical Changes in CXL

CXL has been described to stiffen the keratoconic cornea by instilling riboflavin in combination with exposure to an ultraviolet A light source [31]. In an ex vivo study of the human cornea, the corneal stiffness increased by 328.9% after CXL [32]. An early study from Turkey utilized the ORA to evaluate patients who had undergone CXL but was unable to find a difference in either early (months: 1–6) or late postoperative (months: 10–29) period [33]. In an Iranian population treated with CXL, the Corvis ST showed that the *A*2 length increased and *A*2 velocity decreased; the ORA demonstrated a significant decrease in CRF and increase in waveform scores [20]. Another study showed that CXL improved *A*1 time and *A*2 time [34]. Lastly, a study evaluating SP-A1 changes over 2 years demonstrated efficacy of accelerated CXL [7].

3.3.5 Biomechanics in Refractive Surgery

The patient with a potential risk of developing keratoconus is intended to undergo corneal refractive surgery, where preoperative screening for early stage of keratoconus is important. Corneal topography alone is sometimes not sufficient to diagnose a keratoconus and needs to be combined with biomechanics. At the same time, if too much corneal tissue is removed during the procedure of refractive surgery, the patient may be at risk for postoperative corneal ectasia since the biomechanical stability of the cornea is reduced after surgery. Therefore, before discussing the importance of biomechanics on treatment success, the most important is preventing harm coming to patients for refractive surgery and pay attention to the role of biomechanics as a diagnostic assistance, although abnormal topography and tomography are currently the standard of care for recognizing susceptibility to developing ectasia after LASIK [7].

Biomechanical changes in the cornea as a function of progressive, age-related cross-linking likely affect refractive surgery. One well-known phenomenon would be the varying corneal responses to astigmatic keratotomy eye surgery and LASIK in younger compared to older corneas [12]. Biomechanics are already being used to improve the predictability and efficacy of laser vision correction [5]. One case described a patient who developed ectasia in one eye only after SMILE to both eyes. Preoperatively, he had a normal CBI; retrospective analysis showed an abnormal preoperative TBI in the ectatic eye with corroborating differences in the molecular markers between the two extracted lenticules [35].

3.4 Conclusions

The biomechanics of the eye, the cornea in particular, is a new, rapidly approaching horizon in ophthalmology. The ability to detect biomechanical instability in pathological corneas will allow surgeons to preserve better vision and monitor changes after interventions. High-resolution, three-dimensional mapping of healthy—and more importantly presumably healthy—corneas will aid refractive surgeons in tailoring treatment patterns and screening out patients at risk for ectasia.

Key Points

- The biomechanics of the cornea varies as a function of layer and specific location within the cornea.
- The Corvis ST generates large amounts of data which are in the process of characterizing and interpreting for individual patients. These findings need to be placed in context of the diversity of patients around the world of varying ages and health.
- Biomechanical analysis with biometers such as the ORA and Corvis ST can help distinguish KCN from ffKCN.
- Screening for early stage of keratoconus with the assistance of corneal biomechanics could avoid the postoperative corneal ectasia and keratoconus.
- Interventions such as corneal cross-linking or intrastromal corneal ring segments can improve the biomechanical stability of the cornea and make it approach to a healthy cornea.

References

1. Galvis V, Sherwin T, Tello A, Merayo J, Barrera R, Acera A. Keratoconus: an inflammatory disorder? Eye (Lond). 2015;29(7):843–59.
2. Peris-Martínez C, Díez-Ajenjo MA, García-Domene MC, Pinazo-Durán MD, Luque-Cobija MJ, Del Buey-Sayas MÁ, Ortí-Navarro S. Evaluation of intraocular pressure and other biomechanical parameters to distinguish between subclinical keratoconus and healthy corneas. J Clin Med. 2021;10(9):1905.
3. Auffarth GU, Wang L, Völcker HE. Keratoconus evaluation using the Orbscan Topography system. J Cataract Refract Surg. 2000;26(2):222–8.
4. Bamdad S, Sedaghat MR, Yasemi M, Vahedi A. Sensitivity and specificity of Belin Ambrosio enhanced ectasia display in early diagnosis of keratoconus. J Ophthalmol. 2020;2020:7625659.
5. Wilson SE, Klyce SD. Screening for corneal topographic abnormalities before refractive surgery. Ophthalmology. 1994;101(1):147–52.
6. Yang Y, Pavlatos E, Chamberlain W, Huang D, Li Y. Keratoconus detection using OCT corneal and epithelial thickness map parameters and patterns. J Cataract Refract Surg. 2021;47(6):759–66.
7. Esporcatte LPG, Salomão MQ, Lopes BT, Vinciguerra P, Vinciguerra R, Roberts C, Elsheikh A, Dawson DG, Ambrósio R Jr. Biomechanical diagnostics of the cornea. Eye Vis (Lond). 2020;7:9.
8. Sedaghat MR, Momeni-Moghaddam H, Ambrósio R Jr, Heidari HR, Maddah N, Danesh Z, Sabzi F. Diagnostic ability of corneal shape and biomechanical parameters for detecting frank keratoconus. Cornea. 2018;37(8):1025–34.

9. Vinciguerra R, Ambrósio R Jr, Elsheikh A, Roberts CJ, Lopes B, Morenghi E, Azzolini C, Vinciguerra P. Detection of keratoconus with a new biomechanical index. J Refract Surg. 2016;32(12):803–10.
10. Bao F, Geraghty B, Wang Q, Elsheikh A. Consideration of corneal biomechanics in the diagnosis and management of keratoconus: is it important? Eye Vis (Lond). 2016;3:18.
11. Ambrósio R Jr, Ramos I, Luz A, Faria FC, Steinmueller A, Krug M, Belin MW, Roberts CJ. Avaliação Dinâmica com fotografia de Scheimpflug de alta velocidade para avaliar as propriedades biomecânicas da córnea [Dynamic ultra high speed scheimpflug imaging for assessing corneal biomechanical properties]. Rev Bras Oftalmol. 2013;72(2):99–102.
12. Blackburn BJ, Jenkins MW, Rollins AM, Dupps WJ. A review of structural and biomechanical changes in the cornea in aging, disease, and photochemical crosslinking. Front Bioeng Biotechnol. 2019;7:66.
13. Shetty R, Sathyanarayanamoorthy A, Ramachandra RA, Arora V, Ghosh A, Srivatsa PR, Pahuja N, Nuijts RM, Sinha-Roy A, Mohan RR, Ghosh A. Attenuation of lysyl oxidase and collagen gene expression in keratoconus patient corneal epithelium corresponds to disease severity. Mol Vis. 2015;21:12–25.
14. Meek KM, Tuft SJ, Huang Y, Gill PS, Hayes S, Newton RH, Bron AJ. Changes in collagen orientation and distribution in keratoconus corneas. Invest Ophthalmol Vis Sci. 2005;46(6):1948–56.
15. Dou R, Wang Y, Xu L, Wu D, Wu W, Li X. Comparison of corneal biomechanical characteristics after surface ablation refractive surgery and novel lamellar refractive surgery. Cornea. 2015;34(11):1441–6.
16. Khamar P, Shetty R, Vaishnav R, Francis M, Nuijts RMMA, Sinha RA. Biomechanics of LASIK flap and SMILE cap: a prospective, clinical study. J Refract Surg. 2019;35(5):324–32.
17. Lee H, Kang DSY, Ha BJ, Choi JY, Kim EK, Seo KY, Kim TI. Biomechanical properties of the cornea using a dynamic scheimpflug analyzer in healthy eyes. Yonsei Med J. 2018;59(9):1115–22.
18. Wang W, He M, He H, Zhang C, Jin H, Zhong X. Corneal biomechanical metrics of healthy Chinese adults using Corvis ST. Cont Lens Anterior Eye. 2017;40(2):97–103.
19. Valbon BF, Ambrósio R Jr, Fontes BM, Luz A, Roberts CJ, Alves MR. Ocular biomechanical metrics by CorVis ST in healthy Brazilian patients. J Refract Surg. 2014;30(7):468–73.
20. Salouti R, Khalili MR, Zamani M, Ghoreyshi M, Nowroozzadeh MH. Assessment of the changes in corneal biomechanical properties after collagen cross-linking in patients with keratoconus. J Curr Ophthalmol. 2019;31(3):262–7.
21. Huseynova T, Waring GO IV, Roberts C, Krueger RR, Tomita M. Corneal biomechanics as a function of intraocular pressure and pachymetry by dynamic infrared signal and scheimpflug imaging analysis in normal eyes. Am J Ophthalmol. 2014;157(4):885–93.
22. Reznicek L, Muth D, Kampik A, Neubauer AS, Hirneiss C. Evaluation of a novel scheimpflug-based non-contact tonometer in healthy subjects and patients with ocular hypertension and glaucoma. Br J Ophthalmol. 2013;97(11):1410–4.
23. Tian L, Huang YF, Wang LQ, Bai H, Wang Q, Jiang JJ, Wu Y, Gao M. Corneal biomechanical assessment using corneal visualization Scheimpflug technology in keratoconic and normal eyes. J Ophthalmol. 2014;2014:147516.
24. Salouti R, Bagheri M, Shamsi A, Zamani M. Corneal parameters in healthy subjects assessed by Corvis ST. J Ophthalmic Vis Res. 2020;15(1):24–31.
25. Piñero DP, Alcón N. In vivo characterization of corneal biomechanics. J Cataract Refract Surg. 2014;40(6):870–87.
26. Ye C, Yu M, Lai G, Jhanji V. Variability of corneal deformation response in normal and keratoconic eyes. Optom Vis Sci. 2015;92(7):e149–53.
27. Gupta Y, Sharma N, Maharana PK, Saxena R, Sinha R, Agarwal T, Jhanji V, Titiyal JS. Pediatric keratoconus: topographic, biomechanical and aberrometric characteristics. Am J Ophthalmol. 2021;225:69–75.
28. Fontes BM, Ambrósio R Jr, Jardim D, Velarde GC, Nosé W. Corneal biomechanical metrics and anterior segment parameters in mild keratoconus. Ophthalmology. 2010;117(4):673–9.
29. Rabinowitz YS. Intacs for keratoconus. Curr Opin Ophthalmol. 2007;18(4):279–83.
30. Dauwe C, Touboul D, Roberts CJ, Mahmoud AM, Kérautret J, Fournier P, Malecaze F, Colin J. Biomechanical and morphological corneal response to placement of intrastromal corneal ring segments for keratoconus. J Cataract Refract Surg. 2009;35(10):1761–7.
31. Wollensak G, Spoerl E, Seiler T. Riboflavin/ultraviolet-a-induced collagen crosslinking for the treatment of keratoconus. Am J Ophthalmol. 2003;135(5):620–7.
32. Wollensak G, Spoerl E, Seiler T. Stress-strain measurements of human and porcine corneas after riboflavin-ultraviolet-A-induced cross-linking. J Cataract Refract Surg. 2003;29(9):1780–5.
33. Küçümen RB, Şahan B, Yıldırım CA, Çiftçi F. Evaluation of corneal biomechanical changes after collagen crosslinking in patients with progressive keratoconus by ocular response analyzer. Turk J Ophthalmol. 2018;48(4):160–5.
34. Steinberg J, Katz T, Mousli A, Frings A, Casagrande MK, Druchkiv V, Richard G, Linke SJ. Corneal biomechanical changes after crosslinking for progressive keratoconus with the corneal visualization Scheimpflug technology. J Ophthalmol. 2014;2014:579190.
35. Shetty R, Kumar NR, Khamar P, Francis M, Sethu S, Randleman JB, Krueger RR, Sinha Roy A, Ghosh A. Bilaterally asymmetric corneal ectasia following SMILE with asymmetrically reduced stromal molecular markers. J Refract Surg. 2019;35(1):6–14.

4 Pathophysiology and Histopathology of Keratoconus

Somasheila I. Murthy, Dilip K. Mishra, and Varsha M. Rathi

4.1 Introduction

Historically, keratoconus (KC) is a complex disorder, with multiple etiological factors acting simultaneously to produce its classical signs [1]. The disease is traditionally still considered noninflammatory by many, due to the absence of neovascularization or cellular infiltration. The changes of keratoconus can be noted in all layers, with stromal thinning being the most prominent feature noted both clinically and histopathologically. Early keratoconus is difficult to detect clinically and usually is associated with good vision; however, as the diseases progress, the changes in the corneal structure are evident and go hand in hand with visual deterioration. In this chapter, we describe the pathophysiological processes and histopathological changes in keratoconus to understand the disease in its entirety.

S. I. Murthy (✉)
The Cornea Institute, L V Prasad Eye Institute, Hyderabad, Telangana, India
e-mail: smurthy@lvpei.org

D. K. Mishra
Ophthalmic Pathology Laboratory, L V Prasad Eye Institute, Hyderabad, Telangana, India
e-mail: dilipkumarmishra@lvpei.org

V. M. Rathi
Allen Foster Community Eye Health Research Centre, Gullapalli Pratibha Rao International Centre for Advancement of Rural Eye Care, L V Prasad Eye Institute, Hyderabad, Telangana, India

Indian Health Outcomes, Public Health and Economics (IHOPE) Research Centre, L V Prasad Eye Institute, Hyderabad, Telangana, India
e-mail: varsha@lvpei.org

4.2 Pathophysiology of Keratoconus

Galvis et al. challenged the widely held notion about the noninflammatory origins of the disease, and in their review, they highlighted the dominant role of inflammation as the chief pathway in the development and progression of keratoconus [1]. They proposed five major events supporting inflammation as follows: (a) changes in the composition of corneal stroma, (b) inflammation at the molecular level, (c) imbalance of proteolytic enzymes, (d) oxidative stresses, and (e) cellular hypersensitivity. With the advent of complex molecular techniques to study this disease, new theories on the pathogenesis have been propounded [2–6].

Although these events may take place concurrently, two challenges remain: determining the exact sequence of events that leads to disease progression and establishing the presence of the causative event or events, with certainty.

4.2.1 Composition of the Corneal Stroma in Keratoconus

The cornea is mainly composed of collagen. Therefore, any alterations in volume, charac-

S. Das (ed.), *Keratoconus*, https://doi.org/10.1007/978-981-19-4262-4_4

teristics, shape, and size in collagen would cause changes in the structure of the cornea. Nearly 75% of the collagen present in the cornea is of type I [7]. Collagen types III, V, and VI are interlaced into the lamellae, and collagen type XII is interwoven into the basement membrane epithelium and subepithelial stroma [5, 8].

4.2.2 Alterations in Volume/Stromal Thinning

Studies using mass spectrometric analysis reported the stromal thinning was due to reduction in both the number of collagen lamellae of the stroma and the decrease in the quantity of collagen types I, III, V, and XII and other proteins such as lumican and keratocan [8, 9].

4.2.3 Alterations in Characteristics

As the keratoconus progresses, the distance between the fibers of collagen sheets is reduced, while there is an increase in abnormal proteoglycans, which come into closer contact with the collagen sheets. Slippage of the lamellae occurs due to the abnormal proteoglycans, causing a remodeling of the stromal composition [10]. These findings of slippage and remodeling were confirmed by Meek et al. and were determined by synchrotron X-ray scattering patterns [11].

Second-harmonic imaging studies by Morishige et al. showed reduced interweaving of lamellae as well as reduced inserting into Bowman's layer [12]. Other abnormalities include the presence of fibronectin and tenascin in the anterior portion of corneas with keratoconus, increased type IX collagen, dysregulation of type XVIII collagen expression, and impaired healing response [13]. The interactions between altered stroma, presence of abnormal proteins, and impaired healing response to inflammatory process are associated with the formation of keratoconus [5, 14].

4.2.4 Role of Inflammatory Mediators Including TGF Beta Pathway and Cytokine Dysregulation

An upregulation of transforming growth factor-β (TGFβ) and interleukin (IL)-1 both of which modulate the expression of metalloproteinases was noted by Girard et al. [15] Zhou et al. showed that the expression of TGFβ, IL-1, vimentin, and tenascin was enhanced in keratoconus corneas [16]. Pouliquen et al. reported various molecules such as cytokines, IL-1, tumor necrosis factor-α (TNF-α), TGFβ, IL-6, IL-8, and platelet-derived growth factor (PDGF) which may be putative in the regulation of a protease cascade involving the plasmin system which would eventually lead to the changes noted in the extracellular matrix in keratoconus [17]. They also found a tenfold increase in prostaglandin (PG) E2 synthesis from the keratocytes as compared to normal cornea. Other authors have found decreased corneal sensitivity, shorter tear film breakup times, and increased surface staining and squamous metaplasia and goblet cells in the epithelium suggesting that the pathophysiology can be attributed to an epithelial origin [18]. Another source of inflammatory mediators is the tear film, which showed increased levels of the proinflammatory cytokines IL-6, TNF-α, and elevated levels of matrix metalloproteinase 9 (MMP-9) [19]. This was more evident in unilateral keratoconus (fellow eye being subclinical) where IL-6 and TNF-α were elevated in both eyes, whereas MMP-9 was elevated only in the keratoconic eye [20]. The same authors also found intercellular adhesion molecule (ICAM-1), vascular adhesion molecule 1 (VCAM-1), IL-6, and MMP-9 were overexpressed by 2–40 times in contact lens wearers of keratoconus as compared to myopic controls [21]. It would be appropriate to conclude that this lop-sided balance between proinflammatory and anti-inflammatory cytokines is likely to effect changes in the structure and function of the cornea, stimulating more production of metalloproteinases resulting in keratocyte apoptosis, thus leading to the changes noted in keratoconus [5, 22, 23].

The role of eye rubbing as a predictor for keratoconus progression is well known [24, 25]. Pathophysiological changes due to frequent eye rubbing include friction-induced rise in the corneal temperature, as well as increased levels of tear MMP-13, IL-6, and TNF-α even in normal and keratoconic eyes [26]. Therefore, persistent eye rubbing seemingly causes a sustained increase of proinflammatory cytokines, which may lead to keratoconus or its progression [27].

4.2.5 Imbalance of Proteolytic Enzymes

Several studies have implicated the role of MMPs in the pathophysiology of keratoconus. Studies have shown the increased activity of collagenase and gelatinase, which are produced by corneal epithelial and stromal cells to be much higher in keratoconic corneas [6, 27, 28]. Overexpression of pro-MMP-2, which is a proenzyme of MMP-2, has also been reported in keratoconus, and this could be another mechanism in the pathways regulated by the MMPs [29–31]. Apart from MMP-2, MMP-3 have also been noted to be increased in number and metabolism in the ECM of keratoconic corneas and perhaps contribute to its remodeling [32]. In a similar study, Mackiewicz et al. reported increased expression of several MMPs such as MMP-1, MMP-3, MMP-7, and MMP-13, as well as IL-4, IL-6, and TNF-α [33]. The imbalance between MMPs in terms of oversecretion and decreased expression of its inhibitors has also been implicated for keratoconus progression in pregnancy [34].

4.2.6 Oxidative Stresses

Oxidative stress has been reported as a mechanism in the development of KC [35–39]. However, it was not until 2005 that elevated catalase RNA and activity were demonstrated in human KC corneas [27]. Studies have shown various biochemical factors involved in keratoconus, such as lower levels of glutathione and total antioxidant capacity [36]. Increased oxidative stress can lead to damage to the stromal tissue and the collection of metabolic end products which can directly damage the stromal keratocytes leading to cellular apoptosis [37–39].

4.2.7 Cellular Hypersensitivity to Apoptosis

Pouliquen et al. [17] noted that IL-1 receptors were present in four times the numbers as compared to normal corneas. Other authors too suggested that this increased sensitivity predisposed these corneas to apoptosis as opposed to normal corneas where apoptosis is rare without injury [37, 40, 41].

4.3 Histopathology

The histopathological changes in keratoconus can be very subtle to very prominent and affect all layers of the cornea [42]. The pathological changes in keratoconus are believed to initially affect the anterior stroma and Bowman's layer and epithelium in the early stages with almost normal posterior stroma [43]. Brautaset et al. have reported more global or pan-corneal pathological changes as noted by them [44]. As surgical therapy for this disease has moved from full-thickness transplants to deep anterior lamellar keratoplasty, the types of specimens that reach the pathologist are predominantly lamellar tissue and fragments of tissue. Therefore, the complete histopathological findings are noted in specimens from penetrating keratoplasty only. Hematoxylin and eosin (H&E) and periodic acid-Schiff (PAS) stains are routinely used; however, special stains such as Perls stain can be used specially to demarcate the iron deposition. Overall, the central cornea is thinner, the Bowman's layer (BL) is disrupted, the central stroma is thinned, and the central Descemet membrane (DM) can show fragmentation. The pathological changes are described under the following headings:

(a) Penetrating keratoplasty (PK) specimens: epithelial changes, changes in the BL, stromal changes, Dua's layer, DM, and endothelial cell layer.
(b) Deep anterior lamellar keratoplasty (DALK) specimens and attempted DALK specimens: epithelial changes, BL changes, stromal changes, DM.
(c) Acute and healed hydrops.
(d) Histopathological changes after collagen cross-linking.

4.3.1 Penetrating Keratoplasty Specimens

Histopathologically, under low magnification or scanner view, the specimen shows thinning or elongation, with the central part being the thinnest and scarred due to the loss of lamellar pattern of collagen fibers and increased keratocytes (Fig. 4.1a–d).

4.3.2 Epithelial Changes

The epithelium shows several irregularities that have been extensively described previously [45, 46]. Central epithelial thinning has been found in some cases. Sykakis et al. have described several changes on each layer of the epithelium wherein they noted that the epithelial cells may vary in the number of layers ranging from two to three layers in some areas to more than ten layers especially at the apex of the cone [45]. Millas et al. described three distinctive patterns of epithelial changes in the central cornea. Pattern 1 was defined as central corneal epithelium being focally thicker than the periphery, pattern 2 was described as the central epithelium being thinner than the peripheral epithelium (Fig. 4.2a), and pattern 3 has been described as both the central and the peripheral epithelium with equal thickness [47]. In severe cases, these changes can be very dramatic, with the cone showing hypertrophic epithelium, a very minimal amount of stroma overlying the pre-Descemet-Descemet membrane complex. In addition, there is an elongation of the cells in the superficial layer of the epithelium, which appears

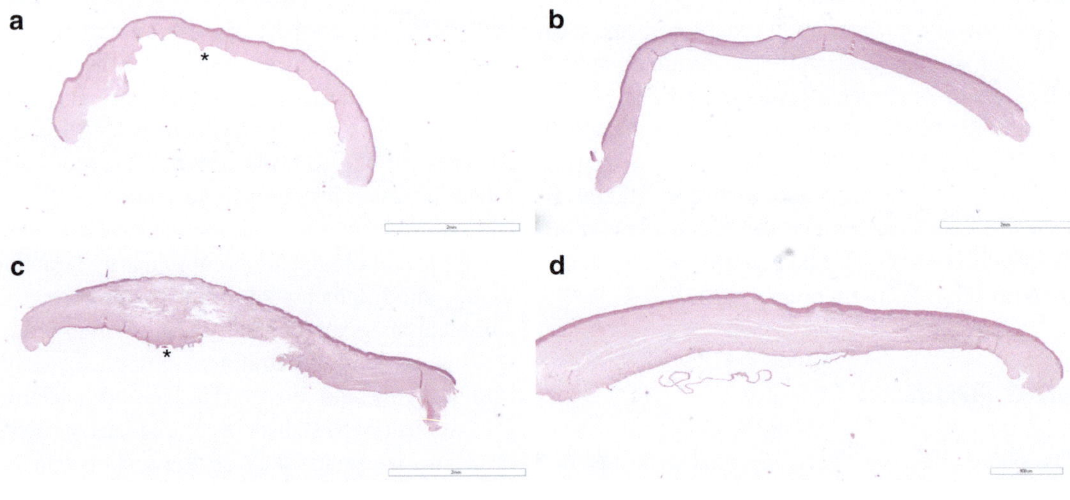

Fig. 4.1 Penetrating keratoplasty specimens: (**a**) histopathology of the entire section of a keratoconic cornea shows a bow-shaped cornea with diffuse thinning throughout except for the peripheral parts of the section. The epithelium showed irregular thickening almost throughout the specimen, and the Bowman's layer has tentlike projections pushing up the epithelium, some of which correspond to protrusion of the posterior stroma and folds in the Descemet membrane (black asterisk), 2× (digital scanner view), hematoxylin and eosin stain. (**b**) Prominent thinning of the central stroma as compared to the periphery, 2× (digital scanner view), hematoxylin and eosin stain. (**c**) Scanner view of a specimen of acute hydrops shows stromal edema and rupture of the Descemet membrane (black asterisk), 2× (digital scanner view), hematoxylin and eosin stain. (**d**) Scanner view of the entire corneal specimen shows a case of chronic hydrops, 2× (digital scanner view), hematoxylin and eosin stain

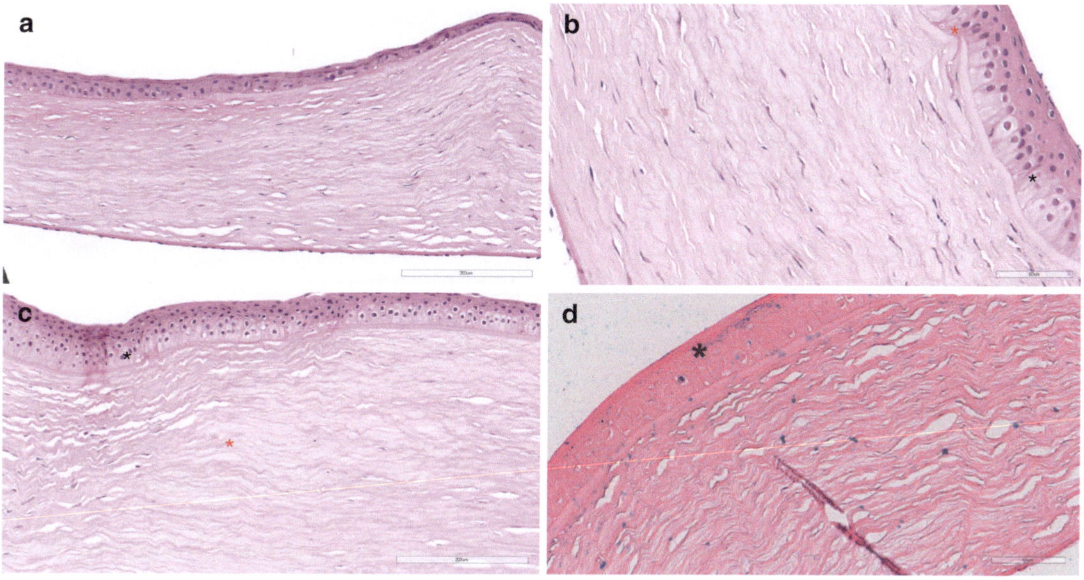

Fig. 4.2 (**a**) The specimen shows central epithelial thinning and irregular arrangement of stromal collagen and intact complement of endothelial cells, 4× (digital scanner view), hematoxylin and eosin stain. (**b**) High magnification shows spindle-shaped appearance of the epithelial cells in the superficial layers and hydropic degeneration in epithelial basal cells (black asterisk). A prominent break in the Bowman's layer is noted as a discontinuity and is bridged by protrusion of stromal collagen (red asterisk), 10× (digital scanner view), hematoxylin and eosin stain. (**c**) Epithelial hypertrophy and enlarged basal cells are noted (black asterisk). Multiple breaks are noted in Bowman's layer with increased keratocytic nuclei at the site corresponding to the break, and the stroma (red asterisk) shows diffuse changes in the collagen, 10× (digital scanner view), hematoxylin and eosin stain. (**d**) Special stain to detect iron at the base of the cone shows faint blue granular staining in the epithelial cells (black asterisk) and Bowman's layer, 10× (digital scanner view), Perls stain

to be spindle-shaped (Fig. 4.2b). The wing cells can have large, irregularly spaced nucleus. The basal epithelial cells also appeared enlarged (Fig. 4.2b, c). Spectral domain optical coherence tomography (OCT) and ultrahigh-resolution OCT studies also show similar findings of marked changes in epithelial thickness [43, 48, 49]. TUNEL staining of the epithelium showed a wider range of positive staining across the epithelium as compared to normal corneas as reported by suggesting that apoptosis may have a role in the loss of epithelial cells and thinning [50].

Fleisher's ring is a hallmark clinical sign in keratoconus and is a brownish pigmented line occurring due to the deposition of iron at the base of the cone. First described by Gass [51], histopathologically, this can be picked as bluish staining using Perls Prussian blue stain for iron (Fig. 4.2d). Electron microscopy has shown that hemosiderin particles accumulate at the level of the basement membrane of the epithelium and within and between the epithelial cells.

4.3.3 Bowman's Layer

The characteristic feature of this layer is the presence of abrupt irregularities or breaks or disruptions (Fig. 4.2b, c) [52]. Degeneration of the basal cell layer can be noted with breaks in this layer leading to the epithelium growing posteriorly into the Bowman's layer and anteriorly into the epithelial layer leading to a Z-shaped configuration. The stroma underlying these breaks is distorted, and these distortions were noted in more than 90% cases in one study [45]. These breaks either can show protrusion of collagen from stroma with abnormal-looking keratocytes and its nuclei or may have protrusion of epithelial cells or of keratocytes [45]. Sykakis et al. described the nuclei in these breaks to often show intense staining, suggesting apoptotic state which was confirmed by TUNEL analysis in their study. In other areas, the stromal keratocytic nuclei appear to line the anterior stroma at the inner edge of the break, suggesting scarring, noted as apical scarring in vivo. Fragmentations noted on scanning electron microscopy of the Bowman's layer is also reported [53, 54]. Scroggs et al. [55] described the histopathological findings in relationship to breaks in the BL and labeled those corneas with breaks as "typical" and those without as "atypical" for keratoconus. They hypothesized that these breaks are features that appear more as the disease advances, with stromal fluctuations being the first signs of the disease.

Shapiro et al. [56] reported clear spaces located in the anterior thinned-out stroma to coincide with the breaks in the Bowman's layer, which may later get filled in by scar tissue according to them. These scar lines could correlate with the small reticular and apical scars noted in keratoconus clinically. In another study, Perry et al. [57] noted these findings to occur more in cases with oval and sagging cones rather than round cones.

4.3.4 Stroma

The central stroma appears thinner than the peripheral area (Fig. 4.1b). Sykakis et al. reported the mean stromal thickness at the periphery was twice the thickness of the area of maximal thinning (477.22 mm compared to 214.11 mm.) [45]. Pouliquen et al. found that while the collagen lamella appeared to be of normal size, the number found within the cone was very small (only 41%) compared to outside the cone [58]. Transmission electron microscopy findings also confirmed that the actual stromal lamella is of normal thickness but the number of lamella is less than in normal corneas [9]. The stromal lamellae show loosely arranged collagen (Fig. 4.2a), degradation of stroma, and poorly differentiated keratocytic nuclei. The anterior stroma shows fewer keratocytic nuclei compared to the posterior stroma. Focal areas especially in the central anterior stroma may show features of scarring which represents scarring noted in vivo and in cases of healed hydrops.

4.3.5 Dua's Layer

In 2003, Dua et al. described a new finding of a pre-Descemet acellular layer which consisted of densely packed collagen fibrils of the posterior most stroma, measuring approximately 10–15 μm in thickness and made up of 5–8 collagen lamella of type 1 collagen bundles running in transverse, oblique, and longitudinal directions [59]. At the corneal periphery, this layer continues as the core of collagen of the trabecular meshwork with the overlying trabecular cells [60].

4.3.6 Descemet's Membrane

This is better assessed with PAS stain. Folds can be noted and sometimes even ruptures can be observed. DM rupture can show curling of the edges away from the break, or the break can get sequestered in the posterior stroma (Fig. 4.3a, b). The area devoid of DM is usually filled in with a new DM-like membrane. In the case of long-standing breaks, the new membrane appears thinner due to stretch. Endothelial cells appear normal morphologically, although their distribution appears sparse. In the case of hydrops, dense and irregular arrangement of fibers within the stroma, with prominent DM break and rolled-up edges of DM, can be noted (Figs. 4.3 and 4.4).

4.3.7 Endothelial Cells

Some degree of polymegathism and pleomorphism can occur which appears to be comparable to normal controls with contact lens usage. Damage to the cells can occur more commonly at the base of the cone and correlates with severity and duration of the disease. However, overall, the endothelial cells are healthy and are often noted to be normal in the keratoplasty specimens (Fig. 4.2a).

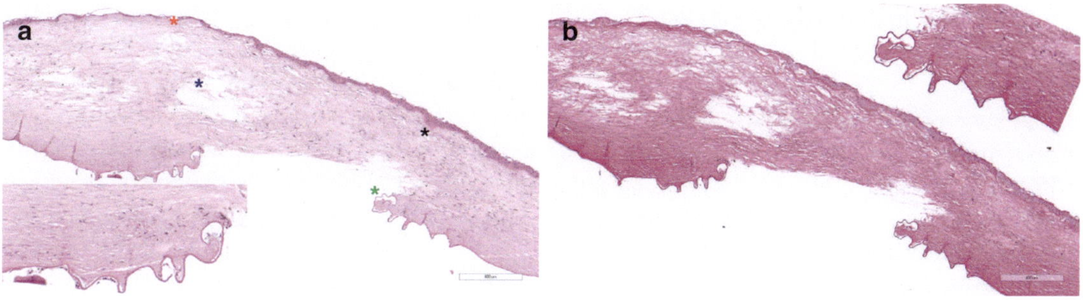

Fig. 4.3 Hydrops specimens: (**a**) histopathology of a specimen of acute hydrops shows attenuated epithelium with vesicle and bullae formation (red asterisk) and irregular thickening of the epithelium with epithelial downgrowths (black asterisk). Bowman's layer is discontinuous and absent in some areas. Stroma showed edema (blue asterisk) which is represented by separated and less stained collagen fibers. Descemet membrane is absent over the central part, and the fragmented ends show irregular folds and coiling inward (green asterisk), 18.5× (digital scanner view), hematoxylin and eosin stain. Inset shows digitally magnified view of the rolled and coiled DM, 40× (digital scanner view), hematoxylin and eosin stain. (**b**) Shows the same specimen with inset showing the other end of the fragmented DM showing irregular folds and coiling inward, 40× (digital scanner view), periodic acid-Schiff stain

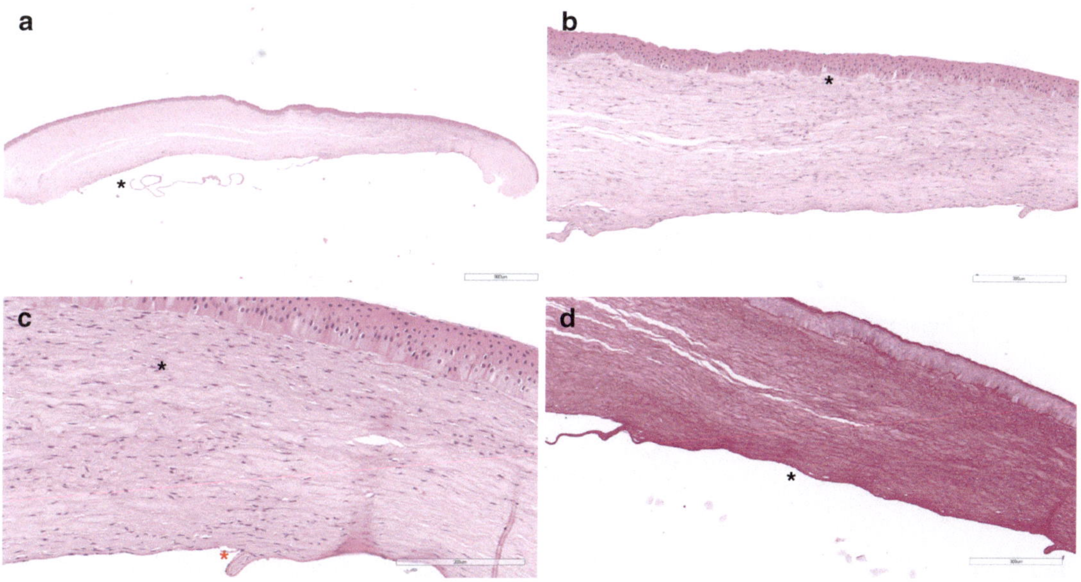

Fig. 4.4 Specimen of healed hydrops showing the following: (**a**) histopathology of a post-hydrops case shows a thickened button with DM lying posteriorly detached from the specimen (black asterisk), 2× (digital scanner view), hematoxylin and eosin stain. (**b**) The epithelium is irregular and thickened; Bowman's layer is discontinuous, shows multiple abrupt breaks (black asterisk), and is replaced by fibrous tissue. Stroma shows scarring, 10× (digital scanner view), hematoxylin and eosin stain. (**c**) The epithelium shows prominent hydropic degeneration in the basal cell layer, stroma shows disorganization, and an increased number of fibroblasts are noted under higher magnification (black asterisk). The edge of the DM rupture is noted as a fold, and the rest of the DM appears to be replaced by a membranous layer (red asterisk), 15× (digital scanner view), hematoxylin and eosin stain. (**d**) The rolled and thickened DM with thin linear basement-like material is noted to be deposited to occupy the gap of absent DM (black asterisk), 10× (digital scanner view), periodic-Schiff stain

4.3.8 DALK and Attempted DALK Specimens

In the case of the lamellar keratoplasty specimens, only tissue fragments are received (Fig. 4.5a–c). In most of the cases, the anterior most 200–300 μm layer is excised and submitted, with no air injection or alterations, and the deeper stroma typically shows air insufflation [61]. Epithelial, BL, and anterior stromal changes can be noted as mentioned earlier; however, the apical thinning is not easily appreciated in these specimens (Fig. 4.5a–d) [62]. Deeper stromal changes are distorted due to air insufflation thought out the stroma (Fig. 4.5d), which may be somewhat more at one periphery [61]. Air is noted as clear spaces separating the stromal lamellae (Fig. 4.5d). Some of the spaces show some granular material of unknown etiology. The areas of stroma which appear scarred typically show less air insufflation. In the case of attempted DALK, DM is also included in the specimen and appears as a separate layer (Fig. 4.5b, d). In some case of DALK where the manual separation was performed rather than big bubble or air insufflation, the pathological findings may be better preserved. Ting et al. studied 136 cases of clinically diagnosed keratoconus that underwent DALK, and they reported most of the conus samples had air artifacts and epithelial edema. In their study,

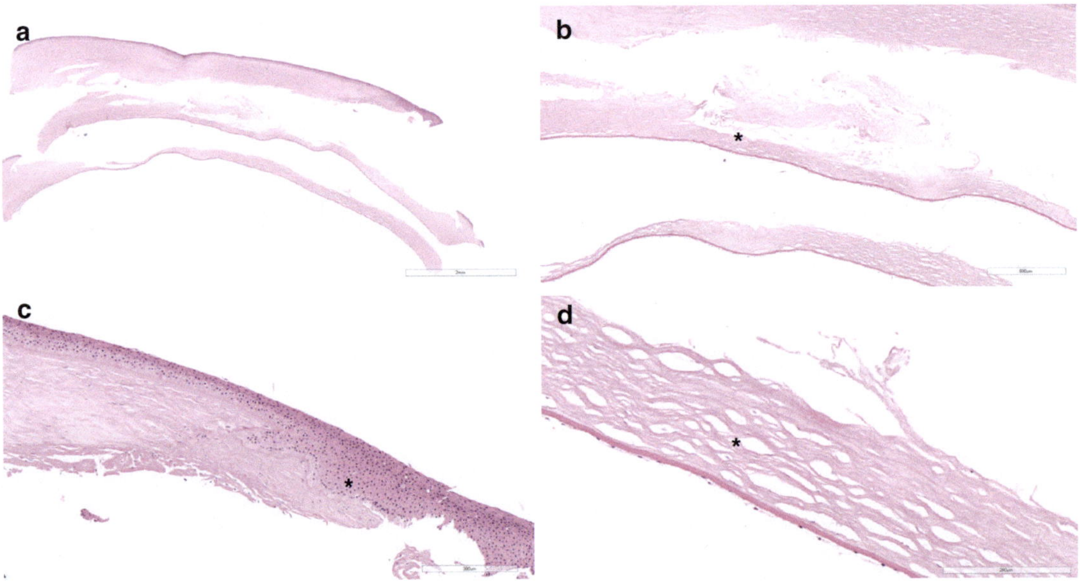

Fig. 4.5 (**a**) Histopathology of a specimen of unsuccessful deep anterior lamellar keratoplasty in a case of keratoconus and status post-radial keratectomy. Multiple linear fragments of the corneal tissue are submitted in this case due to the surgical techniques of lamellar dissection in layers. Note that the changes in these tissue fragments are difficult to interpret, 1.7× (digital scanner view), hematoxylin and eosin stain. (**b**) Several such tissue specimens are submitted in DALK cornea as seen here, and this mount shows the mid and posterior stroma with intact DM (black asterisk), 2× (digital scanner view), hematoxylin and eosin stain. (**c**) The same specimen under higher magnification shows epithelial hyperplasia and prominent epithelial downgrowth at one end (black asterisk). Bowman layer fragmentation at this region is prominent, and the underlying stroma shows generalized disorganization of collagen lamellae as well as oblique stromal scarring (red asterisk) consistent with radial keratotomy incision, 10× (digital scanner view), hematoxylin and eosin stain. (**d**) The deepest part of the specimen shows deep stroma filled with pseudocystic spaces due to air insufflation in vivo (black asterisk). DM and endothelial cells are intact (red asterisk), 20× (digital scanner view), hematoxylin and eosin stain

they were unable to identify conus or breaks in BL, which is an initial pathognomonic feature of keratoconus [63].

4.3.9 Acute Hydrops and Healed Hydrops

Apart from classical features such as epithelial hyperplasia, BL fragmentation and scarring, as well as stromal thinning, what can be additionally noted are acute and healed corneal hydrops [64]. Acute corneal hydrops is mostly seen in males in the second or third decade of life, and its incidence is approximately 2.5–3% of eyes with KC. The histopathology of the cornea in acute hydrops reveals intraepithelial microcyst formation with separation of the epithelium from BL to form bullae (Fig. 4.3a). These bullae are formed due to the accumulation of fluid in the breaks of the BL and come in direct contact with stroma. Stromal changes noted are edema with less pink staining of collagen fibers and pseudocyst formation. The corneal hydrops is a result of the torn DM which allows the anterior chamber aqueous into the cornea. Rupture or torn DM is noted to be coiled or rolled in from the edges because of the elastic property of DM (Fig. 4.3b). Additionally, in those cases where descemetopexy was done as a therapeutic procedure for resolution of the hydrops in the past followed by keratoplasty, unusual compression artifacts have been described by Basu et al. wherein they noted burial of the ruptured end of the DM into the posterior stroma [64]. In healed hydrops of keratoconus, corneal edema regresses, and stoma shows scarring with increased and irregularly placed keratocytes and broken DM retracted, curled, and folded inwardly, forming a scroll-like structure at the edge (Fig. 4.4a–d).

4.3.10 Histopathological Changes After Collagen Cross-linking

Many histopathological findings in post collagen cross-linking specimens are expected to be similar to that noted in other keratoconic corneas. Messmer et al. described light microscopic, ultrastructural, and immunohistochemical findings in 6 corneas obtained 5–30 months post cross-linking procedure and compared them with non-cross-linked keratoconic corneas [65]. The epithelium showed central thinning, the basement membrane was intact, and the Bowman's layer showed breaks. Stroma showed diffuse thinning, more in the central and paracentral regions, with marked reduction of keratocytes. The collagen structure appeared the same in both groups when seen on light microscopy. The Descemet membrane was normal and endothelium cells appeared normal. Overall, most of the findings were similar in the two groups. The only striking difference was a significant decrease in the keratocytes in the anterior stroma in cross-linked corneas, even as late as 30 months post-procedure. Based on this study, noting prominent loss of keratocytes in the anterior stroma on light microscopy in a keratoconic cornea most likely indicates history of cross-linking. The flowchart shown in Fig. 4.6 summarizes the histopathological changes in keratoconus.

4.4 Conclusion

Understanding the primary pathophysiological process resulting in weakening of the corneal collagen has helped to develop an effective therapy against its progression, such as cross-linking. However, the exact mechanism in this multifactorial disease remains elusive and incomplete. The trigger for this disease could be either an external environmental trigger or genetic predisposition, leading to a destructive cycle, as noted by evidence, provided by studies on molecular and genetic elements along with the studies on histopathology [66]. Whether this disease is inflammatory or whether inflammatory mediators aid the pathogenesis as an association remains to be answered, as there is evidence, both for and against inflammation.

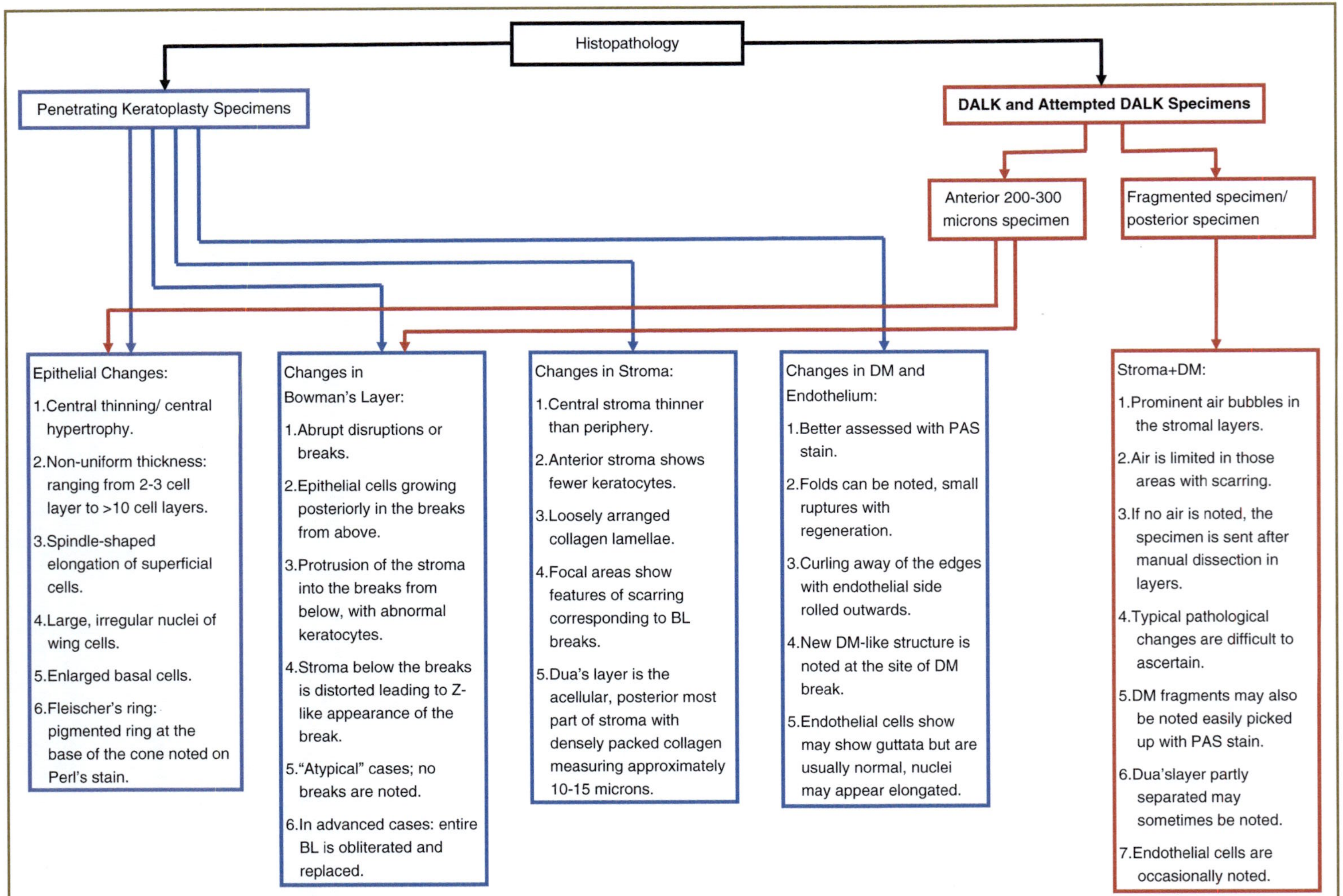

Fig. 4.6 Summary of histopathological changes

Acknowledgments
1. Dr. Vijayalakshmi Idimadakala for editing help.
2. Mr. Chenchu Naidu and Mr. B Sreedhar for histopathology slides.

Funding Support Hyderabad Eye Research Foundation, Hyderabad, India.

References

1. Galvis V, Sherwin T, Tello A, Merayo J, Barrera R, Acera A. Keratoconus: an inflammatory disorder? Eye (Lond). 2015;29(7):843–59.
2. Davidson AE, Hayes S, Hardcastle AJ, Tuft SJ. The pathogenesis of keratoconus. Eye (Lond). 2014;28(2):189–95.
3. Sugar J, Macsai MS. What causes keratoconus? Cornea. 2012;31(6):716–9.
4. Cristina Kenney M, Brown DJ. The cascade hypothesis of keratoconus. Cont Lens Anterior Eye. 2003;26(3):139–46.
5. Cheung IM, McGhee CN, Sherwin T. A new perspective on the pathobiology of keratoconus: interplay of stromal wound healing and reactive species-associated processes. Clin Exp Optom. 2013;96(2):188–96.
6. Nelidova D, Sherwin T. Keratoconus layer by layer–pathology and matrix metalloproteinases. Adv Ophthalmol. 2012;6:105–18.
7. Newsome DA, Gross J, Hassell JR. Human corneal stroma contains three distinct collagens. Invest Ophthalmol Vis Sci. 1982;22(3):376–81.
8. Chaerkady R, Shao H, Scott SG, Pandey A, Jun AS, Chakravarti S. The keratoconus corneal proteome: loss of epithelial integrity and stromal degeneration. J Proteome. 2013;87:122–31.
9. Takahashi A, Nakayasu K, Okisaka S, Kanai A. [Quantitative analysis of collagen fiber in keratoconus]. Nippon Ganka Gakkai Zasshi. 1990;94(11):1068–73.
10. Akhtar S, Bron AJ, Salvi SM, Hawksworth NR, Tuft SJ, Meek KM. Ultrastructural analysis of collagen fibrils and proteoglycans in keratoconus. Acta Ophthalmol. 2008;86(7):764–72.
11. Meek KM, Tuft SJ, Huang Y, Gill PS, Hayes S, Newton RH, Bron AJ. Changes in collagen orientation and distribution in keratoconus corneas. Invest Ophthalmol Vis Sci. 2005;46(6):1948–56.
12. Morishige N, Wahlert AJ, Kenney MC, Brown DJ, Kawamoto K, Chikama T, Nishida T, Jester JV. Second-harmonic imaging microscopy of normal human and keratoconus cornea. Invest Ophthalmol Vis Sci. 2007;48(3):1087–94.
13. Tuori A, Virtanen I, Aine E, Uusitalo H. The expression of tenascin and fibronectin in keratoconus, scarred and normal human cornea. Graefes Arch Clin Exp Ophthalmol. 1997;235(4):222–9.
14. Cheung IM, McGhee CN, Sherwin T. Deficient repair regulatory response to injury in keratoconic stromal cells. Clin Exp Optom. 2014;97(3):234–9.
15. Girard MT, Matsubara M, Fini ME. Transforming growth factor-beta and interleukin-1 modulate metalloproteinase expression by corneal stromal cells. Invest Ophthalmol Vis Sci. 1991;32(9):2441–54.
16. Zhou L, Yue BY, Twining SS, Sugar J, Feder RS. Expression of wound healing and stress-related proteins in keratoconus corneas. Curr Eye Res. 1996;15(11):1124–31.
17. Pouliquen Y, Bureau J, Mirshahi M, Mirshahi SS, Assouline M, Lorens G. Keratocone et processus inflammatoires [Keratoconus and inflammatory processes]. Bull Soc Belge Ophtalmol. 1996;262:25–8.
18. Dogru M, Karakaya H, Ozçetin H, Ertürk H, Yücel A, Ozmen A, Baykara M, Tsubota K. Tear function and ocular surface changes in keratoconus. Ophthalmology. 2003;110(6):1110–8.
19. Lema I, Durán JA. Inflammatory molecules in the tears of patients with keratoconus. Ophthalmology. 2005;112(4):654–9.
20. Lema I, Sobrino T, Durán JA, Brea D, Díez-Feijoo E. Subclinical keratoconus and inflammatory molecules from tears. Br J Ophthalmol. 2009;93(6):820–4.
21. Lema I, Durán JA, Ruiz C, Díez-Feijoo E, Acera A, Merayo J. Inflammatory response to contact lenses in patients with keratoconus compared with myopic subjects. Cornea. 2008;27(7):758–63.
22. Jun AS, Cope L, Speck C, Feng X, Lee S, Meng H, Hamad A, Chakravarti S. Subnormal cytokine profile in the tear fluid of keratoconus patients. PLoS One. 2011;6(1):e16437.
23. Wojcik KA, Blasiak J, Szaflik J, Szaflik JP. Role of biochemical factors in the pathogenesis of keratoconus. Acta Biochim Pol. 2014;61(1):55–62.
24. Bawazeer AM, Hodge WG, Lorimer B. Atopy and keratoconus: a multivariate analysis. Br J Ophthalmol. 2000;84(8):834–6.
25. Ridley F. Eye-rubbing and contact lenses. Br J Ophthalmol. 1961;45(9):631.
26. McMonnies CW, Korb DR, Blackie CA. The role of heat in rubbing and massage-related corneal deformation. Cont Lens Anterior Eye. 2012;35(4):148–54.
27. Balasubramanian SA, Pye DC, Willcox MD. Effects of eye rubbing on the levels of protease, protease activity and cytokines in tears: relevance in keratoconus. Clin Exp Optom. 2013;96(2):214–8.
28. Soiberman U, Foster JW, Jun AS, Chakravarti S. Pathophysiology of keratoconus: what do we know today. Open Ophthalmol J. 2017;11:252–61.
29. Smith VA, Easty DL. Matrix metalloproteinase 2: involvement in keratoconus. Eur J Ophthalmol. 2000;10(3):215–26.
30. Smith VA, El-Rakhawy A, Easty DL. Matrix metalloproteinase 2 activation in cultured corneas. Ophthalmic Res. 2001;33(1):1–6.

31. Smith VA, Hoh HB, Littleton M, Easty DL. Overexpression of a gelatinase a activity in keratoconus. Eye (Lond). 1995;9(Pt 4):429–33.
32. Balasubramanian SA, Mohan S, Pye DC, Willcox MD. Proteases, proteolysis and inflammatory molecules in the tears of people with keratoconus. Acta Ophthalmol. 2012;90(4):e303–9.
33. Mackiewicz Z, Määttä M, Stenman M, Konttinen L, Tervo T, Konttinen YT. Collagenolytic proteinases in keratoconus. Cornea. 2006;25(5):603–10. Erratum in: Cornea. 2006;25(6):760.
34. Bilgihan K, Hondur A, Sul S, Ozturk S. Pregnancy-induced progression of keratoconus. Cornea. 2011;30(9):991–4.
35. Behndig A, Karlsson K, Johansson BO, Brännström T, Marklund SL. Superoxide dismutase isoenzymes in the normal and diseased human cornea. Invest Ophthalmol Vis Sci. 2001;42(10):2293–6.
36. Arnal E, Peris-Martínez C, Menezo JL, Johnsen-Soriano S, Romero FJ. Oxidative stress in keratoconus? Invest Ophthalmol Vis Sci. 2011;52(12):8592–7.
37. Wojcik KA, Kaminska A, Blasiak J, Szaflik J, Szaflik JP. Oxidative stress in the pathogenesis of keratoconus and Fuchs endothelial corneal dystrophy. Int J Mol Sci. 2013;14(9):19294–308.
38. Toprak I, Kucukatay V, Yildirim C, Kilic-Toprak E, Kilic-Erkek O. Increased systemic oxidative stress in patients with keratoconus. Eye (Lond). 2014;28(3):285–9.
39. Buddi R, Lin B, Atilano SR, Zorapapel NC, Kenney MC, Brown DJ. Evidence of oxidative stress in human corneal diseases. J Histochem Cytochem. 2002;50(3):341–51.
40. Kim WJ, Rabinowitz YS, Meisler DM, Wilson SE. Keratocyte apoptosis associated with keratoconus. Exp Eye Res. 1999;69(5):475–81.
41. Wilson S, He Y, Weng J, Li Q, McDowall AW, Vital M, Chwang EL. Epithelial injury induces keratocyte apoptosis: hypothesized role for the interleukin-1 system in the modulation of corneal tissue organization and wound healing. Ophthalmic Lit. 1997;1(50):10.
42. Fernandes BF, Logan P, Zajdenweber ME, Santos LN, Cheema DP, Burnier MN Jr. Histopathological study of 49 cases of keratoconus. Pathology. 2008;40(6):623–6.
43. Mathew JH, Goosey JD, Bergmanson JP. Quantified histopathology of the keratoconic cornea. Optom Vis Sci. 2011;88(8):988–97.
44. Brautaset RL, Nilsson M, Miller WL, Leach NE, Tukler JH, Bergmanson JP. Central and peripheral corneal thinning in keratoconus. Cornea. 2013;32(3):257–61.
45. Sykakis E, Carley F, Irion L, Denton J, Hillarby MC. An in depth analysis of histopathological characteristics found in keratoconus. Pathology. 2012;44(3):234–9.
46. Tsubota K, Mashima Y, Murata H, Sato N, Ogata T. Corneal epithelium in keratoconus. Cornea. 1995;14(1):77–83.
47. Crespo Millas S, López JC, García-Lagarto E, Obregón E, Hileeto D, Maldonado MJ, Pastor JC. Histological patterns of epithelial alterations in keratoconus. J Ophthalmol. 2020;2020:1468258.
48. Yadav R, Kottaiyan R, Ahmad K, Yoon G. Epithelium and Bowman's layer thickness and light scatter in keratoconic cornea evaluated using ultrahigh resolution optical coherence tomography. J Biomed Opt. 2012;17(11):116010.
49. Somodi S, Hahnel C, Slowik C, Richter A, Weiss DG, Guthoff R. Confocal in vivo microscopy and confocal laser-scanning fluorescence microscopy in keratoconus. Ger J Ophthalmol. 1996;5(6):518–25.
50. Kaldawy RM, Wagner J, Ching S, Seigel GM. Evidence of apoptotic cell death in keratoconus. Cornea. 2002;21(2):206–9.
51. Gass JD. The iron lines of the superficial cornea. Arch Ophthalmol. 1964;71:348–58.
52. Naderan M, Jahanrad A, Balali S. Histopathologic findings of keratoconus corneas underwent penetrating keratoplasty according to topographic measurements and keratoconus severity. Int J Ophthalmol. 2017;10(11):1640–6.
53. Sawaguchi S, Fukuchi T, Abe H, Kaiya T, Sugar J, Yue BY. Three-dimensional scanning electron microscopic study of keratoconus corneas. Arch Ophthalmol. 1998;116(1):62–8.
54. Kenney MC, Nesburn AB, Burgeson RE, Butkowski RJ, Ljubimov AV. Abnormalities of the extracellular matrix in keratoconus corneas. Cornea. 1997;16(3):345–51.
55. Scroggs MW, Proia AD. Histopathological variation in keratoconus. Cornea. 1992;11(6):553–9.
56. Shapiro MB, Rodrigues MM, Mandel MR, Krachmer JH. Anterior clear spaces in keratoconus. Ophthalmology. 1986;93(10):1316–9.
57. Perry HD, Buxton JN, Fine BS. Round and oval cones in keratoconus. Ophthalmology. 1980;87(9):905–9.
58. Pouliquen Y. Doyne lecture keratoconus. Eye (Lond). 1987;1(Pt 1):1–14.
59. Dua HS, Faraj LA, Said DG, Gray T, Lowe J. Human corneal anatomy redefined: a novel pre-Descemet's layer (Dua's layer). Ophthalmology. 2013;120(9):1778–85.
60. Dua HS, Faraj LA, Said DG. Dua's layer: discovery, characteristics, clinical applications, controversy and potential relevance to glaucoma. Expert Rev Ophthalmol. 2015;10(6):531–47.
61. Braun JM, Hofmann-Rummelt C, Schlötzer-Schrehardt U, Kruse FE, Cursiefen C. Histopathological changes after deep anterior lamellar keratoplasty using the 'big-bubble technique'. Acta Ophthalmol. 2013;91(1):78–82.
62. Lim P, Bradley JC, Harocopos GJ, Smith ME, Mannis MJ. Histopathology of deep anterior lamellar keratoplasty with pneumatic dissection: the "big-bubble" technique. Cornea. 2009;28(5):579–82.
63. Ting DS, Ramaesh K, Srinivasan S, Sau CY, Mantry S, Roberts F. Deep anterior lamellar keratoplasty:

challenges in histopathological examination. Br J Ophthalmol. 2012;96(12):1510–2.
64. Basu S, Reddy JC, Vaddavalli PK, Vemuganti GK, Sangwan VS. Long-term outcomes of penetrating keratoplasty for keratoconus with resolved corneal hydrops. Cornea. 2012;31(6):615–20.
65. Messmer EM, Meyer P, Herwig MC, Loeffler KU, Schirra F, Seitz B, Thiel M, Reinhard T, Kampik A, Auw-Haedrich C. Morphological and immunohistochemical changes after corneal cross-linking. Cornea. 2013;32(2):111–7.
66. Loukovitis E, Kozeis N, Gatzioufas Z, Kozei A, Tsotridou E, Stoila M, Koronis S, Sfakianakis K, Tranos P, Balidis M, Zachariadis Z, Mikropoulos DG, Anogeianakis G, Katsanos A, Konstas AG. The proteins of keratoconus: a literature review exploring their contribution to the pathophysiology of the disease. Adv Ther. 2019;36(9):2205–22.

Clinical Diagnosis of Keratoconus

5

Zeba A. Syed, Beeran B. Meghpara,
and Christopher J. Rapuano

5.1 Introduction

While the diagnosis of keratoconus is often confirmed with imaging, a meticulous clinical evaluation plays a critical role. A careful discussion about symptoms as well as ocular, family, and medical history should be combined with slit lamp evaluation to guide clinicians toward this diagnosis. It is important for providers to be familiar with these symptoms and signs, as early diagnosis and management can lead to better visual functioning for patients and reduced disease progression.

5.2 Symptoms

The symptoms of keratoconus differ based on disease severity. At early or subclinical stages, keratoconus is often asymptomatic and is typically undiagnosed unless specific topographic or tomographic tests are performed [1]. When symptomatic, patients with keratoconus usually present with slowly progressive blurring or distortion of vision, typically in one eye at early stages but eventually involving both eyes. Often, near visual acuity is preserved initially and better than anticipated given the patient's refraction and distance visual acuity [2]. Patients can often read down the vision chart to a relatively good Snellen acuity if they do it slowly, but if asked to read the letters quickly, the Snellen vision is much worse. As the disease progresses, patients may complain of glare, halos, decreased contrast sensitivity, monocular diplopia, or "shadowed vision." Patients often report difficulty with night driving due to the aforementioned features. Many symptoms occur secondary to the development and progression of irregular astigmatism and higher-order aberrations [3]. Gordon-Shaag et al. measured and compared higher-order aberrations in patients with and without manifest keratoconus and found that all ocular and corneal higher-order aberrations (including trefoil, coma, tetrafoil, and spherical aberration) were significantly higher for keratoconic as compared to normal eyes [4].

The age of onset of symptoms in keratoconus varies significantly across studies. There is a difference in presenting age based on region of investigation, with patients typically presenting at age 31 years at a tertiary referral eye care center in Iran [5], 23–28 years in European studies [6–8], 18–24 years in East Asia and India [9–11], and 25–39 years in the United States [12, 13]. Possible explanations for these geographic variations in age at presentation may include different etiologic factors (see Chap. 2), lack of early detection due to shortage of imaging technology, and socioeconomic reasons causing delayed presentation to medical care. Importantly, the age at

Z. A. Syed (✉) · B. B. Meghpara · C. J. Rapuano
Cornea Service, Wills Eye Hospital, Sidney Kimmel Medical College at Thomas Jefferson University, Philadelphia, PA, USA
e-mail: zsyed@willseye.org; bmeghpara@willseye.org; cjrapuano@willseye.org

S. Das (ed.), *Keratoconus*, https://doi.org/10.1007/978-981-19-4262-4_5

presentation will have major implications for management and course of the disease. Generally, corneas stiffen with age due to natural changes in corneal collagen fibrils [14], which may result in keratoconus stabilization or possibly a decrease in severity of some keratoconus cases [15]. For this reason, progression of keratoconus is typically thought to halt by age 40–45 years or approximately 20 years after the onset of disease [16, 17]. There are certainly exceptions to this general observation, as cases of progression in older patients have been documented [18].

Many of the symptoms of keratoconus occur due to secondary or associated features. For example, signs and symptoms (e.g., eyelid itchiness, ocular surface irritation) of blepharitis occur more often in patients with keratoconus than in healthy individuals [19]. Patients with keratoconus may also exhibit neurotrophic keratopathy and as such may have impaired tear secretion and dry eye symptoms including irritation and photophobia [20]. Changes in corneal sensitivity and tear production in patients with keratoconus are not associated with disease severity, indicating that impaired corneal nerve function may be an early feature of keratoconus [20]. The exact mechanism of neurotrophic keratopathy in keratoconus remains unknown. It is important to counsel patients on the importance of avoiding eye rubbing, especially in the context of severe ocular surface symptoms, as eye rubbing has been associated with keratoconus progression [21].

Several studies have attempted to model visual function based on specific anatomical features of the cornea in patients with keratoconus. One study determined that contrast sensitivity correlated with corneal-shaped parameters (maximum corneal surface point, minimum point, difference between them, and keratoconus apex elevation) and that these parameters defining the corneal surface had stronger correlations with contrast sensitivity as compared to visual acuity [22]. Another study aimed to model visual limitation in patients with keratoconus based on refractive and topographic features and found that visual limitation was strongly associated with maximum curvature and higher-order aberrations. Subsequently, a model was constructed to quantify visual limitation using spherical equivalent, the root mean square of higher-order aberrations, spherical aberration, and interaction between the anterior and the posterior vertical coma, and found that the model was a good fit (sensitivity 91.9%, specificity 83.6%) [23]. A study correlating posterior corneal characteristics with the degree of visual impairment found that posterior surface irregularity, posterior ectasia vertex, and posterior corneal aberrations correlated with visual function deterioration and helped to differentiate normal eyes from mild keratoconus cases [24]. Finally, epithelial thickness measurements in patients with keratoconus demonstrated that patients with poorer visual acuity had thinner 3-mm central ($p = 0.04$), thicker 8-mm superior ($p < 0.001$), and thinner 8-mm inferior ($p < 0.001$) epithelial measurements [25].

Although keratoconus is typically a bilateral disease, there is some variation in published studies, at least partly due to the exact definition of keratoconus and the specific imaging technology used for diagnosis. In one study, bilateral keratoconus was detected in 93.3% of patients, while unilateral keratoconus constituted the remaining minority [5]. The percentage of unilateral keratoconus in various studies has ranged from 4 to 18%, and reports from Asian countries have mostly documented a lower frequency of unilateral keratoconus (4–12%) as compared to assessments from other ethnic populations (13–18%) [9–13, 26]. These differences may be secondary to a selection bias, as many of these reports are clinical studies and therefore include more severe and established cases of keratoconus. Furthermore, there may be a difference in laterality based on average age of studied patients, as higher age is associated with an increased odd of bilateral involvement [17].

5.3 History

5.3.1 Past Ocular History

In early stages of progressive keratoconus, patients may report a need to frequently update spectacles due to their rapidly changing refraction. Specifically, patients may note that their degree of myopia and/or level of astigmatism increase at subsequent ophthalmic evaluations. In these early stages, the patient's vision is generally correctable with new glasses; however, some patients may report that their eye doctor has found their refraction to be increasingly challenging, and it is not uncommon for patients to note that they have had more trouble being corrected to 20/20. School-age children may be referred due to poor scholastic performance in school or pediatrician vision screening exam. Other common historical features in early keratoconus in somewhat older patients include those who failed a driver vision test or a screening for laser refractive surgery due to topographic abnormalities. In cases where keratoconus develops in early childhood, patients may have been diagnosed with anisometropic meridional amblyopia [27].

As keratoconus progresses to more moderate and advanced stages, patients may note that their spectacles no longer provide adequate visual acuity and visual quality. Progression is suspected when a patient presents with a loss of best spectacle-corrected visual acuity [28], and by this stage, patients have typically begun to present with symptoms in both eyes. Patients may describe repeated visits to their eye doctors due to these complaints, however, noting that the revised spectacles do not provide enhanced vision or correct them to 20/20. Some patients may note having to wear contact lenses for visual rehabilitation in the past, either soft toric contact lenses, rigid gas-permeable contact lenses, hybrid lenses, or scleral lenses, and may not recall the reason for needing advanced contact lens technology (see Chap. 13). As their conditions progress, patients may note that they require frequent contact lens evaluations to update lenses; they may rapidly develop intolerance to new contacts as their corneas continue to change shape. In addition to providing information about keratoconus progression, obtaining a contact lens history is important in the evaluation of patients with keratoconus as contact lens wear is an environmental factor that may predispose to keratoconus development or progression [29].

In the most severe cases, patients may report frequent contact lens evaluations but an inability to be fitted with lenses that provide the visual acuity, quality, and comfort that the patient desires. Some patients note that the contacts frequently "pop out" of their eye or that the contacts cause significant irritation or discomfort. Recurrent corneal erosions secondary to poorly fitting contact lenses are another common complaint in contact lens wearing patients with progressive keratoconus. In these severe cases, patients may need to undergo evaluation for lamellar or penetrating keratoplasty (see Chaps. 15 and 16). In all cases of suspected keratoconus progression, patients should also be evaluated for possible corneal collagen cross-linking (see Chap. 14) to stabilize the cornea prior to further refractive rehabilitation.

5.3.2 Family History

A genetic etiology of keratoconus is suggested by the condition's bilateral nature, family aggregation, monozygotic twin concordance, and ethnic disparities in prevalence [30]. While inquiry about family history of keratoconus may shed valuable information, the utility of family history in the diagnosis of keratoconus is inconsistent. A study performed in central China demonstrated that only 3.52% of patients with a clinical diagnosis of keratoconus had a positive family history [31], while another large study noted that approximately 14% of patients with keratoconus have a family history [32]. Naderan et al. studied a large cohort of patients with keratoconus and found that 19.5% had a positive family history [33]. Of these, 54.5% had one family member with keratoconus, and 45.5% had two or more family members with keratoconus. Individuals with a family history of keratoconus displayed more severe disease according to the Amsler-Krumeich classification ($p < 0.05$), and patients with more family members afflicted by keratoconus had lower thinnest corneal thickness, higher steep keratometry, higher astigmatism, and more severe disease using the Amsler-Krumeich classification [33].

Importantly, inquiring about family history only captures data on family members with a known diagnosis of keratoconus. In a study evaluating relatives of patients with keratoconus, at least one corneal topography or tomography parameter was abnormal in 34% of first-degree relatives of keratoconus patients, which was significantly lower for controls (14%, p = 0.01). Furthermore, first-degree relatives of keratoconus patients had significantly more abnormal anterior corneal topography features than controls [34]. In another study that mapped the corneas of 28 family members of 5 patients with keratoconus, the authors found anomalies including central steepening, significant steepening of the cornea inferior to the apex, and substantial central dioptric power asymmetry between the two eyes [35]. These features may represent variable expression in genetic factors contributing to keratoconus risk.

Given that keratoconus is a multifactorial condition resulting from the interaction of environmental, behavioral, and genetic factors, the relationship between genetic predisposition and phenotypic outcome is undoubtedly complex. This is evident by the finding that despite the strong role of family history suggested in the aforementioned reports, other studies have demonstrated that family history has no relationship with keratoconus disease severity [36].

5.3.3 Medical History and Associated Diseases

Keratoconus and atopic disease have been long associated in the medical literature [37–39]. In 2015, the Global Delphi Panel of Keratoconus and Ectatic Diseases, a group of corneal experts from around the world, agreed that atopy, ocular allergy, connective tissue disorders, and Down syndrome all were associated with keratoconus [40]. The Collaborative Longitudinal Evaluation of Keratoconus study found a 53% prevalence of atopic disease in over 1200 keratoconus patients [32]. Bawazeer et al. reported that their univariate analysis revealed both atopic disease and eye rubbing were associated with keratoconus; however, in their multivariate analysis, eye rubbing alone increased the odds of having keratoconus [21]. Eye rubbing itself has long been established as an important risk factor for the progression of keratoconus [21, 41–43]; a recent meta-analysis of the literature revealed that the odds ratio of developing keratoconus was threefold higher in individuals who reported rubbing their eyes daily [44].

Atopy represents a group of conditions, including allergic conjunctivitis, asthma, eczema, and allergic rhinitis, all of which have also been individually implicated to be associated with keratoconus. A recent systematic review reported that atopic disease as a group did not increase the risk of keratoconus; however, individually, asthma, allergy, and eczema did [44]. The Dundee University Scottish Keratoconus study found the prevalence of allergic rhinitis, asthma, and eczema to be higher in keratoconus patients compared to controls [45]. A large study performed in the United States analyzing over 16,000 keratoconus patients using a nationwide insurance claims database revealed asthmatic patients had a 31% higher odds of having keratoconus [46]. Other recent large national population-based studies from Denmark and Taiwan, as well as a study done on Israeli adolescents, all showed an association between asthma and keratoconus [47–49]. These large registry-based studies also reported associations between keratoconus and allergic conjunctivitis [47, 50], allergic rhinitis [47–49], and eczema [49]. Large database-driven studies, either from insurance claim records in the United States or from national health registries in Europe and Asia, have the ability to harness data from a large number of patients. However, registry-based studies have the limitation of misclassification of diagnoses. Without access to clinical records, the diagnosis of keratoconus and the associated diseases cannot be confirmed. Nonetheless, the evidence associating keratoconus with various atopic diseases appears convincing enough that clinicians should inquire about atopy as these patients can benefit from systemic treatment. Treatment of underlying atopy can help decrease the tendency of problematic eye rubbing.

The association between keratoconus and Down syndrome has been widely published [46, 48, 51, 52]. Compared to the general population, the prevalence of keratoconus in patients with Down syndrome has been estimated to be over ten times higher [28, 53]. One plausible explanation for this link is an underlying common genetic abnormality; however, despite such a strong association, a specific mutation linking these conditions has not yet been identified. Another explanation is that excessive eye rubbing is the underlying risk factor. Keratoconus has also been reported among non-Down syndrome developmentally delayed patients. It is prudent to have a high degree of suspicion for keratoconus in this patient population as these individuals often cannot clearly express problems with their vision. With the advent of collagen cross-linking, early detection and treatment of keratoconus are important to prevent later complications of the disease including corneal hydrops, scarring, and the need for corneal transplantation.

There are conflicting reports in the literature regarding an association between keratoconus and diabetes. Seiler et al. first reported a lower rate of keratoconus in patients with type 2 diabetes mellitus compared to age-matched controls in their retrospective case-controlled study of 1142 patients [54]. Woodward et al. also detected a lower rate of keratoconus in diabetic patients in their large study of 32,106 patients using a national insurance claims database. Patients with uncomplicated diabetes had 20% lower odds of having keratoconus compared to nondiabetics. Patients who had complicated diabetes, defined as having end-organ damage, had a 52% lower odds of having keratoconus [46]. Lin et al. demonstrated a reduced odds of having keratoconus in type 1, type 2, and unspecified diabetic patients in their study on 25,275 Taiwanese patients [48]. The proposed pathophysiologic mechanism to explain the protective effect of diabetes on keratoconus is based on research where elevated levels of blood glucose result in glycosylation of collagen fibrils in the cornea, thereby cross-linking and strengthening the corneal tissue [55–57]. However, in a large case control study of 5508 patients, Kosker et al. reported a higher prevalence of type 2 diabetes mellitus in their keratoconus patients compared to controls (6.7% versus 4.8%). There was no statistical difference detected in type 1 diabetes mellitus prevalence between patients with and without keratoconus [58]. The discrepancy between results of this study compared to others could potentially be explained by selection bias, as patients with diabetes potentially underwent more regular ophthalmic examinations and therefore had a higher opportunity to be diagnosed with keratoconus [46].

A variety of other systemic conditions have also been reported to be associated with keratoconus including sleep apnea, noninflammatory connective tissue disorders, collagen vascular disorders, mitral valve prolapse, aortic aneurysm, depression, and obesity [46, 48, 49, 59–66]. A discrepancy in results across various studies, however, may question these associations. Several studies report an association between sleep apnea and keratoconus [46, 59–61]. Gupta et al. surveyed patients with keratoconus and found that 65% either had the diagnosis of sleep apnea or were considered high risk for the condition [59]. Woodward et al. reported that a greater percentage of keratoconus patients had sleep apnea compared to normal controls and patients with sleep apnea had a 13% higher odds of having keratoconus [46]. On the contrary, large population-based studies from Taiwan and Denmark did not report an association between sleep apnea and keratoconus [48, 49]. One proposed explanation for this discrepancy is that sleep apnea may be underdiagnosed in these populations. Given the potential systemic morbidity and mortality associated with sleep apnea, it is our clinical practice to screen for symptoms in keratoconus patients and refer those deemed high risk for further evaluation. Floppy eyelid syndrome has been associated with both sleep apnea and keratoconus [67]. Donnenfeld et al. first described a series of patients with floppy eyelid syndrome and keratoconus and suggested a mechanical etiology for the relationship. In eyes with asymmetric keratoconus, the keratoconus was more severe in the eye with greater lid laxity, and patients reported sleeping on the side with worse disease [68]. Additional reports later confirmed this association as well as a tendency for patients to sleep face down [69]. Mitral valve prolapse has been reported to be associated with keratoconus with one study noting an increased prevalence of 58%, compared to 7% in age-matched controls [62, 63]. However, the sample sizes in these studies were relatively small, and a larger cross-sectional study and multiple large population registry studies did not find an association between keratoconus and mitral valve prolapse [46, 48, 49, 64]. Noninflammatory connective tissue disorders such as Ehlers-Danlos syndrome have been linked to keratoconus [28, 40]. Joint hypermobility has been reported in up to 50% of keratoconus patients [70, 71]. However, a more recent study using topography to diagnose keratoconus in 72 eyes of patients with genetically typed Ehlers-Danlos syndrome found only 1 patient with mild topographic changes suggestive of keratoconus [72]. Large population studies from South Korea and the United States did not find any association between keratoconus and noninflammatory connective tissue disorders [46, 50].

5.4 Clinical Examination

There are many features noted during the ocular examination that point toward the diagnosis of keratoconus. In early cases, using a thin slit beam, practitioners may appreciate that the cornea has subtle central or paracentral posterior protrusion, central or paracentral anterior steepening, and central or paracentral corneal stromal thinning (Fig. 5.1). Typically, the thinnest point of the cornea is outside visual axis at the apex of the cone. Importantly, because keratoconus is a noninflammatory process, there should be no associated stromal vascularization or anterior chamber inflammation. While these subtle features may be present bilaterally, they are often asymmetric between the two eyes. In more severe cases, practitioners may be able to visualize inferior corneal steepening using slit lamp evaluation.

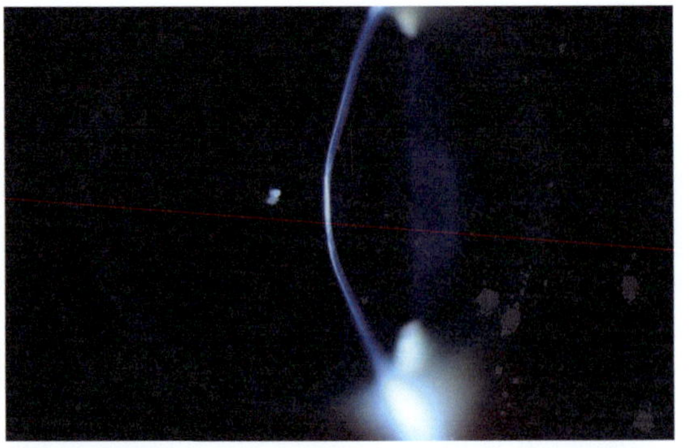

Fig. 5.1 Paracentral corneal stromal thinning and scarring are demonstrated with a thin slit beam

During refraction, patients may be noted to have a high level of astigmatism, which is often asymmetric between the two eyes. As further described (see Chap. 10), this is typically noted to be irregular on corneal topography, and therefore refraction alone often does not get the patient to read 20/20 in moderate and severe cases of keratoconus. In clinical practice, corneal topography and tomography are integral tools for the clinical diagnosis of keratoconus (see Chap. 10). Common topographic features of keratoconus include inferior steepening (Fig. 5.2), asymmetric bowtie astigmatism, and irregular astigmatism. Common tomographic findings in keratoconus include corneal thinning, decentration of the thinnest cornea, and focal elevation on anterior and posterior float maps (Fig. 5.3) [73]. Other diagnostic tools include epithelial thickness mapping with high-resolution ultrasound or anterior segment optical coherence tomography [74–78].

Retinoscopy of patients with keratoconus may demonstrate a very characteristic scissoring retinal reflex (also called as a splitting reflex), which involves two bands moving toward and away from each other like the two blades on a pair of scissors [65]. A scissoring reflex on retinoscopy, which occurs early in the course of the disease, is a highly useful tool to diagnose keratoconus, and one study documented sensitivity, specificity, positive predictive value, and negative predictive value of 97.7%, 79.9%, 70.8%, and 98.4%, respectively, for retinoscopy in the detection of

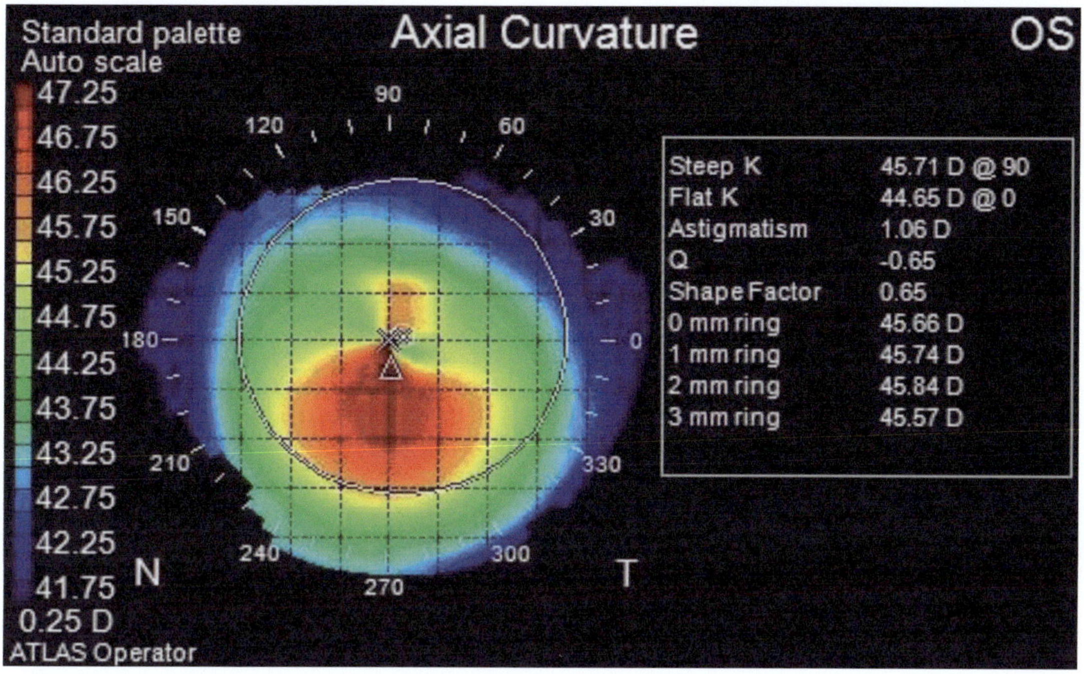

Fig. 5.2 Inferior corneal steepening on corneal topography is a hallmark of keratoconus

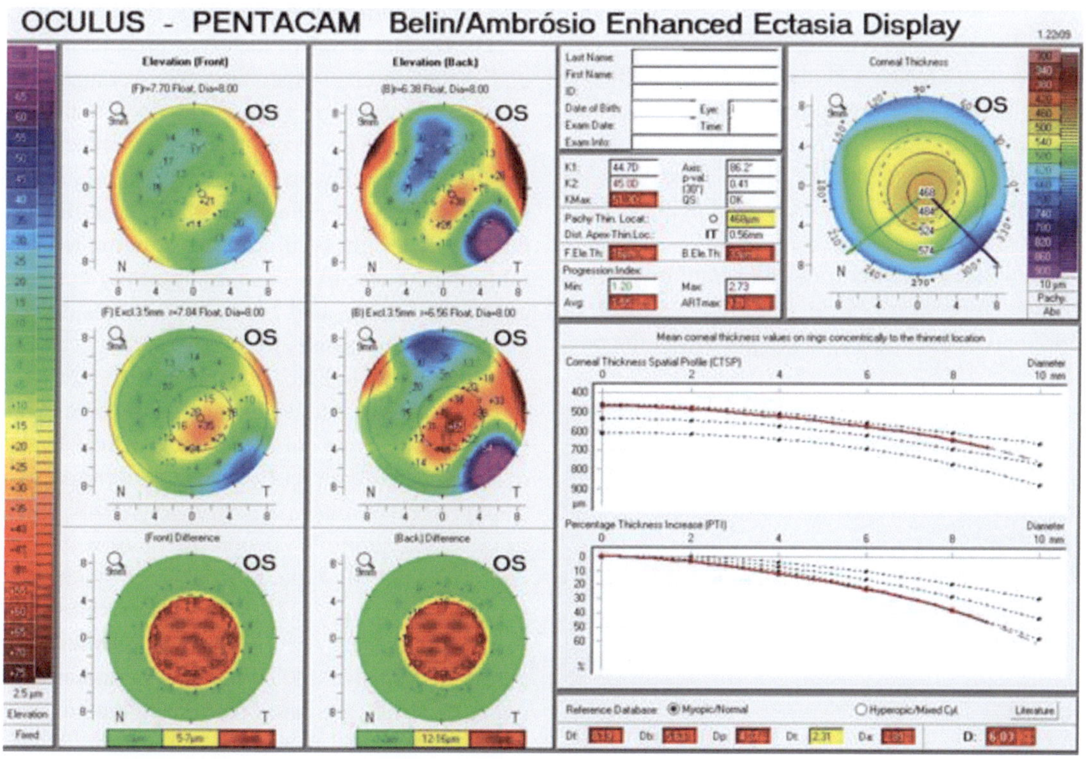

Fig. 5.3 Mildly decentered corneal thinning is evident on corneal tomography. This Belin-Ambrosio enhanced ectasia display on the Oculus Pentacam also demonstrates abnormal anterior and posterior elevation, consistent with keratoconus

keratoconus [79]. The scissoring reflex occurs secondary to the effect of irregular astigmatism on light rays traversing the cornea. Furthermore, the patterns of the retinoscopy reflex may help to identify the general location of the cone's apex and its diameter.

Another finding in clinical examination is the Charleux oil-droplet sign (also called teardrop reflex), which is evident by retroillumination while the pupil is dilated [28]. This finding is characterized by a dark reflex in the area of the cone using diffuse illumination and is caused by the more accentuated central curvature of the cornea acting as a convex mirror.

A common clinical finding in keratoconus is a Fleischer ring, a brown pigmented ring which can be identified as partially or completely encircling the base of the cone (Fig. 5.4). The Fleischer ring is composed of hemosiderin deposits in the basal epithelium, just anterior to Bowman membrane, and represents an accumulation of iron deposits derived from the tear film. Deposition occurs due to significant curvature changes and modifications of normal tear-epithelial dynamics [80]. The process resulting in Fleischer ring formation also creates a Hudson-Stahli line (at the upper border of a normal tear film), Stocker line (at the leading edge of a pterygium), and Ferry line (at the edge of filtering blebs). The Fleischer ring has no visual or clinical significance, as is the case in other epithelial iron lines.

Another clinically relevant feature is Vogt striae. These are vertical (or rarely oblique or horizontal), fine, parallel lines present in the posterior stroma (Fig. 5.5). These findings may be asymmetric depending on the severity of keratoconus in each eye. There is a general association between the orientation of the striae and the steep axis of the cornea. Vogt striae result from mechanical stress forces on collagen lamellae radiating from the cone apex, and the striae typically temporarily disappear with digital compression on the cornea or globe [81].

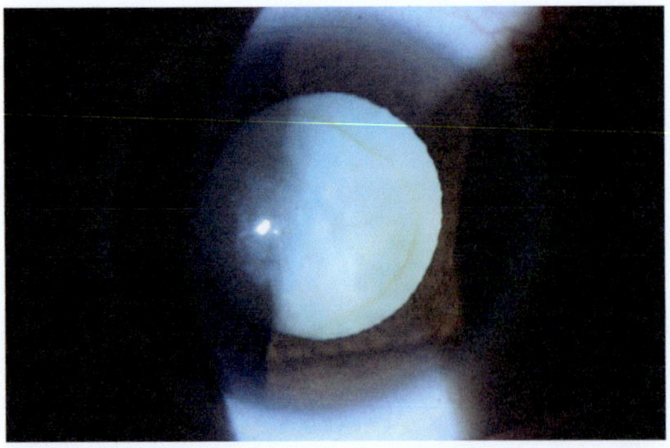

Fig. 5.4 A Fleischer ring is quite apparent in a patient with keratoconus and an advanced cataract

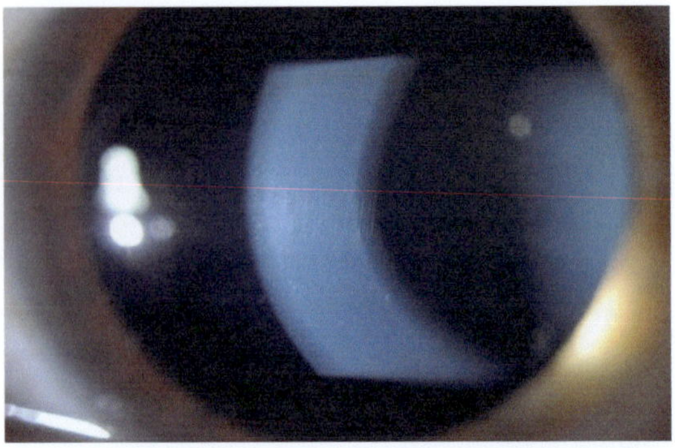

Fig. 5.5 The fine vertical stress lines of Vogt striae can be seen in this wide slit view in this eye with fairly mild keratoconus. A Fleischer ring is also present

The conical shape of the cornea results in several phenomena specific to keratoconus. Specifically, Munson sign represents a V-shaped displacement of the lower eyelid when the cornea is oriented in a downward position. Rizzuti sign involves a conical reflection on the nasal limbal region when light is introduced from the temporal limbus. These two signs are typically noted in advanced disease, and more subtle cones do not produce these findings [81].

An additional clinical feature is increased visibility of corneal nerves. Other diseases that present with prominent corneal nerves include Fuchs dystrophy, posterior polymorphous corneal dystrophy, *Acanthamoeba* keratitis, ichthyosis, multiple endocrine neoplasia type 2b, neurofibromatosis type 1, Riley-Day syndrome, and Refsum disease [82]. The pathophysiology of prominent corneal nerves is not entirely known, but hypotheses include an increase in endoneural collagen fibrils, increased nerve myelination, and degeneration of axons and Schwann cells. Consistent with these findings, clinical evaluation may also demonstrate a decrease in corneal sensitivity to various stimuli in patients with keratoconus. The axonal damage and/or transduction defects seem to affect different types of corneal nerves, as sensitivity to mechanical, chemical, hot, and cold stimuli appears to be altered in patients with keratoconus [20].

In more severe disease, breaks in Descemet membrane may occur. These can result in the acute development of stromal edema, which is known as hydrops (see Chap. 12) [83]. Patients usually present with sudden vision loss and significant pain. Clinical examination demonstrates moderate to severe corneal edema that may be accompanied by intrastromal fluid clefts or blebs overlying the break [84]. Over time, the edema typically resolves and leaves behind a scar, which is often visually significant (Fig. 5.6). Peripheral hydrops may paradoxically improve uncorrected vision upon resolution, as the peripheral scar may result in central flatting of the cornea. Other findings in more severe cases of keratoconus include subepithelial or anterior stromal scars, which may result from breaks in Bowman membrane (Figs. 5.7 and 5.8) [85]. Patients may also present with elevated corneal nodules, and although the pathophysiology of these findings is not entirely known, possible etiologies include changes in the metabolic activity of epithelial cells, disruption of the normal epithelial basement membrane and Bowman layer, and differentiation and anterior migration of stromal fibroblasts (Fig. 5.9) [86].

Clinical evaluation may also demonstrate floppy eyelid syndrome, characterized by an upper eyelid that may be readily everted, tarsal laxity, and diffuse papillary conjunctival changes [68]. While the mechanism of the association remains unclear, an underlying connective tissue condition may link these two diseases [87].

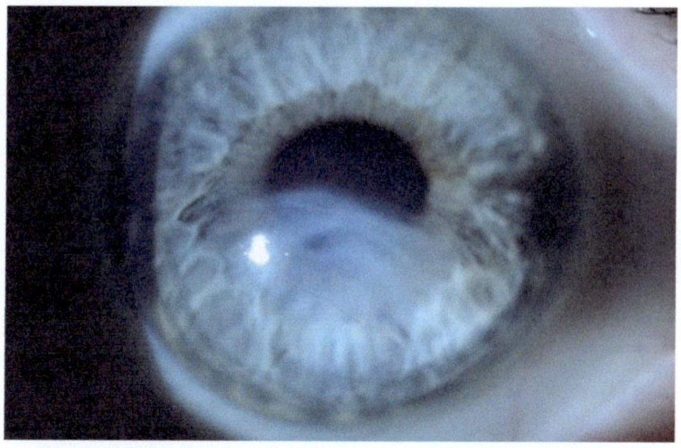

Fig. 5.6 An inferiorly decentered corneal scar is noted in a patient with previous hydrops

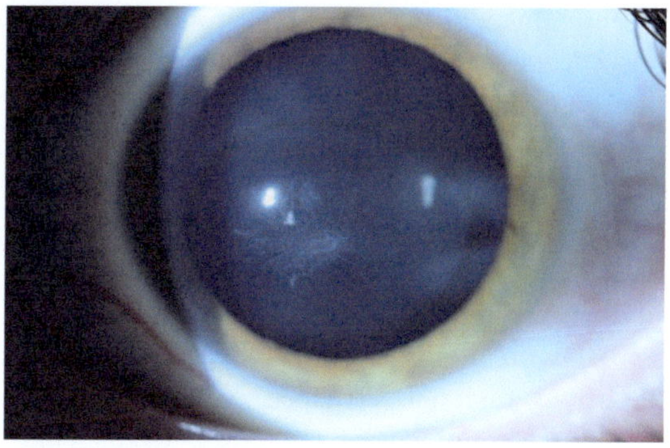

Fig. 5.7 Mild anterior stromal scarring and a Fleischer ring are easily seen in this cornea with keratoconus

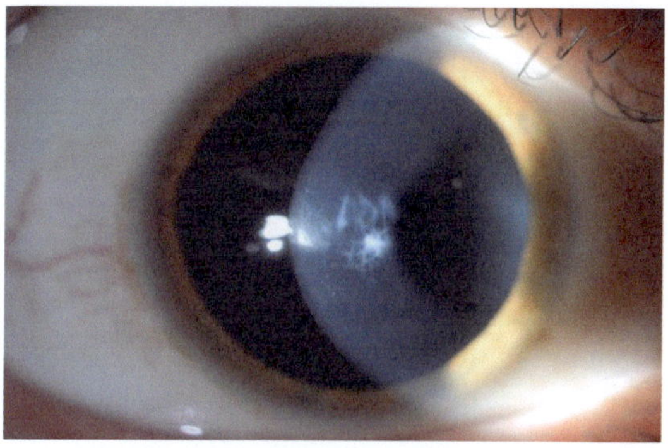

Fig. 5.8 Moderate anterior stromal scarring and a Fleischer ring can be seen in an eye with fairly advanced keratoconus

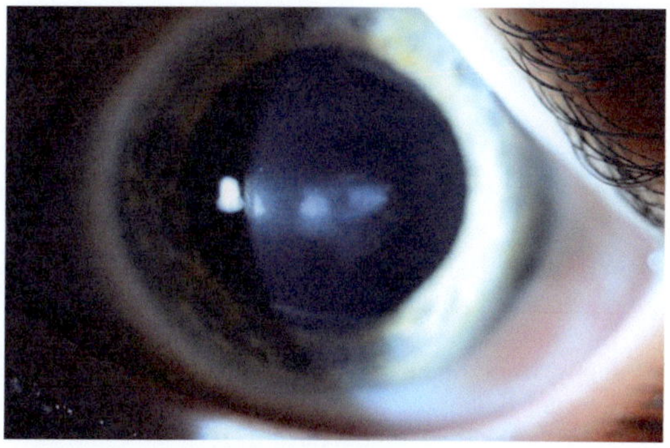

Fig. 5.9 Elevated corneal nodules are present in this eye with keratoconus, which were impeding comfortable contact lens wear

Genetic linkages between keratoconus and early-onset cataract have also been identified, and therefore patients with keratoconus should be evaluated for cataractous changes [88]. Finally, evaluation of binocular visual function in patients with keratoconus may show abnormal results. In one report, 78.6% of keratoconus patients displayed binocular vision anomalies: 48.8% presented with impaired stereopsis, 44% featured abnormal fusional vergence, and 39.3% displayed accommodative infacility [89]. These findings may be secondary to the typical asymmetric nature of keratoconus, as well as its early age of onset that may interfere with visual developmental processes.

The diagnosis of keratoconus involves a combination of history, visual acuity, slit lamp examination, and ancillary testing. A history of eye rubbing and other family members with keratoconus is important, as is searching for associated conditions including atopic disease, Down syndrome, and sleep apnea. Slit lamp examination may be diagnostic, but in early disease, corneal topography and tomography analyses are extremely helpful. The earlier the diagnosis of keratoconus is made, the sooner patients can be advised to stop rubbing their eyes, the sooner their visual function can be improved with appropriate visual correction, and the sooner corneal cross-linking can be performed to stop progressive disease.

References

1. Arntz A, Durán JA, Pijoán JI. Diagnóstico del queratocono subclínico por topografía de elevación [Subclinical keratoconus diagnosis by elevation topography]. Arch Soc Esp Oftalmol. 2003;78(12):659–64.
2. Romero-Jiménez M, Santodomingo-Rubido J, Wolffsohn JS. Keratoconus: a review. Cont Lens Anterior Eye. 2010;33(4):157–66.
3. Applegate RA, Hilmantel G, Howland HC, Tu EY, Starck T, Zayac EJ. Corneal first surface optical aberrations and visual performance. J Refract Surg. 2000;16(5):507–14.
4. Gordon-Shaag A, Millodot M, Ifrah R, Shneor E. Aberrations and topography in normal, keratoconus-suspect, and keratoconic eyes. Optom Vis Sci. 2012;89(4):411–8.
5. Rafati S, Hashemi H, Nabovati P, Doostdar A, Yekta A, Aghamirsalim M, Khabazkhoob M. Demographic profile, clinical, and topographic characteristics of keratoconus patients attending at a tertiary eye center. J Curr Ophthalmol. 2019;31(3):268–74.
6. Nielsen K, Hjortdal J, Aagaard Nohr E, Ehlers N. Incidence and prevalence of keratoconus in Denmark. Acta Ophthalmol Scand. 2007;85(8):890–2.
7. Georgiou T, Funnell CL, Cassels-Brown A, O'Conor R. Influence of ethnic origin on the incidence of keratoconus and associated atopic disease in Asians and white patients. Eye (Lond). 2004;18(4):379–83.
8. Ihalainen A. Clinical and epidemiological features of keratoconus genetic and external factors in the pathogenesis of the disease. Acta Ophthalmol Suppl. 1986;178:1–64.
9. Li SW, Li ZX, Shi WY, Zeng QY, Jin XM. Clinical features of 233 cases of keratoconus. Zhonghua Yan Ke Za Zhi. 2005;41(7):610–3.
10. Tanabe U, Fujiki K, Ogawa A, Ueda S, Kanai A. [Prevalence of keratoconus patients in Japan]. Nippon Ganka Gakkai Zasshi. 1985;89(3):407–11.
11. Jonas JB, Nangia V, Matin A, Kulkarni M, Bhojwani K. Prevalence and associations of keratoconus in rural Maharashtra in central India: the central India eye and medical study. Am J Ophthalmol. 2009;148(5):760–5.
12. Zadnik K, Barr JT, Gordon MO, Edrington TB. Biomicroscopic signs and disease severity in keratoconus. Collaborative Longitudinal Evaluation of Keratoconus (CLEK) Study Group. Cornea. 1996;15(2):139–46.
13. Kennedy RH, Bourne WM, Dyer JA. A 48-year clinical and epidemiologic study of keratoconus. Am J Ophthalmol. 1986;101(3):267–73.
14. Andreassen TT, Simonsen AH, Oxlund H. Biomechanical properties of keratoconus and normal corneas. Exp Eye Res. 1980;31(4):435–41.
15. Krachmer JH. Potential research projects. Cornea. 2007;26(3):243–5.
16. Olivares Jiménez JL, Guerrero Jurado JC, Bermudez Rodriguez FJ, Serrano Laborda D. Keratoconus: age of onset and natural history. Optom Vis Sci. 1997;74(3):147–51.
17. Ertan A, Muftuoglu O. Keratoconus clinical findings according to different age and gender groups. Cornea. 2008;27(10):1109–13.
18. Coco G, Kheirkhah A, Foulsham W, Dana R, Ciolino JB. Keratoconus progression associated with hormone replacement therapy. Am J Ophthalmol Case Rep. 2019;15:100519.
19. Mostovoy D, Vinker S, Mimouni M, Goldich Y, Levartovsky S, Kaiserman I. The association of keratoconus with blepharitis. Clin Exp Optom. 2018;101(3):339–44.
20. Dienes L, Kiss HJ, Perényi K, Nagy ZZ, Acosta MC, Gallar J, Kovács I. Corneal sensitivity and dry eye symptoms in patients with keratoconus. PLoS One. 2015;10(10):e0141621.

21. Bawazeer AM, Hodge WG, Lorimer B. Atopy and keratoconus: a multivariate analysis. Br J Ophthalmol. 2000;84(8):834–6.
22. Liduma S, Luguzis A, Krumina G. The impact of irregular corneal shape parameters on visual acuity and contrast sensitivity. BMC Ophthalmol. 2020;20(1):466.
23. Pérez-Rueda A, Castro-Luna G. A model of visual limitation in patients with keratoconus. Sci Rep. 2020;10(1):19335.
24. Vega-Estrada A, Alio JL. Keratoconus corneal posterior surface characterization according to the degree of visual limitation. Cornea. 2019;38(6):730–6.
25. Vega-Estrada A, Mimouni M, Espla E, Alió Del Barrio J, Alio JL. Corneal epithelial thickness Intrasubject repeatability and its relation with visual limitation in keratoconus. Am J Ophthalmol. 2019;200:255–62.
26. Khor WB, Wei RH, Lim L, Chan CM, Tan DT. Keratoconus in Asians: demographics, clinical characteristics and visual function in a hospital-based population. Clin Exp Ophthalmol. 2011;39(4):299–307.
27. Arora R, Lohchab M. Pediatric keratoconus misdiagnosed as meridional amblyopia. Indian J Ophthalmol. 2019;67(4):551–2.
28. Rabinowitz YS. Keratoconus. Surv Ophthalmol. 1998;42(4):297–319.
29. Barr JT, Wilson BS, Gordon MO, Rah MJ, Riley C, Kollbaum PS, Zadnik K, CLEK Study Group. Estimation of the incidence and factors predictive of corneal scarring in the Collaborative Longitudinal Evaluation of Keratoconus (CLEK) Study. Cornea. 2006;25(1):16–25.
30. Rong SS, Ma STU, Yu XT, Ma L, Chu WK, Chan TCY, Wang YM, Young AL, Pang CP, Jhanji V, Chen LJ. Genetic associations for keratoconus: a systematic review and meta-analysis. Sci Rep. 2017;7(1):4620.
31. Yang K, Xu L, Fan Q, Gu Y, Zhang B, Meng F, Zhao D, Pang C, Ren S. A hospital-based study on clinical data, demographic data and visual function of keratoconus patients in Central China. Sci Rep. 2021;11(1):7559.
32. Zadnik K, Barr JT, Edrington TB, Everett DF, Jameson M, McMahon TT, Shin JA, Sterling JL, Wagner H, Gordon MO. Baseline findings in the Collaborative Longitudinal Evaluation of Keratoconus (CLEK) Study. Invest Ophthalmol Vis Sci. 1998;39(13):2537–46.
33. Naderan M, Rajabi MT, Zarrinbakhsh P, Naderan M, Bakhshi A. Association between family history and keratoconus severity. Curr Eye Res. 2016;41(11):1414–8.
34. Shneor E, Frucht-Pery J, Granit E, Gordon-Shaag A. The prevalence of corneal abnormalities in first-degree relatives of patients with keratoconus: a prospective case-control study. Ophthalmic Physiol Opt. 2020;40(4):442–51.
35. Rabinowitz YS, Garbus J, McDonnell PJ. Computer-assisted corneal topography in family members of patients with keratoconus. Arch Ophthalmol. 1990;108(3):365–71.
36. Szczotka-Flynn L, Slaughter M, McMahon T, Barr J, Edrington T, Fink B, Lass J, Belin M, Iyengar SK, CLEK Study Group. Disease severity and family history in keratoconus. Br J Ophthalmol. 2008;92(8):1108–11.
37. Galin MA, Berger R. Atopy and keratoconus. Am J Ophthalmol. 1958;45(6):904–6.
38. Rahi A, Davies P, Ruben M, Lobascher D, Menon J. Keratoconus and coexisting atopic disease. Br J Ophthalmol. 1977;61(12):761–4.
39. Harrison RJ, Klouda PT, Easty DL, Manku M, Charles J, Stewart CM. Association between keratoconus and atopy. Br J Ophthalmol. 1989;73(10):816–22.
40. Gomes JA, Tan D, Rapuano CJ, Belin MW, Ambrósio R Jr, Guell JL, Malecaze F, Nishida K, Sangwan VS, Group of Panelists for the Global Delphi Panel of Keratoconus and Ectatic Diseases. Global consensus on keratoconus and ectatic diseases. Cornea. 2015;34(4):359–69.
41. Jafri B, Lichter H, Stulting RD. Asymmetric keratoconus attributed to eye rubbing. Cornea. 2004;23(6):560–4.
42. Carlson AN. Expanding our understanding of eye rubbing and keratoconus. Cornea. 2010;29(2):245.
43. Yeniad B, Alparslan N, Akarcay K. Eye rubbing as an apparent cause of recurrent keratoconus. Cornea. 2009;28(4):477–9.
44. Hashemi H, Heydarian S, Hooshmand E, Saatchi M, Yekta A, Aghamirsalim M, Valadkhan M, Mortazavi M, Hashemi A, Khabazkhoob M. The prevalence and risk factors for keratoconus: a systematic review and meta-analysis. Cornea. 2020;39(2):263–70.
45. Weed KH, MacEwen CJ, Giles T, Low J, McGhee CN. The Dundee University Scottish Keratoconus study: demographics, corneal signs, associated diseases, and eye rubbing. Eye (Lond). 2008;22(4):534–41.
46. Woodward MA, Blachley TS, Stein JD. The association between sociodemographic factors, common systemic diseases, and keratoconus: an analysis of a Nationwide Heath Care claims database. Ophthalmology. 2016;123(3):457–465.e2.
47. Merdler I, Hassidim A, Sorkin N, Shapira S, Gronovich Y, Korach Z. Keratoconus and allergic diseases among Israeli adolescents between 2005 and 2013. Cornea. 2015;34(5):525–9.
48. Lin KK, Lee JS, Hou CH, Chen WM, Hsiao CH, Chen YW, Yeh CT, See LC. The sociodemographic and risk factors for keratoconus: nationwide matched case-control study in Taiwan, 1998-2015. Am J Ophthalmol. 2021;223:140–8.
49. Bak-Nielsen S, Ramlau-Hansen CH, Ivarsen A, Plana-Ripoll O, Hjortdal J. A nationwide population-based study of social demographic factors, associ-

ated diseases and mortality of keratoconus patients in Denmark from 1977 to 2015. Acta Ophthalmol. 2019;97(5):497–504.
50. Lee HK, Jung EH, Cho BJ. Epidemiological association between systemic diseases and keratoconus in a Korean population: a 10-year nationwide cohort study. Cornea. 2020;39(3):348–53.
51. Alio JL, Vega-Estrada A, Sanz P, Osman AA, Kamal AM, Mamoon A, Soliman H. Corneal morphologic characteristics in patients with Down syndrome. JAMA Ophthalmol. 2018;136(9):971–8.
52. Shapiro MB, France TD. The ocular features of Down's syndrome. Am J Ophthalmol. 1985;99(6):659–63.
53. Vincent AL, Weiser BA, Cupryn M, Stein RM, Abdolell M, Levin AV. Computerized corneal topography in a paediatric population with Down syndrome. Clin Exp Ophthalmol. 2005;33(1):47–52.
54. Seiler T, Huhle S, Spoerl E, Kunath H. Manifest diabetes and keratoconus: a retrospective case-control study. Graefes Arch Clin Exp Ophthalmol. 2000;238(10):822–5.
55. Goldich Y, Barkana Y, Gerber Y, Rasko A, Morad Y, Harstein M, Avni I, Zadok D. Effect of diabetes mellitus on biomechanical parameters of the cornea. J Cataract Refract Surg. 2009;35(4):715–9.
56. Dyer DG, Dunn JA, Thorpe SR, Bailie KE, Lyons TJ, McCance DR, Baynes JW. Accumulation of Maillard reaction products in skin collagen in diabetes and aging. J Clin Invest. 1993;91(6):2463–9.
57. Spoerl E, Huhle M, Seiler T. Induction of cross-links in corneal tissue. Exp Eye Res. 1998;66(1):97–103.
58. Kosker M, Suri K, Hammersmith KM, Nassef AH, Nagra PK, Rapuano CJ. Another look at the association between diabetes and keratoconus. Cornea. 2014;33(8):774–9.
59. Gupta PK, Stinnett SS, Carlson AN. Prevalence of sleep apnea in patients with keratoconus. Cornea. 2012;31(6):595–9.
60. Saidel MA, Paik JY, Garcia C, Russo P, Cao D, Bouchard C. Prevalence of sleep apnea syndrome and high-risk characteristics among keratoconus patients. Cornea. 2012;31(6):600–3.
61. Pihlblad MS, Schaefer DP. Eyelid laxity, obesity, and obstructive sleep apnea in keratoconus. Cornea. 2013;32(9):1232–6.
62. Sharif KW, Casey TA, Coltart J. Prevalence of mitral valve prolapse in keratoconus patients. J R Soc Med. 1992;85(8):446–8.
63. Lichter H, Loya N, Sagie A, Cohen N, Muzmacher L, Yassur Y, Weinberger D. Keratoconus and mitral valve prolapse. Am J Ophthalmol. 2000;129(5):667–8.
64. Street DA, Vinokur ET, Waring GO III, Pollak SJ, Clements SD, Perkins JV. Lack of association between keratoconus, mitral valve prolapse, and joint hypermobility. Ophthalmology. 1991;98(2):170–6.
65. Krachmer JH, Feder RS, Belin MW. Keratoconus and related noninflammatory corneal thinning disorders. Surv Ophthalmol. 1984;28(4):293–322.
66. Eliasi E, Bez M, Megreli J, Avramovich E, Fischer N, Barak A, Levine H. The association between keratoconus and body mass index: a population-based cross-sectional study among half a million adolescents. Am J Ophthalmol. 2021;224:200–6.
67. Idowu OO, Ashraf DC, Vagefi MR, Kersten RC, Winn BJ. Floppy eyelid syndrome: ocular and systemic associations. Curr Opin Ophthalmol. 2019;30(6):513–24.
68. Donnenfeld ED, Perry HD, Gibralter RP, Ingraham HJ, Udell IJ. Keratoconus associated with floppy eyelid syndrome. Ophthalmology. 1991;98(11):1674–8.
69. Culbertson WW, Tseng SC. Corneal disorders in floppy eyelid syndrome. Cornea. 1994;13(1):33–42.
70. Robertson I. Keratoconus and the Ehlers-Danlos syndrome: a new aspect of keratoconus. Med J Aust. 1975;1(18):571–3.
71. Woodward EG, Morris MT. Joint hypermobility in keratoconus. Ophthalmic Physiol Opt. 1990;10(4):360–2.
72. McDermott ML, Holladay J, Liu D, Puklin JE, Shin DH, Cowden JW. Corneal topography in Ehlers-Danlos syndrome. J Cataract Refract Surg. 1998;24(9):1212–5.
73. Chan E, Chong EW, Lingham G, Stevenson LJ, Sanfilippo PG, Hewitt AW, Mackey DA, Yazar S. Prevalence of keratoconus based on scheimpflug imaging: the Raine study. Ophthalmology. 2021;128(4):515–21.
74. Reinstein DZ, Archer TJ, Gobbe M. Corneal epithelial thickness profile in the diagnosis of keratoconus. J Refract Surg. 2009;25(7):604–10.
75. Reinstein DZ, Gobbe M, Archer TJ, Silverman RH, Coleman DJ. Epithelial, stromal, and total corneal thickness in keratoconus: three-dimensional display with artemis very-high frequency digital ultrasound. J Refract Surg. 2010;26(4):259–71.
76. Li Y, Chamberlain W, Tan O, Brass R, Weiss JL, Huang D. Subclinical keratoconus detection by pattern analysis of corneal and epithelial thickness maps with optical coherence tomography. J Cataract Refract Surg. 2016;42(2):284–95.
77. Rocha KM, Perez-Straziota CE, Stulting RD, Randleman JB. SD-OCT analysis of regional epithelial thickness profiles in keratoconus, postoperative corneal ectasia, and normal eyes. J Refract Surg. 2013;29(3):173–9.
78. Li Y, Tan O, Brass R, Weiss JL, Huang D. Corneal epithelial thickness mapping by Fourier-domain optical coherence tomography in normal and keratoconic eyes. Ophthalmology. 2012;119(12):2425–33.
79. Al-Mahrouqi H, Oraba SB, Al-Habsi S, Mundemkattil N, Babu J, Panchatcharam SM, Al-Saidi R, Al-Raisi

A. Retinoscopy as a screening tool for keratoconus. Cornea. 2019;38(4):442–5.
80. Barraquer-Somers E, Chan CC, Green WR. Corneal epithelial iron deposition. Ophthalmology. 1983;90(6):729–34.
81. Li X, Rabinowitz YS, Rasheed K, Yang H. Longitudinal study of the normal eyes in unilateral keratoconus patients. Ophthalmology. 2004;111(3):440–6.
82. Kim SK, Dohlman CH. Causes of enlarged corneal nerves. Int Ophthalmol Clin. 2001;41(1):13–23.
83. Thota S, Miller WL, Bergmanson JP. Acute corneal hydrops: a case report including confocal and histopathological considerations. Cont Lens Anterior Eye. 2006;29(2):69–73.
84. McGhee CN. 2008 Sir Norman McAlister Gregg Lecture: 150 years of practical observations on the conical cornea—what have we learned? Clin Exp Ophthalmol. 2009;37(2):160–76.
85. Vazirani J, Basu S. Keratoconus: current perspectives. Clin Ophthalmol. 2013;7:2019–30.
86. Paranjpe V, Galor A, Monsalve P, Dubovy SR, Karp CL. Salzmann nodular degeneration: prevalence, impact, and management strategies. Clin Ophthalmol. 2019;13:1305–14.
87. Negris R. Floppy eyelid syndrome associated with keratoconus. J Am Optom Assoc. 1992;63(5):316–9.
88. Hughes AE, Dash DP, Jackson AJ, Frazer DG, Silvestri G. Familial keratoconus with cataract: linkage to the long arm of chromosome 15 and exclusion of candidate genes. Invest Ophthalmol Vis Sci. 2003;44(12):5063–6.
89. Dandapani SA, Padmanabhan P, Hussaindeen JR. Spectrum of binocular vision anomalies in keratoconus subjects. Optom Vis Sci. 2020;97(6):424–8.

Classifications and Patterns of Keratoconus

6

M. Vanathi and Navneet Sidhu

6.1 Introduction

Keratoconus is defined as a chronic, noninflammatory ectatic disorder of the cornea, characterized by steepening, apical thinning, and scarring leading to a decrease in visual acuity [1]. The disease is quite prevalent, especially in the younger population. With the recent advances in diagnostic modalities, the previous prevalence rates seem to have been underestimated since the older systems lacked focus on the subclinical forms of the disease. Clinical diagnosis of moderate to advanced keratoconus is relatively easy on slit-lamp examination. However, the diagnosis of subclinical and early keratoconus, especially in eyes with good visual acuity, becomes challenging. With increase in keratorefractive surgery procedures, the need to identify cases of subclinical or early cases of keratoconus has become imperative to avoid complication of post-LASIK ectasia in these eyes [2].

There are several classification systems of keratoconus in accordance with clinical characteristics and corneal curvature. Many topographical criteria have been developed to identify the early presentation of the disease. This chapter provides an insight into the various classification systems that have been adopted for keratoconus and the topographic patterns prevalent in keratoconus corneas.

M. Vanathi (✉) · N. Sidhu
Cornea, Lens & Refractive Service,
Dr. R. P. Centre for Ophthalmic Sciences, All India Institute of Medical Sciences, New Delhi, India

6.2 Classification Systems in Keratoconus

The normal corneal surface being prolate is aspherical. The following corneal topography findings should arouse a suspicion for the presence of keratoconus [3]:

1. Astigmatism >5 diopters (D)
2. Keratometry values:
   (a) $K_1/K_2 > 48$ D
   (b) Maximum keratometry (K_{max}) >49 D
3. Central corneal thickness (CCT) <470 μm and
4. Corneal asphericity > −0.50 μm

Keratoconus should be suspected in any patient with significant astigmatism, especially in a scenario of irregular astigmatism. It is important to recognize the subclinical forms of the disease, especially in refractive surgery candidates. Such eyes have the risk of development of post-LASIK ectasia if refractive procedures are performed. The term "subclinical keratoconus" can be used to include cases of keratoconus suspect or forme fruste keratoconus [4]. There is a general lack of clarity in existing literature on the definition of terminology of subclinical keratoconus and forme fruste keratoconus [5]. Subclinical

S. Das (ed.), *Keratoconus*, https://doi.org/10.1007/978-981-19-4262-4_6

Table 6.1 Differentiation between the various clinical forms of keratoconus

	Slit-lamp findings of keratoconus	Retinoscopy scissoring reflex	Topography suggestive of keratoconus
Keratoconus	Present	Present	Present
Early keratoconus	Absent	Present	Present
Topographic keratoconus	Absent	Absent	Present
Keratoconus suspect	Absent	Absent	May or may not be present

keratoconus do not show clinical signs of manifest keratoconus and can be diagnosed only using a topographic imaging (Table 6.1) [6]. A recent systematic review of studies on subclinical and forme fruste keratoconus describes the most common definition of subclinical keratoconus definition as an eye with topographic signs of keratoconus and/or suspicious topographic findings under normal slit-lamp examination and keratoconus in the fellow eye and that of forme fruste keratoconus as an eye with normal topography, normal slit-lamp examination, and keratoconus in the fellow eye.

Several classification systems have been proposed for keratoconus [7–15]. Many modifications have been suggested to get a better clarity on diagnosis and severity of the disease. The clinical course of keratoconus has been studied with inclusion of both risk and protective factors influencing the severity and progression of keratoconus in the Collaborative Longitudinal Evaluation of Keratoconus (CLEK) study [16]. Changes in vision, keratometric anterior corneal curvature, biomicroscopic signs, corneal scarring, and vision-specific quality of life were used as measures to define the stage and severity of disease in keratoconus patients in the CLEK study. A major drawback in Amsler-Krumeich classification and CLEK classification was that both did not employ topographic analysis in the classification of keratoconus. Different authors have tried to establish a comprehensive system for the classification of the disease by using different imaging techniques. These include videokeratography [17], corneal higher-order aberration imaging [11], Keratoconus Severity Score (KSS) [12], Fourier-domain optical coherence tomography imaging [15], topometric and tomographic indices [18], OCT corneal epithelial topographic asymmetry [19], scanning slit-beam topographic parameters [20], and anterior segment parameters on Scheimpflug imaging [21].

6.2.1 KISA Index

KISA index has been described by Rabinowitz, which provides an algorithm to quantify results from computerized videokeratography [17]. The topographic parameters required to derive the KISA index include:

- The corneal central keratometry (K value), which indicates central corneal steepening.
- The inferior-superior ($I - S$) dioptric asymmetry value.
- The amount of astigmatism (AST) which quantifies the degree of regular corneal astigmatism based on Sim$K$1 – Sim$K$2. Simulated keratometry (Sim$K$) talks about the dioptric power of the flattest and the steep meridians.
- The skewed radial axis (SRAX) value which measures the skew of the steepest radial axis between the superior and the inferior semi-meridian:

$$\text{KISA}(\%) = \frac{(K)\times(I-S)\times(\text{AST})\times(\text{SRAX})\times 100}{300}$$

The interpretation of KISA index is as follows:

- Normal: KISA index <60%.
- Keratoconus suspect: KISA index of 60–100%.
- Keratoconus: KISA index >100%.

6.2.2 McMahon and Colleagues' Keratoconus Severity Score (KSS)

The severity of keratoconus can be graded using the KSS score as proposed by McMahon and the Collaborative Longitudinal Evaluation of Keratoconus (CLEK) [16]. The KSS score assesses the following to elaborate a one-to-five grading system:

- Clinical signs (Vogt's striae, Fleischer ring, corneal scarring).
- Two corneal topography indices (average corneal power and the root mean square (RMS) error for higher-order aberrations).
- Manual interpretation of the topography map.

Though there are several methods described in literature, these have not found widespread adoption in clinical practice due to their limitations, as posterior corneal data was not considered in these classifications. Until recently, imaging of the posterior cornea has not been satisfactory. The limitation of incorporation of posterior corneal data prohibits a comprehensive understanding of the cornea. This led to the description of the new method of staging keratoconus tomographic data of the cornea which was more precise in reflecting the anatomical and functional changes of the disease.

6.3 Classification of Keratoconus Based on Clinical Characteristics

6.3.1 Based on Severity of the Corneal Curvature

Keratoconus was earlier classified based on the curvature of the cornea (Table 6.2).

Table 6.2 Keratoconus classification based on the severity of corneal curvature

Keratoconus severity	Corneal curvature
Mild	45.00 D
Moderate	45.00–52.00 D
Advanced	52.00–62.00 D
Severe	>62.00 D

Table 6.3 Morphological classification of keratoconus

Cone-type	Characteristics	Size in mm
Nipple	Small size and steep curvature	<5
Oval	Larger and ellipsoid in shape—the most common type	5–6
Globus	Large and globe-like	>6

6.3.2 Classification of Keratoconus Based on Morphological Appearance of the Cone

Classification of keratoconus based on the clinical appearance of the cone on slit-lamp examination describes it as nipple, oval, or globus type of cone (Table 6.3). The cone can be classified as follows depending on the shape and size:

6.4 Amsler–Krumeich Classification

Until recently, Amsler-Krumeich classification (Table 6.4), which is one of the oldest classifications, was the most commonly used clinical classification system for keratoconus. This classification system, initially described by Marc Amsler in 1947, was based entirely on anterior corneal data. Keratoconus was classified into four stages, stage I to stage IV, based on four parameters of keratometry, pachymetry, refraction, and corneal scarring in the central 3-mm curvature [22, 23]. The Placido disc image of the corneal surface was used in this system of classification [24]. The major drawbacks in this classification include the lack of integration of posterior corneal data and failure of incorporation of the complete pachymetry data, the imaging of which was not available at the time this classification was elaborated. This classification system does not take into consideration any other changes in the corneal surface other than on the anterior corneal surface. Overall, this system has the following deficiencies:

- Lack of posterior data.
- Measurements taken at the corneal apex rather than the thinnest point.
- Visual acuity not considered.
- Different parameters of the cornea were not categorized accordingly as per the stage of the disease.

6.4.1 Belin ABCD Classification

The Belin ABCD classification was introduced on the Scheimpflug imaging OCULUS Pentacam (OCULUS GmbH, Wetzlar, Germany) taking into account the shortcomings of the Amsler-Krumeich system [2]. This new classification (Table 6.5) considers the changes in the following four corneal topographic parameters:

A. Anterior radius of curvature (ARC) as measured in the 3.0-mm zone centered on the thinnest pachymetry.
B. Posterior radius of curvature (PRC) as measured in the 3.0-mm zone centered on the thinnest pachymetry.
C. Thinnest pachymetry measured in μm.
D. Distance best corrected visual acuity.

The advantages of the ABCD classification are that its measurements are centered on the thinnest point which is the apex of the cone utilizing the thinnest pachymetry and not the central apical reading. This classification is relatively simple to use in clinical practice. It enables the grading of each component independently, thereby comprehensively reflecting the corneal changes during the progression of the disease or at the time of documentation.

The Belin ABCD Progression Display (Fig. 6.1), incorporated in the software of the image in the OCULUS Pentacam tomography, enables up to eight examination data that can be displayed and compared together to analyze for progression. This helps in monitoring the disease and diagnosing the progression at an earlier stage and planning further line of management accordingly.

Table 6.4 Amsler-Krumeich classification

Stage	Characteristics
I	• Eccentric corneal steepening
	• Induced myopia and/or astigmatism <5 D
	• Corneal radii ≤48 D
	• Vogt's striae, no scars
II	• Induced myopia and/or astigmatism >5, <8 D
	• Corneal radii ≤53 D
	• No central scars
	• Corneal thickness ≥400 μm
III	• Induced myopia and/or astigmatism >8, <10 D
	• Corneal radii >53 D
	• No central scars
	• Corneal thickness 200–400 μm
IV	• Refraction not measurable
	• Corneal radii >55 D
	• Central scars, perforation
	• Corneal thickness <200 μm

Table 6.5 ABCD classification

	Topographic parameters for grading and monitoring keratoconus severity				
	A	B	C	D	
Keratoconus severity	ARC	PRC	Thinnest pachymetry	BDVA	Scarring
Stage 0	>7.25 mm (<46.5 D)	>5.90 mm	>490 μm	≥20/20 (≥1.0)	–
Stage I	>7.05 mm (<48.0 D)	>5.70 mm	>450 μm	<20/20 (<1.0)	–,+,++
Stage II	>6.35 mm (<53.0 D)	>5.15 mm	>400 μm	<20/40 (<0.5)	–,+,++
Stage III	>6.15 mm (<55.0 D)	>4.95 mm	>300 μm	<20/100) (<0.2)	–,+,++
Stage IV	<6.15 mm (>55.0 D)	<4.95 mm	≤300 μm	<20/400 (<0.05)	–,+,++

ARC anterior radius of curvature, *PRC* posterior radius of curvature, *BDVA* best distance corrected visual acuity. Scarring: (–) clear, no scarring, (+): iris details visible, (++) iris obscured

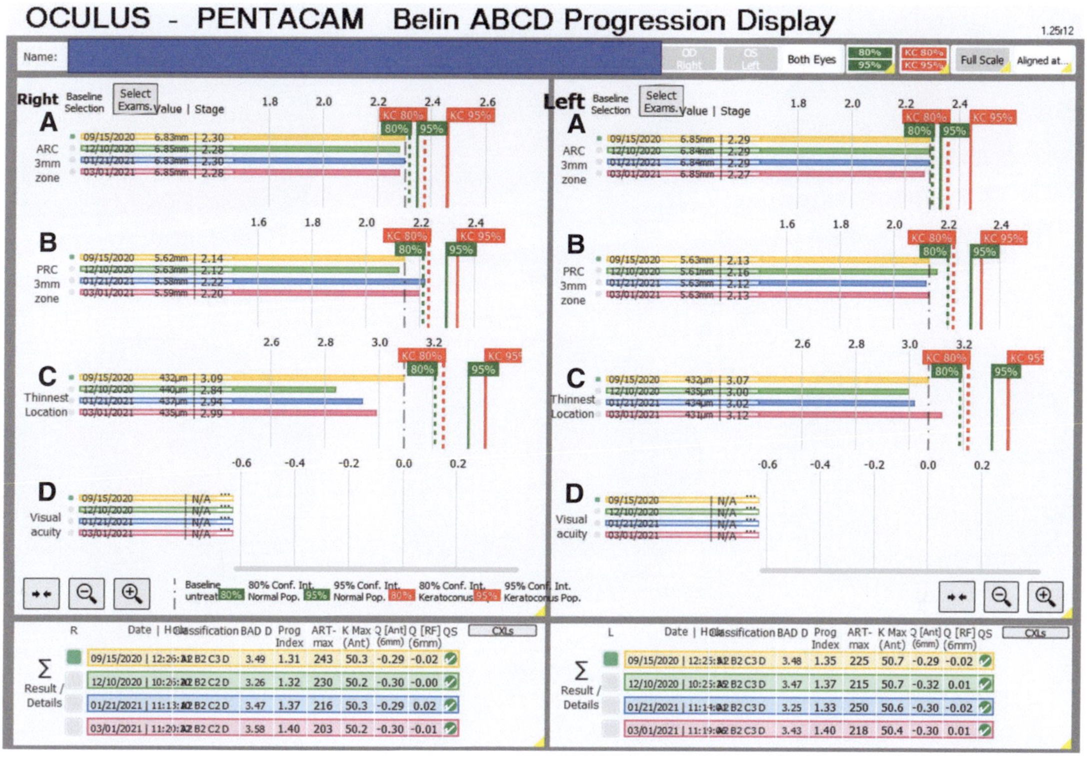

Fig. 6.1 Belin ABCD progression display

6.5 Fourier-Domain OCT Classification

This classification system was devised on Fourier-domain OCT system [with 5-μm axial resolution] [15] imaging across the keratoconus cone (Table 6.6).

Table 6.6 Fourier-domain OCT classification

Severity	OCT characteristics
Stage 1	Thinning of apparently normal epithelial and stromal layers
Stage 2	Hyper-reflective anomalies occurring at the Bowman's layer with epithelial thickening at the conus
Stage 3	Posterior displacement of the hyper-reflective structure occurring at the Bowman's layer level with increased epithelial thickening and stromal thinning
Stage 4	Pan-stromal scar
Stage 5a	Hydrops of acute onset—Descemet's rupture and dilaceration of collagen lamellae with large fluid-filled intrastromal cysts
Stage 5b	Hydrops healing stage—pan-stromal scarring with a remaining aspect of Descemet's membrane rupture

6.6 Topographic Patterns in Keratoconus

Corneal topography is the representation of the corneal shape and curvature which represents the geometrical properties of the corneal surface. Corneal topography can be used to assess epithelial irregularities, stromal abnormalities, corneal astigmatism, refractive stability, or any other undiagnosed corneal ectatic diseases. Topographic maps are reflective of these changes that occur either clinically or subclinically. The corneal parameters are represented in various colors on the topographic maps, warmer colors (toward the red spectrum) indicating steeper curvatures while the cooler color (toward the blue

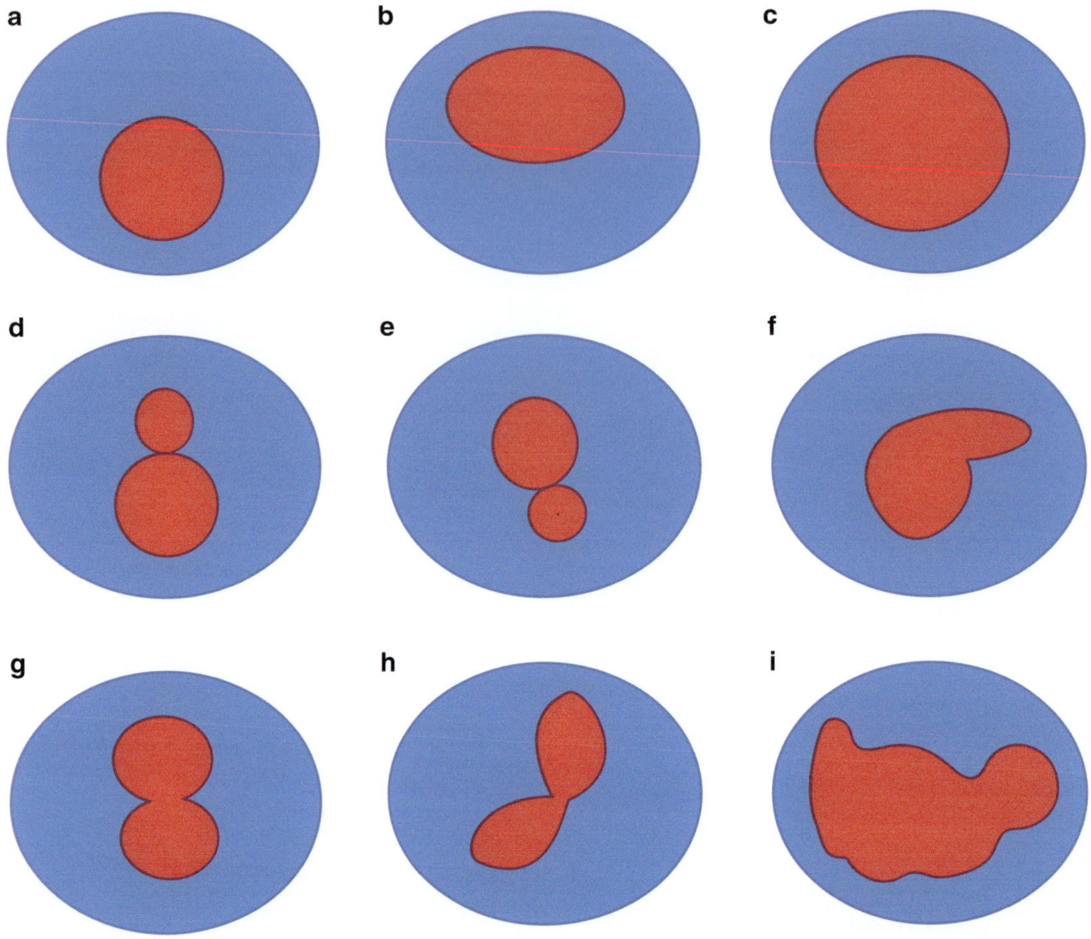

Fig. 6.2 Common topographical patterns of keratoconus. Front sagittal curvature maps showing the nine different sagittal patterns. (**a**) Inferior steepening; (**b**) superior steepening; (**c**) round; (**d**) asymmetric bowtie with inferior steepening; (**e**) asymmetric bowtie with superior steepening; (**f**) asymmetric bowtie with skewed axis; (**g**) symmetric bowtie; (**h**) symmetric bowtie with skewed axis; (**i**) irregular pattern

spectrum) indicating flatter curvatures. Rabinowitz et al. proposed ten topographical patterns in normal corneas [14] (Figs. 6.2 and 6.3). These include:

1. Round
2. Oval
3. Superior steepening
4. Inferior steepening
5. Irregular
6. Symmetric bowtie
7. Symmetric bowtie with skewed radial axes
8. Asymmetric bowtie with inferior steepening (AB/IS)
9. Asymmetric bowtie with superior steepening (AB/SS)
10. Asymmetric bowtie with skewed radial axes (AB/SRAX)

The cone is considered central, paracentral, or peripheral when the apex of the cone is within the central 3-mm zone, within 3–5-mm zone, or outside the central 5-mm zone, respectively, in the analysis of anterior elevation map (with BFS float mode) of the corneal tomography images.

Some authors consider pellucid marginal corneal degeneration (PMCD) to be a peripheral form of keratoconus [25]. PMCD is an idiopathic,

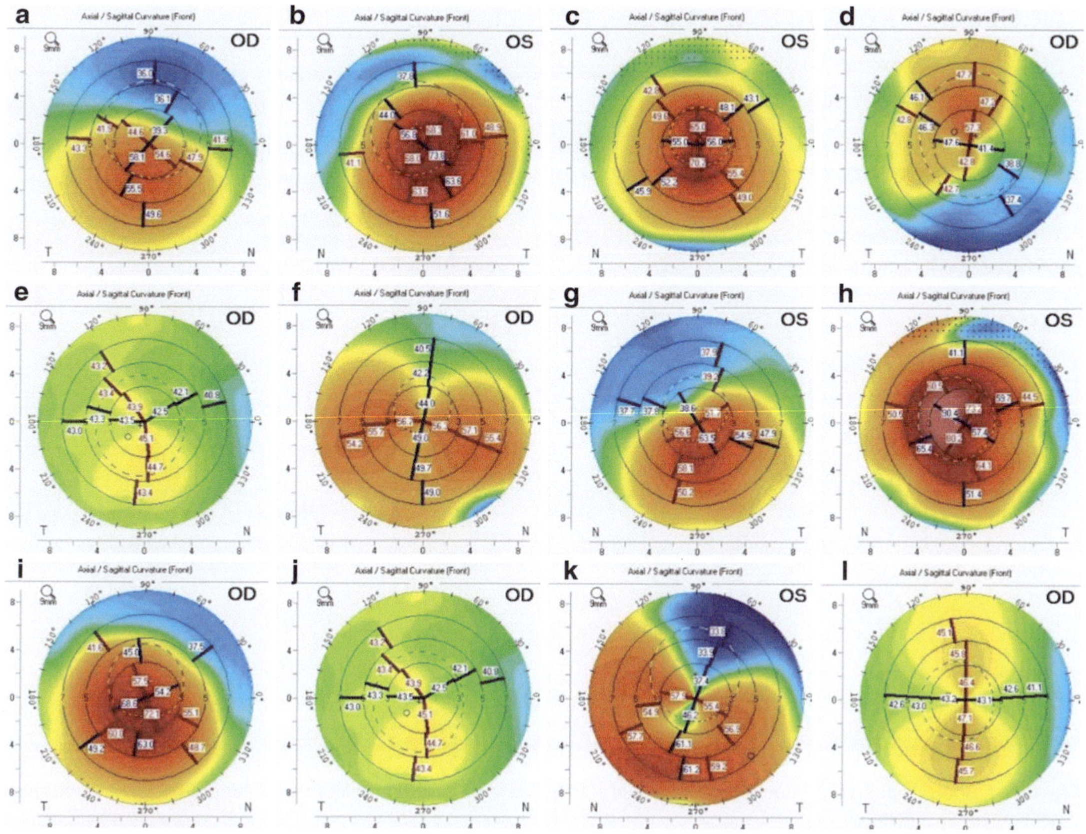

Fig. 6.3 Topography images showing different patterns seen in keratoconus: (**a**) oval, (**b**) round, (**c**) AB-IS, (**d**) AB-SS, (**e**) AB-SRAX, (**f**) butterfly, (**g**) junctional, (**h**) irregular, (**i**) inferior steep, (**j**) asymmetric bowtie-SRAX, (**k**) lobster claw pattern in pellucid marginal degeneration, (**l**) symmetric bowtie

progressive, noninflammatory, ectatic corneal disorder characterized by a peripheral inferior band of corneal thinning in a crescent-shaped pattern. Clinically, the area of maximal thinning and steepening coincide in keratoconus, while in PMCD, the corneal steepening is superior to the inferior region of ectasia in PMCD.

Corneal tomography analysis in PMCD is characterized by flattening in the vertical meridian, inducing a significant against-the-rule (ATR) astigmatism and a significant steepening around the area of maximum thinning [26]. This characteristic corneal tomographic pattern is described as the classical claw pattern (Fig. 6.4) and has also been noted in cases of keratoconus besides PMCD [27]. A similar clawlike pattern appearance, described as the "kissing bird sign" in anterior elevation maps in BFS float mode, in cases of peripheral cones, but without the presence of inferior corneal thinning in pachymetric map (as seen in PMCD) has led to the description of "pellucid-like keratoconus" (PLK) [28].

6.7 Conclusion

Corneal topography is an important diagnostic tool for the assessment of suspected keratoconus patients and in patients planned for refractive surgery. It is also important to differentiate keratoconus from other conditions such as displaced apex syndrome, contact lens-induced warpage, prominent tear meniscus, misalignment, dry eye disease, or accidental external pressure on the globe [29]. Since keratoconus is a bilaterally, asymmetrical disease with variable rates of progression,

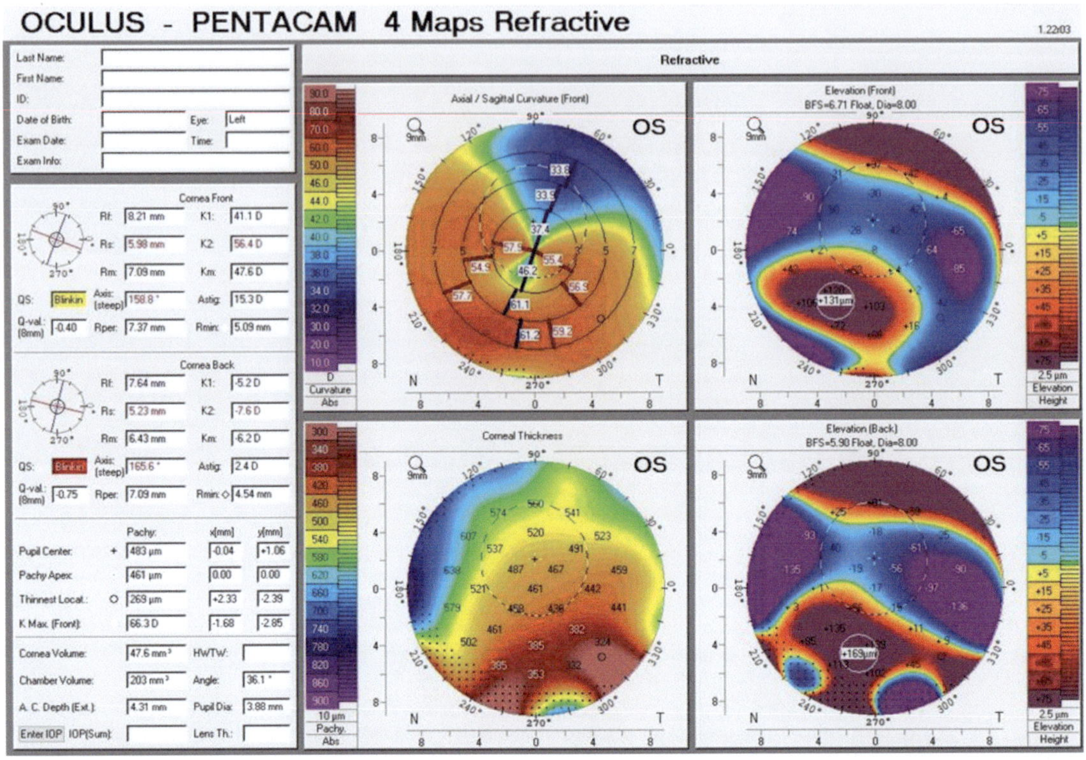

Fig. 6.4 Corneal topography showing the classical lobster claw pattern in curvature map suggestive of pellucid marginal corneal degeneration

early detection and intervention are the key to prevent the development of a significant visual morbidity. The new ABCD system classification depicts both anatomical and functional data that were not described previously in the Amsler-Krumeich classification. This elaborates both anterior and posterior corneal surfaces and is centered on the thinnest pachymetry. It allows for an improved description of the cornea in patients with keratoconus and hence a more tailored treatment approach.

References

1. Rabinowitz YS. Keratoconus. Surv Ophthalmol. 1998;42(4):297–319.
2. Belin MW, Kundu G, Shetty N, Gupta K, Mullick R, Thakur P. ABCD: a new classification for keratoconus. Indian J Ophthalmol. 2020;68(12):2831–4.
3. Mas Tur V, MacGregor C, Jayaswal R, O'Brart D, Maycock N. A review of keratoconus: diagnosis, pathophysiology, and genetics. Surv Ophthalmol. 2017;62(6):770–83.
4. Koc M, Tekin K, Kiziltoprak H, Inanc M, Kosekahya P, Ozulken K, Durukan I. Topometric and tomographic evaluation of subclinical keratoconus. Ophthalmic Epidemiol. 2020;27(4):289–97.
5. Henriquez MA, Hadid M, Izquierdo L Jr. A systematic review of subclinical keratoconus and Forme Fruste keratoconus. J Refract Surg. 2020;36(4):270–9.
6. Matalia H, Swarup R. Imaging modalities in keratoconus. Indian J Ophthalmol. 2013;61(8):394–400.
7. Perry HD, Buxton JN, Fine BS. Round and oval cones in keratoconus. Ophthalmology. 1980;87(9):905–9.
8. Krumeich JH, Daniel J, Knülle A. Live-epikeratophakia for keratoconus. J Cataract Refract Surg. 1998;24(4):456–63.
9. Rabinowitz YS, Rasheed K. KISA% index: a quantitative videokeratography algorithm embodying minimal topographic criteria for diagnosing keratoconus. J Cataract Refract Surg. 1999;25(10):1327–35. Erratum in: J Cataract Refract Surg. 2000;26(4):480.
10. Maeda N, Klyce SD, Smolek MK, Thompson HW. Automated keratoconus screening with corneal topography analysis. Invest Ophthalmol Vis Sci. 1994;35(6):2749–57.

11. Alió JL, Shabayek MH. Corneal higher order aberrations: a method to grade keratoconus. J Refract Surg. 2006;22(6):539–45.
12. McMahon TT, Szczotka-Flynn L, Barr JT, Anderson RJ, Slaughter ME, Lass JH, Iyengar SK, CLEK Study Group. A new method for grading the severity of keratoconus: the Keratoconus Severity Score (KSS). Cornea. 2006;25(7):794–800.
13. Mahmoud AM, Roberts CJ, Lembach RG, Twa MD, Herderick EE, McMahon TT, CLEK Study Group. CLMI: the cone location and magnitude index. Cornea. 2008;27(4):480–7.
14. Rabinowitz YS, Yang H, Brickman Y, Akkina J, Riley C, Rotter JI, Elashoff J. Videokeratography database of normal human corneas. Br J Ophthalmol. 1996;80(7):610–6.
15. Sandali O, El Sanharawi M, Temstet C, Hamiche T, Galan A, Ghouali W, Goemaere I, Basli E, Borderie V, Laroche L. Fourier-domain optical coherence tomography imaging in keratoconus: a corneal structural classification. Ophthalmology. 2013;120(12):2403–12.
16. Wagner H, Barr JT, Zadnik K. Collaborative Longitudinal Evaluation of Keratoconus (CLEK) Study: methods and findings to date. Cont Lens Anterior Eye. 2007;30(4):223–32.
17. Li X, Yang H, Rabinowitz YS. Keratoconus: classification scheme based on videokeratography and clinical signs. J Cataract Refract Surg. 2009;35(9):1597–603.
18. Bae GH, Kim JR, Kim CH, Lim DH, Chung ES, Chung TY. Corneal topographic and tomographic analysis of fellow eyes in unilateral keratoconus patients using Pentacam. Am J Ophthalmol. 2014;157(1):103–109.e1.
19. Kanellopoulos AJ, Asimellis G. OCT corneal epithelial topographic asymmetry as a sensitive diagnostic tool for early and advancing keratoconus. Clin Ophthalmol. 2014;8:2277–87.
20. Sonmez B, Doan MP, Hamilton DR. Identification of scanning slit-beam topographic parameters important in distinguishing normal from keratoconic corneal morphologic features. Am J Ophthalmol. 2007;143(3):401–8.
21. Emre S, Doganay S, Yologlu S. Evaluation of anterior segment parameters in keratoconic eyes measured with the Pentacam system. J Cataract Refract Surg. 2007;33(10):1708–12.
22. Amsler M. Kératocône classique et kératocône fruste; arguments unitaires [Classic keratocene and crude keratocene; unitary arguments]. Ophthalmologica. 1946;111(2–3):96–101.
23. Krachmer JH, Feder RS, Belin MW. Keratoconus and related noninflammatory corneal thinning disorders. Surv Ophthalmol. 1984;28(4):293–322.
24. Gatinel D, Malet J, Hoang-Xuan T, Azar DT. Corneal elevation topography: best fit sphere, elevation distance, asphericity, toricity, and clinical implications. Cornea. 2011;30(5):508–15.
25. Sridhar MS, Mahesh S, Bansal AK, Rao GN. Superior pellucid marginal corneal degeneration. Eye (Lond). 2004;18(4):393–9.
26. Maguire LJ, Klyce SD, McDonald MB, Kaufman HE. Corneal topography of pellucid marginal degeneration. Ophthalmology. 1987;94(5):519–24.
27. Lee BW, Jurkunas UV, Harissi-Dagher M, Poothullil AM, Tobaigy FM, Azar DT. Ectatic disorders associated with a claw-shaped pattern on corneal topography. Am J Ophthalmol. 2007;144(1):154–6.
28. Sinjab MM, Youssef LN. Pellucid-like keratoconus. F1000Res. 2012;1:48.
29. Jiang HJ, Xie PY. The analysis of corneal topography for keratoconus. Chin J Ophthalmol. 2006;42(3):231–5.

Differential Diagnosis of Keratoconus

7

Elias Flockerzi, Loay Daas, Haris Sideroudi, and Berthold Seitz

7.1 Introduction

The differential diagnosis of keratoconus (KC) includes corneal diseases with similar tomographic findings. These must be differentiated from KC to be able to make appropriate and correct treatment decisions. The first group comprises other true corneal ectasias.

The second group includes corneal diseases that may imitate KC with a pseudokeratoconic tomography.

A small, third group includes conditions that could be confused with acute hydrops in KC.

7.2 True Corneal Ectasias

7.2.1 Pellucid Marginal Degeneration (PMD): Keratotorus

Pellucid marginal degeneration (PMD) is a corneal ectatic disease that affects the inferior periphery of the cornea and was first described in 1957 [1]. "Pellucid" means "very clear" which indicates that the cornea generally remains transparent without showing the typical KC signs (Vogt striae, hemosiderin deposits designated as Fleischer ring, corneal scarring) despite advanced thinning [2]. There is consensus that, similar to KC, it is a bilateral disease which can lead to tears in Descemet's membrane and thus to a corneal hydrops in very advanced stages [3].

The thinning area in PMD comprises an arcuate band of thinning in the peripheral cornea that may reach from the 4 to 8 o'clock position [2, 3]. This inferior band of thinning is comparable to the inferior part of a *torus* (doughnut form). It is usually located in a distance of 1–2 mm to the limbus and is separated from it by an area of normal corneal thickness [4]. The cornea above this band is characterized by (a) a normal thickness with (b) a flattening of the vertical meridian and (c) an "against-the-rule" astigmatism [2–4].

The prevalence of PMD has been reported to be higher in comparison to keratoglobus or isolated KC posticus [2, 3]. Estimating the true prevalence of PMD, however, is extremely difficult as PMD was often diagnosed based on topographic criteria in the past that should no longer be used today: A "crab claw," "lobster claw," or "kissing birds" pattern raised by isolated examination of the anterior corneal curvature—corneal topography—was considered to be typical of PMD. But these patterns show only corneal curvature abnormalities and therefore ignore the actual proving criterion of inferior peripheral corneal thinning in PMD [5, 6].

Moreover, the arcuate band of thinning in PMD is located in the periphery of the cornea in

E. Flockerzi (✉) · L. Daas · H. Sideroudi · B. Seitz
Department of Ophthalmology, Saarland University Medical Center, Homburg, Germany
e-mail: Elias.Flockerzi@uks.eu; Loay.Daas@uks.eu; Haris.Sideroudi@uks.eu; Berthold.Seitz@uks.eu

S. Das (ed.), *Keratoconus*, https://doi.org/10.1007/978-981-19-4262-4_7

a distance of 1–2 mm from the limbus. Based on an average corneal diameter of 12 mm [7, 8], the thinned region would be located in the 10-mm zone. However, this area is often not covered by the topographic imaging showing pattern anomalies as described above. Therefore, it is recommended that PMD should nowadays never be diagnosed without a full corneal pachymetry map covering 12 mm in diameter [5]. Accordingly, the diagnosis of PMD must be critically questioned when it is treated with intracorneal ring segments, since in true PMD the area of maximal ectasia would fall outside of any currently available intracorneal ring segments. It can therefore be assumed that some PMD cases that were diagnosed based on the "crab claw," "lobster claw," or "kissing birds" patterns might have been classified as false positives while they actually were cases of inferior KC [9].

Corneal biomechanics were evaluated in PMD based on Ocular Response Analyzer® (ORA, Reichert Instruments, Depew, USA) and Corvis ST® (OCULUS Optikgeräte, Wetzlar, Germany) measurements. A lower corneal hysteresis and a lower corneal resistance factor were found in PMD compared to healthy controls [10, 11]. Corvis ST® measurements showed no differences between PMD and healthy controls [10]. When interpreting biomechanical measurements in PMD, it must, however, always be kept in mind that both devices measure mainly in the corneal center, whereas the pathology in PMD is located inferiorly.

The most common therapeutic options for true PMD is refractive correction with spectacles or contact lenses [3]. Surgically, PMD can be stabilized by corneal cross-linking with riboflavin and ultraviolet-A light irradiation [12] or by implantation of intracorneal ring segments in early cases [13]. In terms of keratoplasty, deep anterior lamellar and penetrating keratoplasty [2] are possible treatment options, the latter decentered inferiorly or with a large graft diameter and fixation with single-knot sutures because of the pronounced peripheral thinning in advanced cases [14].

Brief Case A 62 year-old male patient presented with a best spectacle-corrected distance visual acuity of 20/400 in his right eye (Fig. 7.1). He underwent excimer laser-assisted penetrating keratoplasty because of advanced pellucid marginal degeneration using a 8.6-mm graft fixed with single-knot sutures and achieved a postoperative best spectacle-corrected distance visual acuity of 20/40.

7.2.2 Keratoglobus

In contrast to KC and PMD, keratoglobus is considered to be a bilateral congenital disorder that is nonprogressive or only minimally progressive during lifetime [15]. However, reports exist which describe cases of acquired keratoglobus [16, 17]. It can be associated with connective tissue disorders such as Marfan or Ehlers-Danlos syndrome and is characterized by (a) a global protrusion of the cornea with thinning from limbus to limbus and (b) the maximal thinning located at the periphery [3]. The typical KC signs (Vogt striae, Fleischer ring, scarring) are missing. The thinned and protruding cornea causes myopia with irregular astigmatism and makes the keratoglobus among ectatic corneal diseases the most susceptible to spontaneous or trauma-induced perforation [18].

The normal corneal diameter and the absence of glaucomatous changes in isolated keratoglobus allow to differentiate it from buphthalmos in congenital glaucoma. Megalocornea, which is another differential diagnosis, is of normal corneal thickness as opposed to keratoglobus [15].

Conservative therapy consists of refractive correction with spectacles or contact lenses. However, the use of contact lenses is controversially discussed because of the increased risk of perforation caused even by minimal trauma [17]. Surgically, penetrating keratoplasty is challenging because of the circularly thinned periphery of the cornea resulting in the need of a large graft reaching from limbus to limbus. A surgical method used more frequently in the past was epi-

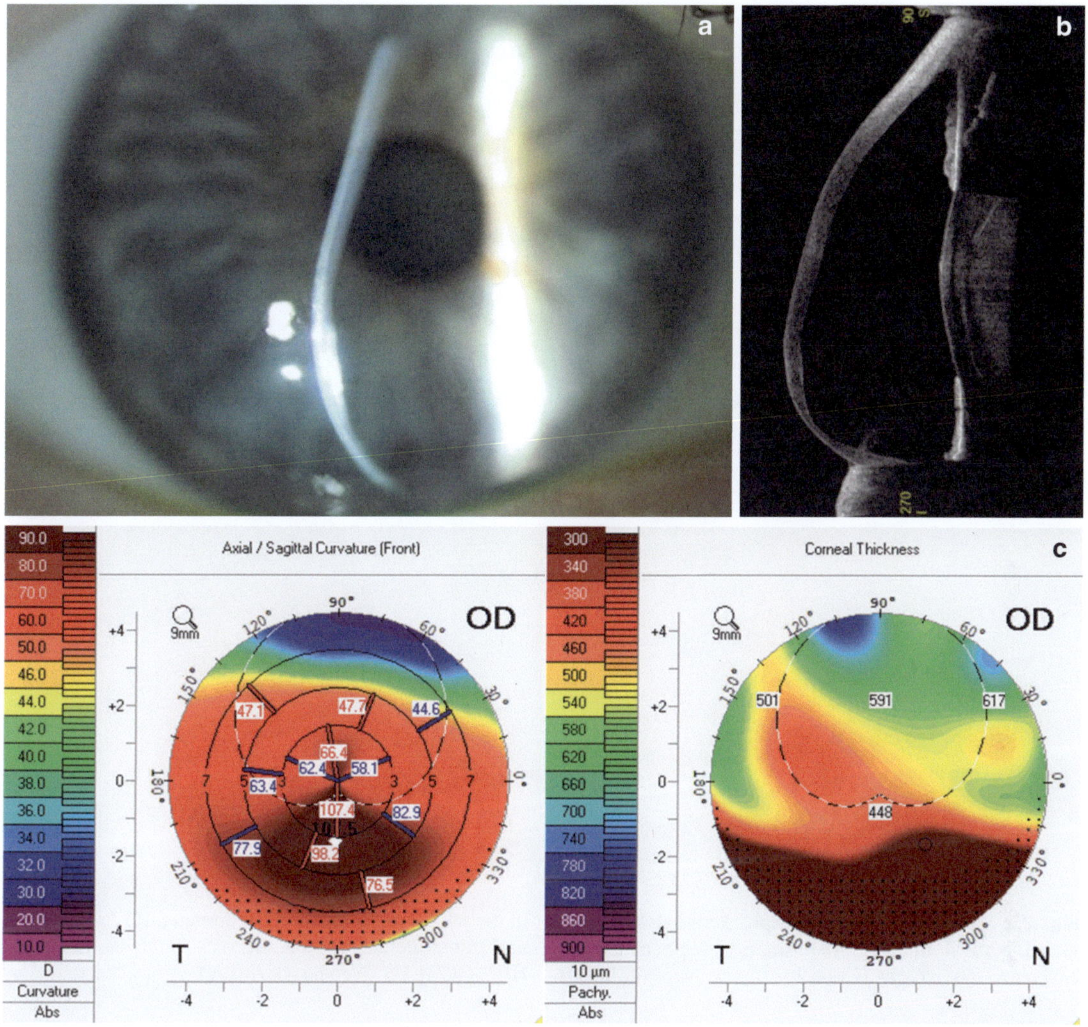

Fig. 7.1 (**a**) Slit-lamp photograph, pellucid marginal degeneration with inferior band of thinning and steepening. (**b**) Anterior segment optical coherence tomography (Casia 2®, Tomey, Nagoya, Japan) of the same eye. *S* superior, *I* inferior. (**c**) Anterior corneal curvature and corneal thickness analysis (Pentacam HR®, OCULUS, Wetzlar, Germany). Inferior band of thinning and steepening

keratophakia, which includes suturing a corneal donor lenticule onto the thinned host cornea [19]. If scarring occurred in the interface between the patient‘s cornea and the donor lenticule, subsequent penetrating keratoplasty was suggested. In recent years, this procedure has been partially replaced by the advent of deep anterior lamellar keratoplasty which nowadays remains an option in the treatment of keratoglobus besides penetrating keratoplasty [14, 15].

Brief Case A 19-year-old female patient presented with a best spectacle-corrected distance visual acuity of 20/400 in her right eye (Fig. 7.2) and 20/40 in her left eye. She was recommended to try contact lenses prior to planning penetrating keratoplasty because of keratoglobus. She did not support contact lenses, and, therefore, penetrating keratoplasty with single-knot sutures and a graft diameter of 8.6 mm was performed in her right eye.

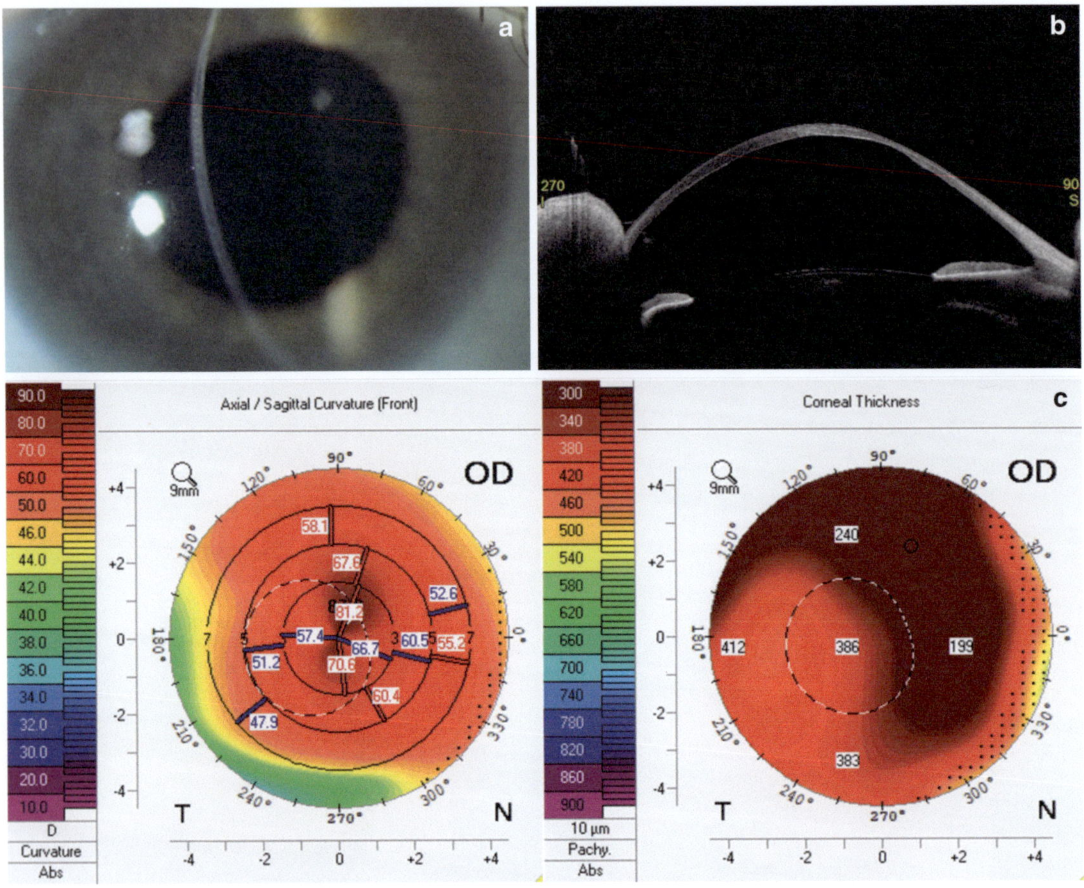

Fig. 7.2 (**a**) Slit-lamp photograph, keratoglobus with global corneal thinning. (**b**) Anterior segment optical coherence tomography (Casia 2®, Tomey, Nagoya, Japan) of the same eye. Global corneal thinning. (**c**) Anterior corneal curvature and corneal thickness analysis (Pentacam HR®, OCULUS, Wetzlar, Germany)

7.2.3 Isolated Keratoconus Posticus

The isolated keratoconus posticus represents a rare entity that is characterized by an abnormal posterior corneal curvature, while the anterior corneal curvature remains unaffected with a regular astigmatism in most cases [20]. Two subtypes exist: (a) the KC posticus generalis or totalis that affects the entire posterior cornea and (b) the KC posticus circumscriptus that can be localized (para-)centrally in most cases and rather rarely in the corneal periphery and may be accompanied by corneal opacity [21]. Both forms can appear unilaterally or bilaterally, and they are etiologically classified as congenital cleavage abnormalities that remain noninflammatory and nonprogressive during lifetime [22]. Most patients with KC posticus, especially those with unilateral occurrence, suffer from impaired visual acuity since childhood because they developed amblyopia [23]. To prevent this, early detection and refractive correction with spectacles or contact lenses are essential. In case of associated corneal opacity, a rotational autologous keratoplasty may also be considered. An internistic workup should be performed as KC posticus can also occur in association with systemic conditions such as growth disorders, cleft formation, genitourethral malformations, or musculoskeletal abnormalities [24]. The consensus is that KC posticus neither does progress to anterior KC nor is associated with anterior KC [22, 23]. When planning cataract surgery, a hyperopic refractive surprise because of overestimation of the total corneal power has to be expected even more in KC posticus than in typical KC [23, 24]. With the advent of corneal posterior surface analysis based on Scheimpflug imaging and anterior segment optical coherence tomography, one could hypothesize that, nowadays, KC posticus might be diagnosed more frequently in daily practice as part of the workup for unclear visual impairment.

Brief Case A 48-year-old female patient presented with a best spectacle-corrected distance visual acuity of 20/40 in the right eye and 20/25 in her left eye with suspicion of KC (Fig. 7.3). While anterior corneal curvature was innocuous, there was a slight posterior corneal elevation indicating a mild form of KC posticus. The patient was recommended to wear contact lenses.

7.2.4 Regular Astigmatism

A characteristic sign of typical KC is the progressive thinning of the cornea that goes along with the development of an irregular astigmatism and visual impairment [25]. Typical KC, however, can also be associated with regular astigmatism [26], and in these cases, the mere presence of regular astigmatism must be distinguished from the combination of regular astigmatism and KC. While uncorrected regular astigmatism may be the cause of amblyopia development in children, it may also be the cause of permanent visual impairment in adults and may be misinterpreted prima vista as KC if there is a high refractive error.

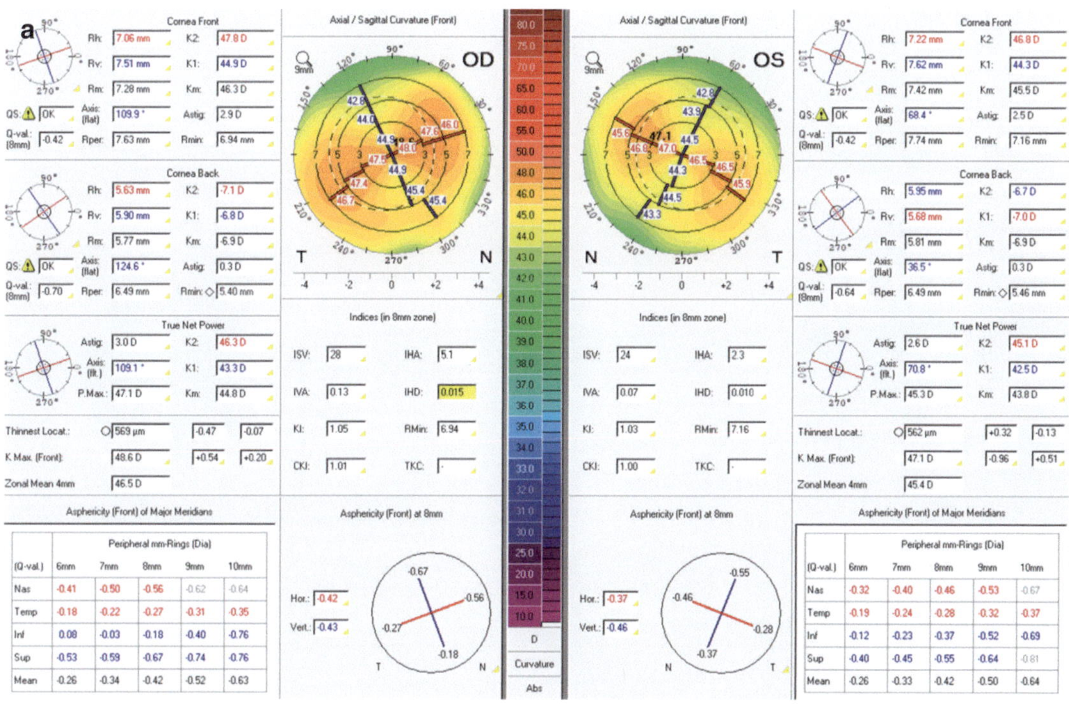

Fig. 7.3 (**a**) Topometric analysis (Pentacam HR®, OCULUS, Wetzlar, Germany) revealing oblique astigmatism more in the right than in the left eye. (**b**) The right eye, Belin/Ambrósio enhanced ectasia screening display (Pentacam HR®, OCULUS, Wetzlar, Germany) with a posterior elevation at the thinnest point ≥13 µm (20 µm, based on a best-fit sphere from 8.0-mm optical zone) and a final Belin/Ambrósio enhanced ectasia screening display deviation "*D*" = 1.73. (**c**) The left eye, Belin/Ambrósio enhanced ectasia screening display (Pentacam HR®, OCULUS, Wetzlar, Germany) with a posterior elevation at the thinnest point ≥13 µm (18 µm, based on a best-fit sphere from 8.0-mm optical zone) and a final Belin/Ambrósio enhanced ectasia screening display deviation "*D*" = 1.83

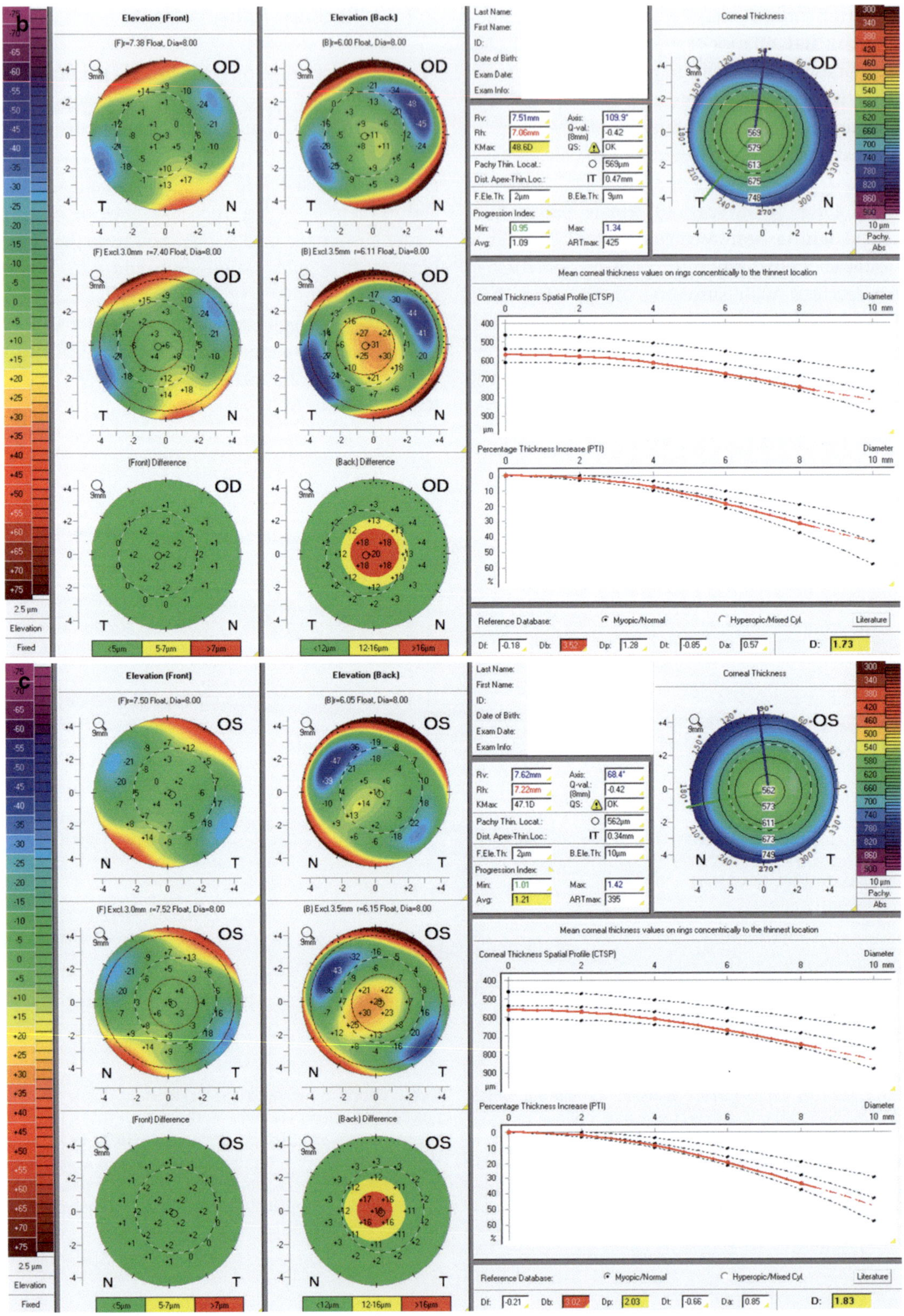

Fig. 7.3 (continued)

There is controversy regarding the distribution of the different types of astigmatism in KC. One study based on 137 KC corneas of 137 patients reported that with-the-rule astigmatism was more prevalent in the anterior corneal surface and against-the-rule astigmatism was more prevalent in the posterior corneal surface [27]. This result could not be confirmed by a larger study on 1273 KC and 1035 healthy corneas: They found that (a) the dominant astigmatism of the anterior corneal surface was against-the-rule astigmatism in KC and with-the-rule astigmatism in normal corneas, while (b) the reverse was found for the posterior cornea [28]. These differences could be due to different age groups or disease stages included, contact lens wear, and, finally, different ethnicities in these studies.

The ABCD KC classification according to Belin and Duncan provides analysis of the anterior (**A**) and the posterior (**B**) corneal curvature (in an optical zone of 3 mm centered on the thinnest corneal point), the thinnest corneal thickness (**C**), and the best spectacle-corrected visual acuity (**D**) including stages 0–4 for each parameter [29–31], and its criteria for KC diagnosis can be used for differentiation: (a) posterior elevation at the thinnest point ≥13 μm (based on a best-fit sphere from 8-mm optical zone), (b) a final Belin/Ambrósio enhanced ectasia screening display deviation "*D*" ≥ 3.0, (c) a minimal corneal thickness < 550 μm, and (d) a spherical equivalent <0 (myopic) [5]. Whereas early stages of regular astigmatism already benefit from spectacles, advanced stages can achieve optimal visual rehabilitation by rigid contact lens fitting.

While the corneal apex in KC corneas is usually located in the temporal inferior quadrant, KC cases with a central apex localization exist, which may show a regular astigmatism. In these cases, it is important to differentiate between a central KC with regular astigmatism and a pure regular astigmatism without KC based on the aforementioned criteria.

Brief Case A 13-year-old girl presented with a best spectacle-corrected distance visual acuity of 20/40 in both eyes and suspicion of KC (Fig. 7.4). After the diagnosis of regular astigmatism, contact lens fitting led to an increase of visual acuity to 20/25.

7.2.5 Post-LASIK Ectasia

The corneal ectasia after laser-assisted in situ keratomileusis (LASIK) designates an iatrogenic keratectasia following corneal refractive surgery, and it is hereafter referred to as "post-LASIK ectasia" [32]. It is characterized by an abnormal posterior corneal elevation [33], progressive corneal thinning, and steepening similar to KC [34]. The steepening occurs mostly inferiorly which leads to an increase of myopia and astigmatism in a period of days to years after LASIK [35]. Although it can usually be diagnosed unambiguously if there is an abnormal tomography with progressive corneal thinning and steepening after a history of refractive surgery, the post-LASIK ectasia remains a tomographic differential diagnosis of KC.

The possible risk factors for developing a post-LASIK ectasia include high myopia with an increased ablation depth, reduced postoperative corneal thickness with a reduced residual stromal bed, and the undetected preoperative presence of ectatic corneal diseases such as KC or PMD [35, 36].

Similar to KC, contact lenses are used in the treatment of early post-LASIK ectasia for visual rehabilitation. Surgical approaches include corneal cross-linking with riboflavin and ultraviolet-A light irradiation to stabilize the ectasia or the off-label implantation of intracorneal ring segments with the aim of modifying the anterior corneal curvature. Both procedures rely on a sufficient residual corneal thickness, which is 400 μm in the center for cross-linking and 450 μm for intracorneal ring segments in the 6-mm zone—the latter are implanted in a depth of 80% within the corneal stroma. Patients with significant myopia regression after LASIK can benefit from the implantation of a phakic intraocular lens for myopia correction if there is sufficient anterior chamber depth (we recommend >3 mm).

A focal anterior stromal weakening measured by optical coherence tomography-based elastography of the cornea together with the outward

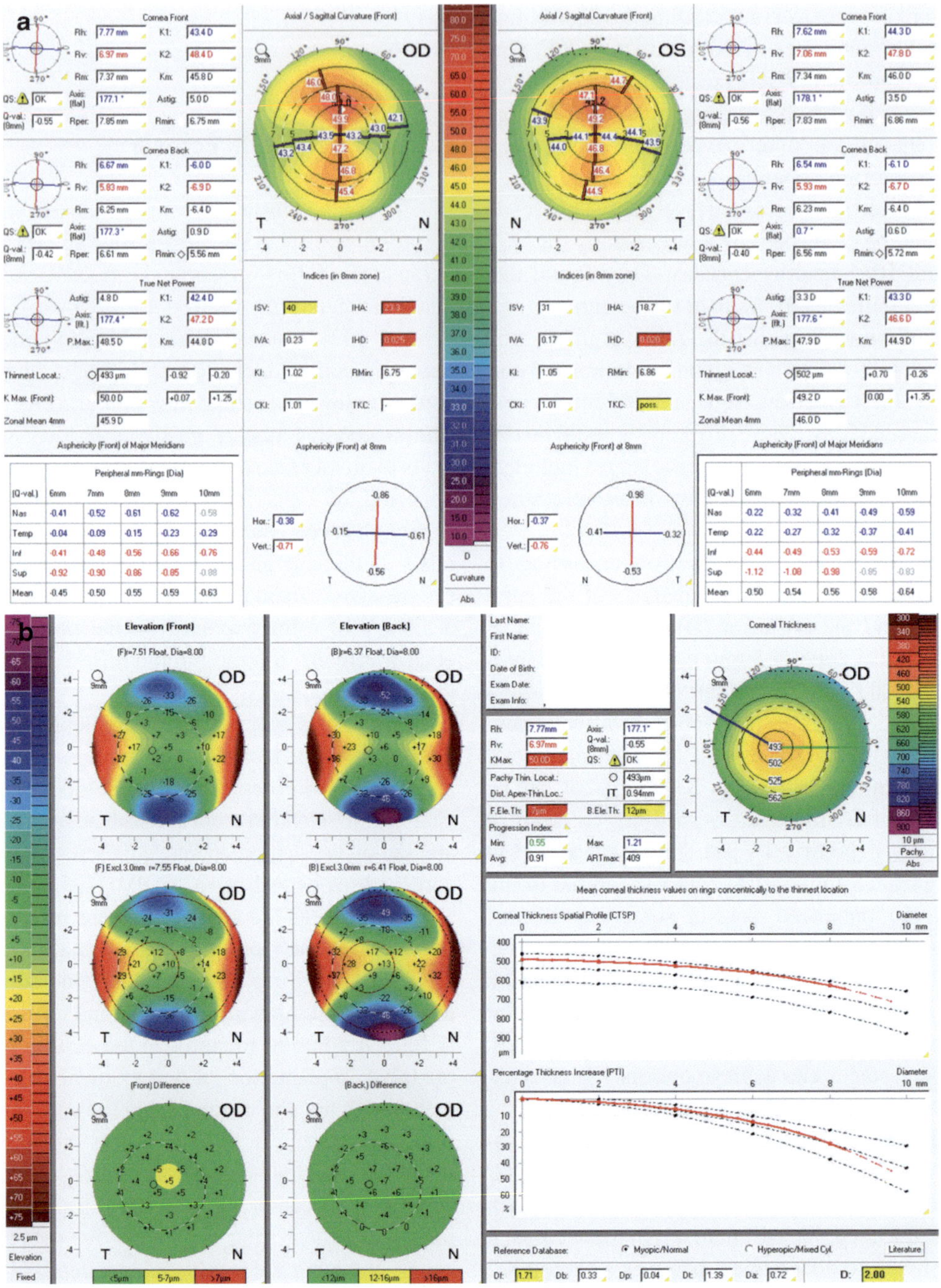

Fig. 7.4 (**a**) Topometric analysis (Pentacam HR®, OCULUS, Wetzlar, Germany) revealing regular astigmatism more in the right than in the left eye. Red, abnormal results for the keratoconus indices IHA (index of height asymmetry) and IHD (index of height decentration). (**b**) The right eye, Belin/Ambrósio enhanced ectasia screening display (Pentacam HR®, OCULUS, Wetzlar, Germany) with innocuous finding considering posterior elevation at the thinnest point (7 μm, based on a best-fit sphere from 8.0-mm optical zone), but a final Belin/Ambrósio enhanced ectasia screening display deviation "*D*" = 2.00. (**c**) The left eye, Belin/Ambrósio enhanced ectasia screening display (Pentacam HR®, OCULUS, Wetzlar, Germany) with innocuous finding considering posterior elevation at the thinnest point (6 μm, based on a best-fit sphere from 8.0-mm optical zone) and a final Belin/Ambrósio enhanced ectasia screening display deviation "*D*" = 1.49

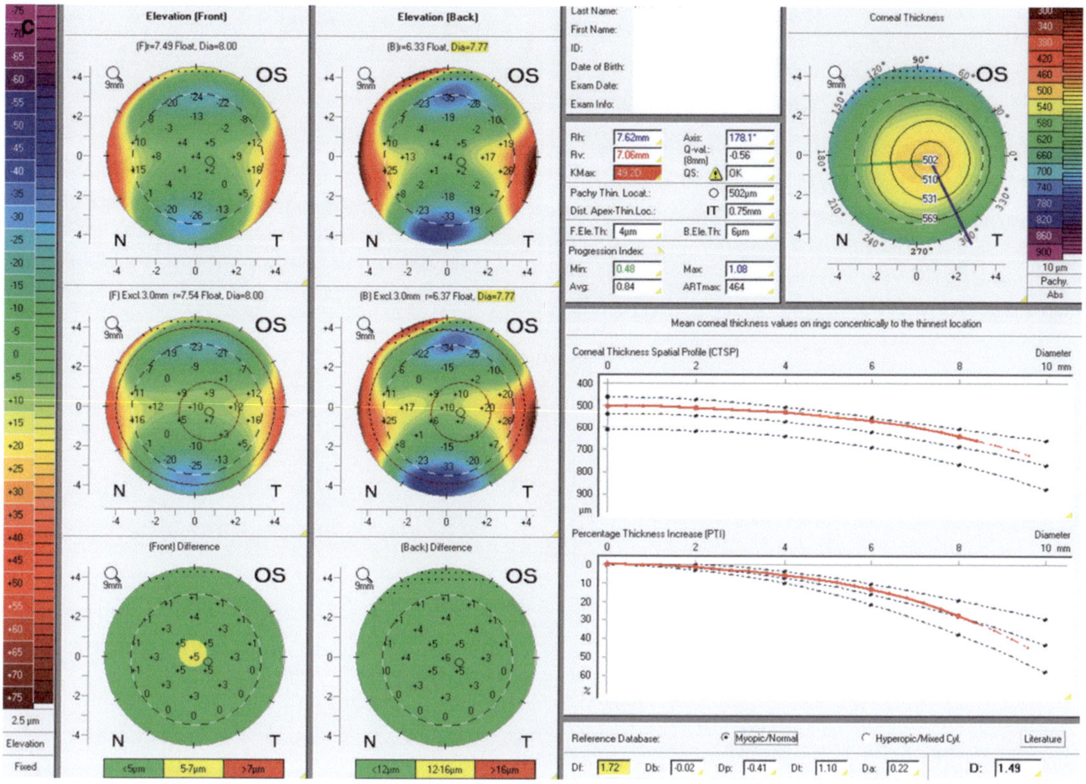

Fig. 7.4 (continued)

force of intraocular pressure has been hypothesized to be contributor to the posterior surface elevation in early KC stages [37]. A similar anterior stromal weakening occurs after LASIK because of the stromal ablation. Very early in its development, there could therefore be a beneficial effect of lowering intraocular pressure, which then would have a favorable effect on the further development [38].

Finally, penetrating keratoplasty or deep anterior lamellar keratoplasty (DALK) remains the ultimate salvation for surgical rehabilitation of very advanced post-LASIK ectasias.

Brief Case A 29-year-old male patient underwent LASIK at the age of 25 in Egypt and presented with impaired spectacle-corrected visual acuity (20/40 in his right and 20/30 in his left eye) because of post-LASIK ectasia. Further follow-up examinations revealed progression of the ectasia in the right eye, and, therefore, subsequent corneal cross-linking was performed, and the patient was thereafter recommended to wear rigid contact lenses or scleral lenses (Fig. 7.5).

7.2.6 Superior Keratoconus and Superior Pellucid Marginal Degeneration (PMD)

The majority of KC corneas are characterized by a temporally inferior apex localization. However, reports of KC cases with a superior apex localization exist. Unilateral superior corneal steepening without other clinical signs of KC was reported in 2 children aged 12 and 15 years [39]. In a 32-year-old patient, a corneal hydrops located superiorly was observed together with a superior steepening and incomplete Fleischer ring in his partner eye [40]. In another 57-year-old patient, there was a superior corneal protrusion in both corneas with an incomplete Fleischer ring in one eye [41]. Also among our patients was a 45-year-old female with clinically manifested KC in the left eye and supe-

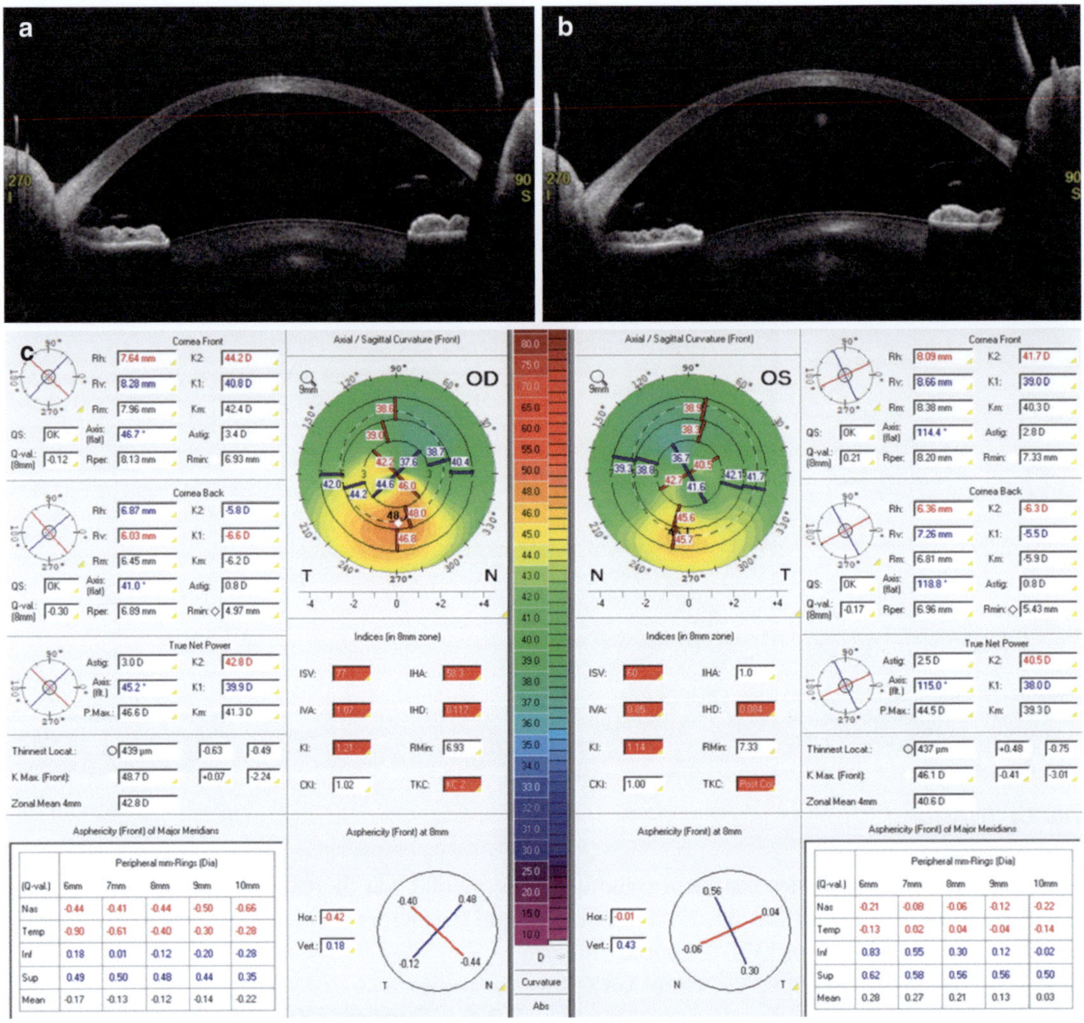

Fig. 7.5 (**a**) Anterior segment optical coherence tomography (Casia 2®, Tomey, Nagoya, Japan) of the right eye. (**b**) Anterior segment optical coherence tomography (Casia 2®, Tomey, Nagoya, Japan) of the left eye. (**c**) Topometric analysis (Pentacam HR®, OCULUS, Wetzlar, Germany) revealing inferior steepening more in the right than in the left eye after laser-assisted in situ keratomileusis (LASIK)

rior nasal steepening in both eyes with abnormal values in the Belin/Ambrósio enhanced ectasia screening display (Fig. 7.6). These forms have to be distinguished from mechanically induced superior KC configuration as reported in a 62-year-old patient with a superior corneal steepening, which resolved during a period of 3 months after surgical treatment of blepharoptosis [42]. All the case reports mentioned above have in common that the diagnosis of superior KC was based solely on topographic corneal diagnostics. However, the various stages that have been described ranging from superior steepening without clinical signs to superior corneal hydrops could lead to the hypothesis that superior KC might exist as a very rare variant of KC.

A superior localization of pellucid marginal degeneration has been reported in analogy to superior KC. While the authors reported that the inferior part of the cornea was normal, the superior hemisphere was characterized by (a) a crescent-shaped area superiorly, (b) a vertical meridian of least power, and (c) a superior loop cylinder [43].

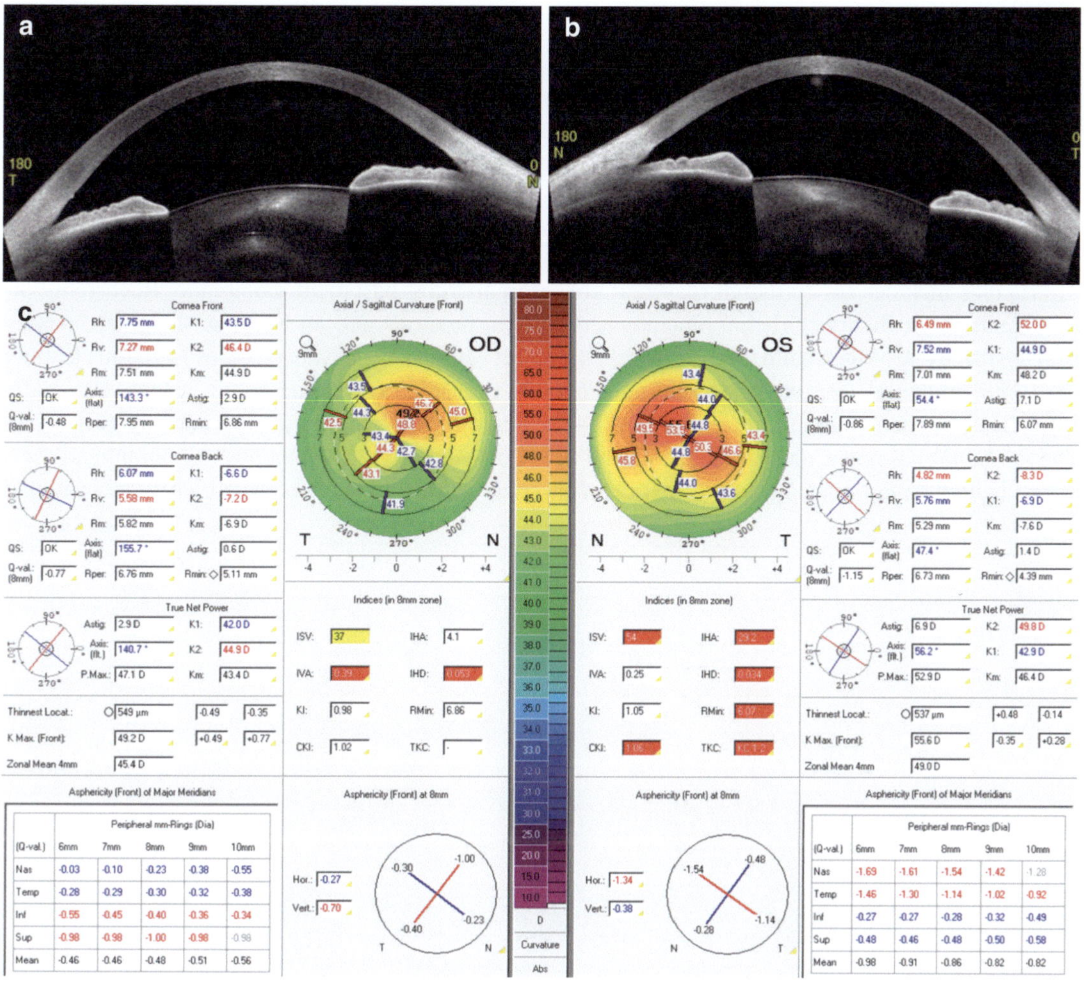

Fig. 7.6 (**a**) Anterior segment optical coherence tomography (Casia 2®, Tomey, Nagoya, Japan) of the right eye. (**b**) Anterior segment optical coherence tomography (Casia 2®, Tomey, Nagoya, Japan) of the left eye. (**c**) Topometric analysis (Pentacam HR®, OCULUS, Wetzlar, Germany) revealing superior nasal steepening in the right and in the left eye. Red, abnormal results for the keratoconus indices IVA (index of vertical asymmetry), IHD (index of height decentration), ISV (index of surface variance), IHA (index of height asymmetry), R_{min} (minimum axial/sagittal curvature), CKI (central keratoconus index), and TKC (topographic keratoconus classification)

Besides these superior ectasias, Fuchs-Terrien marginal corneal degeneration and peripheral ulcerative keratopathy must be considered in the differential diagnosis of superior corneal thinning and protrusion.

Brief Case A 42-year-old female patient presented with a best spectacle-corrected distance visual acuity of 20/40 in her right eye and 20/50 in her left eye and suspicion of KC (Fig. 7.6). Corneal tomography revealed a nasal superior steepening more in her left than in her right eye. There was epithelial hemosiderin deposition (Fleischer ring) in her left eye. These findings led to the diagnosis of atypical superior KC, and the patient was recommended to wear contact lenses.

7.3 Corneal Diseases with Pseudokeratoconic Tomography

7.3.1 Epithelial Basement Membrane Dystrophy (EBMD)

The group of epithelial and subepithelial corneal dystrophies includes (a) epithelial recurrent erosion dystrophies, (b) subepithelial mucinous corneal dystrophy, (c) Meesmann corneal dystrophy, (d) Lisch epithelial corneal dystrophy, and (e) epithelial basement membrane dystrophy [44]. The epithelial basement membrane dystrophy is also called map-dot-fingerprint dystrophy because of its characteristic epithelial patterns. These consist of maps formed by irregular islands, irregular intraepithelial opacities (dots), and parallel curvilinear lines in a fingerprint pattern. The majority of cases have no documented inheritance, and therefore, they are considered to be of degenerative or traumatic origin [44]. The dystrophy is histopathologically characterized by an aberrant basement membrane. Recurrent corneal erosions and an irregular astigmatism may develop in very advanced cases [45], thus leading to conspicuous topographic values especially among the topographic KC indices (Fig. 7.7). Consequently, conspicuous topographical corneal values must be expected when an epithelial

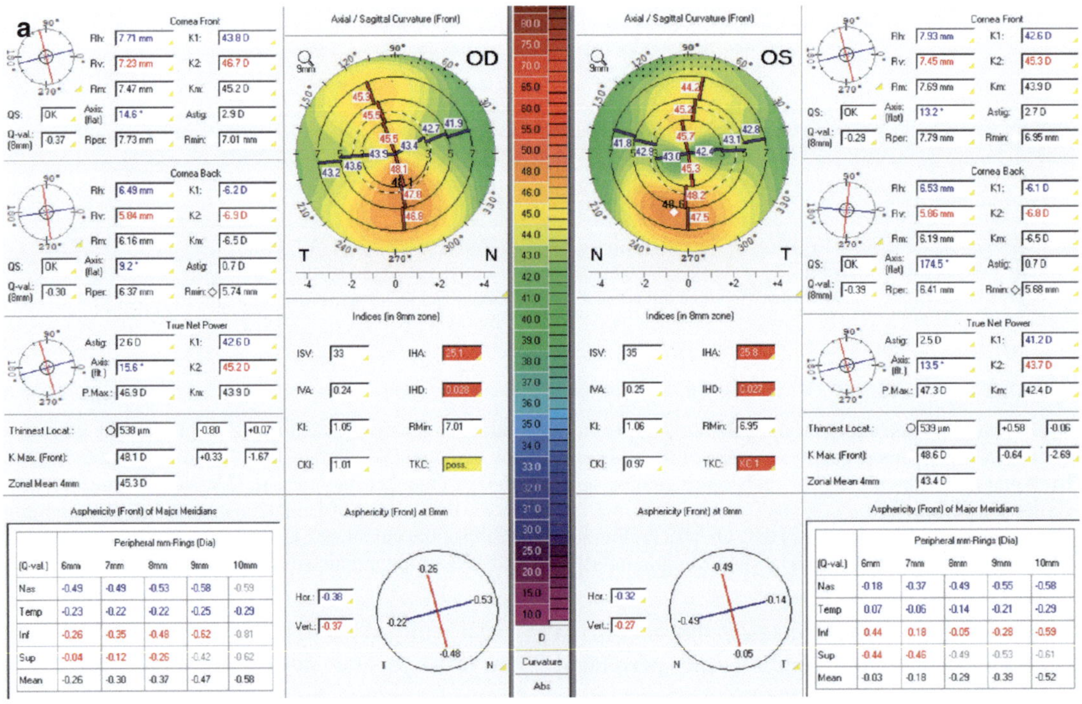

Fig. 7.7 (**a**) Topometric analysis (Pentacam HR®, OCULUS, Wetzlar, Germany) of epithelial basement dystrophy revealing slight inferior nasal steepening in the right and in the left eye. Red, abnormal results for the keratoconus indices IHA (index of height asymmetry), IHD (index of height decentration), and TKC (topographic keratoconus classification). (**b**) Maps and fingerprints, slit-lamp photograph of the left eye. (**c**) Maps and fingerprints, slit-lamp photograph of the left eye, magnification

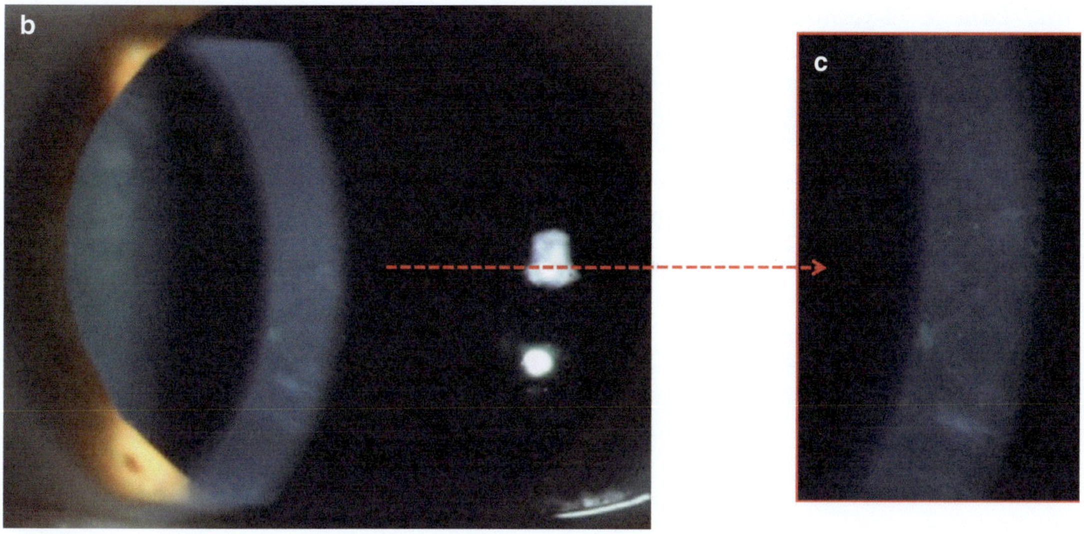

Fig. 7.7 (continued)

basement membrane dystrophy is present. It can be differentiated from KC by the examination and analysis of posterior corneal curvature as enabled by the Belin/Ambrósio enhanced ectasia screening display and corneal biomechanics. The treatment of choice is minimal invasive subepithelial phototherapeutic keratectomy (PTK) using an excimer laser with a low pulse energy and a low number of pulses [46]. This treatment achieves an increase in hemidesmosome density which increases the adherence of the corneal epithelium to its basement membrane, thus putting an end to recurrent corneal erosions [47].

Brief Case A 61-year-old female patient presented with a best spectacle-corrected distance visual acuity of 20/30 in her right eye and 20/50 in her left eye and suspicion of a corneal dystrophy. Epithelial basement membrane dystrophy was diagnosed (Fig. 7.7), and phototherapeutic keratectomy was planned. The patient was recommended contact lenses for optimal postoperative visual rehabilitation.

7.3.2 Scar-Associated Irregular Astigmatism

Corneal scarring may occur after infections, trauma, or corneal surgery and represents the leading cause of visual impairment worldwide besides cataract. Visual impairment results from blocked and scattered light and scar-induced irregular astigmatism [48]. During prolonged corneal wound healing, keratocytes differentiate to myofibroblasts, which in turn proliferate, migrate, and induce extracellular matrix synthesis, thus resulting in contraction of the wound site and scar formation [49].

One corneal disease that typically results in stromal corneal scarring and thinning with an induced irregular astigmatism is stromal herpetic keratitis [50]. Stromal herpetic keratitis may occur in two subtypes: These are (a) the interstitial keratitis with intrastromal inflammation as a complement-mediated response to virus antigen, and (b) the ulcerating necrotizing stromal keratitis which is often associated with deep stromal scar formation [51]. Stromal corneal scars do lead to visual impairment not only by loss of corneal transparency but also by inducing irregular astigmatism similar to KC. Scar-induced astigmatism limits the chances of visual rehabilitation when the scarring is located in the center of the cornea. Additionally, it must be taken into account, especially considering herpetic keratitis, that contact lens-induced complications may occur in the context of postherpetic neurotrophic keratopathy. Scleral contact lenses that allow the formation of a tear film layer between the cornea and the contact lens can be used in these cases [52].

Brief Case A 75-year-old female patient presented with a deep avascular stromal corneal scar in her right eye and a best spectacle-corrected distance visual acuity of 20/200 (Fig. 7.8). After treatment of the scar with topical and systemic acyclovir and steroids, cataract surgery led to a visual recovery up to 20/25 allowing postponement of penetrating keratoplasty.

7.3.3 Central Fuchs Endothelial Corneal Dystrophy

Fuchs endothelial corneal dystrophy (FECD) is one of the most common indications for corneal transplantation worldwide [53, 54]. It is characterized by (a) an abnormal extracellular matrix deposition with guttae formation, (b) Descemet's

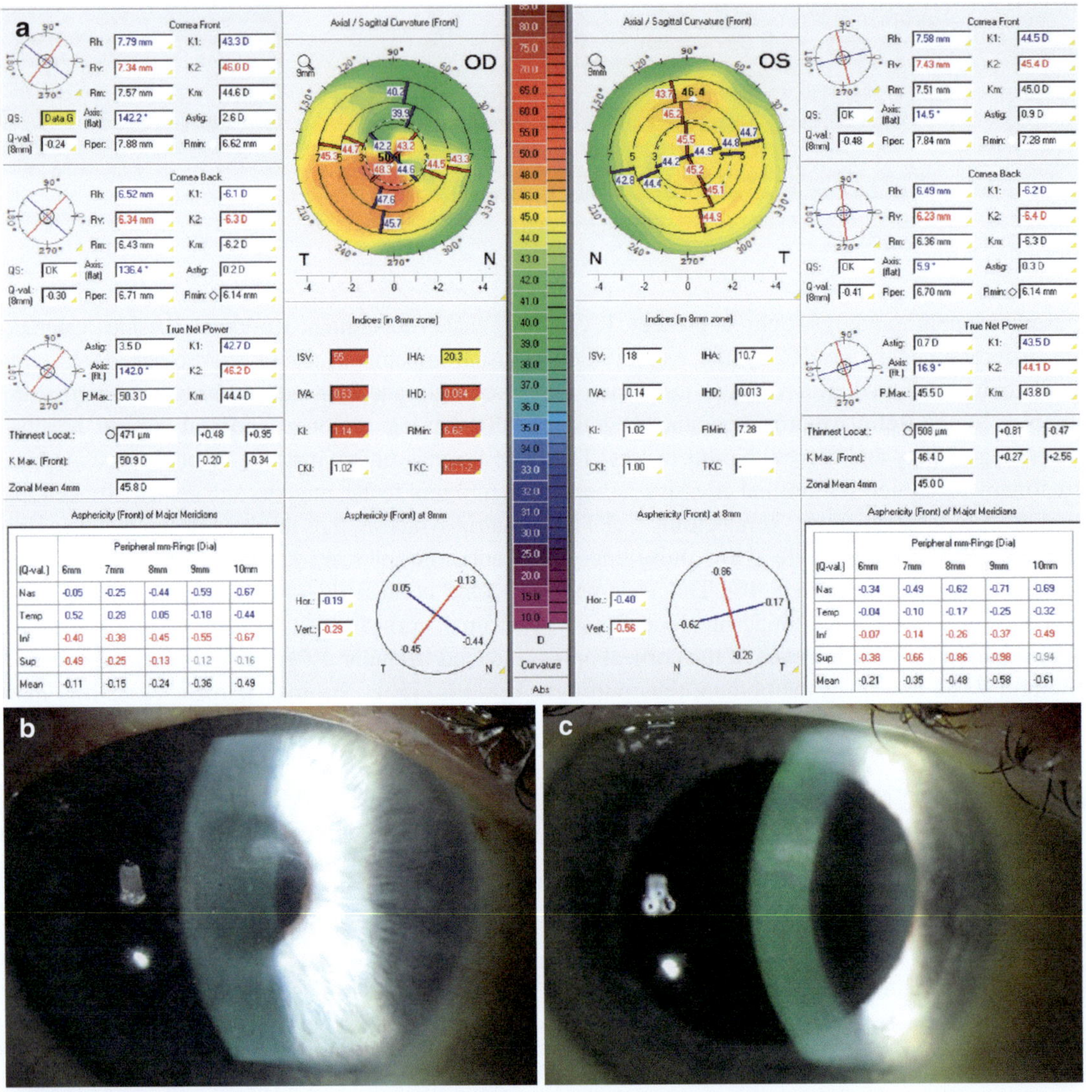

Fig. 7.8 (**a**) Topometric analysis (Pentacam HR®, OCULUS, Wetzlar, Germany). The right eye, temporal inferior steepening with abnormal keratoconus indices in red: ISV (index of surface variance), IVA (index of vertical asymmetry), IHD (index of height decentration), KI (keratoconus index), R_{min} (minimum axial/sagittal curvature), and TKC (topographic keratoconus classification). The left eye with innocuous findings. (**b**) Slit-lamp photographs of the right eye revealing avascular stromal scarring after stromal herpetic keratitis. (**c**) Slit-lamp photographs of the right eye revealing avascular stromal scarring after stromal herpetic keratitis

membrane thickening, and (c) corneal endothelial dysfunction [44] with consecutive stromal and epithelial corneal edema leading to visual impairment. Topical therapy in the form of hyperosmolar eye drops can be prescribed in early stages. In advanced stages, therapy is surgical by conducting posterior lamellar keratoplasty or penetrating keratoplasty in case of stromal scarring [55]. FECD can be classified into stages according to the modified Krachmer scale, but the disadvantage of this classification is that all corneas with edema are classified as stage 6. A recent study proposed a staging based on anterior segment optical coherence tomography designating 0 as normal corneas, 1 as corneas with guttae, 2 as corneas with stromal edema, and 3 as corneas with epithelial and stromal edema [56]. Early FECD stages are tomographically characterized by an inversion of the positive posterior corneal elevation values to a negative bulging toward the anterior chamber [57]. In advanced stages with stromal edema (stage 2) and combined edema of the corneal stroma and epithelium (stage 3), however, a link exists to the differential diagnosis of KC. At the same location of posterior depression, these stages may go along with a focal elevation of the anterior corneal surface leading to irregular astigmatism and inferior steepening, thus simulating KC in tomographic examinations [57]. Even if FECD may be clearly diagnosed clinically and prima vista at the slit lamp in these cases, it has to be distinguished whether there is an additional presence of KC in the same cornea [58]. In this case, the surgical therapy should rather consist of penetrating keratoplasty than posterior lamellar keratoplasty. The diagnosis can be made based on the patients' medical history, earlier tomographic examinations, and posterior elevation analysis as described above within the Belin/Ambrósio enhanced ectasia screening display.

Brief Case A 42-year-old male patient presented with a best spectacle-corrected distance visual acuity of 20/50 in his right eye and 20/60 in his left eye and suspicion of KC (Fig. 7.9). He was

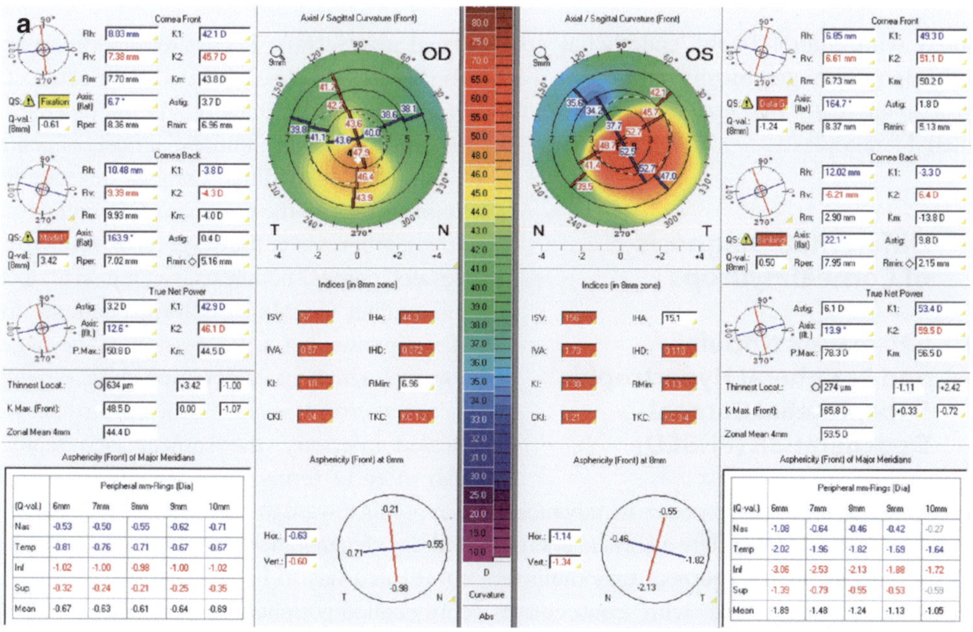

Fig. 7.9 (**a**) Topometric analysis (Pentacam HR®, OCULUS, Wetzlar, Germany). Temporal inferior steepening more in the left than in the right eye with typical keratoconus configuration. Abnormal keratoconus indices in red: ISV (index of surface variance), IHA (index of height asymmetry), IVA (index of vertical asymmetry), IHD (index of height decentration), KI (keratoconus index), R_{min} (minimum axial/sagittal curvature), CKI (central keratoconus index), and TKC (topographic keratoconus classification). (**b**) Central stromal edema in the right eye, anterior segment optical coherence tomography (Casia 2®, Tomey, Nagoya, Japan). (**c**) Central stromal edema and epithelial bulla in the left eye, anterior segment optical coherence tomography (Casia 2®, Tomey, Nagoya, Japan). (**d**) Central stromal edema in the right eye, slit-lamp photograph. (**e**) Central stromal edema and epithelial bulla in the left eye, slit-lamp photograph

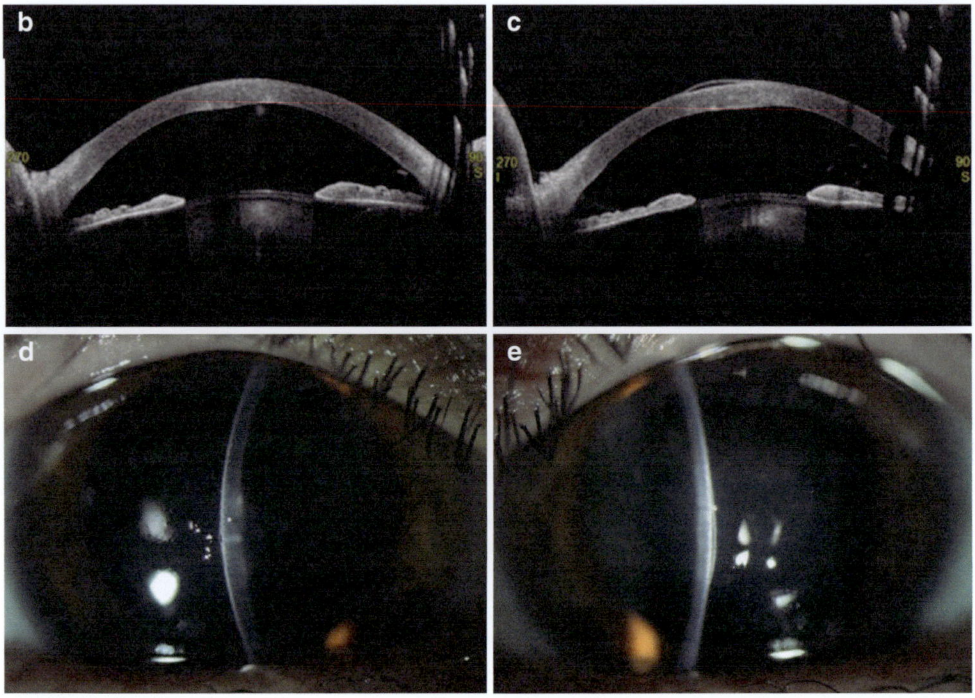

Fig. 7.9 (continued)

diagnosed with central Fuchs endothelial corneal dystrophy tomographically mimicking KC and treated surgically by Descemet's membrane endothelial keratoplasty.

7.4 Differential Diagnosis of Corneal Hydrops

7.4.1 Salzmann's Nodular and Peripheral Hypertrophic Subepithelial Corneal Degeneration (PHSCD)

Acute corneal hydrops may occur in advanced KC cases and is characterized by a corneal edema caused by a break in (the corneal endothelium and) Descemet's membrane with consecutive entering of aqueous in the corneal stroma [59]. The hydrops is typically self-limiting, and the corneal edema may resolve during a period of 2–6 months leaving a stromal scar that impairs visual acuity [60]. There are superficial corneal diseases that can be confused with acute corneal hydrops at least clinically and therefore must be included in the differential diagnosis of acute KC.

Salzmann's nodular corneal degeneration is characterized by the presence of noninflammatory, slowly progressive, bluish-gray, or yellowish-gray elevated corneal nodules varying in size, location, and number [61]. In early forms, patients are free of symptoms, but a progression of the degeneration may result in a decreased surface regularity, recurrent erosions, and visual impairment [62]. If located inferiorly, the corneal topography may also in early forms show an inferior steepening that points toward the presence of KC. Salzmann's nodular degeneration may extend to the central cornea and has to be distinguished from another entity called peripheral hypertrophic subepithelial corneal degeneration (PHSCD), which in turn spares the center of the cornea [61]. It occurs mainly in the nasal superior quadrant of the cornea and consists of peripheral boomerang [61] or sausage roll-shaped elevated subepithelial opacification zones with abnormal limbal vessels and a varying extent of pseudopterygia [63]. While there was a thinning of the epithelium and breaks in Bowman's layer in the histologic examination of Salzmann's nodular degeneration, there was an absence of Bowman's layer in peripheral hypertrophic subepithelial corneal degeneration [61].

Brief Case A 44-year-old female patient presented with a best spectacle-corrected distance visual acuity of 20/30 in her right eye and hand-moving perception in her left eye and suspicion of acute corneal hydrops (Fig. 7.10). There was no diagnosis of KC in her medical history. Anterior segment optical coherence tomography (Casia 2®, Tomey, Nagoya, Japan) revealed a large solid and

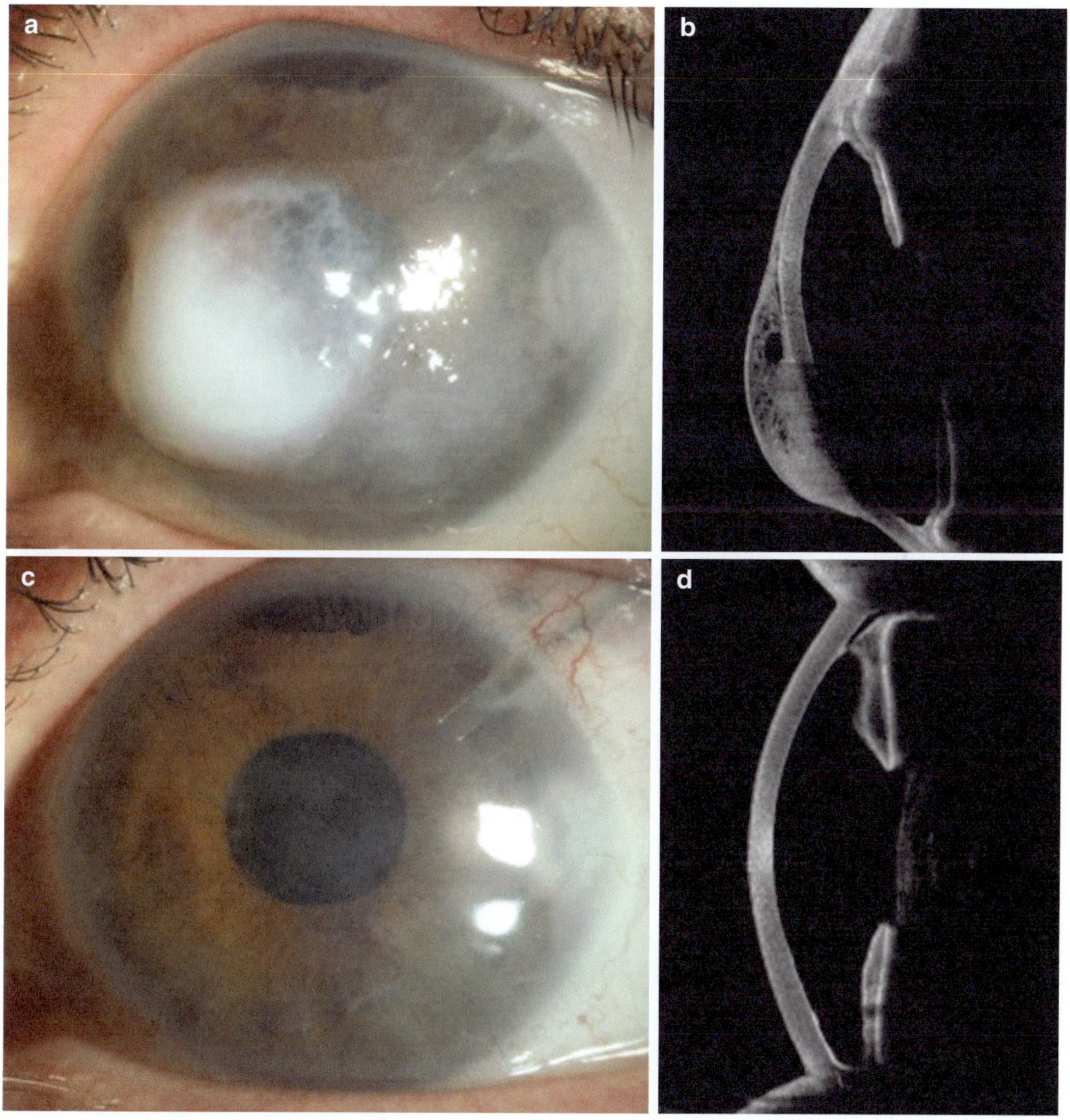

Fig. 7.10 (**a**) Left eye with a whitish prominent opacification referred with suspicion of acute corneal hydrops, slit-lamp photograph. (**b**) Anatomically intact cornea below the whitish mass with solid and cystic parts as revealed by anterior segment optical coherence tomography (Casia 2®, Tomey, Nagoya, Japan). (**c**) The left eye after manual removal of a giant Salzmann's nodular degeneration, slit-lamp photograph. (**d**) Anatomically intact, yet thickened cornea postoperatively, anterior segment optical coherence tomography (Casia 2®, Tomey, Nagoya, Japan)

partially cystoid mass with an anatomically intact cornea below. Assuming a giant Salzmann's nodular degeneration, this mass was removed manually respecting Bowman's layer without subsequent phototherapeutic keratectomy, and histopathological analysis confirmed this diagnosis. Because of underlying glaucoma, this led only to a minor improvement of her visual acuity (20/200).

Thus, the rare variant of a giant Salzmann's nodular degeneration must be included in the differential diagnosis of acute KC and differentiated from the entity of peripheral hypertrophic subepithelial corneal degeneration.

References

1. Schlaeppi V. La dystrophie marginale inférieure pellucide de la cornée [The marginal inferior pelvic cortex dystrophy]. Bibl Ophthalmol. 1957;12(47):672–7.
2. Moshirfar M, Edmonds JN, Behunin NL, Christiansen SM. Current options in the management of pellucid marginal degeneration. J Refract Surg. 2014;30(7):474–85.
3. Jinabhai A, Radhakrishnan H, O'Donnell C. Pellucid corneal marginal degeneration: a review. Cont Lens Anterior Eye. 2011;34(2):56–63.
4. Belin MW, Asota IM, Ambrosio R Jr, Khachikian SS. What's in a name: keratoconus, pellucid marginal degeneration, and related thinning disorders. Am J Ophthalmol. 2011;152(2):157–162.e1.
5. Belin MW. Keratoconus and ectatic disease: evolving criteria for diagnosis. Klin Monatsbl Augenheilkd. 2020;237(6):740–4.
6. Martínez-Abad A, Piñero DP. Pellucid marginal degeneration: detection, discrimination from other corneal ectatic disorders and progression. Cont Lens Anterior Eye. 2019;42(4):341–9.
7. Rüfer F, Schröder A, Erb C. White-to-white corneal diameter: normal values in healthy humans obtained with the Orbscan II topography system. Cornea. 2005;24(3):259–61.
8. Hashemi H, Khabazkhoob M, Emamian MH, Shariati M, Yekta A, Fotouhi A. White-to-white corneal diameter distribution in an adult population. J Curr Ophthalmol. 2015;27(1–2):21–4.
9. Lee BW, Jurkunas UV, Harissi-Dagher M, Poothullil AM, Tobaigy FM, Azar DT. Ectatic disorders associated with a claw-shaped pattern on corneal topography. Am J Ophthalmol. 2007;144(1):154–6.
10. Lenk J, Haustein M, Terai N, Spoerl E, Raiskup F. Characterization of ocular biomechanics in pellucid marginal degeneration. Cornea. 2016;35(4):506–9.
11. Sedaghat MR, Momeni-Moghaddam H, Belin MW, Zarei-Ghanavati S, Akbarzadeh R, Sabzi F, Yekta AA, Sadeghi AJ. Changes in the ABCD keratoconus grade after intracorneal ring segment implantation. Cornea. 2018;37(11):1431–7.
12. Mamoosa B, Razmjoo H, Peyman A, Ashtari A, Ghafouri I, Moghaddam AG. Short-term result of collagen crosslinking in pellucid marginal degeneration. Adv Biomed Res. 2016;5:194.
13. Ertan A, Bahadir M. Intrastromal ring segment insertion using a femtosecond laser to correct pellucid marginal corneal degeneration. J Cataract Refract Surg. 2006;32(10):1710–6.
14. Alfaro Rangel R, Szentmáry N, Lepper S, Daas L, Langenbucher A, Seitz B. 8.5/8.6-mm excimer laser-assisted penetrating keratoplasties in a tertiary corneal subspecialty referral center: indications and outcomes in 107 eyes. Cornea. 2020;39(7):806–11.
15. Wallang BS, Das S. Keratoglobus. Eye (Lond). 2013;27(9):1004–12.
16. Jacobs DS, Green WR, Maumenee AE. Acquired keratoglobus. Am J Ophthalmol. 1974;77(3):393–9.
17. Cameron JA. Keratoglobus. Cornea. 1993;12(2):124–30.
18. Baillif S, Garweg JG, Grange JD, Burillon C, Kodjikian L. Kératoglobe: revue de la littérature [Keratoglobus: review of the literature]. J Fr Ophtalmol. 2005;28(10):1145–9.
19. Kaufman HE, Werblin TP. Epikeratophakia for the treatment of keratoconus. Am J Ophthalmol. 1982;93(3):342–7.
20. Vargas V, Alió J. Posterior keratoconus-clinical aspects and anterior segment optical coherence tomography findings: a case report. Eur J Ophthalmol. 2019;29(1):NP1–5.
21. Süveges I. Histopathologie des Keratoconus posticus circumscriptus [The histopathology of keratoconus posticus circumscriptus]. Klin Monatsbl Augenheilkd. 1986;189(4):323–5.
22. Vajpayee RB, Sharma N. Association between anterior and posterior keratoconus. Aust N Z J Ophthalmol. 1998;26(2):181–3.
23. Silas MR, Hilkert SM, Reidy JJ, Farooq AV. Posterior keratoconus. Br J Ophthalmol. 2018;102(7):863–7.
24. Streeten BW, Karpik AG, Spitzer KH. Posterior keratoconus associated with systemic abnormalities. Arch Ophthalmol. 1983;101(4):616–22.
25. Goebels S, Eppig T, Wagenpfeil S, Cayless A, Seitz B, Langenbucher A. Staging of keratoconus indices regarding tomography, topography, and biomechanical measurements. Am J Ophthalmol. 2015;159(4):733–8.
26. Tanabe T, Tomidokoro A, Samejima T, Miyata K, Sato M, Kaji Y, Oshika T. Corneal regular and irregular astigmatism assessed by Fourier analysis of videokeratography data in normal and pathologic eyes. Ophthalmology. 2004;111(4):752–7.
27. Kamiya K, Shimizu K, Igarashi A, Miyake T. Assessment of anterior, posterior, and total central

corneal astigmatism in eyes with keratoconus. Am J Ophthalmol. 2015;160(5):851–857.e1.
28. Naderan M, Rajabi MT, Zarrinbakhsh P. Distribution of anterior and posterior corneal astigmatism in eyes with keratoconus. Am J Ophthalmol. 2016;167:79–87.
29. Belin MW, Duncan J, Ambrósio R Jr, Gomes JA. A new tomographic method of staging/classifying keratoconus: the ABCD grading system. Int J Kerat Ect Cor Dis. 2015;4(3):55–63.
30. Belin MW, Duncan JK. Keratoconus: the ABCD grading system. Klin Monatsbl Augenheilkd. 2016;233(6):701–7.
31. Flockerzi E, Xanthopoulou K, Goebels SC, Zemova E, Razafimino S, Hamon L, Jullien T, Klühspies U, Eppig T, Langenbucher A, Seitz B. Keratoconus staging by decades: a baseline ABCD classification of 1000 patients in the Homburg Keratoconus Center. Br J Ophthalmol. 2021;105(8):1069–75.
32. Seiler T, Koufala K, Richter G. Iatrogenic keratectasia after laser in situ keratomileusis. J Refract Surg. 1998;14(3):312–7.
33. Zhao W, Shen Y, Jian W, Shang J, Jhanji V, Aruma A, Zhou X. Comparison of corneal biomechanical properties between post-LASIK ectasia and primary keratoconus. J Ophthalmol. 2020;2020:5291485.
34. Alvani A, Hashemi H, Pakravan M, Mahbod M, Seyedian MA, Amanzadeh K, Khabazkhoob M, Jafarzadehpur E, Fotouhi A. Post-LASIK ectasia versus keratoconus: an in vivo confocal microscopy study. Cornea. 2020;39(8):1006–12.
35. Randleman JB. Post-laser in-situ keratomileusis ectasia: current understanding and future directions. Curr Opin Ophthalmol. 2006;17(4):406–12.
36. Binder PS, Lindstrom RL, Stulting RD, Donnenfeld E, Wu H, McDonnell P, Rabinowitz Y. Keratoconus and corneal ectasia after LASIK. J Cataract Refract Surg. 2005;31(11):2035–8.
37. De Stefano VS, Ford MR, Seven I, Dupps WJ Jr. Depth-dependent corneal biomechanical properties in normal and keratoconic subjects by optical coherence elastography. Transl Vis Sci Technol. 2020;9(7):4.
38. Hiatt JA, Wachler BS, Grant C. Reversal of laser in situ keratomileusis-induced ectasia with intraocular pressure reduction. J Cataract Refract Surg. 2005;31(8):1652–5.
39. Weed KH, McGhee CN, MacEwen CJ. Atypical unilateral superior keratoconus in young males. Cont Lens Anterior Eye. 2005;28(4):177–9.
40. Tananuvat N, Leeungurasatien P, Wiriyaluppa C. Superior keratoconus with hydrops. Int Ophthalmol. 2009;29(5):419–21.
41. Prisant O, Legeais JM, Renard G. Superior keratoconus. Cornea. 1997;16(6):693–4.
42. Kim T, Khosla-Gupta B, Debacker C. Blepharoptosis-induced superior keratoconus. Am J Ophthalmol. 2000;130(2):232–4.
43. Sridhar MS, Mahesh S, Bansal AK, Rao GN. Superior pellucid marginal corneal degeneration. Eye (Lond). 2004;18(4):393–9.
44. Weiss JS, Møller HU, Aldave AJ, Seitz B, Bredrup C, Kivelä T, Munier FL, Rapuano CJ, Nischal KK, Kim EK, Sutphin J, Busin M, Labbé A, Kenyon KR, Kinoshita S, Lisch W. IC3D classification of corneal dystrophies--edition 2. Cornea. 2015;34(2):117–59.
45. Sayegh RR, Kouyoumjian PB, Vedula GG, Nottage JM, Nirankari VS. Cocaine-assisted epithelial debridement for the treatment of anterior basement membrane dystrophy. Cornea. 2013;32(6):889–92.
46. Pogorelov P, Langenbucher A, Kruse F, Seitz B. Long-term results of phototherapeutic keratectomy for corneal map-dot-fingerprint dystrophy (Cogan-Guerry). Cornea. 2006;25(7):774–7.
47. Szentmáry N, Seitz B, Langenbucher A, Schlötzer-Schrehardt U, Hofmann-Rummelt C, Naumann GO. Histologic and ultrastructural changes in corneas with granular and macular dystrophy after excimer laser phototherapeutic keratectomy. Cornea. 2006;25(3):257–63.
48. Menda SA, Das M, Panigrahi A, Prajna NV, Acharya NR, Lietman TM, McLeod SD, Keenan JD. Association of postfungal keratitis corneal scar features with visual acuity. JAMA Ophthalmol. 2020;138(2):113–8.
49. Chawla S, Ghosh S. Establishment of in vitro model of corneal scar pathophysiology. J Cell Physiol. 2018;233(5):3817–30.
50. Kaye S, Choudhary A. Herpes simplex keratitis. Prog Retin Eye Res. 2006;25(4):355–80.
51. Seitz B, Heiligenhaus A. Das Chamäleon der Keratitis herpetischer Genese - Diagnose und Therapie [The chameleon of herpetic keratitis—diagnosis and therapy]. Klin Monatsbl Augenheilkd. 2015;232(6):745–53.
52. Hassan OM, Farooq AV, Soin K, Djalilian AR, Hou JH. Management of corneal scarring secondary to herpes zoster keratitis. Cornea. 2017;36(8):1018–23.
53. Matthaei M, Sandhaeger H, Hermel M, Adler W, Jun AS, Cursiefen C, Heindl LM. Changing indications in penetrating keratoplasty: a systematic review of 34 years of global reporting. Transplantation. 2017;101(6):1387–99.
54. Flockerzi E, Maier P, Böhringer D, Reinshagen H, Kruse F, Cursiefen C, Reinhard T, Geerling G, Torun N, Seitz B, all German Keratoplasty Registry Contributors. Trends in corneal transplantation from 2001 to 2016 in Germany: a report of the DOG-section cornea and its keratoplasty registry. Am J Ophthalmol. 2018;188:91–8.
55. Seitz B, Daas L, Flockerzi E, Suffo S. "Descemet membrane endothelial keratoplasty" DMEK – Spender und Empfänger Schritt für Schritt [Descemet membrane endothelial keratoplasty DMEK—donor and recipient step by step]. Ophthalmologe. 2020;117(8):811–28.
56. Yasukura Y, Oie Y, Kawasaki R, Maeda N, Jhanji V, Nishida K. New severity grading system for fuchs endothelial corneal dystrophy using anterior segment optical coherence tomography. Acta Ophthalmol. 2021;99(6):e914–21.

57. Sun SY, Wacker K, Baratz KH, Patel SV. Determining subclinical edema in fuchs endothelial corneal dystrophy: revised classification using scheimpflug tomography for preoperative assessment. Ophthalmology. 2019;126(2):195–204.
58. Cremona FA, Ghosheh FR, Rapuano CJ, Eagle RC Jr, Hammersmith KM, Laibson PR, Ayres BD, Cohen EJ. Keratoconus associated with other corneal dystrophies. Cornea. 2009;28(2):127–35.
59. Fan Gaskin JC, Patel DV, McGhee CN. Acute corneal hydrops in keratoconus—new perspectives. Am J Ophthalmol. 2014;157(5):921–8.
60. Yahia Chérif H, Gueudry J, Afriat M, Delcampe A, Attal P, Gross H, Muraine M. Efficacy and safety of pre-Descemet's membrane sutures for the management of acute corneal hydrops in keratoconus. Br J Ophthalmol. 2015;99(6):773–7.
61. Järventausta PJ, Tervo TM, Kivelä T, Holopainen JM. Peripheral hypertrophic subepithelial corneal degeneration—clinical and histopathological features. Acta Ophthalmol. 2014;92(8):774–82.
62. Das S, Link B, Seitz B. Salzmann's nodular degeneration of the cornea: a review and case series. Cornea. 2005;24(7):772–7.
63. Gore DM, Iovieno A, Connell BJ, Alexander R, Meligonis G, Dart JK. Peripheral hypertrophic subepithelial corneal degeneration: nomenclature, phenotypes, and long-term outcomes. Ophthalmology. 2013;120(5):892–8.

8 Keratoconus in Children

Vineet Joshi and Simmy Chaudhary

8.1 Introduction

Keratoconus (KC) in children or pediatric keratoconus is the manifestation of the disease in children or adolescents <18 years of age. It needs to be discussed separately as the disease tends to be aggressive in nature and progression to advanced stages can happen in early years affecting quality of vision and quality of life. Early diagnosis and intervention are key to maintaining good vision and quality of life in children.

8.2 Epidemiology

Keratoconus is not only more aggressive in pediatric age group but also more severe at the time of diagnosis [1]. The younger the child at the time of diagnosis, the more is the risk of rapid progression [2, 3]. This warrants the need of early diagnosis to prevent severe visual damage. Though literature commonly documents puberty as the age at which keratoconus starts, youngest patient of 4 years of age with Down syndrome has been reported by Sabti et al. [4]. The average age of diagnosis is 15 years [5] with male predominance. Greatest incidence has been noted in Middle-Eastern population and India with incidence of 1/2000 cases a year [6]. The Arabs, Indians, and Polynesians are 4.4 times more likely to get affected by KC. This is likely due to higher rate of consanguinity in their population, especially among Muslim community [7]. Greatest severity and incidence of pediatric KC has been reported from Riyadh (prevalence 1.1%) and Saudi Arabia (prevalence 4.4%) [8]. Pearson et al. [9] reported that compared with White patients, Asians have a fourfold increase in incidence, are younger at presentation, and require corneal grafting at an earlier age. KC in children is known to be bilateral but asymmetrical. In unilateral cases, 50% of the uninvolved fellow eye developed the disease within 16 years [10]. Studies used videokeratography in the Middle East and Asia and estimated a prevalence of 0.9–3.3% [11–17]. Children with male predisposition, associated allergies, habitual eye rubbing, and strong family history of keratoconus were more frequently affected with keratoconus [18].

Earlier, KC was documented as a noninflammatory process [6]. However, recent studies have shown increased levels of inflammatory markers like IL-1, IL-6, IL-8, and TNF-α in the tears of patients of keratoconus [19, 20]. There is increased activity of cyclooxygenase activity with ten times increase in PGE2 production, inhibiting fibroblasts from synthesis of collagen, and proliferation and differentiation of myofibroblasts. Also, inhibitors of cysteine proteases were found to be low in the tears of these patients. It

V. Joshi (✉) · S. Chaudhary
Cornea and Anterior Segment Service, The Cornea Institute, L V Prasad Eye Institute, Hyderabad, Telangana, India
e-mail: vineet@lvpei.org; simmy.chaudhary@lvpei.org

S. Das (ed.), *Keratoconus*, https://doi.org/10.1007/978-981-19-4262-4_8

was the imbalance between activation and inhibition of these cytokines that lead to activation of metalloproteinases and apoptosis of keratocytes [20, 21].

In our experience, we analyzed first visit records of 3316 patients diagnosed with keratoconus based on clinical signs and topography at a tertiary eye center in India, out of which 17.2% were children less than or equal to 16 years. Male-to-female ratio was higher (1.9) compared to individuals more than 16 years of age (1.54). Incidence of allergy and eye rubbing was highest in less than 16 years age group (27.8%) compared to 16–30 years (25%) and more than 30 years age group (17.2%) of patients.

8.3 Genetics

Most of the cases of keratoconus is sporadic, but Kaya et al. has reported incidence of 11% in first-degree relatives of patients with keratoconus [22]. The role of genetics in the disease pathogenesis has been well reflected by ethnic variations [9, 23–25]. Autosomal dominance with incomplete penetrance and autosomal recessive inheritance has also been documented by various studies. Several genetic loci and variants within these genes have been identified to occur in patients with KC. Multiple genome-based studies have been reviewed which mentions at least 19 genes which are associated with development of KC. Of these, LOX at 5q23.2 encoding LOX, lysyl oxidase needs special mention and is implicated in the cross-linking process of elastin and collagen [26]. Authors have also reported association of IL-1 processing and collagen fibril assembly with development of KC [26]. IL1β is implicated in corneal collagen degradation, conversion of plasminogen to plasmin, metalloproteinase 1–3 (MMP-1 and MMP-3), and activation and degradation of collagen in corneal fibroblasts. This further supports an inflammatory etiology for development of KC. Other two loci, Forkhead box protein O1 (FOXO1), and fibronectin type 3 domain containing 3B (FNDC3B) have also been known to increase the risk for KC development [27]. Zinc finger 469 (ZNF469) involved in brittle cornea syndrome type 1, functionally, is known to play a role in the synthesis and/or organization of corneal collagen fibers in conjunction with *PRMD5* [28]. ZNDC3B alleles have been involved in 12.5% European population with KC [29]. Other studies reported contrary results [30]. Thus, the role of ZNDC3B in pathogenesis of KC is controversial. It has been well documented to occur in association with other conditions like Down syndrome, vernal keratoconjunctivitis, Leber congenital amaurosis (LCA), retinitis pigmentosa, Marfan syndrome, and Ehlers-Danlos syndrome.

8.4 Ocular Allergy

Recent studies reported an incidence of 0.61% in children with vernal keratoconjunctivitis [31]. Allergic keratoconjunctivitis and eye rubbing also contribute in increased incidence of corneal hydrops in children with KC [5]. Pediatric patients of KC with VKC undergo more severe and rapid change in corneal topography when compared to children with KC alone suggesting the role of allergic eye condition and eye rubbing with KC progression in children [32]. Eye rubbing and poking have also been postulated to be a cause of KC in children with LCA. Franceschetti's oculodigital sign seen in these children acts as a constant source of corneal trauma and predisposes them to development of KC. Incidence of KC in children with LCA has been reported to be 30% [33]. Habitual eye rubbing has also been blamed to be the cause of KC in children with Down syndrome, with incidence reaching to up to 15% in these patients [34, 35]. When considering atopy, majority of authors have not found significant association of development of KC with atopy, but with eye rubbing [36, 37]. Also, HLA antigen association, particularly HLA-A26, B40, and DR9, has also been found in children with keratoconus as compared to adults [38]. These markers strongly support the genetic association and occurrence of keratoconus in pediatric age group [38]. The effect of androgen in early development and rapid progression of keratoconus has also been described supporting male preponderance in pediatric age group [5].

8.5 Syndromes

Connective tissue disorders with abnormal collagen elasticity like Ehlers-Danlos syndrome and osteogenesis imperfecta and many others show association with KC (Table 8.1). Beckh et al. described three generations of a family with osteogenesis imperfecta to have associated with KC [39]. Various authors have reported the presence of mitral valve prolapse in patients diagnosed with severe KC [40, 41]. Various loci on chromosomes 2, 3, 5, 6, 9, 13, 15, 16, 17, and 20 have been reported to have association with KC [42, 43].

Table 8.1 Keratoconus and syndromic associations

Abnormal collagen elasticity and connective tissue	
Brittle cornea syndrome	Nail patella syndrome
Congenital hip dysplasia	Osteogenesis imperfecta
Joint hypermobility	Ehlers-Danlos syndrome
False chordae tendineae of the left ventricle	Marfan syndrome
Mitral valve prolapse	Pseudoxanthoma elasticum
Oculodigital stimulation with abnormal retinal function	
Albinism	Congenital rubella
Bardet-Biedl syndrome	Leber congenital amaurosis
Neurofibromatosis	Retinitis pigmentosa
Laurence-Moon-Bardet-Biedl syndrome	Cone dystrophy
Tapetoretinal degeneration	Kurz syndrome
Oculodigital stimulation with low mental function	
Apert syndrome	Crouzon syndrome
Angelman syndrome	Hyperornithinemia
Noonan syndrome	
Syndromes associated with eczema and atopy	
Down syndrome	Hyper-IgE syndrome
Ichthyosis	Oculodentodigital syndrome
Turner syndrome	Autographism
Mulvihill-Smith syndrome	

8.6 Risk Factors

In patients with abnormal retinal function, oculodigital stimulation has been reported to be the attributable cause toward development of KC (Table 8.2). This repeated stimulation acts as a source of damage to the corneal epithelium. Expression of lysyl oxidase (LOX) plays a major role in the biogenesis of corneal connective tissue. Its altered activity weakens covalent bonds between collagen and elastin fibrils, causing biomechanical deterioration of the cornea. Abnormal structures were detected within the keratoconic cone, which were reported to be the result of folding or break in the anterior stromal lamellae and eventually led to compromised biomechanical strength of the cornea [44]. On histology, loss of corneal stromal thickness has been reported along with distortion of the cornea due to marked reduction in amount and distribution of collagen fibrils [45]. Takahashi et al. studied quantitative analysis of collagen fibrils and concluded that though these fibrils appeared normal morphologically, the epithelial basement membrane showed fragmentation, Bowman's membrane showed disintegration and fibrillation, and basal epithelial cells showed degenerative changes on electron microscopy [46]. DM ruptures are also seen, and the endothelium, though normal, may have pleomorphism, intracellular dark structures, and elongation of cells in few cases [47].

Gender predilection has been unclear. However, few studies from India concluded male predominance in northern and western part of the country and female prevalence in Central India

Table 8.2 Risk factors in pediatric keratoconus

• Lower thinnest corneal thickness
• Higher average central corneal keratometry
• Increased posterior elevation
• Frequent eye rubbing
• Allergic eye disorders

[11, 48, 49]. The higher prevalence of KC among Indian population has also been attributed to geographical factors like hot weather and sunshine [50]. Also, KC in Indian population tends to present at a younger age, progress rapidly, and are associated with higher need of surgery which can be contributed to rapid progression [48, 50].

Literature also describes factors which reduce the risk of KC. These include smoking and diabetic hyperglycemia [51, 52]. Both of these conditions may increase corneal collagen cross-linking and thus protect the cornea from ectatic changes.

8.7 Clinical Features and Diagnosis

Pediatric KC usually presents as a chronic bilateral progressive corneal ectasia with asymmetric pattern [1]. The clinical features of the disease in children are like that in adults. It is characterized by central or inferior paracentral corneal thinning, loss of biomechanical strength, steepening of the cornea, and irregular corneal astigmatism [53]. Externally, the cone can be visualized as distortion of the lower lid in inferior gaze (Munson's sign) and sharp conical reflection of light on the nasal cornea when light is shone from temporal side (Rizzuti's sign) [54].

On slit lamp, one can identify advanced keratoconus, the margins of the cone with a cobalt blue filter, and the presence of Vogt striae and Fleischer's ring [54, 55]. On retinoscopy, the scissors reflex is a characteristic sign demonstrated due to the irregular astigmatism. Retro illumination can also delineate the size and location of the cone, many times seen as an oil droplet sign (Charleux sign) [54, 55]. There can be associated signs of allergic disease, papillae, giant cobblestone papillae, VKC, conjunctival pigment deposition, Horner-Trantas spots, etc.

Diagnosis can be confirmed by photokeratoscopy or video keratoscopy, showing compression of inferior and central mires, increase in surface corneal keratometry, inferior superior asymmetry, and skewing of steepest radial axes above and below the horizontal meridian [53]. Children with central cones and higher irregular astigmatism leading to blurring of vision tend to present early [56]. They can also present with advanced disease with acute hydrops, which leads to corneal scarring [1, 57]. The cornea tends to flatten after scarring; however, due to the predominant irregular astigmatism, the quality of vision may remain poor despite of the contact lens use. Keratoplasty is the treatment of choice in such cases [58, 59]. It is equally important to differentiate other forms of corneal ectasia or similar clinical features presenting in this age group, for example, keratoglobus which is usually congenital (Table 8.3) [60–65].

According to the Intelligent Sight registry AAO, the prevalence of KC in pediatric population worldwide is 0.16% [66]. The guidelines of AAO Practice Patterns for Pediatric Eye Evaluations and the Corneal Ectasia suggest screening of children for diagnosing keratoconus early [66, 67]. These include children with allergic eye diseases, children with high myopia or myopic astigmatism, children with Down syndrome, children with family history of keratoconus, or children from regions exposed to high UV exposure. A retinoscopy, corneal tomographer, aberrometer, and anterior segment OCT are useful tools that can be used for screening in school children.

In our experience of 3316 patients diagnosed with keratoconus, children in the age group of less than 16 years had an advanced presentation with steeper mean keratometry (50.2 D), thinnest pachymetry (450 μm), and pachymetry at apex (461 μm) compared to other age groups. About 77% of children had asymmetric pattern of presentation at the first visit. The inter-eye asymmetry showed a difference of one to two stages of keratoconus (Amsler-Krumeich classification) at the time of presentation. Overall progression rate of keratoconus in children less than 16 years of age was higher (38.6%) compared to others 16–30 years (22.4%).

Table 8.3 Differential diagnosis for keratoconus and other corneal ectasias

Keratoconus (KC)	Keratoglobus (KG)	Brittle cornea syndrome (BCS)	Terrien's marginal degeneration (TMD)	Pellucid marginal corneal degeneration (PMCD)
Asymmetric bilateral	Symmetric bilateral	Symmetric bilateral	Asymmetric bilateral	Bilateral may be symmetric or asymmetric
Acquired forms—may be associated with congenital and hereditary disorders like Down syndrome	Congenital and acquired forms Acquired forms can represent as a severe manifestation of keratoconus or PMCD	Congenital	Acquired	Acquired Can present along with KC 10% and along with KG 13%. Associated with high astigmatism
First half of second decade, puberty, no gender predilection	Since birth, no gender predilection	Since birth, no gender predilection	Third to fourth decade, no gender predilection	Second to fifth decade, no gender predilection
Inferior paracentral or central corneal stromal thinning	Diffuse corneal involvement	Diffuse corneal involvement with typical blue sclerae and high myopia. Has keratoglobus like corneal picture	Superior stromal thinning with intact epithelium along with pannus and a leading edge of lipid deposition	Crescent-shaped band of inferior corneal thinning approaching 20% of normal thickness that is 1–2 mm in height, 6–8 mm in horizontal extent, and 1–2 mm from the limbus
Isolated or sporadic, multiple genes mapped. For example, LOX at 5q23.2, FOXO1, ZNDC3B	Autosomal recessive	Autosomal recessive. ZNF469 (BCS type 1), PRDM5 gene (BCS type 2)	Isolated	Isolated
Progressive	Nonprogressive	Nonprogressive; associated connective tissue disorders involve musculoskeletal (joint hypermobility), deafness, and cardiovascular manifestations	Usually nonprogressive. The thinning tends to be steeper in the center and slopes toward the periphery	Slowly progressive Unlike KC, area of steepening above the area of ectasia and no Fleischer's ring or Vogt striae
Steepening of the cone, corneal thinning, and irregular astigmatism	Diffuse corneal thinning leading to spontaneous corneal rupture or scarring with trivial trauma	Diffuse corneal thinning leading to spontaneous corneal rupture or scarring with trivial trauma. Scleral rupture and high myopia are also associated	Leads to astigmatism but can be associated with thinning and perforation in rare cases	Progresses slowly leading to irregular astigmatism and corneal protrusion causes vision loss in working age group and is difficult to manage because of the location of ectasia

(continued)

Table 8.3 (continued)

Keratoconus (KC)	Keratoglobus (KG)	Brittle cornea syndrome (BCS)	Terrien's marginal degeneration (TMD)	Pellucid marginal corneal degeneration (PMCD)
Spectacles, contact lenses, collagen cross-linking, keratoplasty (PK, DALK)	Protective glasses or tuck-in/ epi-keratoplasty	Protective glasses	Topical steroids or immunomodulatory treatment, spectacles and contact lenses for astigmatism, patch grafting, or keratoplasty to manage perforations	Treatment is difficult depending on the degree of protrusion. Special contact lenses—toric hydrophilic, hybrid, or RGP
		Epi-keratoplasty		CXL can be done to prevent progression. Needs to be decentered over the inferior band. Large graft (9 mm), keratoplasty, C-shaped lamellar grafts, and crescentric or wedge-shaped resection are some options

8.8 Adult vs. Pediatric Keratoconus

Keratoconus in children tends to present earlier, usually in the later part of first decade of life; is more advanced at presentation; has a higher chance of progression, higher incidence of eye rubbing, allergy, and VKC; and is associated with various syndromes when compared to adults (Table 8.4). Although keratoconus presents asymmetrically, the incidence of asymmetry is higher in children [1, 68]. This can lead to early deprivation of vision and amblyopia. Ocular aberrations generated by the irregular cornea may be partially compensated by internal ocular structures and the high accommodative power resulting in parents reporting their children later to the clinic [58]. The cohort of keratoconus in the age group 18–35 years and in adult populations tends toward natural stabilization in third to fourth decade unlike children <18 years age group where the progression can be aggressive. Pediatric keratoconus also has a high incidence of acute hydrops during the follow-up or even at the first visit to the clinic and may need descemetopexy. Higher rates of corneal collagen remodeling were observed in pediatric corneas due to the weak ectatic lamellae which may exceed the capacity of the cross-linking process leading to more rapid ectasia progression and a sevenfold higher risk of needing corneal transplantation [69–71].

Table 8.4 Challenges in pediatric kheratoconus

• Late diagnosis
• Faster progression
• Allergic eye disorders and eye rubbing
• Accurate diagnosis (tomography)
• Follow-ups
• Poor outcomes of conservative approach
• Need of early surgical intervention

When it comes to management, the protocols of treatment remain the same in adults and children. However, Vinciguerra et al. in their study in collagen cross-linking identified that children had faster healing process and recovery in central corneal thickness. Adults did tend to have better morphological and functional outcomes than children, and the keratometry continued to improve beyond 4 years [72, 73]. Chatzis and Hafezi have reported progression at 36 month follow-up in children after cross-linking, which was not seen in adults, and this could be attributed to the natural cross-linking occurring in corneal stroma in adults [3]. Also in keratoplasty outcomes, pediatric grafts are known to have higher graft failure rates and poor visual outcomes compared to adults [74, 75].

8.9 Treatment

Pediatric KC tends to be advanced and progressive in nature; however, in earlier stages of the disease, spectacles can be prescribed as early as possible to avoid development of amblyopia (if age is <10 years). Due to progression in the irregular astigmatism over time, spectacles fail to deliver the best results, and rigid gas-permeable contact lenses or scleral contact lenses can be tried for visual improvement. However, eye rubbing should be strictly avoided. Eye rubbing, with knuckles, fingertips, sleeping in prone position and side position, dry eyes, screen time, and male sex have been found to be important risk factors in a multivariate analysis study done by Moran et al. and Gatinel et al. [76, 77] VKC and ocular allergy also need to be adequately controlled. Antihistamines (e.g., olopatadine, levocabastine), mast cell stabilizers (e.g., cromolyn sodium, nedocromil), dual-acting agents (e.g., alcaftadine, bepotastine, azelastine, ketotifen), topical immunomodulators (tacrolimus, cyclosporine 0.1% in the USA), and low-dose tapering steroids (loteprednol etabonate, rimexolone, prednisolone) should be given to children, to decrease the severity of allergy and itching [78]. Many physicians prefer to offer early cross-linking as an option in pediatric keratoconus, but ocular allergy should be controlled adequately before planning any surgical intervention or giving a contact lens trial.

8.10 Contact Lens

Various options available for patients with KC include conventional rigid gas-permeable lenses (RGP), piggyback lenses, Rose K lenses, and mini-scleral and scleral lenses. In pediatric KC as the disease tends to be aggressive, one might not be able to achieve correct fit over a long period of time. It is also shown that although it takes additional 15–20 min of sitting time in clinic to train and orient children toward contact lens usage, the complication rate in adults and children associated with CL usage remains the same [79]. Still in the initial stage of disease, soft toric contact lenses (Toric K SiHy) can help improve quality of vision. In the later stages of disease, RGP lenses are preferred [80]. The type of RGP lens to be prescribed depends upon the severity of KC. Mild-to-moderate KC patient can be fitted with monocurve GPs, while more advanced KC does well with bicurve GP lens [81]. In children, RGPs with high oxygen permeability are preferred and need to be replaced frequently.

8.11 Surgical Procedures

8.11.1 Collagen Cross-linking

Collagen cross-linking (CXL) was first described by Wollensak et al. as a technique to arrest the progression of keratoconus in children in 2003. The procedure strengthens collagen fibrils and imparts biomechanical strength by the formation of covalent bonds due to the action of reactive oxygen species like singlet oxygen and superoxide anions released after activation of photosensitive riboflavin with exposure to ultraviolet-A light (UVA) 370 nm. Resultant process leads to photopolymerization of collagen fibrils by increasing bonds between collagen and proteoglycans [82, 83]. Keratoconus tends to progress faster in children, and thus CXL is an important modality in arresting this process. If diagnosed earlier, CXL can halt the disease process in children, save a few lines of best corrected vision, and can also decrease the need of keratoplasty.

8.11.1.1 Indications and Timing of the Procedure in Children vs. Adolescent

Although the strategy in planning CXL in adults/adolescents is to follow up every 6–12 months and wait until progression is documented clinically, when it comes to children, it is better to suspect and diagnose keratoconus earlier, follow up sooner, and better plan CXL earlier as suggested by groups of Chatzis and Hafezi wherein the benefits significantly outweigh the risks. In certain scenarios like severe disease in the other eye, family history of keratoconus, other associated systemic associations like Down syndrome, and family history of keratoplasty, CXL can be considered earlier. The exclusion criteria for CXL in children are similar to adults, thinnest pachymetry of less than 400 μm, corneal opacities, corneal infections, severe dry eyes, severe vernal keratoconjunctivitis, concomitant autoimmune disease, history of previous ocular surgery, and endothelial cell count of less than 1000 cells/mm^2 [3, 6, 56, 73, 84–88].

8.11.2 CXL Standard Dresden Protocol

The standard Dresden protocol described by Wollensak et al. was FDA recognized in 2011. The protocol is still widely used in adults as well as children. This involves epithelial debridement up to 9 mm and application of riboflavin one drop 0.1% solution every 2 min for a total of 30 min, followed by ultraviolet-A light (370 ± 5-nm wavelength, 5.4 J/cm^2 irradiance) exposure with instillation of the riboflavin solution every 2 min for an additional 30-min drop of riboflavin 0.1% solution administered every 2 min for a total of 30 min, followed by ultraviolet-A light (370 ± 5-nm wavelength, 5.4 J/cm^2 irradiance) exposure with instillation of the riboflavin solution every 2 min for an additional 30-min period [82, 83]. This protocol is time tested and has been proven to be safe and efficacious in halting the disease process over several long-term follow-up studies in children. But children are usually uncooperative, and the intraoperative ocular movements occurring in the 1-h-long procedure might affect the radiance and efficacy. Epithelial debridement under topical anesthesia can be cumbersome in children and can lead to postoperative pain; as a result, some novel protocols of delivering the energy and novel techniques of applying riboflavin with no touch technique were explored for better results in children.

8.11.3 Transepithelial CXL (TE CXL)

Epi-On CXL or transepithelial CXL involves administering riboflavin along with 15% dextran supplemented with trometamol + EDTA (Ricrolin TE, Sooft, Montegiorgio, Italy). This enables passage of a heavy riboflavin molecule through the corneal intact epithelium to reach till the stroma, which in normal circumstances acts as a barrier for riboflavin due to its lipophilic nature. The time for riboflavin application and irradiance is similar to the standard protocol [89, 90].

8.11.4 Accelerated Cross-linking Protocol

Accelerated cross-linking protocol involves delivering, a higher irradiance, to reduce exposure time (i.e., 9 mW/cm^2 for 10 min or 30 mW/cm^2 for 4 min instead of 3 mW/cm^2 for 30 min) [56].

8.11.5 Other Methods

CXL has also been tried in other nonstandard methods with the help of cross-hatched grid pattern for epithelial debridement, contact lens-assisted cross-linking, and application of BAK (benzalkonium chloride) and benzoate to improve riboflavin penetration and iontophoresis [91]. There is less literature to prove the efficacy of these methods.

8.11.6 Safety

Overall, CXL has shown to be a safe procedure with long-term follow-up in adults with no significant major complications [92, 93]. In children, not many long-term follow-up studies have been seen. Longest follow-up in one study up to 7.5 years has been observed [85].

8.11.6.1 Epithelial Defect

The epithelium usually heals within 48 h after CXL. A bandage contact lens in place usually aids this. With delayed epithelialization up to 10 days, glare and corneal edema was seen in a few studies [3, 89]. Persistent corneal haze has been reported in two case series in 3.5% patients [56] and in 14.2% patients [94]. More importantly, it is the longer duration of de-epithelialization during the standard protocol procedure that leads to pain and difficult cooperation in children. This can also increase the risk of ulceration, infection, sterile infiltrates, and activation of herpes keratitis [88, 94].

8.11.6.2 Endothelial Cell Loss

The current pachymetry cut-off values of 400 μm primarily prevent endothelial cell damage due to exposure to UVA. Although a few case reports have been noted in adults, there are no significant complications pertaining to endothelial cell loss and corneal decompensation in children; however, more long-term follow-up studies are needed to conclude on this observation [56, 73, 87, 90, 94].

8.11.6.3 Limbal Cell Loss

Recently, few studies have highlighted the aspect of UV-related damage to the limbal stem cells after CXL [95]. De-epithelialization and UV treatment occurs over the central cornea, but being a topical procedure, there is some amount of exposure of riboflavin and UV to the limbal cells. Also, it has shown that de-epithelialized surface ensures better riboflavin concentration even in the peripheral cornea and the limbus which can increase UV exposure. CXL leads to induction of pro-apoptotic genes, inducing oxidative damage to DNA and inhibiting growth of cultured human epithelial stem cells, and cells derived from cadaver eyes have been shown in studies [96–98]. A case of conjunctival intraepithelial neoplasia has been reported [99]. Considering the pediatric age group, these studies do raise a concern of a long-term ocular surface-related complications post-CXL; however, still in majority, the re-epithelialized surface shows normal characteristics, and no long-term ocular surface or limbal stem cell deficiency has been reported so far.

8.11.6.4 Efficacy of Standard Protocol

Multiple studies have proven the efficacy of the standard epi-off protocol in halting the progression of the disease within 12–36 months in children [100]. There have been some instances of failure of CXL with documented progression, and the reported rate has been 5%, 23%, and 88% in some of the reported studies at different follow-up periods [3, 101, 102]. Chatzis and Hafezi reported progression in the disease despite of cross-linking, while Kumar Kodavoor et al. reported the same in three eyes [3, 94]. All of these patients had frequent eye rubbing and documented allergic symptoms or VKC. Henriquez et al. reported CXL failure and progression in 6 out of 26 eyes and highlighted an importance of preoperative high *K* readings more than 54 D as a possible risk factor [102]. In adults, CXL has also shown to improve the flat and steep keratometry, posterior elevation, BCVA, UCVA, and aberrometry over a long period of time. However, in children, the results are variable across multiple studies with different follow-up periods after CXL [3, 72, 87]. Along with stabilization of the disease, BCVA was shown to improve in most of the studies. In the Siena protocol, Caporossi et al. followed 77 and 152 patients (10–18 years) for a period of 36 and 48 months, respectively, in 2 separate studies and highlighted visual improvement in 80% of patients and 90% stabilization achieved in 4 years [92]. Zotta et al.'s long-term results of 20 eyes of (14.34 ± 2.14 years) followed for a period of 89 months noted that *K*1, *K*2, and the topographic cylinder remained stable at 7.5 years [84]. Soeters et al. also reported more corneal flattening and visual improvement in children [56]; however, Vinciguerra reported better visual and functional outcomes of CXL in the age group of 18–39 years [72, 73]. On the other hand, Chatzis and Hafezi observed improvement in keratometry only up to 24 months, with regression to preoperative values by 36 months follow-up suggesting a decrease in efficacy of CXL over a period of time in children <10 years of age [3]. In adults, stabilization of the disease is seen to be long-lasting due to an additive factor contributed by the natural cross-linking occurring in the stromal fibers with increasing age.

8.11.6.5 Efficacy of Transepithelial CXL (EPI-ON) and Accelerated Protocol

Transepithelial CXL did show an advantage in decreasing the postoperative pain, corneal edema in children, and in initial studies by Magli et al. and Salman et al., they found to have no significant difference with the standard protocol with respect to the disease stabilization [86, 89]. However, the sample size of these studies was small, and the follow-up period was shorter. Most of the subsequent studies in children and adults showed progression of keratoconus with the Epi-On technique with a transient improvement in keratometry values. Buzzonetti et al. performed a prospective analysis of TE CXL for pediatric keratoconus (8–18 years age) in 13 eyes of 13 patients and demonstrated that *K* readings and HOA aberrations significantly worsened during follow-up [90]. Confocal microscopy demonstrated a demarcation line at depth of only 105 μm in contrast to the demarcation line typically seen at 300 μm in standard CXL treatment. They concluded that TE CXL appears to be safe but does not effectively halt keratoconus progression as compared with standard CXL. Irregular concentration of riboflavin in the stroma, restricted entry for oxygen due to the intact epithelium, and some amount of riboflavin absorbed by the epithelium could be the causes of its decreased efficacy [103].

Accelerated cross-linking protocol did show an overall improvement in visual acuity and flattening of *K* readings in both children and adults; however, in the long-term follow-up in children at 36 months, increase in K_{max} and posterior elevation values was noted [104]. It was found that the demarcation line post-CXL, which helps us to gauge the depth of treatment in the cornea, was in the range of 100–240 μm compared to 300–350 μm in the standard protocol. This also highlights an area of need for further research to find out the optimal time and irradiance for such accelerated protocols [105].

8.11.7 Intracorneal Ring Segments

Intracorneal ring segments (ICRS) are short PMMA arc/ring segments which when implanted in the peripheral cornea exert an arc-flattening effect and alter the geometry of the cornea leading to central flattening. This effect is inversely proportional to the thickness and size of the ICRS, which means the shorter and thicker segment, implanted in the peripheral cornea, exerts a more flattening effect. There are various normograms to calculate the size and length of ICRS based on the keratometry and refraction: [106]

- Contact lens intolerance.
- Corrected distance visual acuity < 0.6 on the decimal scale.
- Corneal pachymetry > 400 μm in the site of the corneal tunnel (depending on the thickness of ICRS to be implanted).
- Absence of central corneal scarring.
- Alignment of refractive axis and the flattest keratometric meridian *K*1 of the cornea should be such to form an angle between 0° and 15° and is considered properly aligned.

Option of ICRS in children is usually avoided due to a very advanced presentation of the disease, eye rubbing due to allergy, and noncompliance. In patients with VKC, there is a high risk of implant extrusion. Option of ICRS can be considered as a lesser invasive alternative than keratoplasty in children. Very few studies have shown efficacy of intracorneal ring segments in children [107]. A case series in children studied the efficacy of intracorneal ring segments along with CXL and did show regularization of surface and improved visual outcomes [108].

8.11.8 Keratoplasty

Advanced keratoconus, with scarred corneas, irregular corneas not suitable for contact lens fitting, poor compliance with glasses, and contact lenses are common indications for keratoplasty in children with keratoconus. Keratoconus is the most common acquired nontraumatic indication for corneal transplantation in children [1]; however, in India, it is the third most common acquired nontraumatic indication for pediatric keratoplasty after infectious keratitis and adherent leukoma [109]. Although keratoplasty in keratoconus is safer compared to other indications, corneal transplantation in children has its own share of difficulties.

In pediatric keratoconus, it is important to consider various preoperative factors like age of the patient, presence of allergy, VKC, other associated connective tissue disorders, postoperative follow-ups, and compliance with medications. Intraoperatively, it is important to tackle low scleral rigidity and high intravitreal pressure which can be achieved by a general anesthesia, ocular massage, and use of Flieringa ring if needed. Centration of the trephine is important, and it should be around the visual axis or the center of the cone so as to include the entire ectatic region [110]. Intraoperatively, the apex of the cone can be identified in retro-illumination. Usually, a same size donor graft or a 0.25-mm increment is preferred. Postoperative examination of sutures, graft host junction, intraocular pressure, optic disc, and refraction need to be performed under anesthesia. We can anticipate early loosening of the sutures in children especially when there is a history of antecedent allergic disease and VKC, which can also lead to graft host junction dehiscence. Repeated incidents of premature loosening of sutures, followed by suture placements, attract blood vessels and in the long run lead to focal thinning of the graft host junction leading to high post-PK/DALK astigmatism. Immunological graft rejection is more common in PK compared to DALK and is more common in children under the age of 5 years compared to those above 5 years or adolescent [74]. Most common cause of immunological rejection is noncompliance to topical steroids; however, on the other hand, steroid-induced glaucoma and cataract are also known side effects of long-term topical steroid medications [111]. This can be prevented by shifting to steroid-sparing immunomodulators like cyclosporine and tacrolimus. Topical tacrolimus ointment formulation has shown to have great compliance and a great alternative to steroids as a posttransplant maintenance therapy [112].

Deep anterior lamellar keratoplasty (DALK) is preferred over penetrating keratoplasty (PK) for its advantages of structural integrity, endothelium integrity, and lesser chances of immunological rejection [113]. Although surgically more challenging than PK, DALK can be attempted as pre-descemetic DALK with manual dissection or descemetic DALK with the help of a big-bubble technique. Anwar's big-bubble technique is preferable [75]. The likelihood of getting a big bubble to achieve a plane between the Dua's layer and the Descemet membrane is higher in keratoconus corneas, considering weaker ectatic stromal lamellae. Faezi et al. demonstrated successful big-bubble technique in 75% of cases. In the remaining cases, dissection can be completed manually [75]. There is a risk of Descemet's perforation (11.5%) in manual dissection or stromal air injection, which can lead to interface-related complications such as double anterior chamber formation, infection, and vascularization [114, 115].

Visual outcomes of PK for keratoconus in pediatric patients are good as reported by Patel et al. in 65 pediatric patients with logMAR equal to better than 0.3 at the last visit, mean age 10.6 ± 4.3 years [116]. In DALK for keratoconus in children, Ashar et al. noted that more than 75% of patients had best corrected vision better than 20/80 at their last visit, while Karimian et al. compared outcomes of big-bubble DALK vs pre-descemetic DALK and found that the former had better outcomes but the subgroup analysis did not show any significant difference [113, 114]. Buzonetti et al. studied the advantages of a femtosecond laser-assisted DALK over mechanical trephine and found that although corrected distance visual acuity and manifest astigmatism remained comparable, the spherical equivalent was lower in the femtosecond-assisted group [111].

Multiple graft registries and old studies have shown that long-term graft survival for pediatric keratoconus patients is good. The Australian Graft Registry study for keratoconus for all age groups reported best graft survival of 89% for the first PK for the first 10 years [117]. Gulias-Cañizo et al. in their large retrospective series of 574 pediatric patients reported survival of 85% at 60 months follow-up for keratoconus, which was best compared to other indications [118]. In spite of this, graft rejection is a leading cause of graft failure especially in cases undergoing PK. Buzzonetti et al. did show that DALK grafts had better survival than PK and that children under 5 years of age had higher chances of graft failure compared to the older children (75% vs. 31%) [74, 117, 119].

Compared to earlier days, keratoplasty has become a safer procedure and is capable of delivering good anatomical and visual outcomes in children with DALK having definite long-term advantages in children. Thus, pediatric keratoconus is a disease that needs a keen eye to observe and diagnose early for successful early medical and surgical intervention to save significant lines of vision and quality of life.

References

1. Mukhtar S, Ambati BK. Pediatric keratoconus: a review of the literature. Int Ophthalmol. 2018;38(5):2257–66.
2. McMahon TT, Edrington TB, Szczotka-Flynn L, Olafsson HE, Davis LJ, Schechtman KB, CLEK Study Group. Longitudinal changes in corneal curvature in keratoconus. Cornea. 2006;25(3):296–305.
3. Chatzis N, Hafezi F. Progression of keratoconus and efficacy of pediatric [corrected] corneal collagen cross-linking in children and adolescents. J Refract Surg. 2012;28(11):753–8. Erratum in: J Refract Surg. 2013;29(1):72.
4. Sabti S, Tappeiner C, Frueh BE. Corneal cross-linking in a 4-year-old child with keratoconus and Down syndrome. Cornea. 2015;34(9):1157–60.
5. Léoni-Mesplié S, Mortemousque B, Mesplié N, Touboul D, Praud D, Malet F, Colin J. Aspects épidémiologiques du kératocône chez l'enfant [Epidemiological aspects of keratoconus in children]. J Fr Ophtalmol. 2012;35(10):776–85. Erratum in: J Fr Ophtalmol. 2013;36(3):293.
6. Rabinowitz YS. Keratoconus. Surv Ophthalmol. 1998;42(4):297–319.
7. Bittles AH, Hussain R. An analysis of consanguineous marriage in the Muslim population of India at regional and state levels. Ann Hum Biol. 2000;27(2):163–71.
8. Torres Netto EA, Al-Otaibi WM, Hafezi NL, Kling S, Al-Farhan HM, Randleman JB, Hafezi F. Prevalence of keratoconus in paediatric patients in Riyadh, Saudi Arabia. Br J Ophthalmol. 2018;102(10):1436–41.
9. Pearson AR, Soneji B, Sarvananthan N, Sandford-Smith JH. Does ethnic origin influence the incidence or severity of keratoconus? Eye (Lond). 2000;14(Pt 4):625–8.
10. Li X, Rabinowitz YS, Rasheed K, Yang H. Longitudinal study of the normal eyes in unilateral keratoconus patients. Ophthalmology. 2004;111(3):440–6.
11. Jonas JB, Nangia V, Matin A, Kulkarni M, Bhojwani K. Prevalence and associations of keratoconus in rural Maharashtra in central India: the central India eye and medical study. Am J Ophthalmol. 2009;148(5):760–5.
12. Millodot M, Shneor E, Albou S, Atlani E, Gordon-Shaag A. Prevalence and associated factors of keratoconus in Jerusalem: a cross-sectional study. Ophthalmic Epidemiol. 2011;18(2):91–7.
13. Waked N, Fayad AM, Fadlallah A, El Rami H. Dépistage du kératocône dans une population universitaire au Liban [Keratoconus screening in a Lebanese students' population]. J Fr Ophtalmol. 2012;35(1):23–9.
14. Xu L, Wang YX, Guo Y, You QS, Jonas JB, Beijing Eye Study Group. Prevalence and associations of steep cornea/keratoconus in Greater Beijing. The Beijing eye study. PLoS One. 2012;7(7):e39313.
15. Hashemi H, Khabazkhoob M, Fotouhi A. Topographic keratoconus is not rare in an Iranian population: the Tehran eye study. Ophthalmic Epidemiol. 2013;20(6):385–91.
16. Hashemi H, Khabazkhoob M, Yazdani N, Ostadimoghaddam H, Norouzirad R, Amanzadeh K, Miraftab M, Derakhshan A, Yekta A. The prevalence of keratoconus in a young population in Mashhad, Iran. Ophthalmic Physiol Opt. 2014;34(5):519–27.
17. Shneor E, Millodot M, Gordon-Shaag A, Essa M, Anton M, Barbara R, Barbara A. Prevalence of keratoconus among Young Arab students in Israel. Int J Kerat Ect Cor Dis. 2014;3(1):9–14.
18. Wojcik KA, Blasiak J, Szaflik J, Szaflik JP. Role of biochemical factors in the pathogenesis of keratoconus. Acta Biochim Pol. 2014;61(1):55–62.
19. Lema I, Sobrino T, Durán JA, Brea D, Díez-Feijoo E. Subclinical keratoconus and inflammatory molecules from tears. Br J Ophthalmol. 2009;93(6):820–4.
20. Mackiewicz Z, Määttä M, Stenman M, Konttinen L, Tervo T, Konttinen YT. Collagenolytic proteinases in keratoconus. Cornea. 2006;25(5):603–10.
21. Jun AS, Cope L, Speck C, Feng X, Lee S, Meng H, Hamad A, Chakravarti S. Subnormal cytokine profile in the tear fluid of keratoconus patients. PLoS One. 2011;6(1):e16437.
22. Kaya V, Utine CA, Altunsoy M, Oral D, Yilmaz OF. Evaluation of corneal topography with Orbscan II in first-degree relatives of patients with keratoconus. Cornea. 2008;27(5):531–4.
23. Georgiou T, Funnell CL, Cassels-Brown A, O'Conor R. Influence of ethnic origin on the incidence of keratoconus and associated atopic disease in Asians and white patients. Eye (Lond). 2004;18(4):379–83.

24. Caputo R, Versaci F, Pucci N, de Libero C, Danti G, De Masi S, Mencucci R, Novembre E, Jeng BH. Very low prevalence of keratoconus in a large series of vernal keratoconjunctivitis patients. Am J Ophthalmol. 2016;172:64–71.
25. Panahi Y, Azimi A, Naderi M, Jadidi K, Sahebkar A. An analytical enrichment-based review of structural genetic studies on keratoconus. J Cell Biochem. 2019;120(4):4748–56.
26. Bykhovskaya Y, Li X, Epifantseva I, Haritunians T, Siscovick D, Aldave A, Szczotka-Flynn L, Iyengar SK, Taylor KD, Rotter JI, Rabinowitz YS. Variation in the lysyl oxidase (LOX) gene is associated with keratoconus in family-based and case-control studies. Invest Ophthalmol Vis Sci. 2012;53(7):4152–7.
27. Rong SS, Ma STU, Yu XT, Ma L, Chu WK, Chan TCY, Wang YM, Young AL, Pang CP, Jhanji V, Chen LJ. Genetic associations for keratoconus: a systematic review and meta-analysis. Sci Rep. 2017;7(1):4620.
28. Vincent AL, Jordan CA, Cadzow MJ, Merriman TR, McGhee CN. Mutations in the zinc finger protein gene, ZNF469, contribute to the pathogenesis of keratoconus. Invest Ophthalmol Vis Sci. 2014;55(9):5629–35.
29. Davidson AE, Borasio E, Liskova P, Khan AO, Hassan H, Cheetham ME, Plagnol V, Alkuraya FS, Tuft SJ, Hardcastle AJ. Brittle cornea syndrome ZNF469 mutation carrier phenotype and segregation analysis of rare ZNF469 variants in familial keratoconus. Invest Ophthalmol Vis Sci. 2015;56(1):578–86.
30. Gordon-Shaag A, Millodot M, Shneor E, Liu Y. The genetic and environmental factors for keratoconus. Biomed Res Int. 2015;2015:795738.
31. Cingu AK, Cinar Y, Turkcu FM, Sahin A, Ari S, Yuksel H, Sahin M, Caca I. Effects of vernal and allergic conjunctivitis on severity of keratoconus. Int J Ophthalmol. 2013;6(3):370–4.
32. Naderan M, Rajabi MT, Zarrinbakhsh P, Bakhshi A. Effect of allergic diseases on keratoconus severity. Ocul Immunol Inflamm. 2017;25(3):418–23.
33. Stoiber J, Muss WH, Ruckhofer J, Thaller-Antlanger H, Alzner E, Grabner G. Recurrent keratoconus in a patient with Leber congenital amaurosis. Cornea. 2000;19(3):395–8.
34. Courage ML, Adams RJ, Reyno S, Kwa PG. Visual acuity in infants and children with Down syndrome. Dev Med Child Neurol. 1994;36(7):586–93.
35. Watt T, Robertson K, Jacobs RJ. Refractive error, binocular vision and accommodation of children with Down syndrome. Clin Exp Optom. 2015;98(1):3–11.
36. Gasset AR, Hinson WA, Frias JL. Keratoconus and atopic diseases. Ann Ophthalmol. 1978;10(8):991–4.
37. Bawazeer AM, Hodge WG, Lorimer B. Atopy and keratoconus: a multivariate analysis. Br J Ophthalmol. 2000;84(8):834–6.
38. Adachi W, Mitsuishi Y, Terai K, Nakayama C, Hyakutake Y, Yokoyama J, Mochida C, Kinoshita S. The association of HLA with young-onset keratoconus in Japan. Am J Ophthalmol. 2002;133(4):557–9.
39. Beckh U, Schönherr U, Naumann GO. Autosomal dominanter Keratokonus als okuläres Leitsymptom bei Osteogenesis imperfecta tarda Lobstein [Autosomal dominant keratoconus as the chief ocular symptom in Lobstein osteogenesis imperfecta tarda]. Klin Monatsbl Augenheilkd. 1995;206(4):268–72.
40. Beardsley TL, Foulks GN. An association of keratoconus and mitral valve prolapse. Ophthalmology. 1982;89(1):35–7.
41. Sharif KW, Casey TA, Coltart J. Prevalence of mitral valve prolapse in keratoconus patients. J R Soc Med. 1992;85(8):446–8.
42. Bisceglia L, De Bonis P, Pizzicoli C, Fischetti L, Laborante A, Di Perna M, Giuliani F, Delle Noci N, Buzzonetti L, Zelante L. Linkage analysis in keratoconus: replication of locus 5q21.2 and identification of other suggestive loci. Invest Ophthalmol Vis Sci. 2009;50(3):1081–6.
43. Tang YG, Rabinowitz YS, Taylor KD, Li X, Hu M, Picornell Y, Yang H. Genomewide linkage scan in a multigeneration Caucasian pedigree identifies a novel locus for keratoconus on chromosome 5q14.3-q21.1. Genet Med. 2005;7(6):397–405.
44. Sherwin T, Brookes NH, Loh IP, Poole CA, Clover GM. Cellular incursion into Bowman's membrane in the peripheral cone of the keratoconic cornea. Exp Eye Res. 2002;74(4):473–82.
45. Meek KM, Tuft SJ, Huang Y, Gill PS, Hayes S, Newton RH, Bron AJ. Changes in collagen orientation and distribution in keratoconus corneas. Invest Ophthalmol Vis Sci. 2005;46(6):1948–56.
46. Takahashi A, Nakayasu K, Okisaka S, Kanai A. [Quantitative analysis of collagen fiber in keratoconus]. Nippon Ganka Gakkai Zasshi. 1990;94(11):1068–73.
47. Khaled ML, Helwa I, Drewry M, Seremwe M, Estes A, Liu Y. Molecular and histopathological changes associated with keratoconus. Biomed Res Int. 2017;2017:7803029.
48. Sharma R, Titiyal JS, Prakash G, Sharma N, Tandon R, Vajpayee RB. Clinical profile and risk factors for keratoplasty and development of hydrops in north Indian patients with keratoconus. Cornea. 2009;28(4):367–70.
49. Agrawal VB. Characteristics of keratoconus patients at a tertiary eye center in India. J Ophthalmic Vis Res. 2011;6(2):87–91.
50. Saini JS, Saroha V, Singh P, Sukhija JS, Jain AK. Keratoconus in Asian eyes at a tertiary eye care facility. Clin Exp Optom. 2004;87(2):97–101.
51. Spoerl E, Raiskup-Wolf F, Kuhlisch E, Pillunat LE. Cigarette smoking is negatively associated with keratoconus. J Refract Surg. 2008;24(7):S737–40.
52. Kuo IC, Broman A, Pirouzmanesh A, Melia M. Is there an association between diabetes and keratoconus? Ophthalmology. 2006;113(2):184–90.
53. Olivo-Payne A, Abdala-Figuerola A, Hernandez-Bogantes E, Pedro-Aguilar L, Chan E, Godefrooij

D. Optimal management of pediatric keratoconus: challenges and solutions. Clin Ophthalmol. 2019;13:1183–91.
54. Thanos S, Oellers P, Meyer Zu Hörste M, Prokosch V, Schlatt S, Seitz B, Gatzioufas Z. Role of thyroxine in the development of keratoconus. Cornea. 2016;35(10):1338–46.
55. Anitha V, Vanathi M, Raghavan A, Rajaraman R, Ravindran M, Tandon R. Pediatric keratoconus—current perspectives and clinical challenges. Indian J Ophthalmol. 2021;69(2):214–25.
56. Soeters N, van der Valk R, Tahzib NG. Corneal cross-linking for treatment of progressive keratoconus in various age groups. J Refract Surg. 2014;30(7):454–60.
57. Fecarotta CM, Huang WW. Pediatric genetic disease of the cornea. J Pediatr Genet. 2014;3(4):195–207.
58. Schlegel Z, Lteif Y, Bains HS, Gatinel D. Total, corneal, and internal ocular optical aberrations in patients with keratoconus. J Refract Surg. 2009;25(10 Suppl):S951–7.
59. Sray WA, Cohen EJ, Rapuano CJ, Laibson PR. Factors associated with the need for penetrating keratoplasty in keratoconus. Cornea. 2002;21(8):784–6.
60. Maguire LJ. Ectatic corneal degenerations. In: Kaufmann HE, editor. The cornea. 2nd ed. Oxford: Butterworth-Heinemann; 1997. p. 525–43.
61. Wallang BS, Das S. Keratoglobus. Eye (Lond). 2013;27(9):1004–12.
62. Wan Q, Tang J, Han Y, Xiao Q, Deng Y. Brittle cornea syndrome: a case report and review of the literature. BMC Ophthalmol. 2018;18(1):252.
63. Ruutila M, Fagerholm P, Lagali N, Hjortdal J, Bram T, Moilanen J, Kivelä TT. Diagnostic criteria for Terrien marginal degeneration: nordic Terrien degeneration study. Cornea. 2021;40(2):133–41.
64. Sridhar MS, Mahesh S, Bansal AK, Nutheti R, Rao GN. Pellucid marginal corneal degeneration. Ophthalmology. 2004;111(6):1102–7.
65. Shimazaki J, Maeda N, Hieda O, Ohashi Y, Murakami A, Nishida K, Tsubota K, Japan Pellucid Marginal Corneal Degeneration Study Group. National survey of pellucid marginal corneal degeneration in Japan. Jpn J Ophthalmol. 2016;60(5):341–8.
66. Moshirfar M, Heiland MB, Rosen DB, Ronquillo YC, Hoopes PC. Keratoconus screening in elementary school children. Ophthalmol Ther. 2019;8(3):367–71.
67. Omar IAN. Keratoconus screening among myopic children. Clin Ophthalmol. 2019;13:1909–12.
68. Léoni-Mesplié S, Mortemousque B, Touboul D, Malet F, Praud D, Mesplié N, Colin J. Scalability and severity of keratoconus in children. Am J Ophthalmol. 2012;154(1):56–62.e1.
69. Kamiya K, Shimizu K, Ohmoto F. Effect of aging on corneal biomechanical parameters using the ocular response analyzer. J Refract Surg. 2009;25(10):888–93.
70. Rehany U, Rumelt S. Corneal hydrops associated with vernal conjunctivitis as a presenting sign of keratoconus in children. Ophthalmology. 1995;102(12):2046–9.
71. Reeves SW, Stinnett S, Adelman RA, Afshari NA. Risk factors for progression to penetrating keratoplasty in patients with keratoconus. Am J Ophthalmol. 2005;140(4):607–11.
72. Vinciguerra P, Albé E, Frueh BE, Trazza S, Epstein D. Two-year corneal cross-linking results in patients younger than 18 years with documented progressive keratoconus. Am J Ophthalmol. 2012;154(3):520–6.
73. Vinciguerra R, Romano MR, Camesasca FI, Azzolini C, Trazza S, Morenghi E, Vinciguerra P. Corneal cross-linking as a treatment for keratoconus: four-year morphologic and clinical outcomes with respect to patient age. Ophthalmology. 2013;120(5):908–16.
74. Dana MR, Moyes AL, Gomes JA, Rosheim KM, Schaumberg DA, Laibson PR, Holland EJ, Sugar A, Sugar J. The indications for and outcome in pediatric keratoplasty. A multicenter study. Ophthalmology. 1995;102(8):1129–38.
75. Feizi S, Javadi MA, Najafi M, Abolhosseini M, Moshtaghion SM. Outcomes of big-bubble deep anterior lamellar keratoplasty for pediatric keratoconus. Int Ophthalmol. 2020;40(5):1253–9.
76. Moran S, Gomez L, Zuber K, Gatinel D. A case-control study of keratoconus risk factors. Cornea. 2020;39(6):697–701.
77. Gatinel D. Challenging the "no rub, no cone" keratoconus conjecture. Int J Kerat Ect Cor Dis. 2018;7(1):66–81.
78. Kimchi N, Bielory L. The allergic eye: recommendations about pharmacotherapy and recent therapeutic agents. Curr Opin Allergy Clin Immunol. 2020;20(4):414–20.
79. Walline JJ, Jones LA, Rah MJ, Manny RE, Berntsen DA, Chitkara M, Gaume A, Kim A, Quinn N, CLIP STUDY GROUP. Contact lenses in pediatrics (CLIP) study: chair time and ocular health. Optom Vis Sci. 2007;84(9):896–902.
80. Sultan P, Dogan C, Iskeleli G. A retrospective analysis of vision correction and safety in keratoconus patients wearing Toris K soft contact lenses. Int Ophthalmol. 2016;36(6):799–805.
81. Lunardi LH, Arroyo D, Andrade Sobrinho MV, Lipener C, Rosa JM. Descriptive analysis of the type and design of contact lenses fitted according to keratoconus severity and morphology. Arq Bras Oftalmol. 2016;79(2):82–4.
82. Wollensak G, Spoerl E, Seiler T. Riboflavin/ultraviolet-a-induced collagen crosslinking for the treatment of keratoconus. Am J Ophthalmol. 2003;135(5):620–7.
83. Wollensak G. Histological changes in human cornea after cross-linking with riboflavin and ultraviolet A. Acta Ophthalmol. 2010;88(2):e17–8.
84. Zotta PG, Moschou KA, Diakonis VF, Kymionis GD, Almaliotis DD, Karamitsos AP, Karampatakis

VE. Corneal collagen cross-linking for progressive keratoconus in pediatric patients: a feasibility study. J Refract Surg. 2012;28(11):793–9.
85. Bakshi E, Barkana Y, Goldich Y, Avni I, Zadok D. Corneal cross-linking for progressive keratoconus in children: our experience. Int J Kerat Ect Cor Dis. 2012;1(1):53–6.
86. Magli A, Forte R, Tortori A, Capasso L, Marsico G, Piozzi E. Epithelium-off corneal collagen cross-linking versus transepithelial cross-linking for pediatric keratoconus. Cornea. 2013;32(5):597–601.
87. Shetty R, Nagaraja H, Jayadev C, Pahuja NK, Kurian Kummelil M, Nuijts RM. Accelerated corneal collagen cross-linking in pediatric patients: two-year follow-up results. Biomed Res Int. 2014;2014:894095.
88. Arora R, Gupta D, Goyal JL, Jain P. Results of corneal collagen cross-linking in pediatric patients. J Refract Surg. 2012;28(11):759–62.
89. Salman AG. Transepithelial corneal collagen cross-linking for progressive keratoconus in a pediatric age group. J Cataract Refract Surg. 2013;39(8):1164–70.
90. Buzzonetti L, Petrocelli G. Transepithelial corneal cross-linking in pediatric patients: early results. J Refract Surg. 2012;28(11):763–7.
91. Koppen C, Wouters K, Mathysen D, Rozema J, Tassignon MJ. Refractive and topographic results of benzalkonium chloride-assisted transepithelial cross-linking. J Cataract Refract Surg. 2012;38(6):1000–5.
92. Caporossi A, Mazzotta C, Baiocchi S, Caporossi T. Long-term results of riboflavin ultraviolet a corneal collagen cross-linking for keratoconus in Italy: the Siena eye cross study. Am J Ophthalmol. 2010;149(4):585–93.
93. Theuring A, Spoerl E, Pillunat LE, Raiskup F. Hornhautkollagenvernetzung mit riboflavin und UVA-Licht bei Patienten mit progressivem Keratokonus : 10-Jahres-Ergebnisse [Corneal collagen cross-linking with riboflavin and ultraviolet-A light in progressive keratoconus. Results after 10-year follow-up]. Ophthalmologe. 2015;112(2):140–7.
94. Kumar Kodavoor S, Arsiwala AZ, Ramamurthy D. One-year clinical study on efficacy of corneal cross-linking in Indian children with progressive keratoconus. Cornea. 2014;33(9):919–22.
95. Moore JE, Schiroli D, Moore CB. Potential effects of corneal cross-linking upon the limbus. Biomed Res Int. 2016;2016:5062064.
96. Thorsrud A, Nicolaissen B, Drolsum L. Corneal collagen crosslinking in vitro: inhibited regeneration of human limbal epithelial cells after riboflavin-ultraviolet-A exposure. J Cataract Refract Surg. 2012;38(6):1072–6.
97. Matalia H, Shetty R, Dhamodaran K, Subramani M, Arokiaraj V, Das D. Potential apoptotic effect of ultraviolet-A irradiation during cross-linking: a study on ex vivo cultivated limbal epithelial cells. Br J Ophthalmol. 2012;96(10):1339–45.
98. Vimalin J, Gupta N, Jambulingam M, Padmanabhan P, Madhavan HN. The effect of riboflavin-UV-A treatment on corneal limbal epithelial cells--a study on human cadaver eyes. Cornea. 2012;31(9):1052–9.
99. Krumeich JH, Brand-Saberi B, Chankiewitz V, Chankiewitz E, Guthoff R. Induction of neoplasia after deep anterior lamellar keratoplasty in a CXL-treated cornea. Cornea. 2014;33(3):313–6.
100. Caporossi A, Mazzotta C, Baiocchi S, Caporossi T, Denaro R, Balestrazzi A. Riboflavin-UVA-induced corneal collagen cross-linking in pediatric patients. Cornea. 2012;31(3):227–31.
101. Caporossi A, Mazzotta C, Baiocchi S, Caporossi T, Denaro R. Age-related long-term functional results after riboflavin UV a corneal cross-linking. J Ophthalmol. 2011;2011:608041.
102. Henriquez MA, Villegas S, Rincon M, Maldonado C, Izquierdo L Jr. Long-term efficacy and safety after corneal collagen crosslinking in pediatric patients: three-year follow-up. Eur J Ophthalmol. 2018;28(4):415–8.
103. Touboul D, Efron N, Smadja D, Praud D, Malet F, Colin J. Corneal confocal microscopy following conventional, transepithelial, and accelerated corneal collagen cross-linking procedures for keratoconus. J Refract Surg. 2012;28(11):769–76.
104. Tian M, Jian W, Zhang X, Sun L, Zhou X. Three-year follow-up of accelerated transepithelial corneal cross-linking for progressive paediatric keratoconus. Br J Ophthalmol. 2020;104(11):1608–12.
105. Ozgurhan EB, Sezgin Akcay BI, Yildirim Y, Karatas G, Kurt T, Demirok A. Evaluation of corneal stromal demarcation line after two different protocols of accelerated corneal collagen cross-linking procedures using anterior segment optical coherence tomography and confocal microscopy. J Ophthalmol. 2014;2014:981893.
106. Sakellaris D, Balidis M, Gorou O, Szentmary N, Alexoudis A, Grieshaber MC, Sagri D, Scholl H, Gatzioufas Z. Intracorneal ring segment implantation in the management of keratoconus: an evidence-based approach. Ophthalmol Ther. 2019;8(Suppl 1):5–14.
107. Abdelmassih Y, El-Khoury S, Dirani A, Antonios R, Fadlallah A, Cherfan CG, Chelala E, Jarade EF. Safety and efficacy of sequential intracorneal ring segment implantation and cross-linking in pediatric keratoconus. Am J Ophthalmol. 2017;178:51–7.
108. Saleem MIH, Ibrahim Elzembely HA, AboZaid MA, Elagouz M, Saeed AM, Mohammed OA, Kamel AG. Three-year outcomes of cross-linking PLUS (combined cross-linking with femtosecond laser intracorneal ring segments implantation) for management of keratoconus. J Ophthalmol. 2018;2018:6907573.
109. Ganekal S, Gangangouda C, Dorairaj S, Jhanji V. Early outcomes of primary pediatric keratoplasty in patients with acquired, atraumatic corneal pathology. J AAPOS. 2011;15(4):353–5.
110. Gloor P. Pediatric penetrating keratoplasty. In: Krachmer JH, Mannis MJ, Holland EJ, editors.

Cornea: surgery of the cornea and conjunctiva. St Louis: Mosby; 1997. p. 1731–56.

111. Buzzonetti L, Petrocelli G, Valente P, Petroni S, Parrilla R, Iarossi G. Refractive outcome of keratoconus treated by big-bubble deep anterior lamellar keratoplasty in pediatric patients: two-year follow-up comparison between mechanical trephine and femtosecond laser assisted techniques. Eye Vis (Lond). 2019;6:1.
112. Hashemian MN, Latifi G, Ghaffari R, Ghassemi H, Zarei-Ghanavati M, Mohammadi SF, Yasseri M, Fallah Tafti MR, Tafti ZF. Topical tacrolimus as adjuvant therapy to corticosteroids in acute endothelial graft rejection after penetrating keratoplasty: a randomized controlled trial. Cornea. 2018;37(3):307–12. Erratum in: Cornea. 2018;37(10):1345.
113. Ashar JN, Pahuja S, Ramappa M, Vaddavalli PK, Chaurasia S, Garg P. Deep anterior lamellar keratoplasty in children. Am J Ophthalmol. 2013;155(3):570–574.e1.
114. Karimian F, Feizi S. Deep anterior lamellar keratoplasty: indications, surgical techniques and complications. Middle East Afr J Ophthalmol. 2010;17(1):28–37.
115. Elbaz U, Kirwan C, Shen C, Ali A. Avoiding big bubble complications: outcomes of layer-by-layer deep anterior lamellar keratoplasty in children. Br J Ophthalmol. 2018;102(8):1103–8.
116. Patel HY, Ormonde S, Brookes NH, Moffatt LS, McGhee CN. The indications and outcome of paediatric corneal transplantation in New Zealand: 1991-2003. Br J Ophthalmol. 2005;89(4):404–8.
117. Kelly TL, Williams KA, Coster DJ, Australian Corneal Graft Registry. Corneal transplantation for keratoconus: a registry study. Arch Ophthalmol. 2011;129(6):691–7.
118. Gulias-Cañizo R, Gonzalez-Salinas R, Hernandez-Zimbron LF, Hernandez-Quintela E, Sanchez-Huerta V. Indications and outcomes of pediatric keratoplasty in a tertiary eye care center: a retrospective review. Medicine (Baltimore). 2017;96(45):e8587.
119. Buzzonetti L, Ardia R, Petroni S, Petrocelli G, Valente P, Parrilla R, Iarossi G. Four years of corneal keratoplasty in Italian paediatric patients: indications and clinical outcomes. Graefes Arch Clin Exp Ophthalmol. 2016;254(11):2239–45.

9 Allergic Eye Disease and Keratoconus

Prafulla Kumar Maharana, Sohini Mandal, and Namrata Sharma

9.1 Introduction

Keratoconus (KC) is the most common corneal ectatic disorder characterized by progressive asymmetric corneal thinning leading to significant decline in visual functions due to irregular myopic astigmatism and corneal scarring. Patients with this disease tend to develop corneal thinning and ectasia associated with structural aberrations in collagen configuration. Typically, the disease manifests in the second decade of life with blurred vision and frequent change of glasses similar to that of adult population. Corneal thinning with ectasia (Fig. 9.1), prominent corneal nerves, Vogt's striae (Fig. 9.2), Fleischer ring (Fig. 9.3), stromal scarring, Munson sign, scissoring reflex, and oil droplet sign are some of the common presenting signs on slit-lamp and distant direct ophthalmoscopic examination.

A positive association between KC and many conditions has been suggested, and ocular allergy is one of them [1]. The various ocular allergic conditions that have been associated with KC include vernal keratoconjunctivitis (VKC), atopic keratoconjunctivitis, and seasonal or perennial allergic keratoconjunctivitis (Fig. 9.4) [1]. This chapter attempts to elaborately discuss the association of ocular allergy with KC and its implications on the management of KC.

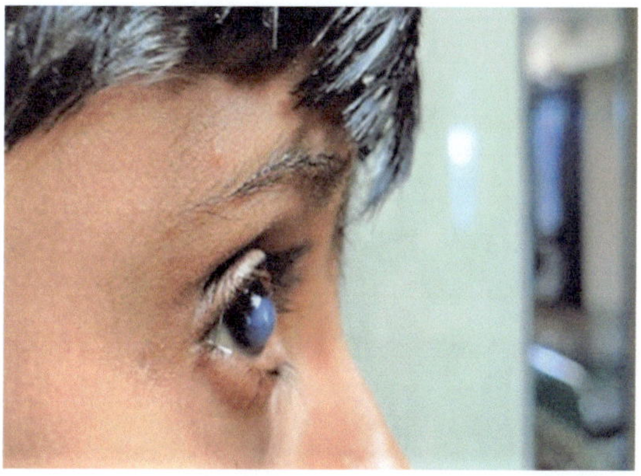

Fig. 9.1 Conical protrusion of the keratoconic cornea in a patient of acute corneal hydrops

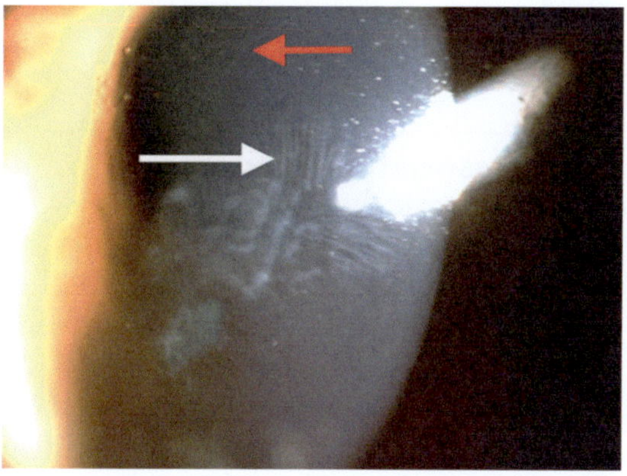

Fig. 9.2 Red arrow, prominent corneal nerves; white arrow, Vogt's striae

P. K. Maharana · S. Mandal · N. Sharma (✉)
Cornea & Refractive Surgery Services,
Dr. Rajendra Prasad Centre for Ophthalmic Sciences,
All India Institute of Medical Sciences,
New Delhi, India

S. Das (ed.), *Keratoconus*, https://doi.org/10.1007/978-981-19-4262-4_9

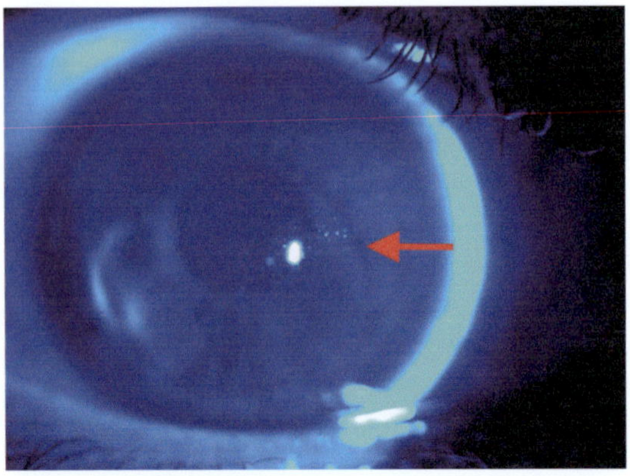

Fig. 9.3 Fleischer ring: iron deposition line at the base of the cone best appreciated under cobalt blue light

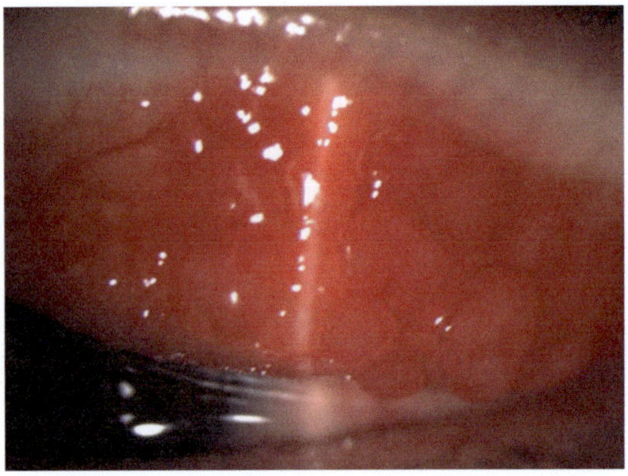

Fig. 9.4 Cobblestone papillae involving upper palpebral conjunctiva

9.2 Association between Allergic Eye Diseases and Keratoconus

Hilgartner had described the association between ocular atopy and KC for the first time in 1937 [2]. Thereafter, few studies have described similar association with incidence ranging from 7% to 35%, whereas others did not show any relationship. However, it's been proven now that there is a strong correlation between these two entities. Bawazeer et al. did a case control study and found a positive correlation between atopy, eye rubbing, and KC [3]. The Dundee University Scottish Keratoconus study reported asthma in 23%, eczema in 14%, and hay fever in 30% out of 200 KC patients [4]. The study by Agrawal et al. evaluated 274 patients of KC and revealed a higher prevalence of allergy in these patients [5]. The presence of skin allergy, symptomatic ocular allergy, and asthma was reported in 26.6%, 24.4%, and 11.3% of patients, respectively [5]. In the CLEK study, 52.9% of patients with KC had hay fever or allergies, 14.9% had asthma, 8.4% had atopic dermatitis, 27% had vernal keratoconjunctivitis (VKC), and 40% had abnormal topography [6]. Several reports have implicated eye rubbing as an important causative factor in the development of KC [7–10]. Eye rubbing increases the level of inflammatory mediators such as tear metalloproteinase-13, IL-6, and TNF-α in normal and keratoconic eyes, the release of which contributes to the development of keratoconus [11]. Persistent and vigorous eye rubbing may further increase the level and activity of these molecules and result in the progression of keratoconus by inducing apoptosis of keratocytes [12]. The reported prevalence ranges from 66% to 73% [10, 13, 14]. Various studies have reported 70% of patients with keratoconus to have history of excessive eye rubbing and 64% to be associated with spring catarrh.

Naderan et al. revealed that KC patients with a higher frequency of eye rubbing have higher mean keratometry and lower corneal thickness, though the differences were not significant. Moreover, the higher frequency of eye rubbing was associated with a more severe clinical disease ($p = 0.01$) [15]. Nemet et al. have reported a strong association between KC and autoimmune diseases [16]. Dry eye indicators, such as reduction in tear secretion, tear film breakup time, and corneal sensitivity, have also been noted [17–19].

9.3 Etiopathogenesis

Keratoconus is a complex multifactorial disorder comprising of genetic, metabolic, and environmental factors [20], and current evidence suggests a significant role of inflammation in its pathogenesis [2, 21]. Due to the altered dynamics of pro- and anti-inflammatory cytokines and apoptosis of keratocytes, there is reduction in collagen cross-linking, resulting in altered corneal rigidity and biomechanical strength [22].

9.3.1 Causative Factors

Various causative factors implicated in the pathogenesis of KC are: [23].

(a)	Genetic	(d)	Role of enzymes
(b)	Environmental	(e)	Role of oxidative stress
(c)	Role of inflammation	(f)	Role of hormones

9.3.2 Genetic Factors

KC, being heterogeneously distributed genetically, can be inherited as either autosomal recessive or dominant or sporadic; however, majority of them are sporadic [24]. About 6–23.5% of keratoconic patients have a positive family history [25]. Wang et al. have reported prevalence of KC in first-degree relatives to be 20.5% and have suggested a major gene defect to be the causative factor [26], while Kriszt et al. have hypothesized KC to be a complex non-Mendelian disease [27]. The suggested pattern of inheritance in these familial cases is mostly autosomal dominant [28]. Monozygotic twins are reported to have higher concordance than dizygotic twins [29].

Moreover, KC is strongly associated with various syndromes such as Down syndrome, Marfan syndrome, osteogenesis imperfecta, Apert syndrome, Ehlers-Danlos syndrome, and Leber congenital amaurosis [26]. Family-based linkage analysis studies have identified at least 17 genomic loci from 12 different studies [30–41]. *MIR184* gene mutation has been shown to predispose this condition, but majority of them still remains unidentified [28]. The genes and mutations associated with KC are explained in Table 9.1 [24, 42].

Table 9.1 Genetic associations of keratoconus

Gene	Chromosome
SOD1 (superoxide dismutase 1)	21q22
ZNF469 (zinc finger protein 469)	16q42
PRMD5 (PR/SET domain 5)	PR domain containing protein 5
TGFBI (transforming growth factor-beta-induced)	5q31 encodes big-h3
DOCK9 (dedicator of cytokinesis 9)	13q32
MiRI184 (microRNA)	13q32
VSX1 (visual system homeobox 1)	20p11-q11

9.3.3 Environmental Factors

Several environmental factors, such as contact lens wear, vigorous eye rubbing, atopy, ultraviolet light exposure, and others related to increased oxidative stress, predispose to KC in patients with or without any family history [4, 15, 16, 43–47]. About 40% of children are affected by systemic allergies [48], and VKC is the most common associated ocular allergy associated with KC [49]. Due to vigorous eye rubbing and associated microtrauma, various pro-inflammatory cytokines (matrix metalloproteinase-1, MMP-13, interleukin-6, and tumor necrosis factor-α) are released from both epithelial and stromal cells. These inflammatory mediators have a significant role in the apoptotic activity of the keratocytes which further results in stromal tissue loss, corneal thinning, and ectasia [12, 44, 50]. These eyes are known to be at a higher risk of developing acute hydrops (40%) when compared to primary KC eyes (2.6%) [51]. Regular topographic evaluations are vital as abnormal patterns such as increased posterior elevation, thinner pachymetry, and increased corneal curvature are detected in these corneas [25, 52]. Studies have shown that eye rubbing for 15 seconds resulted in 18.4% decrease in central and midperipheral corneal epithelial thickness which explains the most common site of ectasia being paracentral and inferonasal [53].

9.3.4 Role of Inflammation

Increased levels of IL-6, IL-1β, TNF-α, TNF- β, TNF-γ, gelatinases, collagenases, metalloproteinases, proteases, and cytokines are noted in keratoconus eyes due to the underexpression of lactoferrin (antimicrobial and anti-inflammatory protein) [12, 44, 50]. The tear biomarkers identified through enzyme-linked immunosorbent assay (ELISA) analysis are TNF-α and TNF-β; MMP-9, MMP-1, MMP-3, MMP-7, and MMP-13; and IL-4, IL-5, IL-6, and IL-8 [54, 55].

9.3.5 Role of Enzymes

Immunohistochemistry labeling has recognized an upregulation of several MMPs, such as MMP-9, MMP-14, MMP-1, MMP-7, and MMP-2. This is responsible for degradation of fibronectin, membrane glycoprotein, and types I and II collagen [56, 57]. Reduced expression of lysyl oxidase (LOX) mRNA is significantly associated with loss of cohesion between collagen fibrils resulting in corneal ectasia [58]. LOX, located on chromosome 5q23.2, oxidizes peptide lysine and hydroxyl lysine residues in collagen to peptidyl alpha amino adipic delta semialdehyde, which naturally combines with vicinal peptidyl aldehydes and forms covalent cross-linkage bonds between collagen and elastin fibers [57, 58]. Besides, copper deficiency has also been hypothesized to be associated with reduced LOX activity [59].

9.3.6 Role of Oxidative Stress

Antioxidants such as superoxide dismutase (SOD) enzymes, ascorbic acid, ferritin, glutathione, catalase, and glutathione peroxidase have a protective role against ocular tissue damage; therefore, an imbalance between free radical production and antioxidant levels results in accumulation of free radicals (aldehydes, peroxynitrites) leading to tissue destruction. IL-1 that is released in tears following eye rubbing also inhibits the synthesis of SOD [17, 60]. Hence, oxidative stress index is considered a reliable indicator for KC progression.

9.3.7 Role of Hormones

Sex hormones and thyroid hormones have a definitive role to play in the pathogenesis of KC [61–63]. The disease has its onset at puberty following altered hormone levels and progresses during pregnancy, following infertility treatment, and in children with vernal keratoconjunctivitis due to increased number of estrogen and progesterone receptors. Moreover, corneal hysteresis (CH) and corneal resistance factor (CRF) have been reported to decrease during different stages of menstrual cycle, whereas corneal thickness increases during ovulation. As T4 (thyroxine) receptors are found in lacrimal gland, T4 levels have been found to be elevated in tears of patients with KC.

Ocular allergy can impact the above-discussed factors and cause KC. The impact of eye rubbing on inflammation and oxidative stress is well documented. Eye rubbing and subsequent inflammation could provide the final blow in a patient already predisposed genetically to KC.

9.4 Role of Early Topography in Allergic Eye Diseases

Since allergic eye disorders are often associated with corneal ectasia, routine corneal topography is indicated in all cases (Fig. 9.5). Totan et al. in their study noted KC to be present in 26.8% of VKC patients by quantitative evaluation on videokeratography [64]. Male gender, long-standing disease, mixed/palpebral form, and advanced corneal lesions were the most common predisposing factors associated. The higher incidence of KC was attributed toward early detection of KC (on topography), stressing its importance in VKC patients. Léoni-Mesplié et al. [21] in their epidemiological study found allergy (67.3% versus 47.3%, respectively) and eye rubbing (91.8% and 70%, respectively) to be more common in children compared to adults. Therefore, corneal topography is routinely recommended in all younger age group with history of eye rubbing and recent-onset corneal astigmatism.

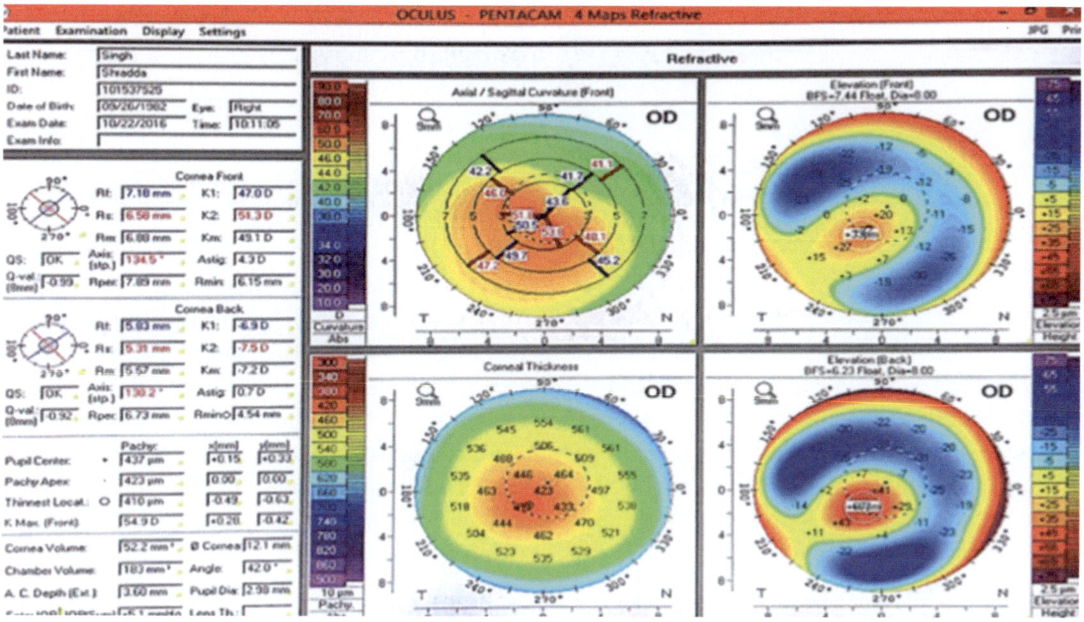

Fig. 9.5 Pentacam quad map showing inferior corneal steepening depicted by warmer colors in the axial/sagittal map with corresponding thinning at the same point on the pachymetry map and increase in posterior elevation

9.5 Role of Allergic Eye Diseases in KC Progression

The effect of allergy on KC progression is controversial. Study by Lapid-Gortzak et al. found VKC patients to have more abnormal corneal topographic patterns than non-VKC controls [65]. In a similar study by Barreto Jr. et al. who had compared the slit-scanning topography (SST) of eyes with VKC (n = 50) and normal eyes (n = 54), they found that VKC patients have more abnormal corneal SST patterns than controls [52]. Taneja et al. evaluated KC progression in VKC patients (22 eyes) and observed the rate of ectasia progression to remain unaffected by the clinical course of VKC [66]. Although atopy may not accelerate KC progression, it certainly increases the chances of developing acute corneal hydrops. Sharma et al. in their study found that the patients of KC with associated VKC required keratoplasty earlier as compared to primary KC cases. Besides, patients with earlier age of onset, history of eye rubbing, and atopy had higher risk for developing acute hydrops [67].

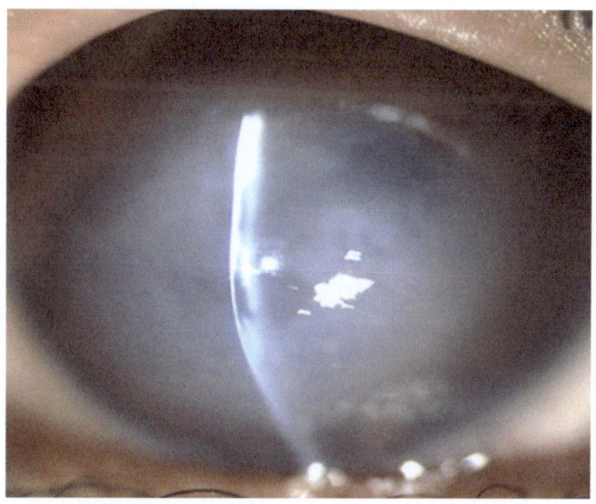

Fig. 9.6 Slit-lamp examination shows corneal edema and large intrastromal fluid clefts in a child with advanced keratoconus

9.6 Role of Allergic Eye Diseases in Acute Corneal Hydrops and Perforation

Corneal thinning diseases may end up in complications such as acute corneal hydrops (ACH) with or without subsequent perforation (Figs. 9.6

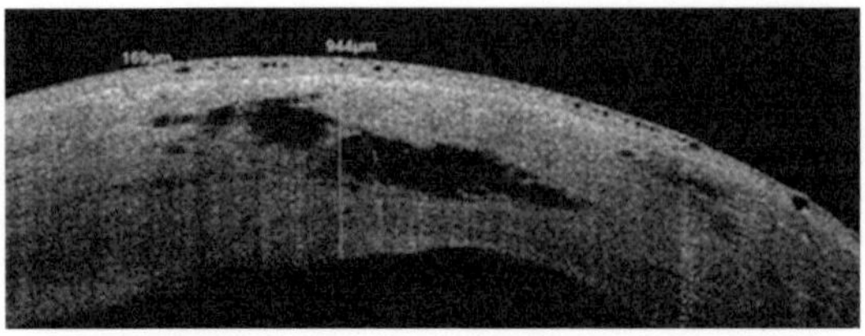

Fig. 9.7 Anterior segment optical coherence tomography [ASOCT] shows intrastromal fluid clefts with increased corneal thickness

and 9.7). This occurs due to reduced resistance to IOP forces which may be further aggravated by eye rubbing or trivial trauma [44]. ACH is characterized by corneal edema, which following natural course of healing leaves a visually significant corneal scar. Therefore, triggers for IOP elevation, such as coughing, sneezing, nose blowing, sneeze suppression, and eye rubbing/wiping/massaging/touching may reduce the risk for associated complications [44].

9.7 Management of Allergic Eye Disorders

Treatment of ocular allergy is usually tailored to fit the severity of signs and symptoms. If symptoms are mild, no treatment is necessary. Many patients tolerate mild itching and redness of the eyes during the allergy season without resorting to medication. When avoidance of non-pharmacologic strategy does not provide adequate symptom relief, pharmacologic treatments may be applied topically or given systemically to diminish the allergic response.

9.7.1 Treatment Options for Ocular Allergy

9.7.1.1 Avoidance of Allergen

Avoidance of the offending antigen is the primary behavioral modification for all types of allergic conjunctivitis.

9.7.1.2 Cold Compresses

It helps in alleviating the symptoms of itching.

9.7.1.3 Artificial Tear Substitutes

Artificial tear substitutes provide a barrier function and help to improve the first-line defense at the level of conjunctival mucosa. These agents help to dilute various allergens and inflammatory mediators that are present on the ocular surface and flush the ocular surface.

9.7.1.4 Topical Antihistamine

Topical antihistamines competitively and reversibly block histamine receptors and relieve itching and redness temporarily. They do not have any effect on other inflammatory mediators, such as prostaglandins and leukotrienes. A limited duration of action necessitates frequent dosing (of up to four times per day) and may cause ocular irritation with prolonged use.

9.7.1.5 Topical Vasoconstrictors

Vasoconstrictors are effective in reducing hyperemia; however, adverse effects include burning and stinging on instillation, mydriasis, and rebound hyperemia or conjunctivitis medicamentosa with chronic use. Therefore, they are suitable only for short-term symptom relief only.

9.7.1.6 Topical Mast Cell Stabilizers

Mast cell stabilizers increase calcium influx into the cell by preventing membrane changes and/or they may reduce membrane fluidity prior to mast cell degranulation. The end result is a decrease in degranulation of mast cells, which prevents release of histamine and other chemotactic factors that are present in the preformed and newly formed state. They require a loading period during which they must be applied before the antigen exposure.

9.7.1.7 Multimodal Anti-Allergic Agents

Several multimodal anti-allergic agents, such as olopatadine, ketotifen, azelastine, epinastine, and bepotastine, have been introduced in the market, which exert multiple pharmacological effects such as histamine receptor antagonist action, stabilization of mast cell degranulation, and suppression of activation and infiltration of eosinophils. Ketotifen inhibits eosinophil activation, generation of leukotrienes, and cytokine release. Azelastine is a selective second-generation H1 receptor antagonist that also acts by inhibiting platelet-activating factor and blocking expression of intercellular adhesion molecule 1. Epinastine has effect on both H1 and H2 receptors and also has mast cell-stabilizing and anti-inflammatory effects. These drugs have become the drug of choice for providing immediate symptomatic relief for patients with allergic conjunctivitis.

9.7.1.8 Topical Corticosteroids

Corticosteroids remain among the most potent pharmacologic agents in severe cases of ocular allergy. They possess immunosuppressive and antiproliferative properties as they can block the transcription factor that regulates the transcription of Th2-derived cytokine genes and differentiation of activated T-lymphocytes into Th2-lymphocytes. Owing to their ocular side effects, they are recommended only for short courses (up to 2–3 weeks).

9.7.1.9 Topical Immunomodulatory Agents

Cyclosporine A (CsA) is effective in controlling VKC-associated ocular inflammation by blocking Th2-lymphocyte proliferation and interleukin-2 (IL-2) production. It inhibits histamine release from mast cells and basophils through a reduction in IL-5 production and may reduce eosinophil recruitment and effects on the conjunctiva and cornea. Since CsA is lipophilic, it must be dissolved in an alcohol-oil base. Lower concentrations (1%, 0.5%, and 0.05%) have been used and shown to be effective.

Tacrolimus is a potent drug, similar to CsA in its mode of action. A tacrolimus skin ointment is used for the treatment of atopic eyelid diseases, which also may have secondary benefits for allergic keratoconjunctivitis. In a multicenter, randomized, double-masked, placebo-controlled clinical trial, 0.1% tacrolimus ophthalmic suspension was shown to be effective in treating severe allergic conjunctivitis. In the same study, it is also reported that the dose of tacrolimus was based on the results from a previous dose-ranging study in which tacrolimus ophthalmic suspensions 0.01%, 0.03%, and 0.1% were tested. Since 0.1% showed stronger improvement and similar safety profile compared with 0.01% and 0.03%, the 0.1% was considered an optimal dose [68].

A prospective double-masked randomized comparative trial comparing the efficacy of 0.1% tacrolimus ophthalmic ointment with 2% CsA showed that both were equally effective in the treatment of VKC [69].

9.7.1.10 Systemic Agents

Traditionally, immunotherapy is delivered via subcutaneous injection. However, sublingual (oral) immunotherapy (SLIT) is gaining momentum. SLIT has been shown to control ocular signs and symptoms, although ocular symptoms may respond less well than nasal symptoms [70–75]. Oral antihistamines are commonly used for the therapy of nasal and ocular allergy symptoms. These newer second-generation antihistamines are recommended in preference to first-generation antihistamines because they have a reduced propensity for adverse effects such as somnolence [76]. Second-generation antihistamines can, however, induce ocular drying, which may impair the protective barrier provided by the ocular tear film and thus actually worsen allergic symptoms [77, 78]. It has therefore been suggested that the concomitant use of an eye drop may treat ocular allergic symptoms more effectively. Intranasal corticosteroids are highly effective for treating nasal symptoms of allergic rhinitis, but the evidence that they may also be effective for the treatment of ocular symptoms is inconsistent [77, 79, 80].

9.8 Prevention of Eye Rubbing

Avoidance of rubbing may decrease the likelihood of associated adverse responses following keratoplasty. McMonnies proposed an approach for preventing this habit of eye rubbing. The stage-wise strategy for the habit modification consists of four stages:

Stage 1	:	Rubbing habit awareness
Stage 2	:	Competing responses (finding activities that could substitute for rubbing and/or distract from the urge to rub)
Stage 3	:	Developing high motivation (take-home written information in the form of an abnormal rubbing guide as the basis for the development of motivation)
Stage 4	:	Social support (responsibility for avoiding eye rubbing widens to include all family members)

Sharing the responsibility with the family members for avoiding eye rubbing may help reduce the stress. Besides, avoiding eye rubbing in adolescence may have the greatest impact on halting the progression of keratoconus, especially in patients with mental retardation. Such patients are known to have worse outcomes following keratoplasty such as globe rupture, corneal ulceration, and graft rejection owing to the vigorous habit of eye rubbing postoperatively.

9.9 Surgical Treatment

Supratarsal injection of either a short- or intermediate-acting corticosteroid has been proposed as a therapeutic approach to treating patients with refractory VKC. Surgical removal of corneal plaques is recommended to alleviate severe symptoms and to allow for corneal re-epithelialization. Giant papillae excision with intraoperative 0.02% mitomycin C followed by CsA topical treatment may be indicated in cases of mechanical pseudoptosis or the presence of coarse giant papillae and continuous active disease.

Cryotherapy and/or excision of giant papillae should otherwise be avoided because these measures treat only the complications and not the underlying disease and may induce unnecessary scarring. Amniotic membrane transplantation (AMT) following keratectomy has been described as a successful treatment for deep ulcers, in cases with slight stromal thinning. The treatment algorithm for corneal complication can be based on the Cameron clinical grading of shield ulcers: Grade 1, ulcers receive medical therapy alone; Grade 2 and Grade 3, ulcer receives either medical therapy alone or medical therapy combined with debridement, AMT, or both. Grade 2 ulcers occasionally may require additional debridement or AMT; Grade 3 ulcers are frequently refractory to medical therapy and require debridement and AMT for rapid re-epithelialization.

Significant limbal stem cell deficiency might occur as a complication of severe and persistent limbal inflammation [81, 82].

9.9.1 Surgical Outcome in Cases with Allergic Eye Diseases and KC

Several studies have inferred on the fact that even though the final outcome may not differ after keratoplasty in cases of KC with or without ocular allergy, close follow-up is required in the postoperative period to detect epithelial breakdown and steroid-induced complications. Egrilmez et al. found that the clinical outcomes of penetrating keratoplasty in eyes with KC and VKC are comparable to that in eyes with KC alone; however, complications such as loose sutures and steroid-induced cataracts were more common in the former group [83]. Wagoner et al. found that the graft survival, postoperative complications, and visual outcomes are comparable in both cohorts [84]. Thomas et al. found no difference in the prevalence of endothelial graft rejections or graft survival between both groups [85].

9.10 Conclusion

Allergic eye disorder is one of the important predisposing factors for KC. Subtle cases are unmasked on corneal topography, and therefore, all cases with ocular allergy should undergo these investigations. Eye rubbing both triggers the onset and exacerbates the progression of KC; hence, patients should be strictly counseled against eye rubbing. They always remain at an increased risk of acute corneal hydrops that may require early keratoplasty. The surgical outcome in cases of ocular allergy with KC is similar to the primary cases of KC, but a close follow-up is required to avoid complications related to epithelial healing or steroid use.

References

1. Gorskova EN, Sevost'ianov EN. Epidemiologiia keratokonusa na Urale [epidemiology of keratoconus in the Urals]. Vestn oftalmol. 1998;114(4):38–40.
2. Hilgartner HL, Hilgartner HL Jr, Gilbert JT. A preliminary report of a case of keratoconus, successfully treated with organotherapy, radium, and short-wave diathermy. Am J Ophthalmol. 1937;20(10):1032–9.
3. Bawazeer AM, Hodge WG, Lorimer B. Atopy and keratoconus: a multivariate analysis. Br J Ophthalmol. 2000;84(8):834–6.
4. Weed KH, MacEwen CJ, Giles T, Low J, McGhee CN. The Dundee university Scottish keratoconus study: demographics, corneal signs, associated diseases, and eye rubbing. Eye (Lond). 2008;22(4):534–41.
5. Agrawal VB. Characteristics of keratoconus patients at a tertiary eye center in India. J Ophthalmic Vis Res. 2011;6(2):87–91.
6. Zadnik K, Barr JT, Edrington TB, Everett DF, Jameson M, McMahon TT, Shin JA, Sterling JL, Wagner H, Gordon MO. Baseline findings in the collaborative longitudinal evaluation of keratoconus (CLEK) study. Invest Ophthalmol Vis Sci. 1998;39(13):2537–46.
7. Owens H, Gamble G. A profile of keratoconus in New Zealand. Cornea. 2003;22(2):122–5.
8. Duke-Elder S, Leigh AG. System of ophthalmology. Vol.8, disease of the outer eye. Part-2. London: Henry Kimpton; 1965. p. 964–76.
9. Hanna C, O'brien JE. Cell production and migration in the epithelial layer of the cornea. Arch Ophthalmol. 1960;64:536–9.
10. Gasset AR, Hinson WA, Frias JL. Keratoconus and atopic diseases. Ann Ophthalmol. 1978;10(8):991–4.
11. Cingu AK, Cinar Y, Turkcu FM, Sahin A, Ari S, Yuksel H, Sahin M, Caca I. Effects of vernal and allergic conjunctivitis on severity of keratoconus. Int J Ophthalmol. 2013;6(3):370–4.
12. Balasubramanian SA, Pye DC, Willcox MD. Effects of eye rubbing on the levels of protease, protease activity and cytokines in tears: relevance in keratoconus. Clin Exp Optom. 2013;96(2):214–8.
13. Karseras AG, Ruben M. Aetiology of keratoconus. Br J Ophthalmol. 1976;60(7):522–5.
14. Copeman PW. Eczema and keratoconus. Br Med J. 1965;2(5468):977–9.
15. Naderan M, Shoar S, Rezagholizadeh F, Zolfaghari M, Naderan M. Characteristics and associations of keratoconus patients. Cont Lens Anterior Eye. 2015;38(3):199–205.
16. Nemet AY, Vinker S, Bahar I, Kaiserman I. The association of keratoconus with immune disorders. Cornea. 2010;29(11):1261–4.
17. Lema I, Durán JA. Inflammatory molecules in the tears of patients with keratoconus. Ophthalmology. 2005;112(4):654–9.
18. Carracedo G, Recchioni A, Alejandre-Alba N, Martin-Gil A, Crooke A, Morote IJ, Pintor J. Signs and symptoms of dry eye in keratoconus patients: a pilot study. Curr Eye Res. 2015;40(11):1088–94.
19. Dienes L, Kiss HJ, Perényi K, Nagy ZZ, Acosta MC, Gallar J, Kovács I. Corneal sensitivity and dry eye symptoms in patients with keratoconus. PLoS One. 2015;10(10):e0141621.
20. Gokhale NS. Epidemiology of keratoconus. Indian J Ophthalmol. 2013;61(8):382–3.
21. Léoni-Mesplié S, Mortemousque B, Touboul D, Malet F, Praud D, Mesplié N, Colin J. Scalability and severity of keratoconus in children. Am J Ophthalmol. 2012;154(1):56–62.e1.
22. Hovakimyan M, Guthoff RF, Stachs O. Collagen cross-linking: current status and future directions. J Ophthalmol. 2012;2012:406850.
23. Wojcik KA, Blasiak J, Szaflik J, Szaflik JP. Role of biochemical factors in the pathogenesis of keratoconus. Acta Biochim Pol. 2014;61(1):55–62.
24. Burdon KP, Vincent AL. Insights into keratoconus from a genetic perspective. Clin Exp Optom. 2013;96(2):146–54.
25. Karimian F, Aramesh S, Rabei HM, Javadi MA, Rafati N. Topographic evaluation of relatives of patients with keratoconus. Cornea. 2008;27(8):874–8.
26. Wang Y, Rabinowitz YS, Rotter JI, Yang H. Genetic epidemiological study of keratoconus: evidence for major gene determination. Am J Med Genet. 2000;93(5):403–9.
27. Kriszt A, Losonczy G, Berta A, Vereb G, Takács L. Segregation analysis suggests that keratoconus is a complex non-Mendelian disease. Acta Ophthalmol. 2014;92(7):e562–8.
28. Wheeler J, Hauser MA, Afshari NA, Allingham RR, Liu Y. The genetics of keratoconus: a review. Reprod Syst Sex Disord. 2012;(Suppl 6):001.
29. Bechara SJ, Waring GO 3rd, Insler MS. Keratoconus in two pairs of identical twins. Cornea. 1996;15(1):90–3.
30. Gajecka M, Radhakrishna U, Winters D, Nath SK, Rydzanicz M, Ratnamala U, Ewing K, Molinari A, Pitarque JA, Lee K, Leal SM, Bejjani BA. Localization of a gene for keratoconus to a 5.6-Mb interval on 13q32. Invest Ophthalmol Vis Sci. 2009;50(4):1531–9.
31. Hughes AE, Dash DP, Jackson AJ, Frazer DG, Silvestri G. Familial keratoconus with cataract: linkage to the long arm of chromosome 15 and exclusion of candidate genes. Invest Ophthalmol Vis Sci. 2003;44(12):5063–6.
32. Hughes AE, Bradley DT, Campbell M, Lechner J, Dash DP, Simpson DA, Willoughby CE. Mutation

altering the miR-184 seed region causes familial keratoconus with cataract. Am J Hum Genet. 2011;89(5):628–33.
33. Bisceglia L, De Bonis P, Pizzicoli C, Fischetti L, Laborante A, Di Perna M, Giuliani F, Delle Noci N, Buzzonetti L, Zelante L. Linkage analysis in keratoconus: replication of locus 5q21.2 and identification of other suggestive loci. Invest Ophthalmol Vis Sci. 2009;50(3):1081–6.
34. Li X, Rabinowitz YS, Tang YG, Picornell Y, Taylor KD, Hu M, Yang H. Two-stage genome-wide linkage scan in keratoconus sib pair families. Invest Ophthalmol Vis Sci. 2006;47(9):3791–5.
35. Tyynismaa H, Sistonen P, Tuupanen S, Tervo T, Dammert A, Latvala T, Alitalo T. A locus for autosomal dominant keratoconus: linkage to 16q22.3-q23.1 in Finnish families. Invest Ophthalmol Vis Sci. 2002;43(10):3160–4.
36. Tang YG, Rabinowitz YS, Taylor KD, Li X, Hu M, Picornell Y, Yang H. Genomewide linkage scan in a multigeneration Caucasian pedigree identifies a novel locus for keratoconus on chromosome 5q14.3-q21.1. Genet Med. 2005;7(6):397–405.
37. Hutchings H, Ginisty H, Le Gallo M, Levy D, Stoësser F, Rouland JF, Arné JL, Lalaux MH, Calvas P, Roth MP, Hovnanian A, Malecaze F. Identification of a new locus for isolated familial keratoconus at 2p24. J Med Genet. 2005;42(1):88–94.
38. Brancati F, Valente EM, Sarkozy A, Fehèr J, Castori M, Del Duca P, Mingarelli R, Pizzuti A, Dallapiccola B. A locus for autosomal dominant keratoconus maps to human chromosome 3p14-q13. J Med Genet. 2004;41(3):188–92.
39. Liskova P, Hysi PG, Waseem N, Ebenezer ND, Bhattacharya SS, Tuft SJ. Evidence for keratoconus susceptibility locus on chromosome 14: a genome-wide linkage screen using single-nucleotide polymorphism markers. Arch Ophthalmol. 2010;128(9):1191–5. Erratum in: Arch Ophthalmol 2010;128(11): 1431
40. Hameed A, Khaliq S, Ismail M, Anwar K, Ebenezer ND, Jordan T, Mehdi SQ, Payne AM, Bhattacharya SS. A novel locus for Leber congenital amaurosis (LCA4) with anterior keratoconus mapping to chromosome 17p13. Invest Ophthalmol Vis Sci. 2000;41(3):629–33.
41. Fullerton J, Paprocki P, Foote S, Mackey DA, Williamson R, Forrest S. Identity-by-descent approach to gene localisation in eight individuals affected by keratoconus from north-west Tasmania. Australia Hum Genet. 2002;110(5):462–70.
42. Loukovitis E, Sfakianakis K, Syrmakesi P, Tsotridou E, Orfanidou M, Bakaloudi DR, Stoila M, Kozei A, Koronis S, Zachariadis Z, Tranos P, Kozeis N, Balidis M, Gatzioufas Z, Fiska A, Anogeianakis G. Genetic aspects of keratoconus: a literature review exploring potential genetic contributions and possible genetic relationships with comorbidities. Ophthalmol Ther. 2018;7(2):263–92.
43. Romero-Jiménez M, Santodomingo-Rubido J, Wolffsohn JS. Keratoconus: a review. Cont Lens Anterior Eye. 2010;33(4):157–66.
44. McMonnies CW. Mechanisms of rubbing-related corneal trauma in keratoconus. Cornea. 2009;28(6):607–15.
45. Merdler I, Hassidim A, Sorkin N, Shapira S, Gronovich Y, Korach Z. Keratoconus and allergic diseases among Israeli adolescents between 2005 and 2013. Cornea. 2015;34(5):525–9.
46. Cristina Kenney M, Brown DJ. The cascade hypothesis of keratoconus. Cont Lens Anterior Eye. 2003;26(3):139–46.
47. Kenney MC, Nesburn AB, Burgeson RE, Butkowski RJ, Ljubimov AV. Abnormalities of the extracellular matrix in keratoconus corneas. Cornea. 1997;16(3):345–51.
48. Abelson MB, Granet D. Ocular allergy in pediatric practice. Curr Allergy Asthma Rep. 2006;6(4):306–11.
49. Gordon-Shaag A, Millodot M, Shneor E, Liu Y. The genetic and environmental factors for keratoconus. Biomed Res Int. 2015;2015:795738.
50. Seppälä HP, Määttä M, Rautia M, Mackiewicz Z, Tuisku I, Tervo T, Konttinen YT. EMMPRIN and MMP-1 in keratoconus. Cornea. 2006;25(3):325–30. Erratum in: Cornea 2006; 25(6): 760
51. Tuft SJ, Gregory WM, Buckley RJ. Acute corneal hydrops in keratoconus. Ophthalmology. 1994;101(10):1738–44.
52. Barreto J Jr, Netto MV, Santo RM, José NK, Bechara SJ. Slit-scanning topography in vernal keratoconjunctivitis. Am J Ophthalmol. 2007;143(2):250–4.
53. Baum J. On the location of the cone and the etiology of keratoconus. Cornea. 1995;14(2):142–3.
54. Collier SA. Is the corneal degradation in keratoconus caused by matrix-metalloproteinases? Clin Exp Ophthalmol. 2001;29(6):340–4.
55. Nishtala K, Pahuja N, Shetty R, Nuijts RM, Ghosh A. Tear biomarkers for keratoconus. Eye Vis (Lond). 2016;3:19.
56. Mackiewicz Z, Määttä M, Stenman M, Konttinen L, Tervo T, Konttinen YT. Collagenolytic proteinases in keratoconus. Cornea. 2006;25(5):603–10. Erratum in: Cornea 2006; 25(6): 760
57. Dudakova L, Jirsova K. The impairment of lysyl oxidase in keratoconus and in keratoconus-associated disorders. J Neural Transm (Vienna). 2013;120(6):977–82.
58. Shetty R, Sathyanarayanamoorthy A, Ramachandra RA, Arora V, Ghosh A, Srivatsa PR, Pahuja N, Nuijts RM, Sinha-Roy A, Mohan RR, Ghosh A. Attenuation of lysyl oxidase and collagen gene expression in keratoconus patient corneal epithelium corresponds to disease severity. Mol Vis. 2015;21:12–25.
59. Avetisov SE, Mamikonian VR, Novikov IA. The role of tear acidity and cu-cofactor of lysyl oxidase activity in the pathogenesis of keratoconus. Vestn oftalmol. 2011;127(2):3–8.

60. Olofsson EM, Marklund SL, Pedrosa-Domellöf F, Behndig A. Interleukin-1alpha downregulates extracellular-superoxide dismutase in human corneal keratoconus stromal cells. Mol Vis. 2007;13:1285–90.
61. Thanos S, Oellers P, Hörste MMZ, Prokosch V, Schlatt S, Seitz B, Gatzioufas Z. Role of thyroxine in the development of keratoconus. Cornea. 2016;35(10):1338–46.
62. Ayan B, Yuksel N, Carhan A, Gumuşkaya Ocal B, Akcay E, Cagil N, Asik MD. Evaluation estrogen, progesterone and androgen receptor expressions in corneal epithelium in keratoconus. Cont Lens Anterior Eye. 2019;42(5):492–6.
63. Rabinowitz YS. Keratoconus. Surv Ophthalmol. 1998;42(4):297–319.
64. Totan Y, Hepşen IF, Cekiç O, Gündüz A, Aydin E. Incidence of keratoconus in subjects with vernal keratoconjunctivitis: a videokeratographic study. Ophthalmology. 2001;108(4):824–7.
65. Lapid-Gortzak R, Rosen S, Weitzman S, Lifshitz T. Videokeratography findings in children with vernal keratoconjunctivitis versus those of healthy children. Ophthalmology. 2002;109(11):2018–23.
66. Taneja M, Ashar JN, Mathur A, Vaddavalli PK, Rathi V, Sangwan V, Murthy S. Measure of keratoconus progression in patients with vernal keratoconjunctivitis using scanning slit topography. Cont Lens Anterior Eye. 2013;36(1):41–4.
67. Sharma R, Titiyal JS, Prakash G, Sharma N, Tandon R, Vajpayee RB. Clinical profile and risk factors for keratoplasty and development of hydrops in north Indian patients with keratoconus. Cornea. 2009;28(4):367–70.
68. Ohashi Y, Ebihara N, Fujishima H, Fukushima A, Kumagai N, Nakagawa Y, Namba K, Okamoto S, Shoji J, Takamura E, Hayashi K. A randomized, placebo-controlled clinical trial of tacrolimus ophthalmic suspension 0.1% in severe allergic conjunctivitis. J Ocul Pharmacol Ther. 2010;26(2):165–74.
69. Labcharoenwongs P, Jirapongsananuruk O, Visitsunthorn N, Kosrirukvongs P, Saengin P, Vichyanond P. A double-masked comparison of 0.1% tacrolimus ointment and 2% cyclosporine eye drops in the treatment of vernal keratoconjunctivitis in children. Asian Pac J Allergy Immunol. 2012;30(3):177–84.
70. Abelson MB, Butrus SI, Weston JH. Aspirin therapy in vernal conjunctivitis. Am J Ophthalmol. 1983;95(4):502–5.
71. Anzaar F, Gallagher MJ, Bhat P, Arif M, Farooqui S, Foster CS. Use of systemic T-lymphocyte signal transduction inhibitors in the treatment of atopic keratoconjunctivitis. Cornea. 2008;27(8):884–8.
72. de Klerk TA, Sharma V, Arkwright PD, Biswas S. Severe vernal keratoconjunctivitis successfully treated with subcutaneous omalizumab. J AAPOS. 2013;17(3):305–6.
73. Calderon MA, Penagos M, Sheikh A, Canonica GW, Durham SR. Sublingual immunotherapy for allergic conjunctivitis: Cochrane systematic review and meta-analysis. Clin Exp Allergy. 2011;41(9):1263–72.
74. Mahdy RA, Nada WM, Marei AA. Subcutaneous allergen-specific immunotherapy versus topical treatment in vernal keratoconjunctivitis. Cornea. 2012;31(5):525–8.
75. Holsclaw DS, Whitcher JP, Wong IG, Margolis TP. Supratarsal injection of corticosteroid in the treatment of refractory vernal keratoconjunctivitis. Am J Ophthalmol. 1996;121(3):243–9.
76. Tabbara KF. Ocular complications of vernal keratoconjunctivitis. Can J Ophthalmol. 1999;34(2):88–92.
77. Tanaka M, Takano Y, Dogru M, Fukagawa K, Asano-Kato N, Tsubota K, Fujishima H. A comparative evaluation of the efficacy of intraoperative mitomycin C use after the excision of cobblestone-like papillae in severe atopic and vernal keratoconjunctivitis. Cornea. 2004;23(4):326–9.
78. Fujishima H, Fukagawa K, Satake Y, Saito I, Shimazaki J, Takano Y, Tsubota K. Combined medical and surgical treatment of severe vernal keratoconjunctivitis. Jpn J Ophthalmol. 2000;44(5):511–5.
79. Cameron JA. Shield ulcers and plaques of the cornea in vernal keratoconjunctivitis. Ophthalmology. 1995;102(6):985–93.
80. Reddy JC, Basu S, Saboo US, Murthy SI, Vaddavalli PK, Sangwan VS. Management, clinical outcomes, and complications of shield ulcers in vernal keratoconjunctivitis. Am J Ophthalmol. 2013;155(3):550–559.e1.
81. Sangwan VS, Jain V, Vemuganti GK, Murthy SI. Vernal keratoconjunctivitis with limbal stem cell deficiency. Cornea. 2011;30(5):491–6.
82. Sangwan VS, Murthy SI, Vemuganti GK, Bansal AK, Gangopadhyay N, Rao GN. Cultivated corneal epithelial transplantation for severe ocular surface disease in vernal keratoconjunctivitis. Cornea. 2005;24(4):426–30.
83. Egrilmez S, Sahin S, Yagci A. The effect of vernal keratoconjunctivitis on clinical outcomes of penetrating keratoplasty for keratoconus. Can J Ophthalmol. 2004;39(7):772–7.
84. Wagoner MD, Ba-Abbad R, King Khaled Eye Specialist Hospital Cornea Transplant Study Group. Penetrating keratoplasty for keratoconus with or without vernal keratoconjunctivitis. Cornea. 2009;28(1):14–8.
85. Thomas JK, Guel DA, Thomas TS, Cavanagh HD. The role of atopy in corneal graft survival in keratoconus. Cornea. 2011;30(10):1088–97.

Topography and Tomography of Keratoconus

10

Shizuka Koh

10.1 Introduction

In the human eye, aberrations and light scattering are the primary factors in the degradation of optical quality. In eyes with diseases of the ocular surface or anterior segment, the irregularity of the refractive surfaces, such as anterior/posterior corneal surfaces or the precorneal tear film, can cause increased irregular astigmatism, higher-order aberrations (HOAs), or increased light scattering. Corneal haze with decreased corneal transparency is associated with increased ocular scattering. Clinically, corneal haze is typically estimated as corneal backward light scattering, as observed via slit-lamp examination. In contrast, the detection of a subtle distortion of the corneal shape in a clear cornea without abnormal clinical slit-lamp signs is challenging. Corneal topography is mandatory in such cases.

Thus, corneal topography in clinical practice aims (a) to measure corneal power, (b) to diagnose preexisting corneal irregular astigmatism, and (c) to assess the effect of increased irregular astigmatism or HOAs on the optical quality of the entire eye.

10.2 Topography Vs. Tomography

Topography derives from the Greek words *topos* ("place") and *-graphia* ("writing"), which refer to writing about a place. Tomography is derived from the Greek words *tomos* ("section" or "slice") and *-graphia* ("writing"), which refer to writing about a section (slice). In ophthalmic medicine, corneal topography only provides two-dimensional information about the frontal surface of the cornea, whereas corneal tomography visualizes a three-dimensional section of the cornea [1, 2].

10.2.1 Historical Background

Computerized video keratography for the diagnosis of keratoconus was first introduced in the 1980s. Early systems relied on the analysis of Placido disk images to compute the anterior corneal curvature [3]. It has represented a true revolution in the diagnosis and management of corneal diseases, including keratoconus. The advent of refractive surgery and the coincident risk of iatrogenic ectasia or unmasking of keratoconus spurred the development of newer diagnostic devices aimed at the early detection of subclinical keratoconus. The Orbscan (Bausch and Lomb, Rochester, NY, USA) utilized slit-scanning technology to provide wide-field pachymetry, anterior and posterior elevation, and keratometry maps. In a later iteration, Orbscan II

S. Koh (✉)
Department of Innovative Visual Science, Osaka University Graduate School of Medicine, Osaka, Japan
e-mail: skoh@ophthal.med.osaka-u.ac.jp

S. Das (ed.), *Keratoconus*, https://doi.org/10.1007/978-981-19-4262-4_10

combines slit scanning with Placido-based topography analysis. The Scheimpflug principle has been exploited in corneal tomographers to provide a three-dimensional mapping of the cornea, including direct measurement of anterior and posterior corneal surfaces, pachymetry, and anterior chamber angle characterization. Swept-source/Fourier domain optical coherence tomography devices have been introduced with higher speed and sensitivity, allowing anterior and posterior corneal topography as well as cross-sectional corneal images.

As previously mentioned, corneal topography is used to characterize the shape of the anterior surface of the cornea. Currently, even when the data of the corneal shape are obtained using corneal "tomography"-based devices, terms such as "corneal topography" can be found in the literature. In this way, "corneal topography" is used broadly to mean the characterization of the shape of the cornea, close to "corneal shape imaging" (Fig. 10.1). Therefore, it is always important to make sure whether "topography" or "tomography" is used when observing the description of "corneal topography."

This chapter focuses on the basics of the most commonly used three "corneal topography" techniques: Placido-based corneal topographer, Scheimpflug-based tomography, and anterior segment optical coherence tomography (OCT).

10.3 Placido-Based Corneal Topographer

10.3.1 Principle

A Placido-based corneal topographer, previously referred to as a videokeratoscope, analyzes the contours of the anterior corneal surface [4]. It is based on the Placido disk principle. A Placido disk is a device made of concentric rings drawn on a device of different colors. The name Placido is derived from the name of a Portuguese ophthal-

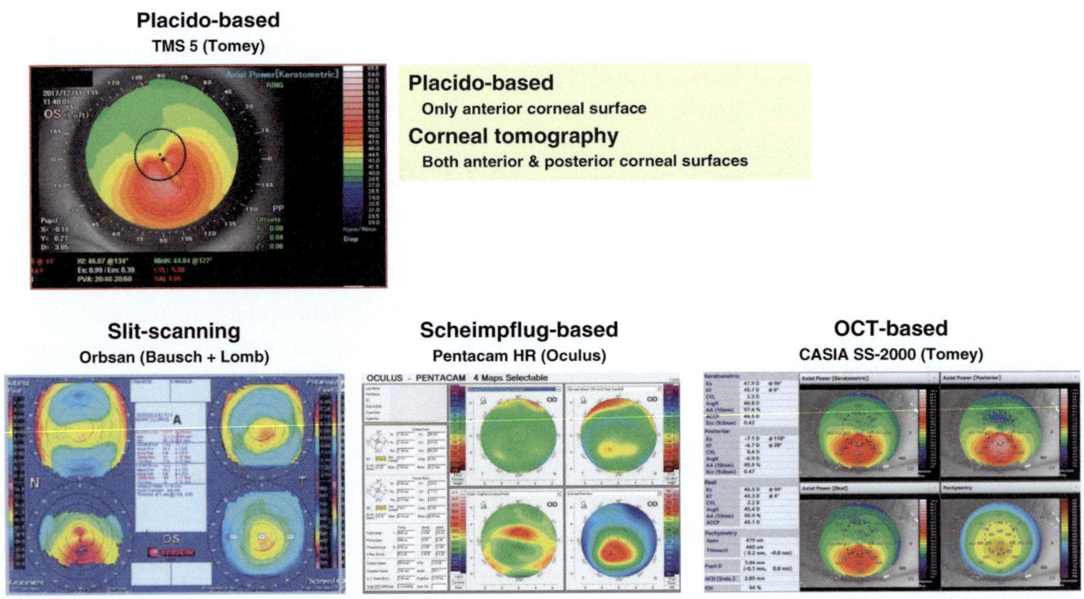

Fig. 10.1 Principles used for the characterization of the shape of the cornea

mologist, Dr. Antonio Placido, who developed this in the late 1800s [5]. It was developed to overcome the shortcomings of the keratometers, which typically measure the average curve of the central 3 mm of the cornea in two meridians. This includes at least three limitations with the keratometer: (a) measures curves that are not equivalent to shape, (b) evaluates the average central curves instead of a true measurement, and (c) implies a very small area compared to the ocular surface. Computerized Placido-based topographers assess the reflection of a circular mire of concentric lighted rings projected onto the air-tear film interface. The radii of the anterior corneal curvature and the axis of astigmatism were determined by analyzing the size and toricity of the mire, similar to the keratometers. Placido-based topographers provide a qualitative and quantitative description of the morphology of the cornea in a color-coded topographical map based on the power across an extensive area of the cornea based on the mires [4, 6].

10.3.2 Features

- Since it uses the same principle as a keratometer, simulated K readings can be indicated as the compatible index of K readings; however, these two indices are not always interchangeable.
- Placido-based corneal topographers quickly obtain the image created at the precorneal tear film in a single shot, which contributes to the good reproducibility of the data. In contrast, Placido-based topographic maps are subject to fluctuations in tear film stability. Therefore, caution is needed when measuring dry eyes or eyes with decreased tear film stability. Previous researchers have reversely used this phenomenon as sequential measurements of corneal topographic data [7, 8].
- It is challenging for the videokeratoscope to digitize heavily distorted mire images in eyes with severe irregular astigmatism.
- Since it can provide information on only the anterior corneal surface, Placido-based corneal topographers cannot identify highly mild forms of keratoconus (generally defined as forme fruste keratoconus), which would require identification, assessing at least the corneal thickness and posterior curvature measurements with corneal tomography described later.

10.3.3 Application Tools for Keratoconus Management

- **Keratoconus Screening Program.**
  A variety of indices were developed for discriminating keratoconus from normal eyes, such as superior-inferior asymmetry value (I-S value) of less than 1.4 at 6 mm (3-mm radii), keratoconus percentage index, Klyce/Maeda keratoconus index, and Smolek/Klyce keratoconus severity index [9–12].

In Fig. 10.2, the keratoconus screening display obtained in a patient with keratoconus is also demonstrated. While her right eye exhibited clinical keratoconus, there was no abnormal finding on the slit-lamp examination of her left eye. However, the keratoconus screening program using Placido-based corneal topography detected keratoconus in her left eye. Although specialty clinics or the screening of refractive surgical patients require further corneal assessment using corneal tomography, the early detection of keratoconus or corneal ectasia is possible using Placido-based corneal topographers in general clinics or primary care.

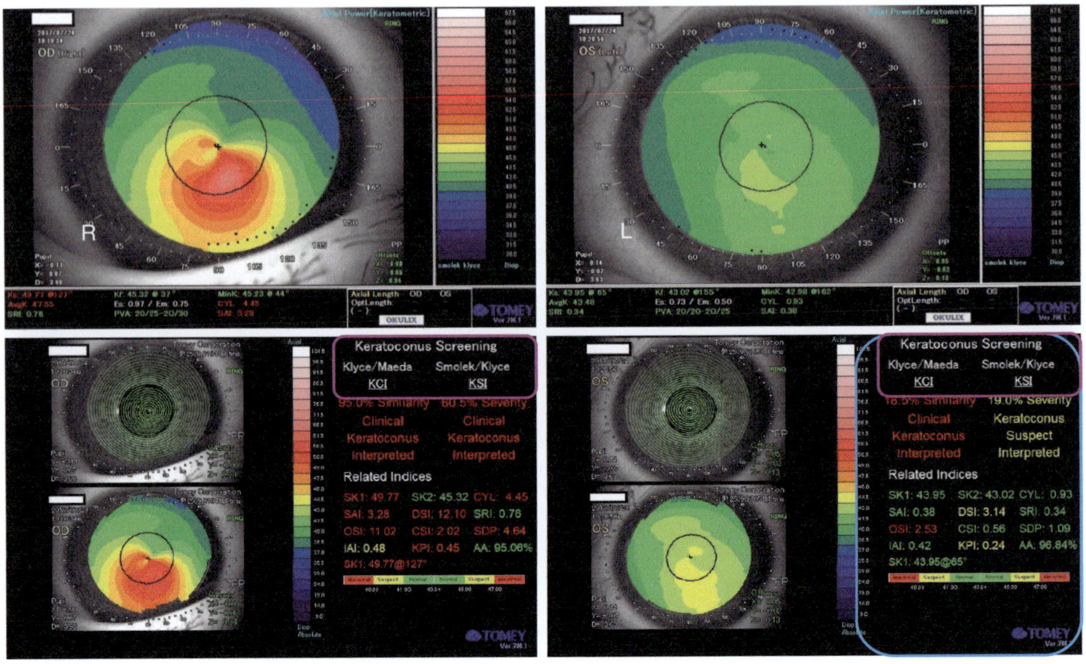

Fig. 10.2 Color-coded topographical map obtained with Placido-based corneal topographer (TMS-5, Tomey). Ring Topo Mode, a Placido-based topography method is used. Upper row panels, original map. Lower row panels, keratoconus screening display

10.4 Scheimpflug-Based Tomography

10.4.1 Principle

Scheimpflug principle [13] eliminates the problem noted with centrally located slit-scanning technology cameras, that there was poor/unreliable capture of the peripheral corneal data, caused by the nonplanar shape of the cornea. The Scheimpflug principle states that when a planar subject is not parallel to the image plane, an oblique tangent can be drawn from the image, object, and lens planes and the point of intersection is called Scheimpflug intersection [2]. The commonly used Scheimpflug-based devices are described in Table 10.1.

The Pentacam HR (OCULUS) is described as an example. A representative color-coded map of keratoconus obtained using Pentacam HR is shown in Fig. 10.3.

10.4.2 Features

- Assessment of clinically relevant parameters such as corneal wavefront aberrations, backward scattering, anterior segment analysis, biometry, and calculation of intraocular lens power is possible.
- Refractive components of the posterior corneal surface and corneal thickness profile can be obtained in addition to the anterior corneal topography.
- The calculation of the total corneal power is possible. For eyes with abnormal corneal shape, appropriate intraocular lens (IOL) power calculation formulae can be applied.
- Corneal scars or haze may scatter visible light (475 nm for Pentacam) in the Scheimpflug-based corneal topographer. Thus, the scattered scanning beam may make it challenging to digitize the corneal surfaces precisely.

Table 10.1 The commercially available, commonly used "corneal tomography" instruments

Technology	Type	Product (manufacturer)
Scheimpflug-based devices	Rotating Scheimpflug	Pentacam Series (OCULUS, Wetzlar, Germany)
		WaveLight® OCULYZER II (Alcon, Texas, USA)
	Hybrid system	Galilei (Ziemer, Port, Switzerland)
		TMS-5 (Tomey, Aichi, Japan)
		Sirius (Costruzione Strumenti Oftalmici, Florence, Italy)
Anterior segment OCT	Time-domain OCT	Visante (Carl Zeiss Meditec, Dublin, California, USA)
	Spectral-domain OCT	RTVue (Optovue Inc., Fremont, California, USA)
	Swept-source OCT	CASIA SS-1000, 2000 (Tomey, Aichi, Japan)
		ANTERION (Heidelberg Engineering, Heidelberg, Germany)

10.4.3 Application Tools for Keratoconus Management

- **Enhanced Ectasia Detection Program**
  The Belin/Ambrósio enhanced ectasia display [14] can be employed for the detection of clinical or subclinical keratoconus (Fig. 10.4). It combines both elevation and pachymetric parameters in a regression analysis. Anterior and posterior elevation data relative to the standard best-fit sphere calculated at a fixed optical zone of 8.0 mm are shown on the left side (orange-lined box). The different elevation maps at the bottom part (navy-lined box) show the relative change in elevation from the standard (baseline). Based on the amount of elevation change, colors in the anterior (front) or posterior (back) corneal surfaces indicate signs such as green (normal), yellow (suspicious), and red (abnormal). In the bottom right of the display (pink-lined box), a series of indices are characterized by a "d" value, which reflect the standard deviation from the mean of a reference population for the following five parameters: Df (front elevation), Db (back elevation), Dp (pachymetric progression), Dt (corneal thickness at thinnest point), and Da (thinnest point displacement). In the BAD D, the final "D" reading represents overall map-reading taken each of these five D parameters into account. If each parameter value exceeds 1.6, it is indicated in yellow (suspicious) and red (abnormal) when the value exceeds 2.6. All D parameters are shown in red in the case of keratoconus (Fig. 10.4).
- **ABCD Keratoconus Grading System**
  This newest classification [15] utilizes four parameters (A to D): anterior (A) and posterior (B) radius of curvature in the 3.0-mm zone centered on the thinnest location of the cornea, thinnest corneal pachymetry (C), and distance best-corrected visual acuity (D). It would be useful to monitor the changes (progression) in keratoconus and assess the efficacy of corneal cross-linking.
- **Tomographic Biomechanical Assessment.**
  Combining Scheimpflug-based corneal tomography with biomechanical data obtained with dynamic Scheimpflug biomechanical analysis (Corvis ST, OCULUS), Tomographic Biomechanical Index (TBI) was calculated using an artificial intelligence approach to optimize ectasia detection [16]. Several studies have demonstrated a higher capability of detecting subclinical (fruste) ectasia among eyes with normal topography in highly asymmetric patients when compared to tomographic analysis alone. The ARV (Ambrósio, Roberts & Vinciguerra) Biomechanical and Tomographic Display showing BAD D (derived from only Pentacam), the Corvis Biomechanical Index (CBI) (derived from only Corvis ST), and TBI. The case shown in Fig. 10.5 is a fellow eye with highly asymmetric ectasia with clinical ectasia in the one eye and a fellow eye with normal topography with-

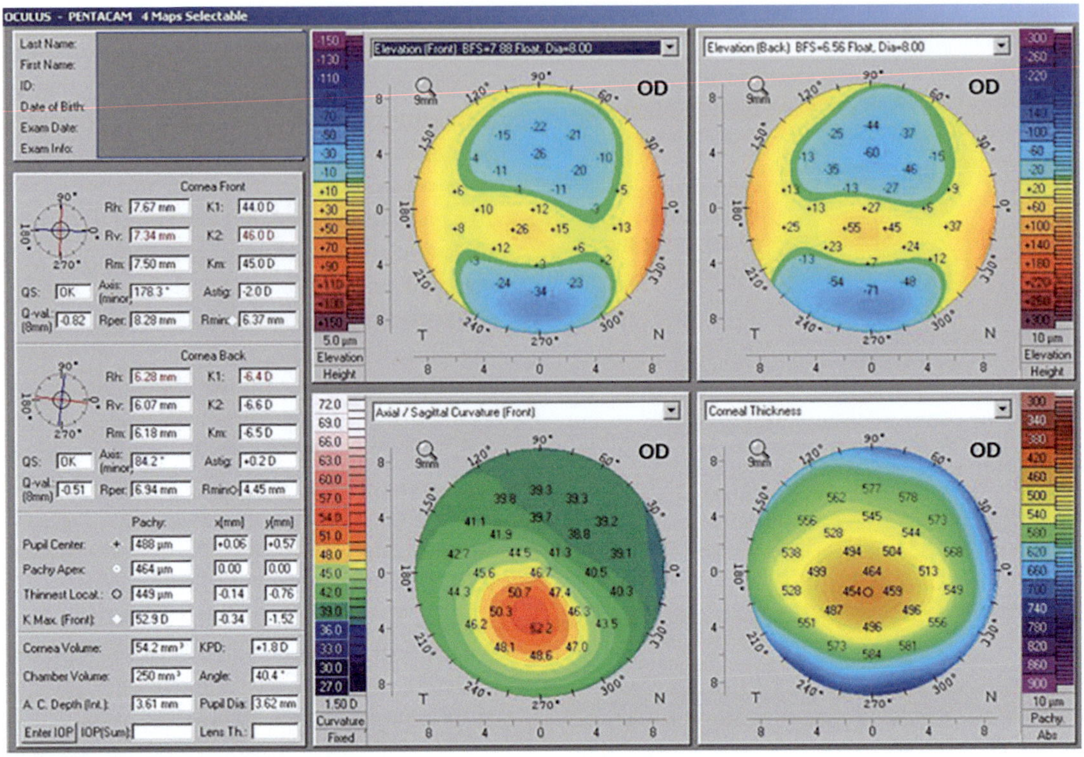

Fig. 10.3 Color-coded map of keratoconus obtained using a rotating Scheimpflug camera (Pentacam HR, OCULUS). Four maps are shown: anterior and posterior elevation maps, axial power maps, and pachymetry maps

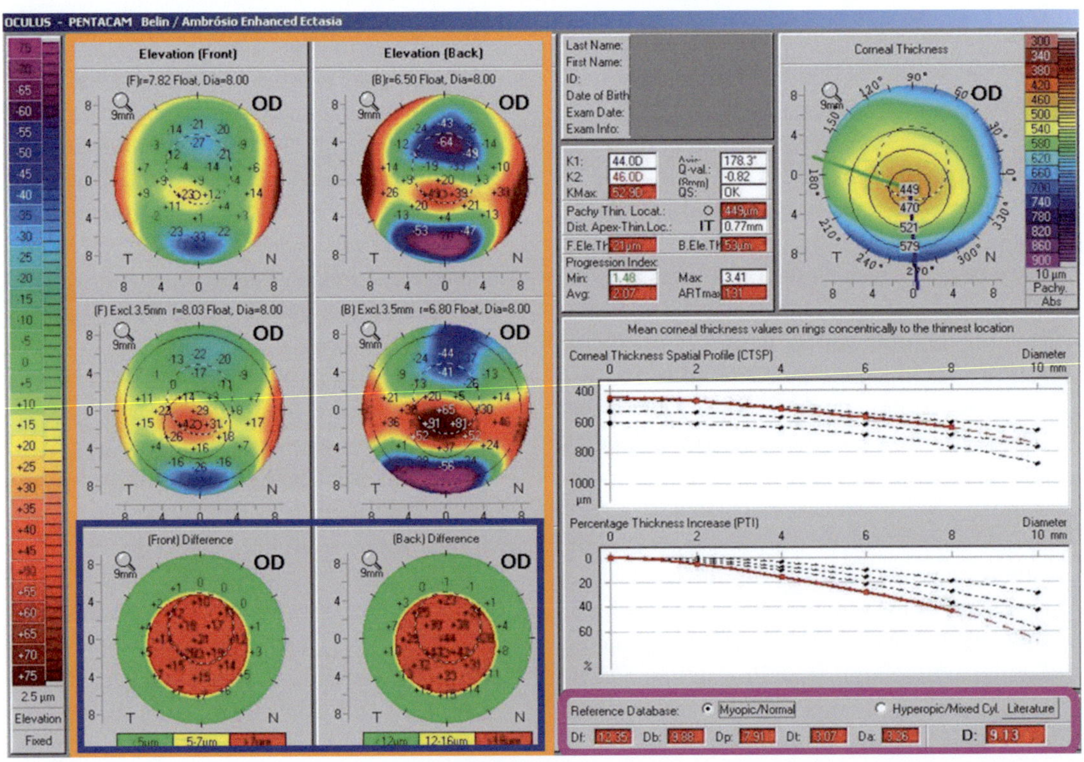

Fig. 10.4 The Belin/Ambrósio Enhanced Ectasia Display (Pentacam HR, OCULUS) for the same data (Fig. 10.3)

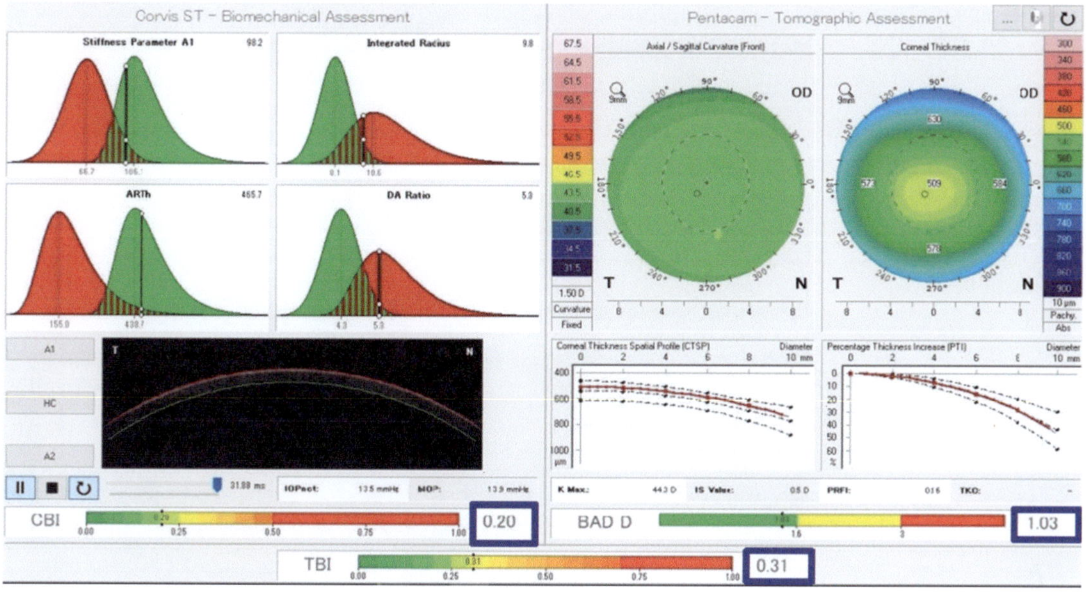

Fig. 10.5 The ARV (Ambrósio, Roberts & Vinciguerra) Biomechanical and Tomographic Display from dynamic Scheimpflug biomechanical analysis (Corvis ST, OCULUS)

out clinical signs [17]. Based on the reported cutoff values (BAD D, 1,6; CBI, 0.5; TBI, 0.29) [16, 18, 19], both BAD D (1.03) and CBI (0.20) values are normal; however, the TBI value (0.31) is suspicious. Thus, subclinical ectasia is detected only in patients with TBI.

10.5 Anterior Segment OCT

10.5.1 Principle

The first report of OCT imaging of the cornea and anterior segment was published in 1994 [20]. OCT can be categorized into two types: time-domain OCT and Fourier-domain OCT. Similar to OCT for retinal imaging, time-domain OCT at 1310 nm was initially introduced for cross-sectional images of the anterior segment of the eye. With the commercial introduction of the 840-nm spectral-domain OCT, imaging of the anterior segment at much higher speeds (>25,000 A-scans/s), and better axial resolution (5 μm) became feasible. However, spectral-domain OCTs use shorter wavelength light sources, optimized for posterior segment imaging, resulting in a more limited image depth range and area [21]. Later, 1310-nm swept-source OCT based on the Fourier-domain OCT type has become commercially available, making it feasible to reconstruct the three-dimensional images of the anterior segment of the eye more precisely and faster [22]. The current generation of spectral-domain OCT devices widely used by clinicians to image the posterior segment can also acquire anterior segment images using anterior segment lenses or attachments. The commonly used Scheimpflug devices are listed in Table 10.1.

CASIA SS-2000 (Tomey) is described as an example. A representative color-coded map of keratoconus obtained using CASIA SS-2000 is shown in Fig. 10.6.

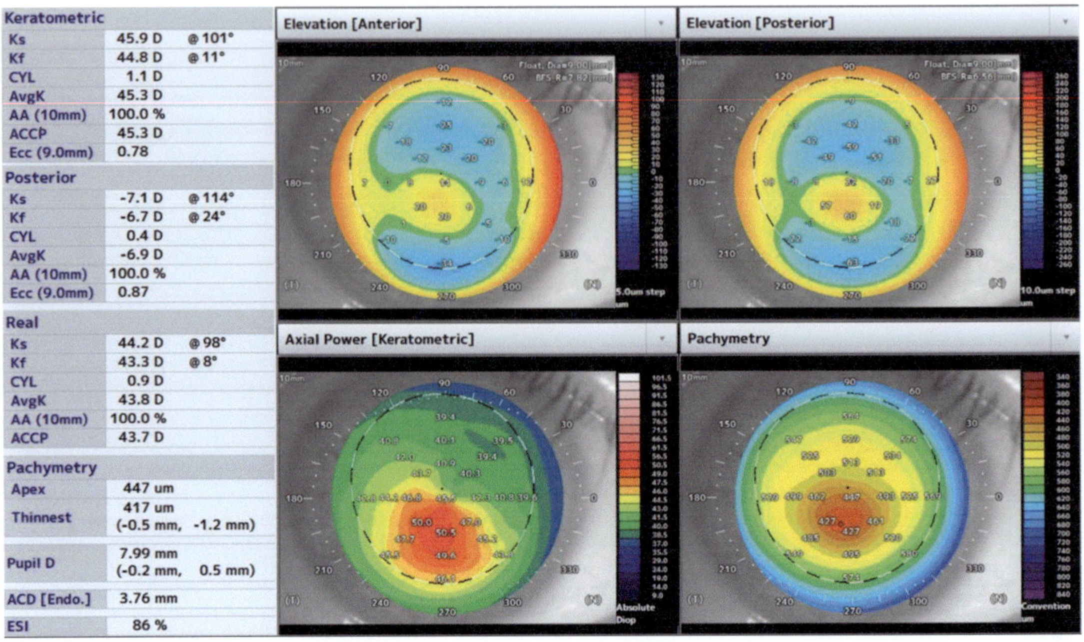

Fig. 10.6 Color-coded map of keratoconus obtained using optical coherence tomography (CASIA SS-2000, Tomey). The same case as in Figs. 10.3 and 10.4. Four maps are shown: anterior and posterior elevation maps, axial power maps, and pachymetry maps

10.5.2 Feature

- The assessment of clinically relevant parameters such as corneal curvature, corneal wavefront aberrations, anterior segment analysis, biometry, and calculation of intraocular lens power is possible.
- With the use of OCT, topographic analysis can be performed even in the area of a severe scar/haze or even when edema exists in the corneal stroma (Fig. 10.7) [23]. This may be a potential advantage of the OCT corneal topographer over other devices for evaluating various types of corneal diseases or eyes, including pre-and post-corneal surgeries.

10.5.3 Application Tools for Keratoconus Management

The application of OCT in clinical practice has been steadily increasing. Herein, unique application tools for keratoconus management are introduced.

- **Fourier Series Harmonic Analysis**
  It can separate and quantify the refractive components of the cornea [24]. Dioptric data from the original color-coded map is expanded into spherical, regular astigmatism, asymmetry, and higher-order irregularity components using Fourier analysis (Fig. 10.8). Among them, asymmetry and higher-order irregularity are components of irregular astigmatism. Fourier indices from the anterior corneal surface in the upper panel, posterior corneal surface in the middle panel, and total cornea in the lower panel are shown in this display. The magnitudes of the Fourier indices of the central 3 and 6 mm of the cornea were indicated and colored as green meaning within the normal range, yellow meaning borderline, and red meaning abnormal. The case presented in Fig. 10.8 is a representative Fourier map captured using OCT in a keratoconic eye.

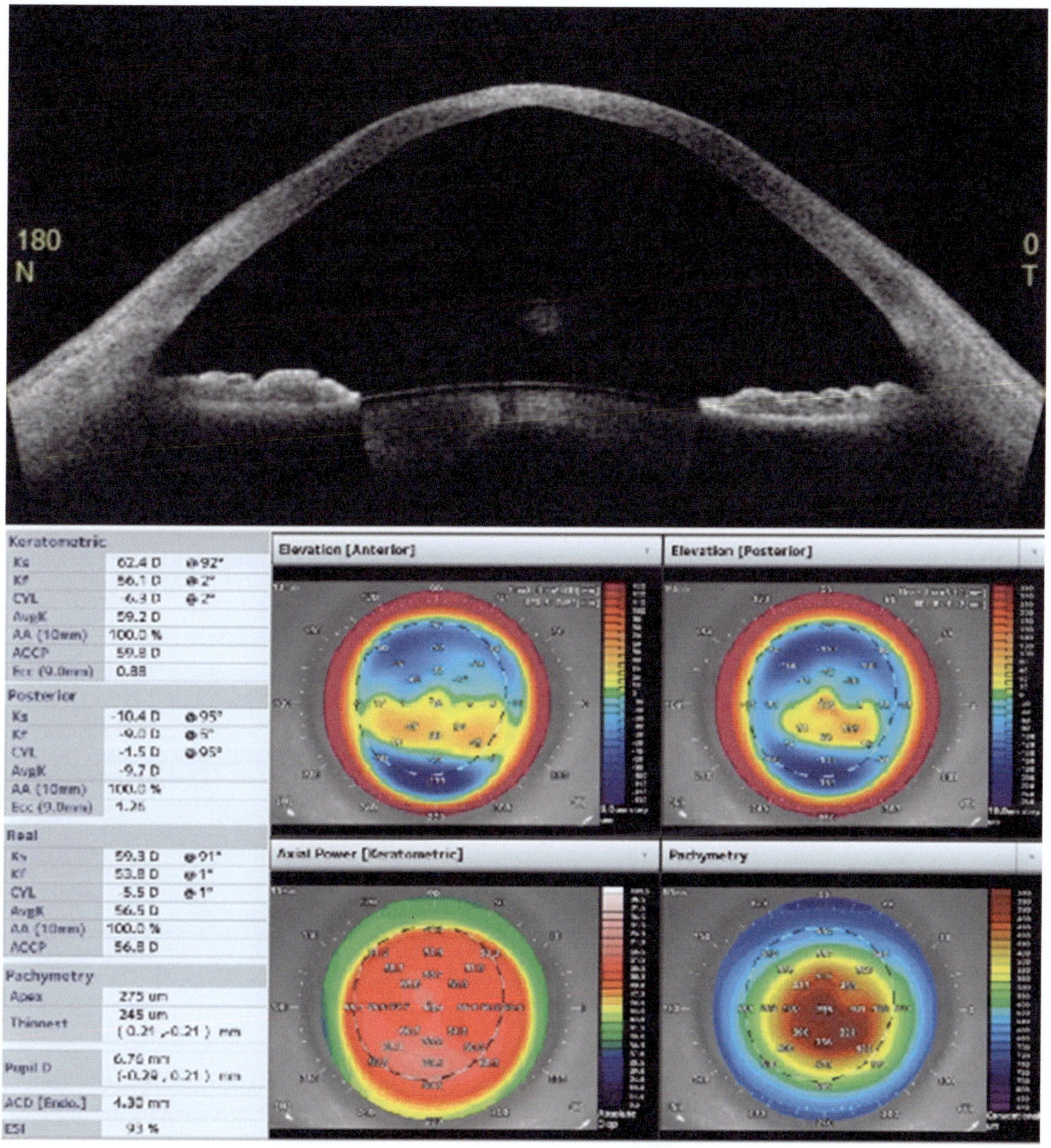

Fig. 10.7 Optical coherence tomography (OCT) image obtained using OCT (CASIA SS-2000, Tomey) for keratoconus with corneal haze after acute hydrops

Moreover, corneal topographical analysis during contact lens wear is possible using OCT (Fig. 10.9). Posterior corneal surface flattening associated with alteration of corneal biomechanics in the corneal stroma during corneal rigid gas-permeable contact lens wear has been reported recently [24].

- **Trend Analysis**
  This application can perform trend analysis of the time course changes patients' corneas based on topographic quantitative parameters [25]. It is useful as a trend analysis tool for keratoconus progression evaluation, corneal cross-linking preoperative indication judgment, and preoperative and postoperative assessment.

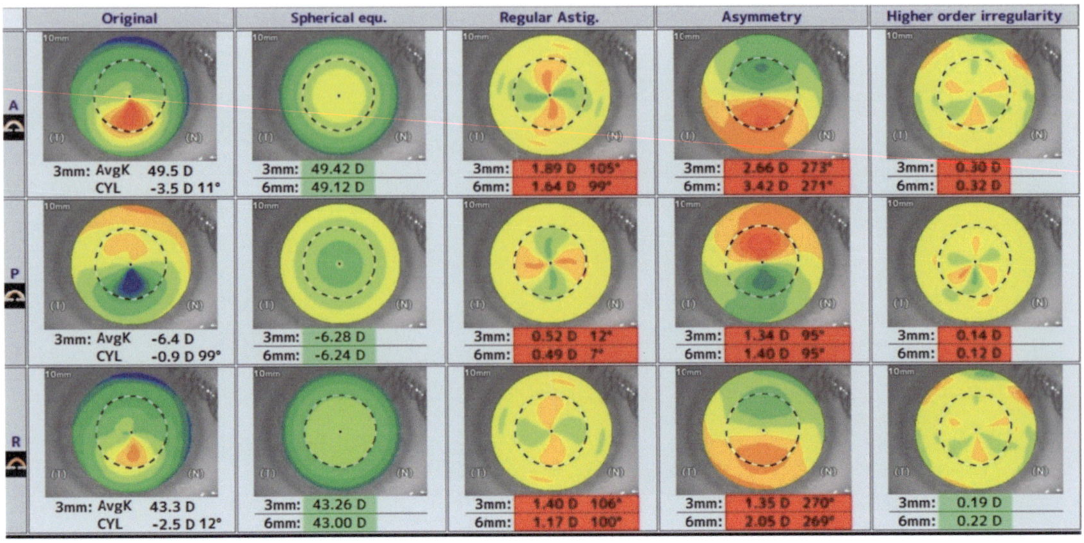

Fig. 10.8 Fourier maps from optical coherence tomography (OCT) (CASIA SS-2000, Tomey) in a keratoconic eye

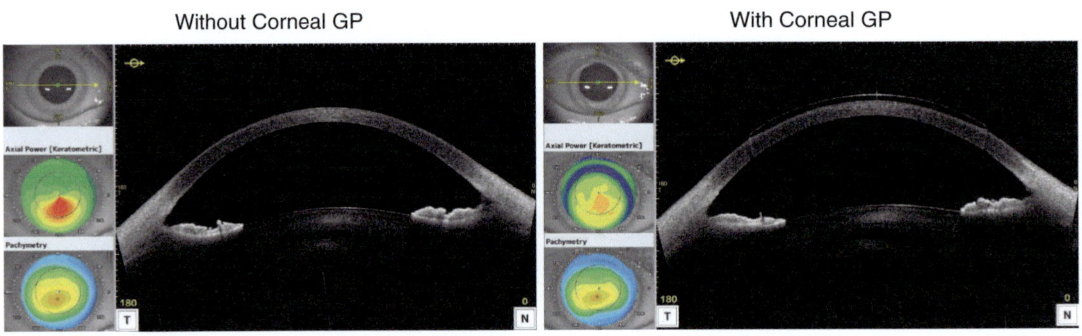

Fig. 10.9 Optical coherence tomography (OCT) images obtained using OCT (CASIA SS-2000, Tomey) for keratoconus with and without corneal rigid gas-permeable contact lens. The same case as in Fig. 10.8

- **Corneal Rigid Gas-Permeable Contact Lenses Fitting Software**
  "Itoi Method of HCL Fitting Software" of CASIA SS-2000 displays can suggest the appropriate base curve values for keratoconus with respect to the lens diameter, based on the corneal tomographic data.

10.6 Combined Systems with a Wavefront Aberrometer

Combined systems of corneal topographers or tomographers with wavefront aberrations that can measure wavefront aberrations of the whole eye are available. KR-1 W (Topcon, Tokyo, Japan) and OPD-Scan (Nikon, Aichi, Japan) integrated a Placido-based topography system and a wavefront aberrometer. The Pentacam AXL Wave (OCULUS) is a combination system that contains a rotating Scheimpflug-based corneal tomography system and a wavefront aberrometer.

10.7 Tips for the Measurements

- The patient fixation during the measurement should be considered.
- The ocular surface and tear film should be ensured to be stable. The patient should

be asked to blink naturally before the measurements.

- The patient should be instructed to open his or her eyes wide, and the upper eyelids or eyelashes should be ensured to be unaffected.
- The measurements should be repeated, and the repeatability should be verified.

10.8 Tips at Reading the Maps

- The quality of the measurements should be checked. In advanced keratoconus or keratoconus with corneal opacity, it is challenging to precisely digitize the corneal surfaces using a Placido-based corneal topographer or Scheimpflug-based tomography, leading to the low reliability of the measurements.
- The color-coded scale [26] for the maps should be checked. Generally, a color palette can be chosen such that lower corneal powers are represented by cooler colors (blue shades), while higher corneal powers are represented by warmer colors (red shades). Green shades represent the corneal powers associated with normal corneas. When comparing the different maps, the same scale must be used; otherwise, even when the change is the same, it can be overestimated or underestimated.
- It is important to observe the topography images of normal eyes without corneal diseases, as there are variations even in normal eyes.

10.9 Final Practical Comment from Specialists

Ophthalmology is a rapidly advancing field with new technologies for diagnosis and treatment. As more advanced techniques develop, the utility of advanced corneal imaging techniques continues to grow. Multimodal imaging should be always applied in detection and diagnosis of subclinical or clinical keratoconus [27]. However, understanding the fundamental tools is always important, and we have to respect previous researchers.

References

1. Ambrósio R Jr, Belin MW. Imaging of the cornea: topography vs tomography. J Refract Surg. 2010;26(11):847–9.
2. Fan R, Chan TC, Prakash G, Jhanji V. Applications of corneal topography and tomography: a review. Clin Exp Ophthalmol. 2018;46(2):133–46.
3. American Academy of Ophthalmology. Corneal topography. Ophthalmology. 1999;106(8):1628–38.
4. Klyce SD. Computer-assisted corneal topography. High-resolution graphic presentation and analysis of keratoscopy. Invest Ophthalmol Vis Sci. 1984;25(12):1426–35.
5. Placido A. Neue Instrumente. Centralbl Prakt Augenheilkd. 1882;6:30–1.
6. Wilson SE, Klyce SD. Quantitative descriptors of corneal topography. A clinical study. Arch Ophthalmol. 1991;109(3):349–53.
7. Németh J, Erdélyi B, Csákány B, Gáspár P, Soumelidis A, Kahlesz F, Lang Z. High-speed videotopographic measurement of tear film build-up time. Invest Ophthalmol Vis Sci. 2002;43(6):1783–90.
8. Goto T, Zheng X, Klyce SD, Kataoka H, Uno T, Karon M, Tatematsu Y, Bessyo T, Tsubota K, Ohashi Y. A new method for tear film stability analysis using videokeratography. Am J Ophthalmol. 2003;135(5):607–12.
9. Maeda N, Klyce SD, Smolek MK, Thompson HW. Automated keratoconus screening with corneal topography analysis. Invest Ophthalmol Vis Sci. 1994;35(6):2749–57.
10. Maeda N, Klyce SD, Smolek MK. Comparison of methods for detecting keratoconus using videokeratography. Arch Ophthalmol. 1995;113(7):870–4.
11. Smolek MK, Klyce SD. Current keratoconus detection methods compared with a neural network approach. Invest Ophthalmol Vis Sci. 1997;38(11):2290–9.
12. Rabinowitz YS, Rasheed K. KISA% index: a quantitative videokeratography algorithm embodying minimal topographic criteria for diagnosing keratoconus. J Cataract Refract Surg. 1999;25(10):1327–35.
13. Wegener A, Laser H. Imaging of the spatial density distribution on the capsule of the lens with Scheimpflug photography. Ophthalmic Res. 1996;28(Suppl 2):86–91.
14. Lopes BT, Ramos IC, Dawson DG, Belin MW, Ambrósio R Jr. Detection of ectatic corneal diseases based on Pentacam. Z Med Phys. 2016;26(2):136–42.
15. Belin MW, Duncan J, Ambrósio R Jr, Gomes JAP. A new tomographic method of staging/classifying keratoconus: the ABCD grading system. Int J Kerat Ect Cor Dis. 2015;4(3):85–93.
16. Ambrósio R Jr, Lopes BT, Faria-Correia F, Salomão MQ, Bühren J, Roberts CJ, Elsheikh A, Vinciguerra R, Vinciguerra P. Integration of Scheimpflug-based corneal tomography and biomechanical assessments for enhancing ectasia detection. J Refract Surg. 2017;33(7):434–43.

17. Koh S, Ambrósio R Jr, Inoue R, Maeda N, Miki A, Nishida K. Detection of subclinical corneal ectasia using corneal tomographic and biomechanical assessments in a Japanese population. J Refract Surg. 2019;35(6):383–90.
18. Villavicencio OF, Gilani F, Henriquez MA, Izquierdo L, Ambrósio RR. Independent population validation of the Belin/Ambrósio enhanced ectasia display: implications for keratoconus studies and screening. Int J Kerat Ect Cor Dis. 2014;3(1):1–8.
19. Vinciguerra R, Ambrósio R Jr, Elsheikh A, Roberts CJ, Lopes B, Morenghi E, Azzolini C, Vinciguerra P. Detection of keratoconus with a new biomechanical index. J Refract Surg. 2016;32(12):803–10.
20. Izatt JA, Hee MR, Swanson EA, Lin CP, Huang D, Schuman JS, Puliafito CA, Fujimoto JG. Micrometer-scale resolution imaging of the anterior eye in vivo with optical coherence tomography. Arch Ophthalmol. 1994;112(12):1584–9.
21. Maeda N. Optical coherence tomography for corneal diseases. Eye Contact Lens. 2010;36(5):254–9.
22. Yasuno Y, Madjarova VD, Makita S, Akiba M, Morosawa A, Chong C, Sakai T, Chan KP, Itoh M, Yatagai T. Three-dimensional and high-speed swept-source optical coherence tomography for in vivo investigation of human anterior eye segments. Opt Express. 2005;13(26):10652–64.
23. Nakagawa T, Maeda N, Higashiura R, Hori Y, Inoue T, Nishida K. Corneal topographic analysis in patients with keratoconus using 3-dimensional anterior segment optical coherence tomography. J Cataract Refract Surg. 2011;37(10):1871–8.
24. Koh S, Inoue R, Maeda N, Oie Y, Jhanji V, Miki A, Nishida K. Corneal tomographic changes during corneal rigid gas-permeable contact lens wear in keratoconic eyes. Br J Ophthalmol. 2022;106(2):197–202.
25. Fujimoto H, Maeda N, Shintani A, Nakagawa T, Fuchihata M, Higashiura R, Nishida K. Quantitative evaluation of the natural progression of keratoconus using three-dimensional optical coherence tomography. Invest Ophthalmol Vis Sci. 2016;57(9):OCT169-175.
26. Wilson SE, Klyce SD, Husseini ZM. Standardized color-coded maps for corneal topography. Ophthalmology. 1993;100(11):1723–7.
27. Ambrósio R Jr. Multimodal imaging for refractive surgery: *quo vadis?* Indian J Ophthalmol. 2020;68(12):2647–9.

Newer Diagnostic Technology for Diagnosis of Keratoconus

11

Rohit Shetty, Sneha Gupta, Reshma Ranade, and Pooja Khamar

11.1 Introduction

Keratoconus is a disease characterized by central or paracentral progressive corneal thinning or bulging resulting in a region of abnormally high curvature and reduced corneal thickness. A combination of genetic and environmental risk factors along with excessive eye rubbing, systemic diseases, floppy eyelid syndrome, allergies, and eczema plays an important role in the evolution of keratoconus. During progression, there is worsening of apical thinning of the cornea causing extreme degree of myopic irregular astigmatism which eventually leads to visual impairment and corneal ectasia if left untreated. It is a debilitating condition that affects the vision and potentially the lifestyle and hence needs to be addressed.

The introduction of Placido disc-based corneal topography has increased the ability to identify ectasia before the development of clinical signs or visual symptoms. But the evolution of 3D corneal tomography along with the ability to image epithelial thickness and Bowman's curvature mapping, biomechanical imaging, confocal imaging, PS-OCT, and Brillouin microscopy has aided in an accurate and objective assessment of the disease. It was possible only through the recent advances in imaging systems identifying each layer of the cornea. This chapter deals with the various imaging techniques that aid in the diagnosis of keratoconus.

11.2 Corneal Topography

Changes in corneal topography due to keratoconus (study of the corneal contour) become evident long before they can be detected clinically, hence enabling prompt identification of ectasia [1]. Topographic indices find several applications in the study of keratoconus:

(a) Diagnosing keratoconus and monitoring its progression.
(b) Ruling out other corneal pathologies that simulate keratoconus like pellucid marginal degeneration, contact lens warpage, and Terrien's marginal degeneration.
(c) Determining the type of procedure to manage progression.
(d) Studying the outcomes of collagen cross-linking on the cornea.

As a result, the need arose to develop topographic indices to diagnose and quantify keratoconus. Corneal topography in keratoconus has been described in detail in Chap. 10. The following is an overview of the corneal topographical indices useful in diagnosing the disease (Table 11.1): [2–9].

R. Shetty · P. Khamar (✉)
Department of Cornea and Refractive Services, Narayana Nethralaya, Bengaluru, Karnataka, India

S. Gupta · R. Ranade
Department of Cataract and Refractive Services, Narayana Nethralaya, Bengaluru, Karnataka, India

S. Das (ed.), *Keratoconus*, https://doi.org/10.1007/978-981-19-4262-4_11

Table 11.1 Types of topographic indices

Local indices	Global indices	Composite indices
Simulated keratometry (SimK)	Amsler-Krumeich staging [3][‡]	Rabinowitz and McDonnell index [8, 9]
Normal: 43.53 ± 1.02D [2]		
Central keratometry [4]	KISA% [9]	Belin/Ambrosio enhanced ectasia display (BAD-D) [9]
Normal: <47.2D	KISA% = [(K) × (I-S) (AST) × (SRAX) × 100]/300	Normal: <1.6 SD
Suspect KC: 47.2–48.7D		Borderline: ≥1.6 SD
Clinical KC: >48.7D		Abnormal: ≥2.6 SD
Surface asymmetry index (SAI) [5]	Keratoconus severity index (KSI) [6]	Roush criterion – Orbscan [9][‡‡]
	Normal: <15%	
	Suspect KC: 15–30%	
	Clinical KC: >30%	
Surface regularity index (SRI) [7]		Pentacam-based Indices [9]
		(1) Corneal thickness spatial profile (CTSP)
		(2) PTI
		(3) Pachymetry progression index (PPI)
		• Mean and SD of PPI-Avg, PPI-max, and PPI-min in a normal population are 0.13 ± 0.33, 0.85 ± 0.18, and 0.58 ± 0.30, respectively. A rapid drop differentiates ectatic corneas from normal corneas
		(4) Ambrosio's relational thickness (ART)
		• Cutoff value for KC is 412 for ART-max
		(5) Index of surface variance (ISV)
		• >37 – Abnormal
		• >41 – Pathological
		(6) Index of vertical asymmetry (IVA)
		• >0.28 – Abnormal
		• >0.32 – Pathological
		(7) Keratoconus index (KI)
		• >1.07 – Abnormal
		(8) Central keratoconus index (CKI)
		• >1.03 – Abnormal and/or pathological
		(9) Index of height asymmetry (IHA)
		• >19 – Abnormal
		• >21 – Pathological
		(10) Index of height decentration (IHD)
		• >0.014 – Abnormal
		• >0.016 – Pathological
		(11) R min
		• <7.71 mm – Abnormal/pathological
Inferior-superior value (I-S) [8]		Sirius-based indices [9]
Suspect KC: 1.4–1.8D		(1) Root mean square (RMS)
Clinical KC: >1.8D		◆ RMSf/A:
		• 0.088 – Suspect
		• 0.13 – Keratoconus
		◆ RMSf/B:
		• 0.212 – Suspect
		• 0.269 – Keratoconus
		(2) Symmetry index of curvature
		(3) Keratoconus vertex – front (KVf) and back (KVb), anterior and posterior keratoconus vertex
		(4) Baiocchi-Calossi-Versaci index – front (BCVf) and back (BCVb)

Table 11.1 (continued)

Local indices	Global indices	Composite indices	
Skew of steepest radial axis (SRAX) [9]		Galilei-based indices [9]	
Suggestive of KC: SRAX>20°		(1) Asphericity asymmetry index (AAI)	
		• Posterior AAI should be within 20–25 μ	
		(2) Center/surround index (CSI)	
		• 0.7	– Keratoconus
		• 0.9	– Pre-keratoconus
		(3) Differential sector index (DSI)	
		• 3.26	– Keratoconus
		• 1.73	– Pre-keratoconus
		(4) Opposite sector index (OSI)	
		• 2.04	– Keratoconus
		• 1.85	– Pre-keratoconus
		(5) Surface regularity index (SRI)	
		• SRI < 1.55	– Normal
		(6) Irregular astigmatism index (IAI)	
		• 0.58	– Cutoff value for KC
		(7) Surface asymmetry index (SAI)	
		• 1.25	– Cutoff value for KC
		(8) Keratoconus prediction index (KPI)	
		• 0–10%	– Normal or suspicious corneas
		• 20–30%	– Keratoconic/ suspicious cornea
		• >30%	– Pellucid marginal degeneration
		(9) Cone location and magnitude index (CLMI)	
		• ≥1.82	– Clinical keratoconus
		(10) Keratoconus probability (Kprob)	
		• 25.55	– Clinical keratoconus
		• 11.60	– Pre-keratoconus
		(11) Percentage probability of KC (PPK)	
		• 45.0%	– Clinical KC
		• 20.0%	– Pre-keratoconus
Calossi-Foggi apex curvature gradient (ACG) [9]			
Keratoconus: >2 D			
Suspect KC: 1.5–2D			
Normal: <1.5D			
Calossi-Foggi top bottom (ACG) [9]			
Normal: <1.5D			
Suspect KC: 1.5–2D			
Clinical KC: >2D			

(continued)

Table 11.1 (continued)

Local indices		Global indices	Composite indices	
[‡]	**Amsler-Krumeich staging**			
Stage	**Corneal surface**	**Induced myopia and/or astigmatism**	**Average *K* value**	**Corneal thickness**
1.	Eccentric corneal steepening	<5D	<48D	>400 microns
2.	No central scars	5–8D	<53D	>400 microns
3.	No central scars	8–10D	>53D	300–400 microns
4.	Central corneal scarring	Not measurable	>55D	<200 microns
[‡‡]	**Roush criterion – Orbscan**			
a.	Thinnest pachymetry <470 μm			
b.	Difference of >100 μm from the thinnest point to the 7-mm optic zone values			
c.	A posterior high point >50 μm above best-fit sphere (BFS) on posterior elevation maps			
d	BFS power > 55D on the posterior corneal surface			
e.	Relative difference > 100 μm between highest and lowest points on posterior elevation map			
f	Keratometric mean power map >46D			
g	Bow tie pattern or lazy C on axial power map with astigmatism shift of >20° from a straight line			
h.	A change within the central 3-mm optic zone of the cornea of >3D from superior to inferior can be correlated to vertical coma being present. Vertical coma is the most common aberration seen in keratoconus			
i.	Composite integrated information which includes the highest point on posterior elevation coincides with the highest point on anterior elevation, the thinnest point on pachymetry, and the point of steepest curvature on the power map			

11.2.1 Types of Topographic Indices

(a) *Local indices*: These are calculated from partial or local topographic data. However, these have low specificity with adequate sensitivity, thus necessitating the development of global and composite indices.
(b) *Global indices*: These indices are calculated from all the topographic data derived from the measured corneal surface.
(c) *Composite indices*: These are calculated from values of several indices.

11.3 Epithelial Mapping in Keratoconus

Anterior segment optical coherence tomography (ASOCT) is a noninvasive and noncontact tool based upon the principle of low-coherence interferometry and used to obtain high-resolution cross-sectional images of the anterior segment of the eye [10].

11.3.1 Classification of OCT-Based Devices

Time-domain OCT helps obtain cross-sectional images by varying the position of the reference mirror as against the Fourier-domain OCT in which the position of the reference mirror is fixed.

1. **Time-domain OCT/swept-source OCT**
   - AS-OCT Visante [Carl Zeiss Meditec, Inc., Dublin, CA, USA]
2. **Fourier-domain OCT/spectral domain**
   - 3D OCT [Topcon Medical Systems Inc., Paramus, NJ, USA]
   - Slit-lamp OCT [Heidelberg Engineering GmbH, Heidelberg, Germany]
   - RTVue [Optovue, Inc., Fremont, California]

11.3.1.1 RTVUE®

It is a Fourier-domain OCT, which gives high-resolution cross-sectional images of the anterior segment. It measures a scan width of 4–6 mm providing a transverse resolution of 10–15 μm. It measures the anterior and posterior corneal curvatures and power with eight high-definition meridional scans acquired in 0.31 s [11].

11.3.1.2 CASIA 2

CASIA 2 Optical Tomography system employs a Fourier-domain method at a wavelength of 1310 nm and measures from the anterior cornea to the posterior lens in a single scan, with a scanning depth of 13 mm and an axial resolution of 10 μm at a lightning speed of 50,000 scans per second.

11.3.1.3 MS-39: A Hybrid Tomographer

The MS-39 combines the advantage offered by a spectral-domain ASOCT with a Placido-based corneal tomography. It provides 16-mm scans, with an axial resolution of 3.5 μm and an imaging depth of 7.5 mm.

11.3.2 Importance of Epithelial Mapping in Diagnosis of Subclinical Keratoconus

Currently, the diagnosis of subclinical or early keratoconus relies primarily upon corneal topography. Previous studies [12, 13] reported cases with seemingly normal corneal topography preoperatively, which developed iatrogenic ectasia after laser vision correction. Elevation in the posterior corneal surface, stromal thinning, and changes in the posterior corneal curvature are one of the earliest signs observed in KC [11]. In early keratoconus, apical steepening is masked by compensatory corneal epithelial thinning [14, 15]. Thus, detecting focal epithelial thinning may aid in identifying early keratoconus. Reinstein et al. observed that epithelial remodeling may mask the alterations of corneal stroma, which may go undetected on topography [15]. This underlines the need for analyzing the corneal epithelium and the corneal stroma as individual entities, to aid early diagnosis and intervention [16, 17].

11.3.3 Imaging the Bowman's Layer in Subclinical and Clinical Keratoconus

Bowman's layer (BL) lies underneath the epithelium and is characterized by significant thinning in keratoconus as well as subclinical keratoconus and disruption or splitting in advanced keratoconus which is due to the alteration in the lamellar structure of the collagen fibers in the Bowman's layer. These structural changes may be noted in the absence of an obvious stromal involvement suggesting the role of imaging of the Bowman's layer for diagnosing early keratoconus. Abou Shousha et al. observed a localized thinning of the Bowman's layer in the inferior cornea of the keratoconus patients [18]. However, the total Bowman's layer thickness could not depict the localized thinning in the inferior cornea. Bowman's ectasia index (BEI) is the minimum thickness of the BL on the inferior cornea divided by the average thickness of the BL on the superior cornea multiplied by 100. BEI-Max is described as minimum thickness of the BL on the inferior cornea divided by the maximum BL thickness on the superior cornea multiplied by 100. They recommended a cutoff value of 80 for BEI and 60 for BEI-Max [18].

11.3.4 Epithelial Changes in Keratoconus

The corneal epithelium is the outermost layer, contributing to 0.85 D of refraction. The cornea is not a rigid tissue and has a tendency to alter thickness to compensate for stromal irregularities. It is capable of altering itself in order to establish a homogeneous symmetrical anterior surface, more so in the presence of stromal changes [19, 20].

11.3.5 True Progression in Keratoconus

Shetty et al. defined progression as either a 0.5 diopter (D) or more of increase in two or more keratometry values in the cone area or a decrease in corneal thickness of 10% or more at the thinnest point between two visits, minimum of 6 months apart [21]. Keratoconus is associated with thinning of the epithelium over the cone area and epithelial thickening in the area of decreased corneal curvature, noted most commonly in the inferior paracentral area. A classical donut-shaped pattern has been introduced consisting of an area of stromal thinning in the region of the cone surrounded by a rim of epithelial thickening (Fig. 11.1a, b) [13]. Progression on tomography as described above in the presence of stromal or posterior elevation is suggestive of true progression (Fig. 11.2a, b) [22]. In cases of advanced keratoconus, there might be a breakdown of the epithelium over the cone area.

11.3.6 Pseudoprogression in Keratoconus

Change in the epithelial thickness can mask the true curvature of the cornea. The stromal elevation can be calculated by subtracting the epithelial thickness changes from the corneal elevation data from the front surface. Recent advances like the MS 39 have made mapping of the pure stromal elevation possible. A change in the keratometry values, in the absence of a true stromal/posterior elevation, may be attributed to epithelial remodeling. Such an increase in the keratometry values on the steep meridian without a true stromal or posterior elevation is termed as pseudoprogression (Fig. 11.3a, b) [23].

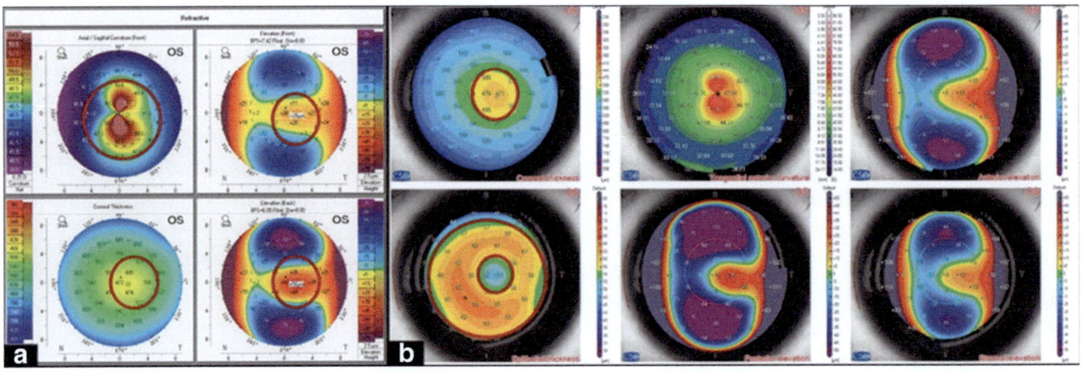

Fig. 11.1 (**a**) Pentacam HR refractive four maps showing grade 2 KC (ABCD classification) in the left eye. (**b**) Corneal pachymetry map of the patient showing by the inferotemporal thinning of the cornea, with the corresponding thinning of the overlying epithelium in cone area, surrounded by compensatory epithelial hypertrophy around the area of thinning known as the "donut sign"

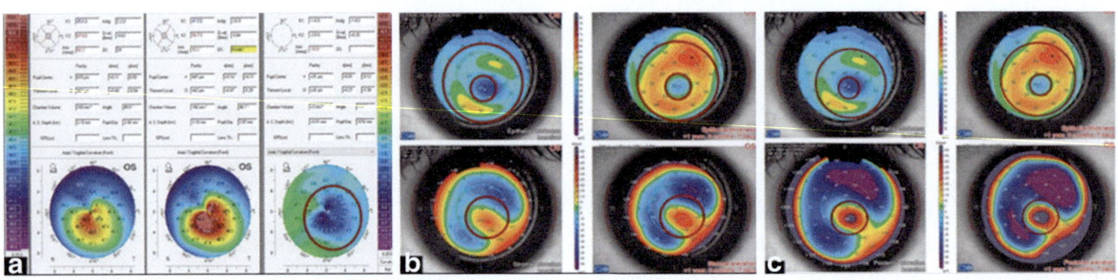

Fig. 11.2 (**a**) OS comparative map on the Pentacam showing progression in the left eye (three points of steepening in the cone area > 1D). (**b**) OS MS 39 comparative epithelial map shows evidence of progression on the stromal or posterior elevation comparative map suggestive of true progression

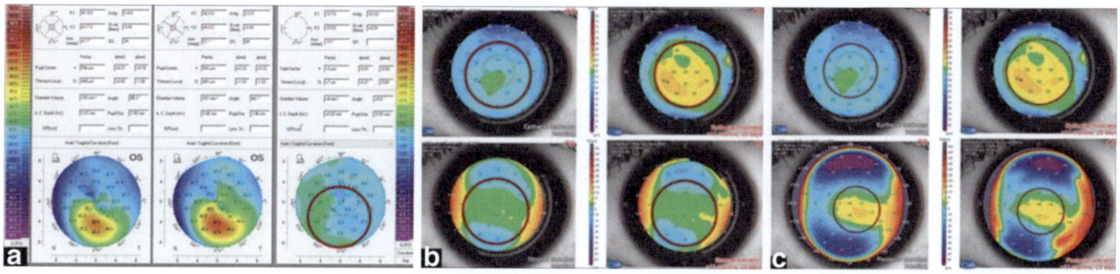

Fig. 11.3 (**a**) OD comparative map on the Pentacam showing progression in the left eye (three points of steepening in the cone area > 1D). (**b**) OD MS 39 comparative epithelial map shows an obvious epithelial remodeling with no evidence of progression on the stromal or posterior elevation comparative map suggestive of pseudoprogression

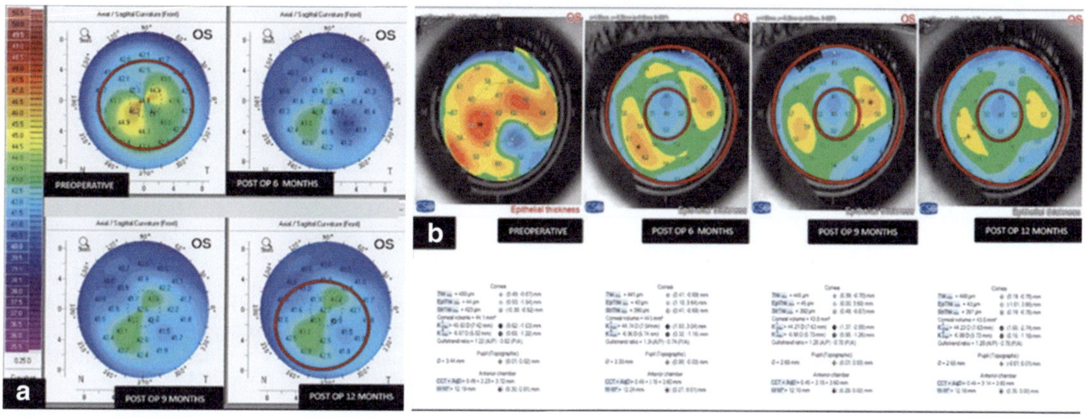

Fig. 11.4 (**a**) OS comparative 4 map on Pentacam HR showing flattening after collagen cross-linking. (**b**) OS comparative maps on MS 39 showing thinning of the peripheral epithelium and epithelium in the cone area after cross-linking

11.3.7 Epithelial Remodeling Post-Cross-Linking

The corneal epithelium has a tendency to change its thickness profile in order to establish a smooth and regular surface. These epithelial changes include elongation of the basal epithelial cells and epithelial hyperplasia. Collagen cross-linking in keratoconic eyes causes epithelial remodeling. Haberman et al. found that there was epithelial thinning in most of the corneal regions at 1 month, followed by epithelial remodeling between 1 and 3 months. They also reported a focal thinning from the baseline in the center, outer nasal, and outer inferonasal regions and a corresponding thickening and thickening in the inner temporal and outer inferotemporal regions. The most significant remodeling takes place over the nasal, temporal, and inferior aspects of the cornea (Fig. 11.4a, b) [24]. Studies suggest better visual outcomes after CXL can be attributed to the epithelial remodeling, due to a more uniform anterior corneal curvature [25].

11.3.8 Importance of Epithelial Imaging in Identifying Keratoconus Masquerades

Epithelial mapping aids in revealing epithelial dysplasia with no stromal or posterior elevation which may masquerade as suspicious topography (Fig. 11.5a, b). This is made possible by mapping the epithelium and the stroma separately. Thus, it

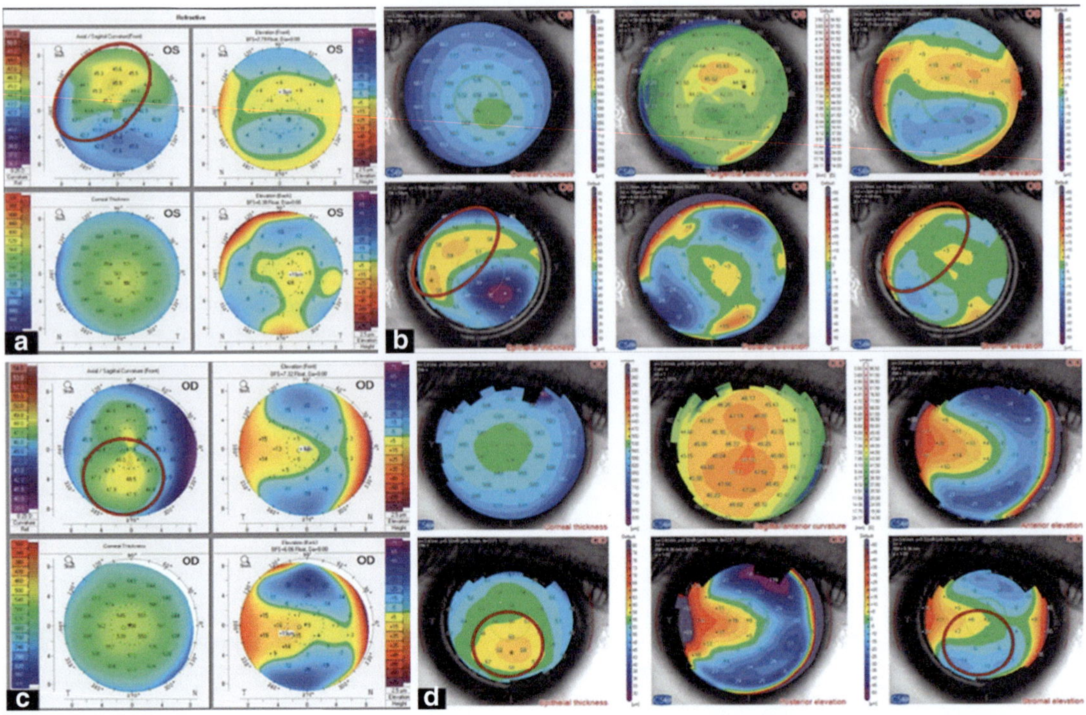

Fig. 11.5 (**a**) OS 4 map refractive on Pentacam HR suggestive of keratoconus suspect. (**b**) OS MS-39 epithelial map showing hyperplasia with no evidence of elevation on the stromal elevation map. This is an example of epithelial hyperplasia masquerading as keratoconus. (**c**) OD 4 map refractive on Pentacam HR showing an asymmetric bow tie pattern (suspicious corneal topography). (**d**) OD MS-39 epithelial map showing epithelial hyperplasia with no evidence of stromal elevation

helps in confirming pure epithelial dysplasia and avoiding the misdiagnosis as suspicious topography [22].

11.3.9 Clinical Applications

(a) To detect early (subclinical) ectasia (Fig. 11.5c, d).
(b) To differentiate true progression from pseudoprogression in ectatic corneas.
(c) To assess epithelial remodeling after cross-linking treatments.
(d) To unmask keratoconus masquerades.

11.4 Corneal Biomechanics

11.4.1 Introduction

Biomechanical property is defined as the response of a biomechanical tissue to a force. Corneal biomechanics is the study of equilibrium and deformation of the corneal tissue to the external and the internal forces. It is the link between structure and function of the cornea. The epithelial cell layers indirectly play a role in biomechanics by regulating corneal hydration. The collagen fibers in the Bowman's membrane and the stroma and ground matrix or the extracellular matrix determine the biomechanical properties.

Ectasia is characterized by progressive distortion of corneal curvature due to a weaker cornea [26]. There is progressive reduction in collagen producing keratocytes as well as disruption of well-organized and arranged collagen, decrease in mean fibril diameter and interfibrillar spacing of individual collagen, and undulation of collagen lamellae. This is due to keratocyte apoptosis with abnormal regulation of collagenase, protease, and tissue inhibitors of MMP1 and MMP3. Biomechanical stability of the cornea is affected by all these factors [26, 27].

The pathophysiology of ectatic disease is primarily associated with changes in the microstructure and biomechanical properties. The architectural and morphological instability (curvature, elevation, and pachymetry changes) is secondary to it. Thus, biomechanical assessment is essential to improve the ability to identify the susceptibility of the cornea to develop keratoconus. Therefore, understanding the corneal biomechanical behavior is essential for detection of subclinical keratoconus as well as keratoconus [27].

11.4.2 Ocular Response Analyzer

Ocular Response Analyzer (ORA) (Reichert Technologies, Depew, NY) analyzes corneal response to bidirectional applanation induced by an air jet pressurizing the cornea. The assessment of deformation takes 25 milliseconds. Corneal deformation is monitored by infrared reflex of the corneal apex of the 3-mm zone (approximately).

11.4.2.1 Application in Keratoconus

Corneal hysteresis (CH) quantifies the viscoelastic mechanical damping effect of the cornea [28]. The mean normal value is 10.0–11.0 mmHg [28]. CH is significantly altered after refractive surgical procedures. The optimal cutoff point for CH is 8.75 with 75% sensitivity and 89% specificity for frank keratoconus [29]. The cutoff for subclinical or pre-keratoconus is 9.80 with 88.5% sensitivity and 88%specificity [30]. Corneal resistance factor (CRF) quantifies the overall viscoelastic resistance of the cornea with an emphasis on its elastic properties. The mean normal value of CRF is 10.0–11.0 mmHg [28]. The optimal cutoff for CRF is 8.45 with 90% sensitivity and 93% specificity for frank keratoconus [29]. The cutoff for subclinical or pre-keratoconus is 8.90 with 89% sensitivity and 93.2% specificity [30]. CRF was found to be better suited for discrimination of frank KC than CH. CH and CRF have lower values in keratoconus as compared to the healthy eyes indicating biomechanical softening of the stroma. As the sensitivity and specificity are poor, ORA needs to be complimented with other diagnostic imaging tools for a more reliable diagnosis of keratoconus. New waveform-derived variables and their integration with the tomographical data have led to better results [31].

11.4.3 Corvis ST

The Corvis ST (OCULUS, Wetzlar, Germany) is a novel noncontact tonometer system. The air puff that is applied concentrically on the corneal apex (first Purkinje reflex) deforms the cornea. The corneal deformation is visualized using an ultrahigh-speed (UHS) Scheimpflug camera with UV-free 455-nm blue light. It takes 4300 frames per second with 8.5-mm horizontal area.

11.4.3.1 Vinciguerra Screening Report

The Vinciguerra screening report shows the following parameters (Fig. 11.6a, b):

(a) IOPnct – uncorrected pressure.
(b) IOP – biomechanically corrected IOP. It has been derived from an inbuilt algorithm which

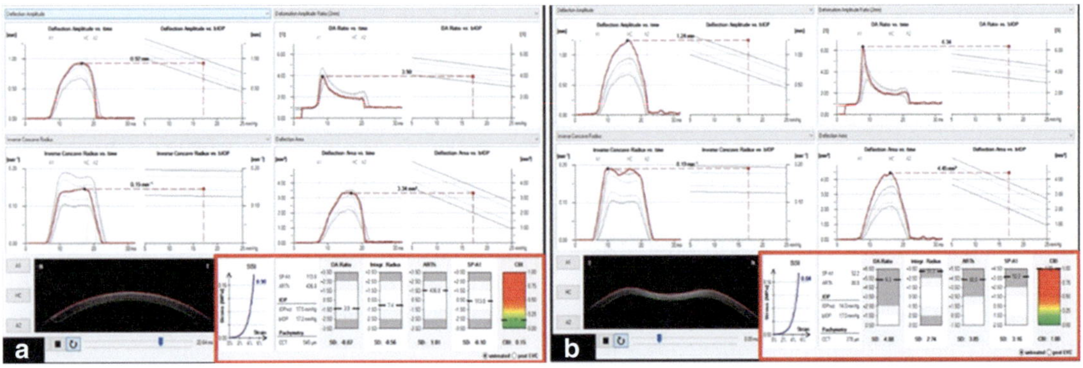

Fig. 11.6 (**a**) Vinciguerra Screening Report from the right eye evidencing normal biomechanical parameters. (**b**) Vinciguerra Screening Report evidencing abnormal biomechanical parameters (abnormal CBI value) in a keratoconic eye

gives the corrected IOP independent of the CCT and corneal biomechanics. It helps in reducing the confounding effects of stiffness parameters and age [32].

(c) Corvis Biomechanical Index (CBI) – The CBI is based on a linear regression analysis of dynamic corneal response parameters measured by Corvis ST in combination with corneal horizontal thickness profile. CBI is calculated using a logistic regression analysis with DA ratio at 1 and 2 mm, first applanation velocity, standard deviation of deformation amplitude at highest concavity, Ambrosio's relational thickness (ARTh) to the horizontal profile, and a novel stiffness parameter at first applanation (SP-A1). DAR2mm, integrated radius (IR), stiffness parameter A1 (SPA1), and CBI have been reported to show high sensitivity and specificity for distinguishing healthy eyes from keratoconus eyes [33].

Cutoff values for frank keratoconus [34, 35]

Parameters	Cutoff values (frank keratoconus)	Sensitivity	Specificity
DA (deformation amplitude) ratio max1	1.61	88%	88%
DA ratio max2	4.82	88%	98%

Cutoff values for frank keratoconus [34, 35]

Parameters	Cutoff values (frank keratoconus)	Sensitivity	Specificity
Integrated radius (IR)	9.41	90%	93%
Stiffness parameter A1 (SPA1)	83.5	86.2%	94.9%
CBI	0.78 [36]	96.6%	99.3%

CBI has also shown sensitivity for the discrimination of normal eyes and KC eyes and the detection of subclinical KC. For preclinical keratoconus, the cutoff value is 0.49 with 68.1% sensitivity and 82.3% specificity [33, 34].

11.4.3.2 TBI (Tomographic/Biomechanical Index)

TBI has been developed using artificial intelligence and is a combination of data derived from Scheimpflug-based corneal tomographic and biomechanical analysis from Pentacam HR and Corvis ST. [37] The cutoff for TBI for frank keratoconus was 0.79 with 100% sensitivity and 100% specificity compared to others [37]. It has presented a better performance in diagnosing ectatic corneal disease and has increased ability to detect early ectasia [31, 38]. It is also useful to detect subclinical ectasia with cutoff value of 0.29 with 90.4% sensitivity and 96% specificity

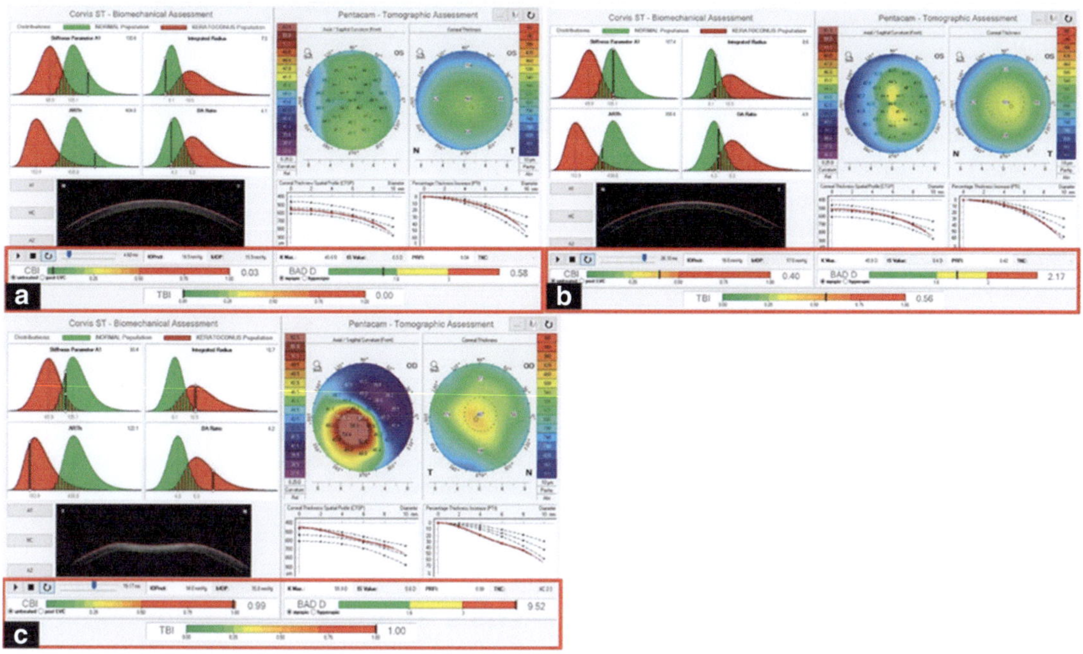

Fig. 11.7 (**a**) Tomographical biomechanical display (ARV) in a normal eye revealing a normal TBI value. (**b**) Tomographical biomechanical display (ARV) revealing a borderline (suspicious) TBI value. (**c**) Tomographical biomechanical display (ARV) revealing an abnormal TBI value with anterior curvature map demonstrating keratoconus grade 3

[37]. TBI, when compared to CBI and Belin/Ambrósio enhanced ectasia total deviation value (BAD_D), demonstrated superior diagnostic accuracy (Fig. 11.7a, b, c) [39].

11.4.3.3 Biomechanics Comparative Display

SSI (stress-strain index) is generated using finite element models simulating the effects of IOP and the Corvis ST air puff. It describes the intrinsic elastic properties of the cornea and shifts to the right in softer corneas whereas to left in stiffer corneas [40].

Normal value is 1. SSI value less than 1 indicates softer cornea, whereas SSI more than 1 indicates stiffer cornea [37]. SSI is relatively stable before the age of 35 and increases significantly with age. Previous studies showed that SSI correlated positively with age, IOP, and anterior radius of curvature and negatively with axial length. There was no significant effect in gender, anterior chamber volume (ACV), CCT, or bIOP [41].

It is a parameter that estimates the overall stress-strain behavior of the cornea and helps in measuring the corneal stiffness. SSI provides a direct method to quantify the deterioration of stiffness within the cone area in keratoconus and how it worsens with progression or improves with cross-linking. Thus, it's a tool to improve fundamental understanding of biomechanics of keratoconus progression in individual patients and helps in better understanding of the effect of the disease and management [42].

The comparative display also helps to study the effect of collagen cross-linking and is helpful in providing documentation of the biomechanical changes post-cross-linking. The blue line represents the preoperative SSI, and the red represents the postoperative SSI. The difference is suggested by the SSI display (Fig. 11.8a, b) [39].

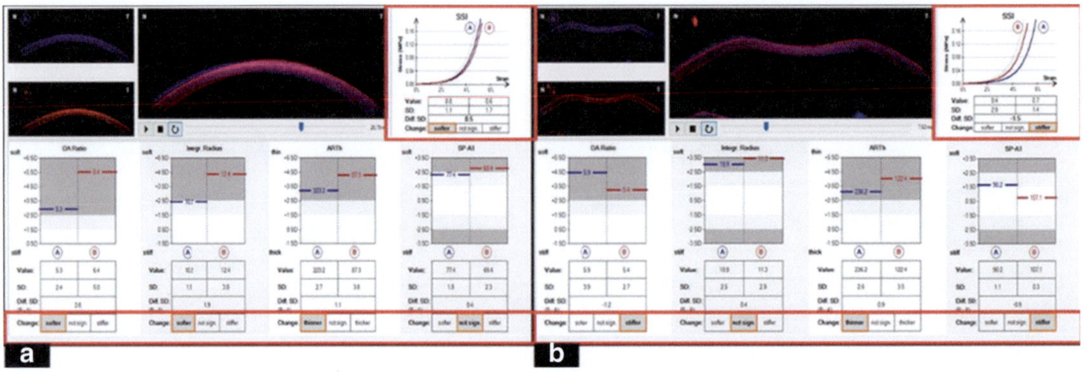

Fig. 11.8 (**a**) Biomechanical comparison displayed from the left eye in 2019 (Exam A) and 2021 (Exam B). Note that the cornea becomes softer and thinner considering the first and second consultations indicating progression of keratoconus. (**b**) Biomechanical comparison displayed from the right eye in 2019 (Exam A) before cross-linking and 2021 (Exam B) after cross-linking. Note that the cornea becomes stiffer considering the first and second consultations

11.4.4 Clinical Applications

(a) It enhances the evaluation of patients with keratoconus and adds to the multimodal diagnostic tools.
(b) The integration of biomechanical data and corneal tomography with artificial intelligence data augments the sensitivity and specificity for screening and early diagnosis of ectasia (subclinical ectasia).
(c) It also helps in determining the prognosis and staging the disease [31].

11.5 Confocal Microscopy

11.5.1 Introduction

One of the major challenges in the clinical assessment and research has been the microscopic examination of the different ocular tissues. The slit-lamp examination technique which has been used for the microscopic examination of the cornea is limited by the magnification factor of 40x. This obstacle was overcome with the invention of the IVCM (in vivo confocal microscopy) which allows a noninvasive high-resolution examination of the layers of the cornea and the nerves.

11.5.2 Principle

The principle of confocal microscopy was first described by Goldmann in 1940 [43].

Marvin Minsky developed the first confocal microscope using the principle in 1957 [43], following which it was first used for studying the neural pathways in the living brain. Since both illumination (condenser) and observation (objective) systems were focused on a single point, the technique was named as confocal microscopy [43]. The IVCM provides a lateral resolution of 1–2 μm and an axial resolution to 5–10 μm and magnifies the image up to 600 times, depending on the aperture of the objective lens used. The IVCM can be divided into three subtypes:

11.5.2.1 Tandem Scanning Confocal Microscope (TSCM)

The TSCM was first described by Petran et al. in 1968 [44]. It was used for both ex vivo [45] and in vivo corneal imaging [46]. TSCM uses a rotating Nipkow disc with multiple pinhole apertures arranged in Archimedean spirals [44]. TSCM has a limited depth of field on account of the small pinhole apertures used. The multiple pinhole openings also result in increased scattering of light. This can be overcome by using a strong source of light and a low light camera. This design however has now become obsolete.

11.5.2.2 Scanning Slit Confocal Microscope (SSCM)

The SSCM was first described by Svishchev in 1969 [47] and used by Masters and Thaer [48] for in vivo corneal imaging in 1994. This technique uses multiple vertical slit apertures for illumination and examination of the tissue. Since the slit apertures allow more light to reach the tissue as compared to the pinhole apertures used in TSCM, even low-intensity light source suffices to provide a clear sharp image of the tissue. The SSCM made possible the in vivo imaging of the subepithelial corneal neural plexus [49]. However, the SSCM provides a lower axial and lateral resolution of the tissue.

11.5.2.3 Confocal Laser Scanning Microscope (CLSM)

The first confocal laser beam scanning microscope was developed by William Bradshaw Amos and John Graham White in the mid-1980s [50]. The CLSM uses two to three mirrors to scan the laser across the sample along x and y axis linearly. A pinhole inside the optical pathway blocks the signals that are out of focus and allows only the fluorescence signals from the illuminated spot to enter the light detector. The CLSM generates high contrast, very sharp, and high-quality images, thereby allowing a better imaging of the subbasal corneal nerve plexus [51].

11.5.3 Confocal Microscopy in Normal

In vivo confocal microscopy (IVCM), a noninvasive imaging modality, allows examination of the microstructure of human cornea [52, 53]. Confocal microscopy provides high-resolution imaging of the five basic layers: corneal epithelium, Bowman's layer, stroma, Descemet's membrane, and corneal endothelium.

11.5.3.1 Corneal Epithelium

Microscopically, it consists of three types of cells: superficial cells, wing cells, and basal cells. Several studies have reported a decrease in the epithelial cell density, with a concurrent increase in the cell surface area in keratoconus [54, 55].

Superficial Cells

These are polygonal, 40–50 μm in diameter with small bright round nuclei, surrounded by a dark cytoplasm with well-defined cell borders (Fig. 11.9a) [56].

Wing Cells

These are the intermediate epithelial cells about 30–45 μm in diameter though they show a significant variability in shape and size. They exhibit bright cell borders with a bright nucleus and a few organelles [56].

Basal Cells

These are 10–15 μm in diameter with bright cell borders and a dark cytoplasm [57].

11.5.3.2 Bowman's Membrane

Bowman's layer is 10-μm-thick amorphous membrane located posterior to the basal epithelium made of collagen fibers and contains unmyelinated c-nerve fibers [54, 58]. On confocal microscopy, the Bowman's membrane appears featureless and gray, with discrete beaded nerve bundles of the subbasal nerve plexus crossing the field of view.

11.5.3.3 Corneal Stroma

The stroma contributes to 90% of the thickness of the cornea and consists of collagen fibers, interstitial substance, and keratocytes. Transparent collagen fibers and interstitial substance form the gray amorphous background of the confocal images. Keratocyte nuclei are 5–30 μm in diameter, variable in shape (Fig. 11.9c, e, g).

11.5.3.4 Descemet's Membrane

Descemet's membrane is the endothelium basement membrane which appears as a general-

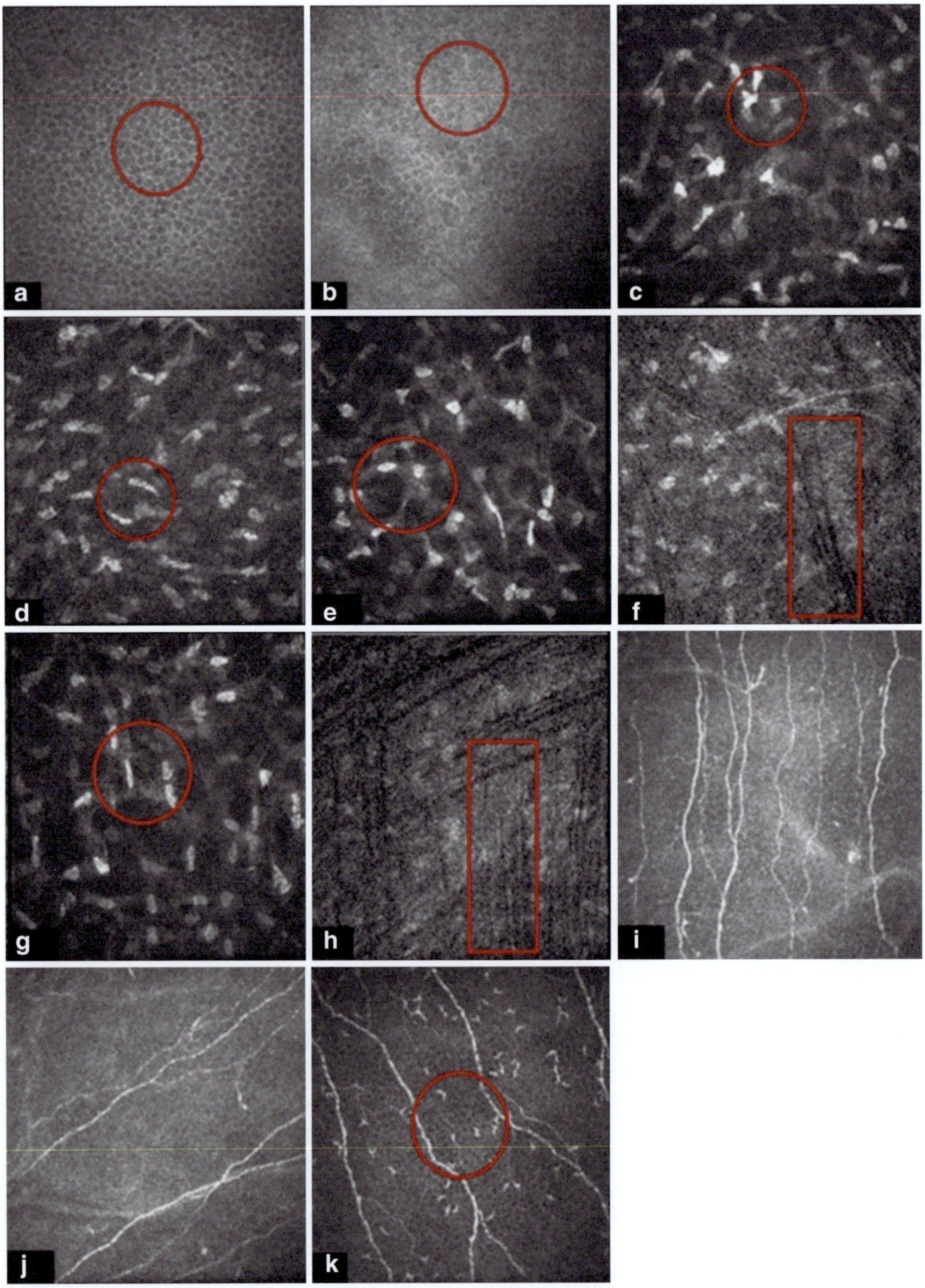

Fig. 11.9 (**a**) Normal epithelium – small bright round nuclei, surrounded by a dark cytoplasm with well-defined cell borders. (**b**) Epithelial cells with hyperreflective borders and desquamation in keratoconus. (**c**) The collagen fibers and interstitial substance are transparent and form the gray amorphous background with keratocytes showing variable shape in normal patients. (**d**) Hyperreflective and elongated anterior stromal keratocytes in keratoconus. (**e**) Showing the collagen fibers and interstitial substance forming the gray amorphous background with variable shape of keratocytes. (**f**) Showing folds in anterior stroma (117 μm). (**g**) Showing normal deep stroma. (**h**) Showing folds in deep stroma (414 μm). (**i**) Normal architecture of nerves. (**j**) Showing diminished nerve density with abnormal architecture. (**k**) Diminished nerve density with the presence of dendritic cells

ized hazy entity with no identifiable cellular structures.

11.5.4 Confocal Microscopy in Keratoconus

11.5.4.1 Corneal Epithelium

Superficial Cells

In severe keratoconus, the superficial epithelial cells may appear desquamating and elongated (Fig. 11.9b) [55].

Basal Cells

Previous studies [52] have shown the deposition of hyperreflective material within the basal epithelial cells. This material is thought to be hemosiderin accumulation correlating to the Fleischer ring in these eyes.

11.5.4.2 Bowman's Membrane

Thinning, breakage, or disruption of the Bowman's membrane may be seen in patients with keratoconus [57].

11.5.4.3 Corneal Stroma

In keratoconus, hyperreflectivity, elongation, and irregular arrangement of anterior stromal keratocyte nuclei may be observed in the anterior stroma in patients with severe KC (Fig. 11.9d) [52]. This hyperreflectivity and disorganization of the keratocyte nuclei may be suggestive of the varying degrees of haze and stromal scarring in these areas. Somodi [56] et al. have observed the elongation of the keratocyte nuclei in the posterior stroma. In addition, folds in the anterior, mid-anterior, and posterior stroma have been noted in patients with severe keratoconus as compared to early KC (Fig. 11.9f, h) [52].

11.5.4.4 Corneal Nerves in Keratoconus

Nerve bundles arising from the trigeminal nerve penetrate Bowman's membrane throughout the central and peripheral cornea. These nerve bundles further divide and form the subbasal nerve plexus between Bowman's layer and basal epithelium (Fig. 11.9i). Corneal nerves are known to regulate multiple pathways, which play crucial roles in several conditions including KC [59].

Decreased corneal subbasal plexus nerve density with increased tortuosity and abnormal architecture has been identified in the cone area in patients with keratoconus (Fig. 11.9j) [60, 61]. The diminished nerve density correlates with reduced corneal sensations in these patients, particularly so in contact lens wearers [54]. CXL treatment causes destruction of subbasal and anterior stromal nerves following mechanical epithelial debridement [62]. Regeneration of nerves has been observed between 6 months and 1 year after CXL, though corneal sensitivity returns earlier between 3 months and 1 year [63].

The Langerhans cells are normally located at the level of the subbasal nerve plexus. These cells can be classified into three types: cell bodies without any processes, cells with short processes, and cells with long processes. The cells without processes are immature Langerhans cells (also known as dendritic cells) that are capable of antigen capture but are able to stimulate the T cells poorly. The mature dendritic cells on the other hand develop processes and are potent T-cell stimulators.

The mature Langerhans cells are seen in the peripheral cornea, whereas immature cells are seen both in the central and in the peripheral cornea. Altered morphology and density of dendritic cells on confocal microscopy have been noted in inflammatory ocular diseases. The presence of mature Langerhans cells in the central cornea suggests the inflammatory etiology of keratoconus (Fig. 11.9k) [64].

11.5.4.5 Descemet's Membrane

Alternating dark and light bands referred to as Vogt's striae have been observed with IVCM in patients with keratoconus [64]. Descemet's folds with polymegathism and polymorphism of endothelial have been noted in keratoconus by Uçakhan et al. [55]

11.5.5 Clinical Applications

It is a noninvasive tool to study the ultrastructure of the corneal layers.

11.6 Polarization-Sensitive Optical Coherence Tomography (PS-OCT)

11.6.1 Introduction

Optical coherence tomography (OCT) is a noncontact noninvasive imaging modality based on the principle of low-coherence interferometry [65]. Over a span of 25-long years since its invention, OCT has undergone a gamut of newer advances leading to faster imaging speed, better resolution, and new contrast mechanisms. PS-OCT is a swept-source OCT based on a fiber-based interferometer. The standard OCT primarily relies upon the intensity of backscattered light or that reflected by the sample; however, PS-OCT also detects polarization state of the sample and gives better image contrast. These properties enable the ultrastructure imaging of the sample which may be below the optical resolution limit of OCT. [66]

11.6.2 Principle of PS-OCT

The unpolarized light waves vibrate in perpendicular planes with respect to the direction of propagation of light. Light is said to be polarized, when all the waves are made to vibrate in a single plane. Interaction between the tissues and the light waves brings about a change in the light polarization. These mechanisms of light-tissue interaction include birefringence, diattenuation, and depolarization. This is how the PS-OCT generates a tissue-specific contrast.

11.6.3 Corneal Imaging Using PS-OCT

The cornea is an optically birefringent structure [67]. This is mainly due to the anatomical structure of the corneal stroma which consists of lamellae. Each lamella contains parallel fibrils that cause form birefringence. PS-OCT provides qualitative assessment of the fibrous arrangement in corneal stroma by phase retardation imaging [68]. Phase retardation is a phase shift introduced by birefringence and axis orientation of the sample.

11.6.4 Clinical Applications

11.6.4.1 Normal Patients

Previous studies [69] show the en face phase retardation maps in blue color, suggestive of homogeneous birefringence (Fig. 11.10a).

11.6.4.2 Keratoconus

Abnormal inhomogeneous birefringence has been noted in advanced keratoconus [67]. The presence of abnormal birefringence in these cases is caused by modifications in the lamellar arrangement of collagen fibers in keratoconus. Such alterations in the lamellar structure of collagen fibers influence corneal shape and mechanical stability of the cornea. Since PS-OCT identifies ultrastructural changes in the collagen fibrils, it may be beneficial in predicting the pre-topographic deformation of corneal shape (Fig. 11.10b).

11.6.4.3 Post-Corneal Collagen Cross-Linking

PS-OCT was used to study the morphological changes in the corneal stroma after CXL treatment. A reduction in corneal thickness, a hyperscattering area in the anterior portion, a slow increase in the phase retardation image, and a discriminable characteristic in the degree of polarization uniformity have been identified, which also provides an estimate of effective depth of cross-linking. Thus, PS-OCT could be a promising optical imaging modality for evaluation of progression and effectiveness of the CXL procedure [70]. While PS-OCT is a promising tool for studying the ultrastructural changes in established keratoconus, additionally, its role in identifying suspect or subclinical keratoconus patients cannot be neglected.

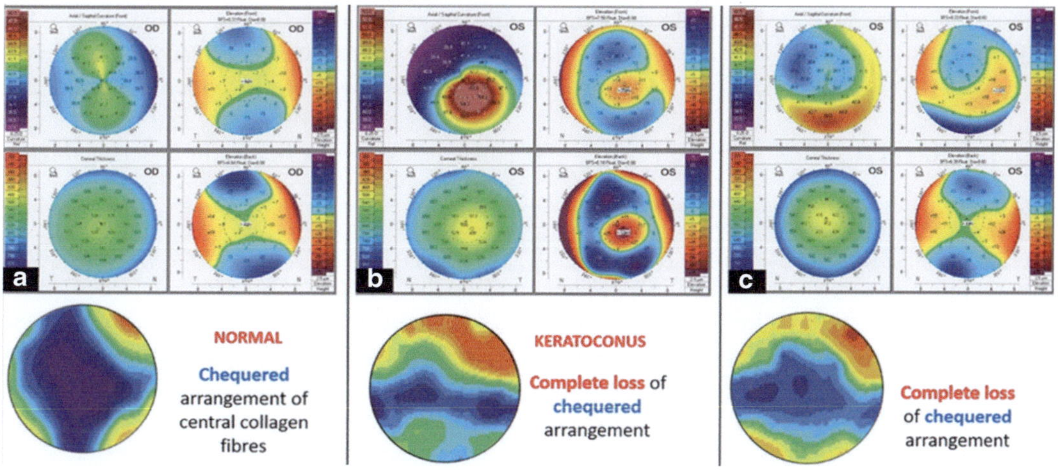

Fig. 11.10 (**a**) In vivo imaging of collagen using polarization-sensitive OCT in the normal cornea. (**b**) Keratoconic cornea. (**c**) Post-refractive surgery (SMILE) ectasia

11.7 Brillouin Microscopy

11.7.1 Introduction

Indicators of corneal health are at present largely derived from analysis of the structural stability of the cornea, through modalities such as pachymetry, tomography, and epithelial mapping. These provide us with a general assessment of the corneal status. However, there is an unmet need for the determination of corneal biomechanics reflected in recent literature, which emphasizes upon the impact of corneal biomechanics on disease and response to treatment. For instance, loss of corneal rigidity has been demonstrated in keratoconus eyes. Furthermore, corneal collagen cross-linking, the current gold standard for arresting progression of keratoconus, is also known to increase the elastic modulus of the cornea and thereby stall the disease [71].

The Ocular Response Analyzer (ORA) and Corvis ST (Oculus) remain the most predominantly used techniques for the evaluation of corneal biomechanics. Although both devices have proven useful in diagnosis of keratoconus, they do not provide direct measurement of corneal biomechanics. The data is instead derived from the measurements made, based on multiple assumptions. Focal regions of corneal weakening or increased elasticity therefore cannot be determined.

11.7.2 Principle of Brillouin Microscopy

Brillouin microscopy helps overcome this limitation. It is a type of optical elastography [72] which relies on the interaction of light waves and acoustic waves intrinsic to the corneal tissue. These acoustic waves are generated due to thermal fluctuations of the molecules. This results in modulation of the refractive index, and reflection of light from this modulation causes a Doppler frequency shift, also known as the Brillouin frequency. The Brillouin microscopy employs a focused laser beam (near-infrared – 780 nm) and a confocal spectrometer to measure the Brillouin frequency at the focal point. This frequency is directly proportional to the speed of acoustic propagation in the tissue at the focal point, thus providing a direct measurement of the longitudinal modulus of the tissue at that point. In short, the technique analyzes the spectral shift of the laser beam when it is reflected from a focal point of the tissue. This shift is directly proportional to the longitudinal modulus or mechanical compressibility of tissue. On the basis of this, confocal imaging is used to create a volumetric map of the elastic properties of the cornea.

11.7.3 Clinical Applications [73]

11.7.3.1 Screening/Diagnosis of Corneal Disease

Early research has shown that Brillouin measurements vary in the cone region as compared to other corneal foci. The average Brillouin frequency of keratoconus eyes has been found to be lower compared to normal eyes, with increasing variation with increase in the severity of disease. This is particularly evident in the cone region. Thus, alterations in biomechanical properties detected through Brillouin measurements may aid in early detection of keratoconus [74].

11.7.3.2 Monitoring Response to Corneal Cross-Linking

Changes in biomechanical properties post-cross-linking may further guide the course of treatment in these patients. Studies conducted have demonstrated return of longitudinal moduli of cross-linked corneas to the normal range. As assessment of depth of penetration after treatment is difficult and cannot be accurately measured by slit-lamp exam or optical coherence tomography (OCT), Brillouin spectroscopy may assist in more precise measurements of the treated area. This may help provide more customized treatment to the patient instead of relying on a nonspecific protocol [75].

11.7.3.3 Advantages

(a) Direct assessment of localized tissue.
(b) Evaluation of focal points.
(c) No physical contact.

11.8 MMP-9 Kit Useful in the Diagnosis of Molecular Markers for Keratoconus

Tear fluid is an important source of information to understand ocular physiology through various disease-specific molecular signatures that help in understanding the etiology of the disease and thus help in prognosis. Molecular markers of keratoconus have been identified in the tear film. Thus, these biomarkers in the tear film of keratoconus patients have helped in understanding the etiopathogenesis as well as the prognosis of the disease.

Keratoconus is characterized by tissue degradation that involves extracellular matrix remodeling and collagen deficiency. There are increased roles of pro-inflammatory cytokines, cell adhesion molecules, and matrix metalloproteinases in the pathogenesis of the disease [76]. Interleukin-6, TNF-α, and MMP-9 are overexpressed in the tears of patients with keratoconus, indicating that the pathogenesis of keratoconus may involve chronic inflammatory events [77]. Thus, a variety of matrix metalloproteinases (MMP-1, MMP-3, MMP-7, MMP-13), interleukins (IL-4, IL-5, IL-6, IL-8), and tumor necrosis factor (TNF-α and TNF-β) are elevated in keratoconus tears, and the extent of increase has been associated with the severity of the disease. The MMP-9 kits are lateral flow immunoassays (LFIA), which aim to detect both active and latent forms of human MMP-9, amounting to more than 40 ng/ml in a 10 μl sample, and provide both quantitative and quantitative results [78]. Owing to the ease of collection of samples in a noninvasive manner as well as diagnostic and prognostic value of biomarkers present, tear fluid is considered as the ideal biological fluid to provide insight into the pathology. Thus, biomarker detection kits with diagnostic and prognostic value aid in the diagnosis, prognosis, and treatment of keratoconus [78].

There are other tear biomarker test kits available that help in diagnosing various ocular conditions. The total tear IgE test kit is a useful auxiliary method for diagnosis of allergic conjunctival diseases (ACD) [79].

The Human Cytokine Kit (EMD Millipore Corporation, Billerica, MA), which comprises of a 96-well plate and assesses the level of tear cytokines, has proven to be useful in the diagnosis, classification, and analysis of treatment efficacy in a variety of inflammatory conditions afflicting the ocular surface [80].

The FluroProfile Protein Quantification Kit has been used in measurement of total tear protein. The ELISA (enzyme-linked immunosorbent assay) Kit has also been devised to measure SFRP1 in the tears of patients as these tear protein profiles are altered in KC [81].

References

1. Krachmer JH, Feder RS, Belin MW. Keratoconus and related noninflammatory corneal thinning disorders. Surv Ophthalmol. 1984;28(4):293–322.
2. Smolek MK, Klyce SD. Current keratoconus detection methods compared with a neural network approach. Invest Ophthalmol Vis Sci. 1997;38(11):2290–9.
3. Amsler M. The "forme fruste" of keratoconus. Wien Klin Wochenschr. 1961;73:842–3.
4. Maeda N, Klyce SD, Smolek MK, Thompson HW. Automated keratoconus screening with corneal topography analysis. Invest Ophthalmol Vis Sci. 1994;35(6):2749–57.
5. Dingeldein SA, Klyce SD, Wilson SE. Quantitative descriptors of corneal shape derived from computer-assisted analysis of photokeratographs. Refract Corneal Surg. 1989;5(6):372–8.
6. Cavas-Martínez F, De la Cruz SE, Nieto Martínez J, Fernández Cañavate FJ, Fernández-Pacheco DG. Corneal topography in keratoconus: state of the art. Eye Vis (Lond). 2016;3:5.
7. Wilson SE, Lin DT, Klyce SD. Corneal topography of keratoconus. Cornea. 1991;10(1):2–8.
8. Rabinowitz YS, McDonnell PJ. Computer-assisted corneal topography in keratoconus. Refract Corneal Surg. 1989;5(6):400–8.
9. Doctor K, Vunnava KP, Shroff R, Kaweri L, Lalgudi VG, Gupta K, Kundu G. Simplifying and understanding various topographic indices for keratoconus using Scheimpflug based topographers. Indian J Ophthalmol. 2020;68(12):2732–43.
10. Izatt JA, Hee MR, Swanson EA, Lin CP, Huang D, Schuman JS, Puliafito CA, Fujimoto JG. Micrometer-scale resolution imaging of the anterior eye in vivo with optical coherence tomography. Arch Ophthalmol. 1994;112(12):1584–9.
11. Matalia H, Swarup R. Imaging modalities in keratoconus. Indian J Ophthalmol. 2013;61(8):394–400.
12. Mas Tur V, MacGregor C, Jayaswal R, O'Brart D, Maycock N. A review of keratoconus: diagnosis, pathophysiology, and genetics. Surv Ophthalmol. 2017;62(6):770–83.
13. Reinstein DZ, Gobbe M, Archer TJ, Silverman RH, Coleman DJ. Epithelial, stromal, and total corneal thickness in keratoconus: three-dimensional display with Artemis very-high frequency digital ultrasound. J Refract Surg. 2010;26(4):259–71.
14. Sandali O, El Sanharawi M, Temstet C, Hamiche T, Galan A, Ghouali W, Goemaere I, Basli E, Borderie V, Laroche L. Fourier-domain optical coherence tomography imaging in keratoconus: a corneal structural classification. Ophthalmology. 2013;120(12):2403–12.
15. Reinstein DZ, Silverman RH, Sutton HF, Coleman DJ. Very high-frequency ultrasound corneal analysis identifies anatomic correlates of optical complications of lamellar refractive surgery: anatomic diagnosis in lamellar surgery. Ophthalmology. 1999;106(3):474–82.
16. Silverman RH, Urs R, Roychoudhury A, Archer TJ, Gobbe M, Reinstein DZ. Epithelial remodeling as basis for machine-based identification of keratoconus. Invest Ophthalmol Vis Sci. 2014;55(3):1580–7.
17. Reinstein DZ, Archer TJ, Gobbe M. Corneal epithelial thickness profile in the diagnosis of keratoconus. J Refract Surg. 2009;25(7):604–10.
18. Abou Shousha M, Perez VL, Fraga Santini Canto AP, Vaddavalli PK, Sayyad FE, Cabot F, Feuer WJ, Wang J, Yoo SH. The use of Bowman's layer vertical topographic thickness map in the diagnosis of keratoconus. Ophthalmology. 2014;121(5):988–93.
19. Gauthier CA, Holden BA, Epstein D, Tengroth B, Fagerholm P, Hamberg-Nyström H. Factors affecting epithelial hyperplasia after photorefractive keratectomy. J Cataract Refract Surg. 1997;23(7):1042–50.
20. Lohmann CP, Reischl U, Marshall J. Regression and epithelial hyperplasia after myopic photorefractive keratectomy in a human cornea. J Cataract Refract Surg. 1999;25(5):712–5.
21. Shetty R, D'Souza S, Srivastava S, Ashwini R. Topography-guided custom ablation treatment for treatment of keratoconus. Indian J Ophthalmol. 2013;61(8):445–50.
22. Khamar P, Rao K, Wadia K, Dalal R, Grover T, Versaci F, Gupta K. Advanced epithelial mapping for refractive surgery. Indian J Ophthalmol. 2020;68(12):2819–30.
23. Li Y, Chamberlain W, Tan O, Brass R, Weiss JL, Huang D. Subclinical keratoconus detection by pattern analysis of corneal and epithelial thickness maps with optical coherence tomography. J Cataract Refract Surg. 2016;42(2):284–95.
24. Haberman ID, Lang PZ, Broncano AF, Kim SW, Hafezi F, Randleman JB. Epithelial remodeling after corneal crosslinking using higher fluence and accelerated treatment time. J Cataract Refract Surg. 2018;44(3):306–12.
25. Hwang ES, Schallhorn JM, Randleman JB. Utility of regional epithelial thickness measurements in corneal evaluations. Surv Ophthalmol. 2020;65(2):187–204.
26. Roberts CJ, Dupps WJ Jr. Biomechanics of corneal ectasia and biomechanical treatments. J Cataract Refract Surg. 2014;40(6):991–8.
27. Bao F, Geraghty B, Wang Q, Elsheikh A. Consideration of corneal biomechanics in the diagnosis and management of keratoconus: is it important? Eye Vis (Lond). 2016;3:18.

28. Lau W, Pye D. A clinical description of ocular response Analyzer measurements. Invest Ophthalmol Vis Sci. 2011;52(6):2911–6.
29. Mohammadpour M, Etesami I, Yavari Z, Naderan M, Abdollahinia F, Jabbarvand M. Ocular response analyzer parameters in healthy, keratoconus suspect and manifest keratoconus eyes. Oman J Ophthalmol. 2015;8(2):102–6.
30. Labiris G, Giarmoukakis A, Gatzioufas Z, Sideroudi H, Kozobolis V, Seitz B. Diagnostic capacity of the keratoconus match index and keratoconus match probability in subclinical keratoconus. J Cataract Refract Surg. 2014;40(6):999–1005.
31. Salomão MQ, Hofling-Lima AL, Gomes Esporcatte LP, Lopes B, Vinciguerra R, Vinciguerra P, Bühren J, Sena N Jr, Luz Hilgert GS, Ambrósio R Jr. The role of corneal biomechanics for the evaluation of ectasia patients. Int J Environ Res Public Health. 2020;17(6):2113.
32. Vinciguerra R, Elsheikh A, Roberts CJ, Ambrósio R Jr, Kang DS, Lopes BT, Morenghi E, Azzolini C, Vinciguerra P. Influence of pachymetry and intraocular pressure on dynamic corneal response parameters in healthy patients. J Refract Surg. 2016;32(8):550–61.
33. Koh S, Inoue R, Ambrósio R Jr, Maeda N, Miki A, Nishida K. Correlation between corneal biomechanical indices and the severity of keratoconus. Cornea. 2020;39(2):215–21.
34. Ambrósio R Jr, Lopes BT, Faria-Correia F, Salomão MQ, Bühren J, Roberts CJ, Elsheikh A, Vinciguerra R, Vinciguerra P. Integration of Scheimpflug-based corneal tomography and biomechanical assessments for enhancing ectasia detection. J Refract Surg. 2017;33(7):434–43.
35. Herber R, Ramm L, Spoerl E, Raiskup F, Pillunat LE, Terai N. Assessment of corneal biomechanical parameters in healthy and keratoconic eyes using dynamic bidirectional applanation device and dynamic Scheimpflug analyzer. J Cataract Refract Surg. 2019;45(6):778–88.
36. Sedaghat MR, Momeni-Moghaddam H, Ambrósio R Jr, Heidari HR, Maddah N, Danesh Z, Sabzi F. Diagnostic ability of corneal shape and biomechanical parameters for detecting frank keratoconus. Cornea. 2018;37(8):1025–34.
37. Ambrósio R Jr, Correia FF, Lopes B, Salomão MQ, Luz A, Dawson DG, Elsheikh A, Vinciguerra R, Vinciguerra P, Roberts CJ. Corneal biomechanics in Ectatic diseases: refractive surgery implications. Open Ophthalmol J. 2017;11:176–93.
38. Masiwa LE, Moodley V. A review of corneal imaging methods for the early diagnosis of pre-clinical keratoconus. J Optom. 2020;13(4):269–75.
39. Kataria P, Padmanabhan P, Gopalakrishnan A, Padmanaban V, Mahadik S, Ambrósio R Jr. Accuracy of Scheimpflug-derived corneal biomechanical and tomographic indices for detecting subclinical and mild keratectasia in a south Asian population. J Cataract Refract Surg. 2019;45(3):328–36.
40. Eliasy A, Chen KJ, Vinciguerra R, Lopes BT, Abass A, Vinciguerra P, Ambrósio R Jr, Roberts CJ, Elsheikh A. Determination of corneal biomechanical behavior *in-vivo* for healthy eyes using CorVis ST tonometry: stress-strain index. Front Bioeng Biotechnol. 2019;7:105.
41. Liu G, Rong H, Pei R, Du B, Jin N, Wang D, Jin C, Wei R. Age distribution and associated factors of cornea biomechanical parameter stress-strain index in Chinese healthy population. BMC Ophthalmol. 2020;20(1):436.
42. Zhang H, Eliasy A, Lopes B, Abass A, Vinciguerra R, Vinciguerra P, Ambrósio R Jr, Roberts CJ, Elsheikh A. Stress-strain index map: a new way to represent corneal material stiffness. Front Bioeng Biotechnol. 2021;9:640434.
43. Minsky M. Memoir on inventing the confocal scanning microscope. Scanning. 1988;10(4):128–38.
44. Petráň M, Hadravský M, Boyde A. The tandem scanning reflected light microscope. Scanning. 1985;7(2):97–108.
45. Lemp MA, Dilly PN, Boyde A. Tandem-scanning (confocal) microscopy of the full-thickness cornea. Cornea. 1985-1986;4(4):205–9.
46. Petroll WM, Cavanagh HD, Jester JV. Three-dimensional imaging of corneal cells using in vivo confocal microscopy. J Microsc. 1993;170(Pt 3):213–9.
47. Svishchev GM. Microscope for the study of transparent light-scattering objects in incident light. Opt Spectrosc. 1969;26:171.
48. Masters BR, Thaer AA. Real-time scanning slit confocal microscopy of the in vivo human cornea. Appl Opt. 1994;33(4):695–701.
49. Auran JD, Koester CJ, Kleiman NJ, Rapaport R, Bomann JS, Wirotsko BM, Florakis GJ, Koniarek JP. Scanning slit confocal microscopic observation of cell morphology and movement within the normal human anterior cornea. Ophthalmology. 1995;102(1):33–41.
50. White JG, Amos WB, Fordham M. An evaluation of confocal versus conventional imaging of biological structures by fluorescence light microscopy. J Cell Biol. 1987;105(1):41–8.
51. Cruzat A, Qazi Y, Hamrah P. In vivo confocal microscopy of corneal nerves in health and disease. Ocul Surf. 2017;15(1):15–47.
52. Patel DV, McGhee CN. Mapping of the normal human corneal sub-basal nerve plexus by in vivo laser scanning confocal microscopy. Invest Ophthalmol Vis Sci. 2005;46(12):4485–8.
53. Patel DV, McGhee CN. In vivo confocal microscopy of human corneal nerves in health, in ocular and systemic disease, and following corneal surgery: a review. Br J Ophthalmol. 2009;93(7):853–60.
54. Wilson SE, Hong JW. Bowman's layer structure and function: critical or dispensable to corneal function? A hypothesis Cornea. 2000;19(4):417–20.

55. Uçakhan OO, Kanpolat A, Ylmaz N, Ozkan M. In vivo confocal microscopy findings in keratoconus. Eye Contact Lens. 2006;32(4):183–91.
56. Somodi S, Hahnel C, Slowik C, Richter A, Weiss DG, Guthoff R. Confocal in vivo microscopy and confocal laser-scanning fluorescence microscopy in keratoconus. Ger J Ophthalmol. 1996;5(6):518–25.
57. Harrison DA, Joos C, Ambrósio R Jr. Morphology of corneal basal epithelial cells by in vivo slit-scanning confocal microscopy. Cornea. 2003;22(3):246–8.
58. Patel S, Reinstein DZ, Silverman RH, Coleman DJ. The shape of Bowman's layer in the human cornea. J Refract Surg. 1998;14(6):636–40.
59. Pahuja NK, Shetty R, Nuijts RM, Agrawal A, Ghosh A, Jayadev C, Nagaraja H. An in vivo confocal microscopic study of corneal nerve morphology in unilateral keratoconus. Biomed Res Int. 2016;2016:5067853.
60. Patel DV, Tavakoli M, Craig JP, Efron N, McGhee CN. Corneal sensitivity and slit scanning in vivo confocal microscopy of the subbasal nerve plexus of the normal central and peripheral human cornea. Cornea. 2009;28(7):735–40.
61. Mocan MC, Yilmaz PT, Irkec M, Orhan M. In vivo confocal microscopy for the evaluation of corneal microstructure in keratoconus. Curr Eye Res. 2008;33(11):933–9.
62. Al-Aqaba M, Calienno R, Fares U, Otri AM, Mastropasqua L, Nubile M, Dua HS. The effect of standard and transepithelial ultraviolet collagen cross-linking on human corneal nerves: an ex vivo study. Am J Ophthalmol. 2012;153(2):258–266.e2.
63. Spoerl E, Huhle M, Seiler T. Induction of cross-links in corneal tissue. Exp Eye Res. 1998;66(1):97–103.
64. Hollingsworth JG, Efron N. Observations of banding patterns (Vogt striae) in keratoconus: a confocal microscopy study. Cornea. 2005;24(2):162–6.
65. Fercher AF, Mengedoht K, Werner W. Eye-length measurement by interferometry with partially coherent light. Opt Lett. 1988;13(3):186–8.
66. Tuchin VV. Polarized light interaction with tissues. J Biomed Opt. 2016;21(7):71114.
67. Bueno JM, Jaronski J. Spatially resolved polarization properties for in vitro corneas. Ophthalmic Physiol Opt. 2001;21(5):384–92.
68. Lim Y, Yamanari M, Fukuda S, Kaji Y, Kiuchi T, Miura M, Oshika T, Yasuno Y. Birefringence measurement of cornea and anterior segment by office-based polarization-sensitive optical coherence tomography. Biomed Opt Express. 2011;2(8):2392–402.
69. Fukuda S, Yamanari M, Lim Y, Hoshi S, Beheregaray S, Oshika T, Yasuno Y. Keratoconus diagnosis using anterior segment polarization-sensitive optical coherence tomography. Invest Ophthalmol Vis Sci. 2013;54(2):1384–91.
70. Ju MJ, Tang S. Usage of polarization-sensitive optical coherence tomography for investigation of collagen cross-linking. J Biomed Opt. 2015;20(4):046001.
71. Scarcelli G, Pineda R, Yun SH. Brillouin optical microscopy for corneal biomechanics. Invest Ophthalmol Vis Sci. 2012;53(1):185–90.
72. Prevedel R, Diz-Muñoz A, Ruocco G, Antonacci G. Brillouin microscopy: an emerging tool for mechanobiology. Nat Methods. 2019;16(10):969–77.
73. Yun SH, Chernyak D. Brillouin microscopy: assessing ocular tissue biomechanics. Curr Opin Ophthalmol. 2018;29(4):299–305.
74. Scarcelli G, Besner S, Pineda R, Kalout P, Yun SH. In vivo biomechanical mapping of normal and keratoconus corneas. JAMA Ophthalmol. 2015;133(4):480–2.
75. Shao P, Eltony AM, Seiler TG, Tavakol B, Pineda R, Koller T, Seiler T, Yun SH. Spatially-resolved Brillouin spectroscopy reveals biomechanical changes in early ectatic corneal disease and post-crosslinking in vivo. arXiv. 2018:1802.01055.
76. Nishtala K, Pahuja N, Shetty R, Nuijts RM, Ghosh A. Tear biomarkers for keratoconus. Eye Vis (Lond). 2016;3:19.
77. Lema I, Durán JA. Inflammatory molecules in the tears of patients with keratoconus. Ophthalmology. 2005;112(4):654–9.
78. Bang SP, Son MJ, Kim H, Lee YH, Jun JH. In vitro validation of the tear matrix metalloproteinase 9 in-situ immunoassay. Sci Rep. 2020;10(1):15126.
79. Shojio J, Uchio E, Ebihara N, Ohashi Y, Ohno S, Okamoto S, Kumagai N, Satake Y, Namba K, Fukagawa K, Fukushima A, Fujishima H, Takamura E. Evaluation of the efficacy of subjective symptoms, objective findings, and of a total tear IgE detection kit in diagnosis of allergic conjunctival diseases. Nippon Ganka Gakkai Zasshi. 2012;116(5):485–93.
80. Wei Y, Gadaria-Rathod N, Epstein S, Asbell P. Tear cytokine profile as a noninvasive biomarker of inflammation for ocular surface diseases: standard operating procedures. Invest Ophthalmol Vis Sci. 2013;54(13):8327–36.
81. You J, Hodge C, Wen L, McAvoy JW, Madigan MC, Sutton G. Tear levels of SFRP1 are significantly reduced in keratoconus patients. Mol Vis. 2013;19:509.

Acute Corneal Hydrops: Etiology, Risk Factors, and Management

12

Tanvi Mudgil, Ritu Nagpal, Sahil Goel, and Sayan Basu

12.1 Introduction

The word "hydrops" is derived from the ancient Greek word *húdōr* simply meaning "water" and is used in medicine to denote any abnormal collection of serous fluid in a tissue or cavity. Acute corneal hydrops is the clinical condition characterized by a rapid development of corneal edema, with or without intrastromal fluid clefts, due to a sudden loss of the physiological endothelial cell barrier, owing to tearing of the Descemet's membrane (DM). The sudden DM tear allows seepage of the aqueous humor from the anterior chamber into the corneal stroma and epithelium, resulting is bullous corneal edema (Fig. 12.1) [1]. Acute corneal hydrops was initially described in relation to keratoconus [1], but subsequently several other corneal ectatic pathologies like keratoglobus [2], pellucid marginal corneal degeneration (PMCD) [3], and Terrien's marginal corneal degeneration (TMD) [4] have been reported to be associated with it. Recent advances in corneal imaging have improved our understanding of this condition and its pathophysiology. The last few decades have also seen several surgical innovations in managing the condition. This chapter aims to summarize the etiology and possible risk factors, the clinical presentation and natural history, and the management of acute corneal hydrops including all recent innovations in imaging and surgery.

T. Mudgil
The Cornea Institute, L V Prasad Eye Institute, Visakhapatnam, Andhra Pradesh, India

R. Nagpal
Dr. Rajendra Prasad Centre for Ophthalmic Sciences, All India Institute of Medical Sciences, New Delhi, India

S. Goel
Dayanand Medical College and Hospital, Ludhiana, Punjab, India

S. Basu (✉)
The Cornea Institute, L V Prasad Eye Institute, Hyderabad, Telangana, India

Centre for Ocular Regeneration (CORE), Prof Brien Holden Eye Research Centre, L V Prasad Eye Institute, Hyderabad, Telangana, India
e-mail: sayanbasu@lvpei.org

12.2 Etiology

The age of patients at the onset of corneal hydrops ranges from 12 to 66 years, with a peak incidence in second to third decade. Men are affected two to three times more commonly than women, and rarely bilateral cases have also been reported, although simultaneous occurrence is extremely rare [1, 5, 6]. It is now understood that any condition leading to excessive or sudden stretching of the DM can lead to acute corneal hydrops. Based on this understanding, Fig. 12.2 classifies the various etiologies of hydrops as primary and secondary corneal ectasias and as other ocular conditions where corneal ectasia is not the primary predisposing factor [7–19].

S. Das (ed.), *Keratoconus*, https://doi.org/10.1007/978-981-19-4262-4_12

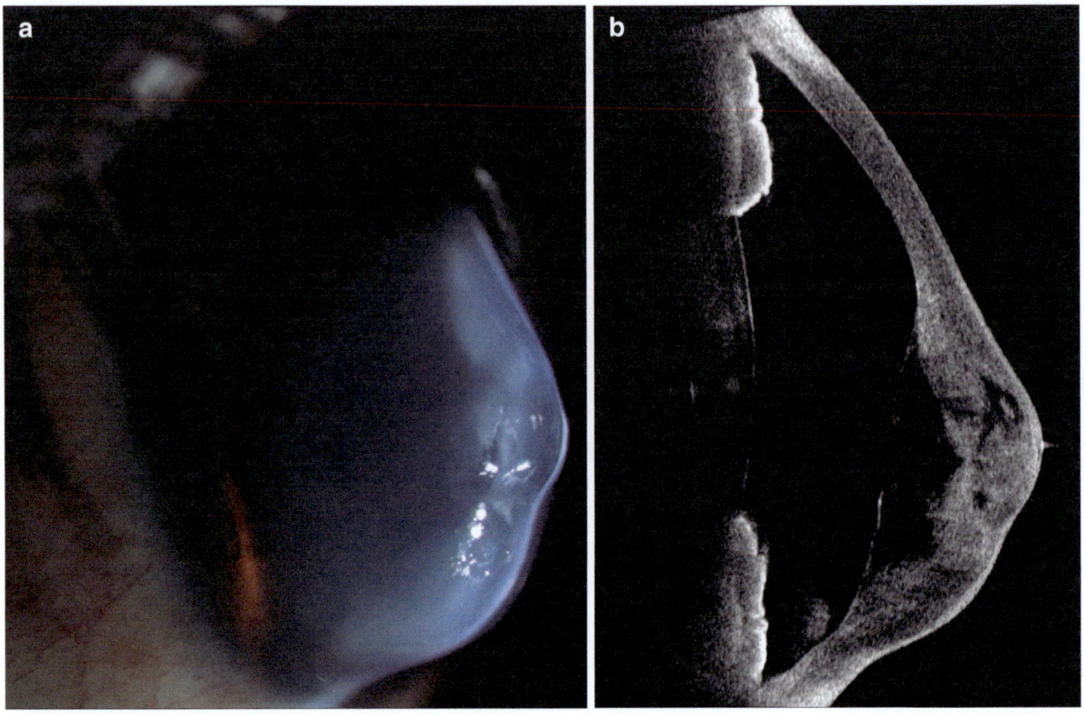

Fig. 12.1 Classic clinical appearance of acute corneal hydrops: (**a**) side view on slit-lamp photography shows inferior paracentral bullous corneal edema. (**b**) The corresponding high-resolution anterior segment optical coherence tomography (AS-OCT) image clearly shows the intrastromal fluid clefts and the Descemet's membrane break with detachment and rolled edges

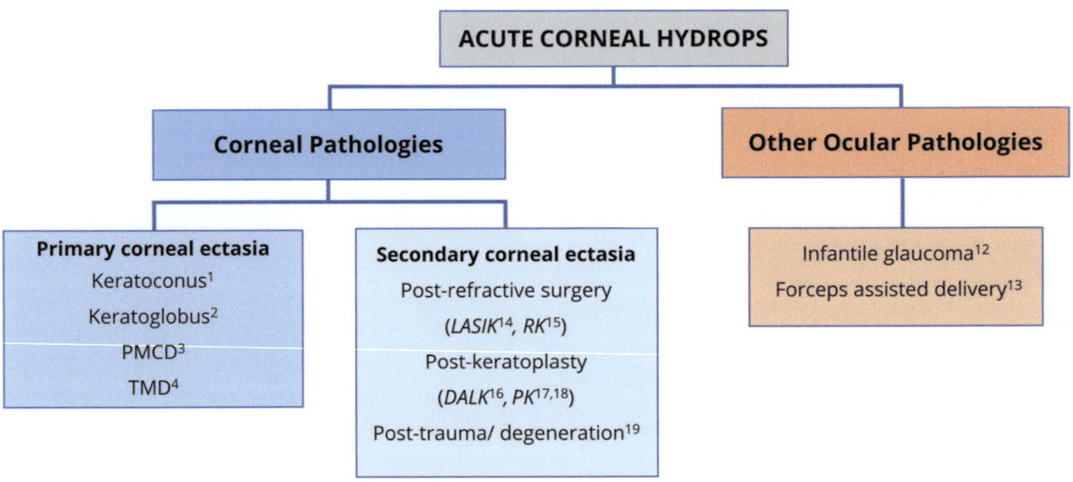

Fig. 12.2 Etiological classification of acute corneal hydrops based on the nature of corneal involvement

12.2.1 Primary Corneal Ectasia

Acute hydrops is most commonly described in association with various primary corneal ectasias such as keratoconus, PMCD, keratoglobus, TMD, and Fuchs' superficial marginal keratitis [20]. The progressive ectasia distorts the corneal architecture and leads to detachments or breaks in the DM irrespective of the etiology of the primary corneal ectasia. The prevalence has been reported as 2.6–2.8%

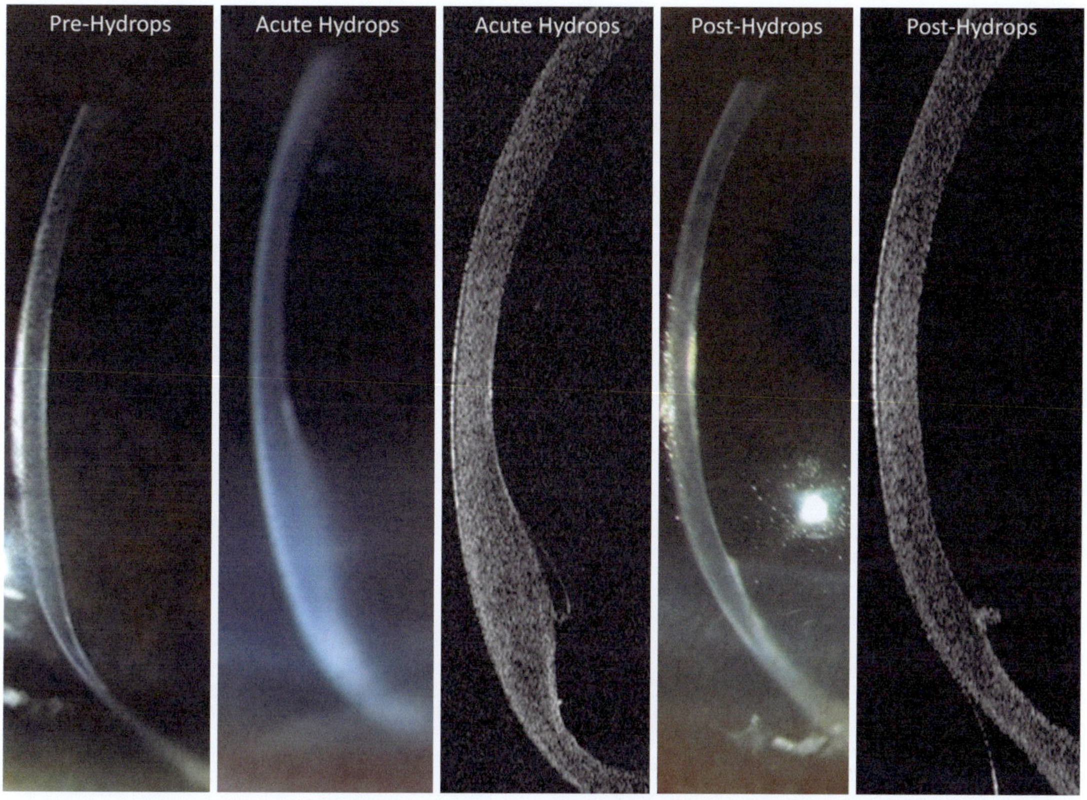

Fig. 12.3 Acute corneal hydrops in a middle-aged adult with pellucid marginal corneal degeneration (PMCD). The serial photographs and AS-OCT images show the spontaneous development and resolution of inferior corneal edema

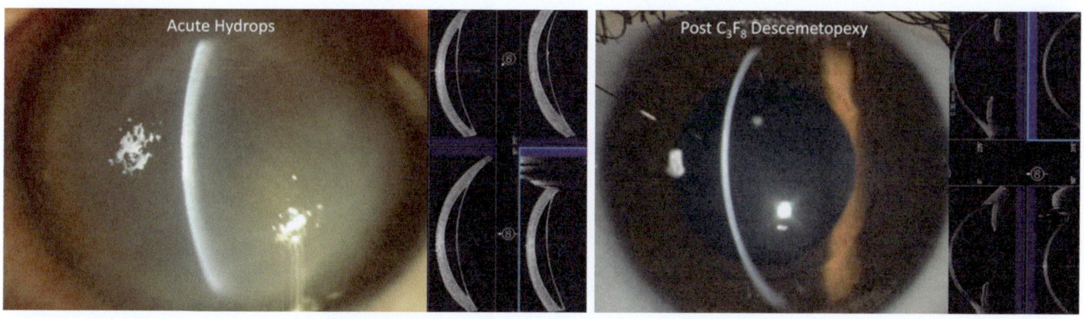

Fig. 12.4 Acute corneal hydrops in a young boy with keratoglobus which resolved with C_3F_8 descemetopexy. Note the global thinning on AS-OCT after resolution

in keratoconus, 6–11.5% in PMCD, and 11% in keratoglobus (Figs. 12.3 and 12.4) [6]. The various risk factors of acute corneal hydrops include younger age at onset [3], habit of eye rubbing [5–8], presence of vernal keratoconjunctivitis [8, 9], atopy [5, 8], advanced corneal ectasia [1], a poor corrected Snellen visual acuity at presentation [1, 5], and Down syndrome [5, 10]. Among these, eye rubbing appears to be the most important risk factor [5, 11].

Fuentes et al. describe anatomic risk factors predisposing to acute corneal hydrops [21] based on high-resolution Fourier-domain corneal optical coherence tomography (OCT) performed in eyes with advanced keratoconus for a period of 24 months. Higher incidence of hydrops was noted in patients with increased epithelial thickening with stromal thinning at the apex of the cone and the presence of anterior hyper-reflectivity at the level of Bowman's layer. Corneal scarring was found to be preventive for the development of hydrops. Epithelial thickening in advanced keratoconus cases seems to be an important indirect predictive factor of corneal fragility and therefore hydrops. Structural classification of keratoconus was established by the same authors based on Fourier-domain OCT imaging in a large series of patients of keratoconus with various stages of severity. This classification is based on structural corneal changes occurring at the conus during the evolution of the disease [21, 22].

12.2.2 Secondary Corneal Ectasia

Acute hydrops has also been reported in secondary keratectasia following kerato-refractive procedures as well as in eyes following corneal transplantation.

12.2.2.1 Post-Laser in Situ Keratomileusis (LASIK)

Post-LASIK corneal ectasia, first reported in 1998, has an incidence of 0.04–0.6% [14, 23–25]. Mechanical corneal weakening due to tissue subtraction after LASIK predisposes to corneal ectasia even in eyes with an advocated minimal residual stromal bed thickness of 250 μm (Fig. 12.5). Enhancement procedures, performed

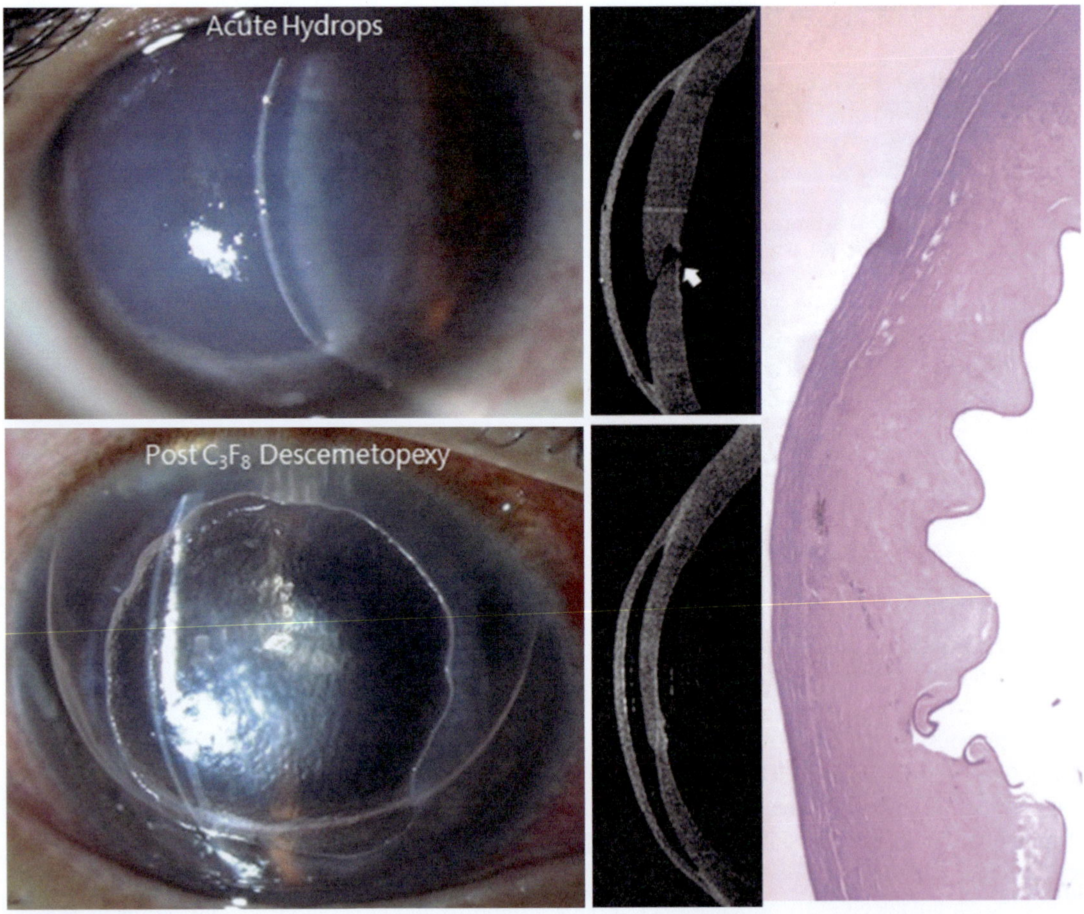

Fig. 12.5 Acute corneal hydrops 16 years after LASIK, in a middle-aged lady. AS-OCT revealed a DM break along with a fistula tract connecting the flap interface with the AC. C_3F_8 Descemetopexy closed the break and PK was done later to restore vision. Histopathology also showed the DM break

for regression, have also been correlated with the progression of keratectasia [26–29].

Corneal hydrops in these eyes is extremely rare; the exact prevalence is unknown and can occur even in the absence of a secondary keratectasia with or without preexisting risk factors. Table 12.1 summarizes the various clinical scenarios where hydrops has been seen to develop with varying intervals post-LASIK [26, 30].

12.2.2.2 Post-Radial Keratotomy (RK)

Corneal hydrops has also been described to occur following RK performed for myopia (Fig. 12.6). The occurrence of corneal hydrops has been attributed to preoperative undiagnosed keratoconus in view of inferotemporal location of the stromal cleft as well as tomographic abnormalities in the fellow eye [15]. Although RK is practically obsolete, the relevance of this potential complication remains relevant because of the renewed interest in corneal-incisional procedures for the correction of refractive errors following the advent of the femto-second laser.

12.2.2.3 Post-Penetrating Keratoplasty

Corneal hydrops has been reported following both anterior lamellar keratoplasty [31] and full-thickness keratoplasty [32] performed for ectatic [16, 17, 33, 34] as well as non-ectatic corneal pathologies [35]. Acute hydrops in a graft should be differentiated from acute graft rejection. The distribution of localized corneal edema crossing the graft interface and involving both the donor and the host with the presence of focal intrastromal clefts favor the diagnosis of corneal hydrops (Fig. 12.7). On the other hand, a diffuse distribution of edema involving only the graft with sparing of host with anterior chamber reaction and keratic precipitates points toward rejection or an endothelial failure [36].

Various mechanisms proposed for the recurrence of ectasia in a keratoconic eye following a full-thickness graft include the failure to excise the cone completely [37], use of donor material with undiagnosed keratoconus, and recurrence of keratoconus in donor corneas which is usually

Table 12.1 Acute corneal hydrops following LASIK with or without associated keratectasia

Author/year	Type of study	Preoperative topography	Retreatment (+/−)	Post-LASIK ectasia (+/−)	Presentation (+/− perforation)	Surgery to hydrops onset interval (years)	Management
Gupta et al. [31], (2015)	CR	Probable forme fruste KCN	−	+	Intrastromal clefts with flap dehiscence and aqueous leak	10	BCL application for 2 weeks followed by PK
Cooke et al. [30] (2015)	CR	Normal	+	+	Intrastromal clefts with flap separation without dehiscence or aqueous leak	11	Conservative
Meyer et al. [26], (2009)	CR	Normal	+	−	Acute hydrops without perforation	3	PK
Chen et al. [14] (2007)	CR	Normal	−	−	Acute hydrops with aqueous leak	9	PK
Chung et al. [29] (2005)	CR	Asymmetric bow-tie pattern with inferior steepening	+	+	Acute hydrops with fluid in the interface	6	PK

CR case report, *BCL* bandage contact lens, *KCN* keratoconus, *PK* penetrating keratoplasty

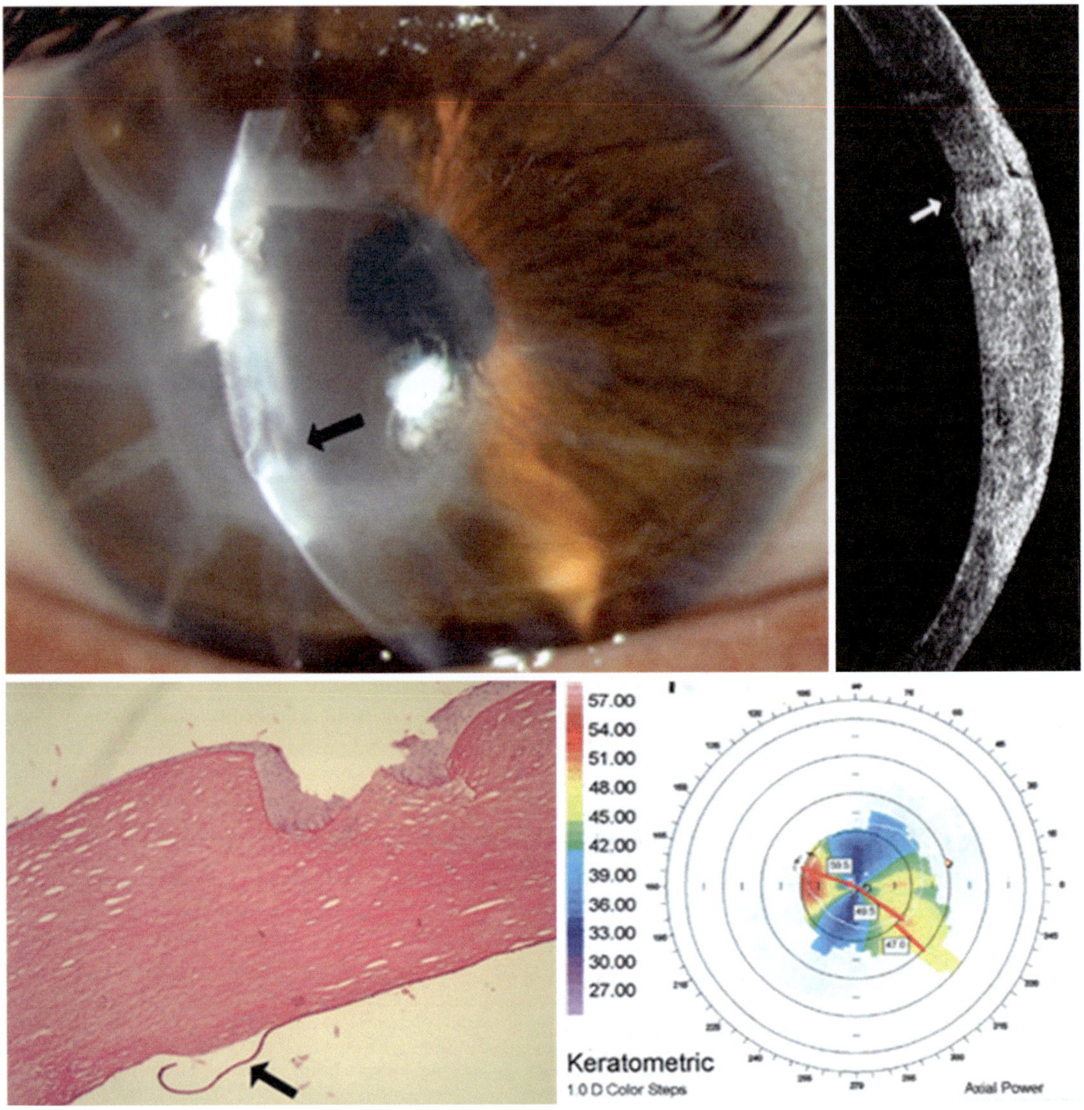

Fig. 12.6 Acute corneal hydrops 14 years after extensive radial keratotomy (RK) for high myopia in a middle-aged lady. Clinical examination showed epithelial and stromal edema, and topography showed ectasia in both eyes. AS-OCT revealed a DM break suggestive of acute corneal hydrops. PK was done to restore vision, and histopathology of the corneal button also showed DM detachment corresponding with the AS-OCT findings

seen around two decades after penetrating keratoplasty (PK) [38]. Migration of cells from the pathologic recipient cornea, including epithelium, keratocytes, and endothelium, is speculated to contribute toward this recurrence [17]. This hypothesis is also supported by the findings of abnormal epithelium and fragmented Bowman layer observed in donor grafts on histopathology several years after PK [33]. Since these structural and topographic changes progress slowly, therefore, the development of a clinically identifiable ectasia after PK is seen predominantly in longstanding grafts [17, 34].

12.2.2.4 Post-Anterior Lamellar Keratoplasty

Contrary to PK, recurrence of ectasia following an anterior lamellar keratoplasty is usually seen

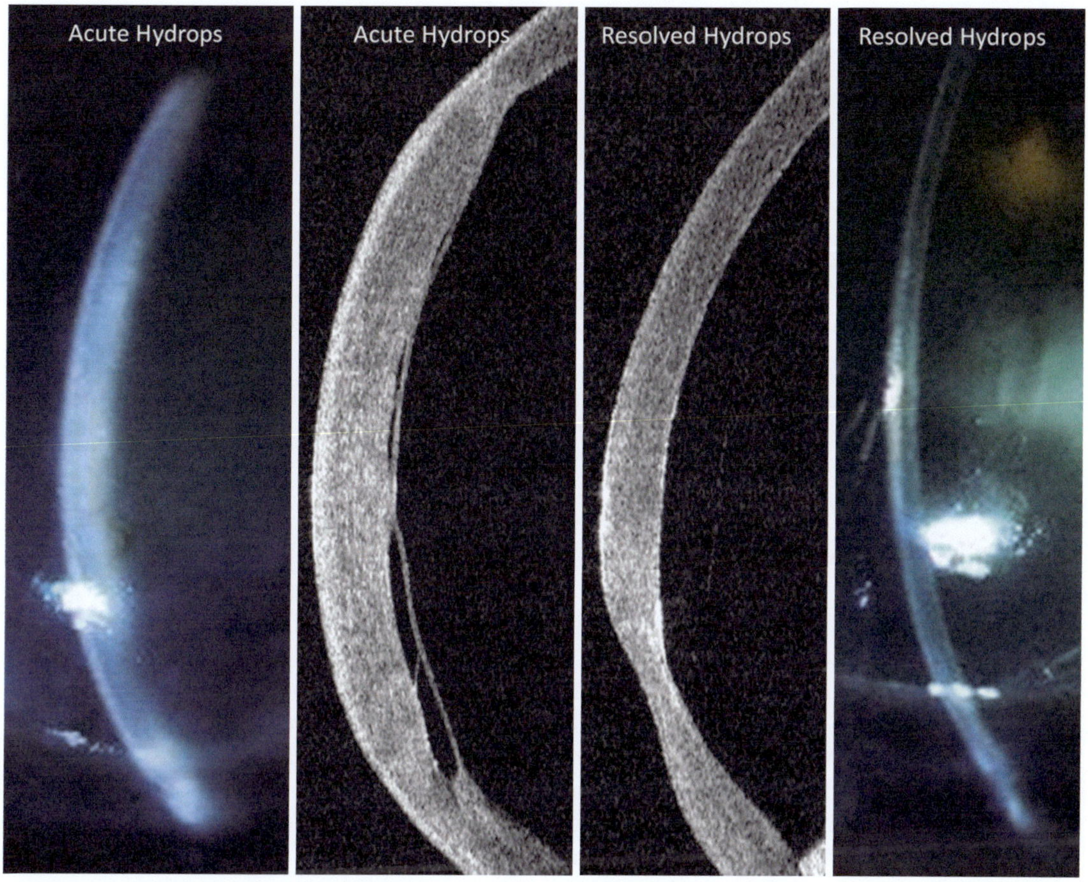

Fig. 12.7 Acute corneal hydrops in an elderly with bilateral corneal grafts and post-PK ectasia developed sudden whitening in the right eye. Clinically, there was diffuse graft edema in the left eye. AS-OCT showed DM detachment without any break. C_3F_8 Descemetopexy was done, and the DM attached with resolution of corneal edema within a span of 1 month

early and is expected to occur at a higher rate than following a full-thickness graft. Proposed mechanisms include invasion of donor tissue by keratocytes retained in the posterior stroma and the retention of abnormal DM and endothelial cells within the host [39]. The management of acute hydrops following deep anterior lamellar keratoplasty (DALK) is more challenging than that after PK because aqueous can easily dissect the potential space between the recipient DM and the donor stroma, leading to the complete separation of host DM-endothelial complex. In contrast, DM detachment is expected to be more localized and resolves spontaneously within 6–8 weeks, leaving only minimal scarring in acute hydrops after PK [36]. Hydrops in corneal grafts done for non-ectatic pathologies has also been reported, attributable to the dislocation of intraocular devices with subsequent damage to the DM caused by mechanical trauma of eye rubbing [32].

12.2.2.5 Post-Corneal Trauma or Degeneration

Rarely corneal thinning and ectasia due to trauma or chronic degeneration can also lead to acute corneal hydrops (Fig. 12.8).

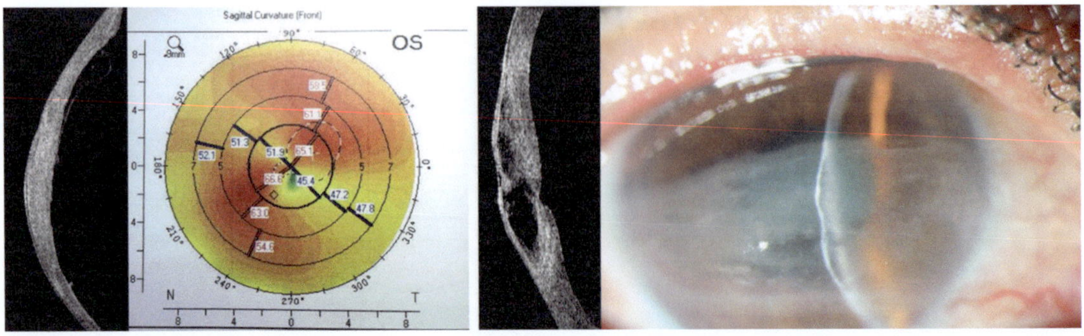

Fig. 12.8 Acute corneal hydrops without and with intrastromal fluid clefts in two cases of advanced corneal thinning and degeneration. Corneal topography revealed the irregular surface in the first case, and AS-OCT confirmed the presence of fluid clefts in the second case. Both these cases had an old history of trauma, and the corneas in the fellow eyes were normal

12.2.3 Primary Infantile Glaucoma

Acute corneal hydrops both unilateral and bilateral forms has been described to occur in infants presenting with glaucoma between ages 1 month and 3 years of life. The occurrence of acute hydrops in these eyes with preexisting megalocornea or buphthalmos has been attributed to the occurrence of breaks in the DM under the influence of raised intraocular pressure. Acute corneal hydrops is often the presenting manifestation in these children since the occurrence of sudden corneal clouding, and consequent bluish appearance of the cornea has been described to prompt the parents of these children to seek medical care [12]. Mandal described successful resolution of corneal edema following adequate lowering of the IOP with a primary combined trabeculotomy-trabeculectomy procedure [12]. The final visual outcome however was limited by the presence of Haab's striae involving the pupillary area in most eyes resulting in high corneal astigmatism and corneal scarring.

12.3 Natural History of Disease

The development of marked corneal edema in acute corneal hydrops is caused by a break in the DM, allowing aqueous fluid to enter the corneal stroma and epithelium. This causes separation of the collagen lamellae and can result in the formation of large fluid-filled intrastromal clefts or cysts [40]. The onset of acute hydrops is usually foreshown by marked epiphora, followed by intense photophobia and pain, associated with markedly reduced visual acuity [41]. After the rupture of the DM, it may retract and curl anteriorly to form scrolls, ridges, or strands around the attached fragments of stroma (Fig. 12.9) [40]. This is thought to be the reason why acute corneal hydrops takes longer to resolve than localized corneal edema caused by a breach of the DM during cataract surgery on a keratoconic eye [40].

Basu et al. postulated that the exact re-approximation of the displaced margins, either spontaneously or with perfluoropropane gas (C_3F_8), is not possible and the resolution of corneal hydrops probably involves two steps. Firstly, the detached DM must reattach to the posterior stroma; the time for this depends on the depth of the DM detachment. Secondly, the endothelium must migrate over the gap between the two broken edges of DM; the interval for this depends on the dimensions of the DM break. Thus, insertion of C_3F_8 can hasten the first step but not the second, which greatly depends on the preexisting severity of the ectasia and the corneal thickness in general [42].

Although acute corneal hydrops is usually self-limiting and clinical signs of edema typically

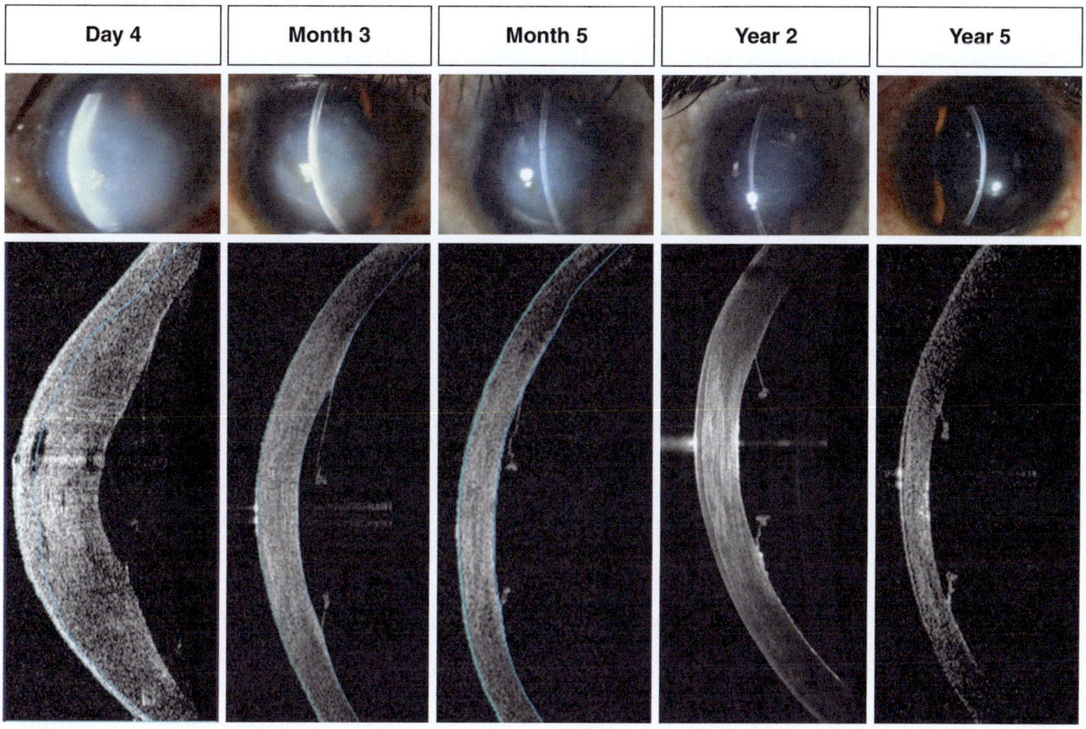

Fig. 12.9 Natural history of acute corneal hydrops in a young teenage boy with active vernal keratoconjunctivitis. Serial clinical photographs and AS-OCT sections reveal the gradual resolution of corneal edema and improvement in corneal clarity. The unaided vision improved from hand motions to 20/100 over the course of 5 years

resolve after 5–36 weeks [1, 5, 6, 43], it may leave behind a vision-impairing scar. Secondary flattening of the cornea may facilitate improved contact lens fitting, but the central corneal scarring can mandate a corneal transplantation to restore visual function [38]. Inevitably, the greater the area of corneal involvement during hydrops, the longer is the duration for the edema to resolve, the higher the risk of neovascularization, and the poorer is the visual outcome [44]. Other complications of acute hydrops include infection, pseudocyst formation, malignant glaucoma, and corneal perforation [1, 6]. A history of hydrops may also predispose patients to greater likelihood of episodes of endothelial graft rejection after penetrating keratoplasty [1, 45, 46].

12.4 Histopathology of Corneal Hydrops

Basu et al. studied the histopathology of post-hydrops eyes which underwent PK and described the presence of broken and rolled edges of the DM, which on higher magnification exhibited endothelial cell migration along with relayering of the basement membrane on periodic acid Schiff stain [42, 46]. Interestingly, the appearance of the DM varied based on whether the eyes had received C_3F_8 injections in the past. In post-C_3F_8 cases, the broken ends of DM were rolled or folded at one end and flattened at the other end, both ends being attached to the posterior corneal stroma. Whereas in cases not receiving C_3F_8 there was either persistent detachment of one end of DM, or the other end was seen lying rolled or flat against the posterior stroma or rolling of both ends of DM with attachment to the posterior corneal stroma. Injection of C_3F_8 gas seemed to cause a characteristic folding or burial of DM in the corneal stroma, suggestive of the pressure tamponade by the gas bubble [43, 46].

Thota et al. [47] suggested that the fluid accumulates more easily between lamellae rather than within them. Hence, corneal hydrops may rather be interlamellar in nature. The histopathology of corneal hydrops indicates that over time the cornea responds to the fluid invasion by developing a cellular lining around the perimeter of these fluid pockets and, thus, making this feature cystic [48, 49].

12.5 Clinical Presentation

Patients typically present to the emergency room complaining of sudden loss of vision with whitish discoloration of the eye, which may be associated with photophobia and pain [6]. On eliciting the history, patients may reveal an antecedent episode of vigorous eye rubbing or coughing [5, 6, 50]. Slit-lamp examination reveals marked stromal and epithelial microcystic edema, intrastromal cyst/clefts, and conjunctival hyperemia. The location and area of the involved cornea are variable. Depending on the extent of corneal edema, it can be graded as follows: grade 1 within a circle of 3 mm diameter, grade 2 between circles of 3 and 5 mm diameters, and grade 3 larger than a circle of 5 mm diameter [50]. The time for resolution of edema and subsequent final best corrected visual acuity achieved are inversely related to the area of involvement [6].

12.6 Investigative Modalities

Acute corneal hydrops is a clinical diagnosis which can be easily established based on the history and slit-lamp examination. But the investigations are essential to determine the size, depth, and extent of DM tear and corneal edema. Thus, the investigations can help us in formulation of the treatment plan, assess the response to the treatment, as well as identify any early complication.

12.6.1 Ultrasound Biomicroscopy (UBM)

On ultrasound biomicroscopy, in the acute phase, the characteristic continuous curvilinear and brightly intense spike of an intact DM is not seen. The DM tear can be clearly seen as an area of deficiency under the area of maximum corneal edema [40, 50]. The number (single or multiple), site, size, and communication of the intrastromal cysts/clefts can also be discerned. One can also measure the length of DM tear which directly corresponds to the extent of corneal edema. The corneal thickness at various locations can be measured quantitatively, which is useful to document the resolution of the hydrops. In addition, hydrops resolving index (HyRI) defined as the ratio between the area of maximum thickness of corneal edema at presentation (CT0) and corneal thickness at a site 2.5 mm from the center (CT2.5) helps in monitoring the resolution of hydrops [50]. The disadvantages of the UBM are the contact nature of the method, low resolution of images, and difficulty in being used in young children [51].

12.6.2 Anterior Segment Optical Coherence Tomography (AS-OCT)

AS-OCT helps in clearly delineating the size and depth of DM detachment in eyes with acute hydrops (Fig. 12.1). These factors significantly correlate with the duration of corneal edema. Eyes with deeper detachments and large DM breaks have a prolonged recovery time even after intracameral gas injection [42]. Basu et al. described morphological patterns of detached DM in 24 keratoconic eyes with acute corneal hydrops. Three patterns of DM detachment were observed: DM detachment with break and rolled ends being the most common pattern, followed by detachment with break and flat ends and detachment without the presence of break [42]. The study showed that the duration of corneal edema (E, in weeks) could be predicted by the equation $E = 5.4 - (3 \times C) + (2.2 \times S) + (3.6 \times D)$, where $C = 1$ for C_3F_8 and $C = 0$ for no C_3F_8, S = average size of the DM break in millimeters, and D = depth of the DM detachment in millimeters. The AS-OCT features have also been found to correlate with the histopathological findings observed in full-thickness keratoplasty specimens obtained from eyes with healed hydrops, giving an insight to the pattern of resolution of disease [42]. The advantages of AS-OCT are that it is noncontact and rapid and provides high-resolution images of the DM that are often not visible on slit-lamp biomicroscopy [51, 52].

12.6.3 In Vivo Confocal Microscopy

In vivo confocal microscopy helps in demonstrating excess fluid seen in both the stroma and the epithelium. Epithelial edema presents as prominent cellular borders between cells of the basal epithelium, whereas the stromal edema is identified as surrounding hyperreflective areas. The keratocyte densities are lower in the edematous area and have oddly shaped nuclei [53]. Notably, although IVCM has increased our understanding of hydrops at the microstructural level, currently, IVCM has a minimal role in management because of being highly operator-dependent and time-consuming. Since many of the acute corneal hydrops patients are children, AS-OCT has obvious advantages over UBM or IVCM, both of which are contact techniques and operator-dependent.

12.7 Management

Acute corneal hydrops is a condition that generally resolves without intervention over weeks to months, but during this time, the sight and comfort of the patient are significantly compromised. Longer duration of edema is also more likely to lead to complications such as neovascularization [44]. Therefore, many therapeutic options are aimed at safely facilitating speedier recovery and thus minimizing or eliminating complications of hydrops. These treatment regimens can be classified as conservative medical management and surgical options.

12.7.1 Conservative Management

Most conservative treatment includes observation and topical lubrication for comfort. Pressure patching and temporary discontinuation of contact lens have also been advocated to reduce edema [6]. Patient comfort may be achieved with the use of topical therapeutic agents (Table 12.2); however, these do not decrease the duration of hydrops. Hyperosmotic agents, such as 5% sodium chloride, may be prescribed to help draw fluid out of the epithelium [1, 54]. To prevent secondary infection, broad-spectrum topical antibiotics may be recommended if the epithelium is compromised [1, 54]. A bandage contact lens may be indicated to counter the discomfort or pain but is often difficult to fit or retain [55, 56]. Therefore, the use of contact lenses is limited after the edema has subsided [1, 56]. A cycloplegic agent and dark glasses can also be used to reduce pain and photophobia [1, 55, 56]. Antiglaucoma medications can be prescribed to lessen the hydrodynamic force on the posterior cornea [1], while topical steroids [1, 55, 56] or nonsteroidal anti-inflammatory drugs (NSAIDs) may be used for easing inflammation and pain on rare occasions [56]. Theoretically, topical corticosteroids may reduce the risk of corneal neovascularization or lessen the extent of progression should neovascularization occur. However, there is little evidence in the literature to support this theory. Indeed, widely used in clinical practice, some studies have found topical corticosteroids to be entirely ineffective in arresting the progression of stromal neovascularization in corneal hydrops [44].

Table 12.2 Topical therapeutic agents used in acute hydrops

Class	Mechanism
Hypertonics	Draw fluid from the epithelium to reduce pain [1, 54]
Antibiotics	Prevent secondary infection when the epithelium is compromised [1, 54]
Antiglaucoma	Reduce hydrodynamic force on the posterior cornea [1]
Cycloplegics	Reduce photophobia and pain [1, 55, 56]
NSAIDs	Decrease inflammation and pain [1, 56]
Steroids	Decrease inflammation and pain [1, 55, 56]

12.7.2 Surgical Management

Surgical management of acute hydrops has evolved over the last few decades, especially with improvement in the understanding of the pathophysiology and better imaging techniques. Table 12.3 compares the outcomes of various treatment modalities for the management of acute corneal hydrops.

12.7.2.1 Thermokeratoplasty (TKP)

This modality dates to the year 1977, where a thermokeratophore (with a temperature setting of 100–110 Celsius) was applied to the area of maximum corneal edema. The use of TKP in the treatment of keratoconus is based on the property of collagen to shrink when proper hydrothermal temperature is reached. This shrinkage causes a flattening in the corneal curvature and increase in corneal thickness. Clinically, it is not unusual for the post-TKP patient to have small vertical folds in the DM along with a slight thickening of the cornea [57].

12.7.2.2 Intracameral Air or Gas Injection

Intracameral air/gas injection shortens the period of persistence of corneal edema in acute hydrops. Various agents that have been used are air [58], 20% sulfur hexafluoride (SF_6) [59], and 14% perfluropropane (C_3F_8) [5]. The main difference between these agents is in their duration of action. Air stays for a shorter time; hence, repeated injections are required [58]. SF_6 is long-acting compared to air (around 2 weeks); however, repeat injections may still be required [59]. C_3F_8 is the longest-acting among all, and usually repeat injections are not required [5]. Faster recovery occurs following intracameral injection due to tamponade effect of air or gases. The injection of air/gas stretches both ends of the ruptured DM, which roll up in acute corneal hydrops. Air/gas injection in the anterior chamber brings the two ruptured edges in the DM closer, facilitating faster wound healing of corneal endothelial cells over the exposed stroma, with deposition of the new DM (Fig. 12.10). As patient keeps a supine position, air/gas prevents aqueous penetration into the stroma [5, 58, 59].

Among the available options, perfluorocarbons (C_3F_8) appear to be the intracameral agent of choice due to a longer half-life, thus requiring lesser number of repeat injections [5], and are proven to be safe in terms of endothelial preservation [60]. Intracameral gas injection achieved faster resolution of edema in cases of acute hydrops occurring in keratoconus, where the tear in the DM is usually central or paracentral in location and the gas bubble can effectively tamponade the detached DM, even when the patient is unable to maintain a strict supine position in the early postoperative period [5]. However, in eyes with PMCD, the peripheral and inferior location of the tear and in eyes with keratoglobus and the large extent of the Descemet's membrane tear are the reasons for suboptimal outcome [5].

The complications of intracameral air/gas injection include intrastromal migration of the gas, elevation of IOP (pupillary block glaucoma), Urrets-Zavalia syndrome, endothelial damage, cataract formation, and infection [5, 59–61]. Intraoperative inadvertent intrastromal migration of the C_3F_8 gas may prevent the closure of the intrastromal cleft and impede the resolution of acute hydrops [50, 61]. The occur-

Table 12.3 Outcomes of various treatment modalities for the management of acute corneal hydrops

Author/year	Type of study	N	Etiology	Treatment	Duration of persistence of corneal edema	Duration of persistence of injected gas	Repeat injections (number of eyes)	Complications
Miyata et al. [58] (2002)	R, cm, NRn	30	KCN	• 9/30 – I/C *air* • 21/30 – Cons	• I/C air 20.1 ± 9 days • Cons 64.7 ± 34.6 days ($p = 0.0008$)	3 days	7/9	None
Panda et al. [59] (2009)	NCm	9	KCN	*20% SF_6*	• 4 weeks	NA	6/9	None
Basu et al. [5] (2011)	R, cm, NRn,	152	KCN PMCD KG	• 62/152 – I/C 0.1 ml *14% C_3F_8* • 90/152 – Cons	• I/C C_3F_8 90.5 ± 55.8 days • Cons 125 ± 68.9 days ($p = 0.0001$)	NA	None	• Pupillary block (10/62) • Stromal vascularization (7/62; 18/90)
Basu et al. [42] (2012)	R	24	KCN	• 13/24–*14% C_3F_8* • 11/24 – Cons • 2/24 – PKP	• I/C C_3F_8 7.6 ± 3.8 weeks • Cons 11.4 ± 4.1 weeks	NA	None	• None
Sharma et al. [50] (2011)	P, NCm	14	KCN	I/C 0.15 ml *14% C_3F_8*	• 6 weeks (12/13; 92.3%)	3 weeks	3/13	• Raised intraocular pressure (2/13) • Intrastromal migration due to fish egging (2/13)
Ting et al. [81] (2014)	R, NCm	8	KCN	*14% C_2F_6*	• 60.0 ± 32.1 days	6–8 days	None	None
Rajaraman et al. [62] (2009)	R	17	16 - KCN 1 - PMCD	• 15 - C_3F_8 + *Cm sutures* • 2 - C_3F_8	• C_3F_8 with sutures 8.87 ± 4.98 days • C_3F_8 alone 27.5 days	10.75 ± 2.62 days	None	None
Cherif et al. [82] (2015)	R	7	KCN	• 6 – Air + *Cm sutures* • 1 - C_3F_8 + air + Cm sutures	15–30	NA	None	None
Vajpayee et al. [83] (2013)	P	5	4 - KCN 1 - KG	I/C air with *venting incisions*	14–21	NA	None	None

R retrospective, *KCN* keratoconus, *BCVA* best corrected visual acuity, *Cm* comparative, *PMCD* pellucid marginal corneal degeneration, *CL* contact lens, *NCm* non-comparative, *KG* keratoglobus, *P* prospective, *NRn* nonrandomized, *Cons* conservative, *DM* Descemet's membrane, *N* number of eyes, *I/C* intracameral, *ASOCT* anterior segment optical coherence tomography, *I/S* intrastromal

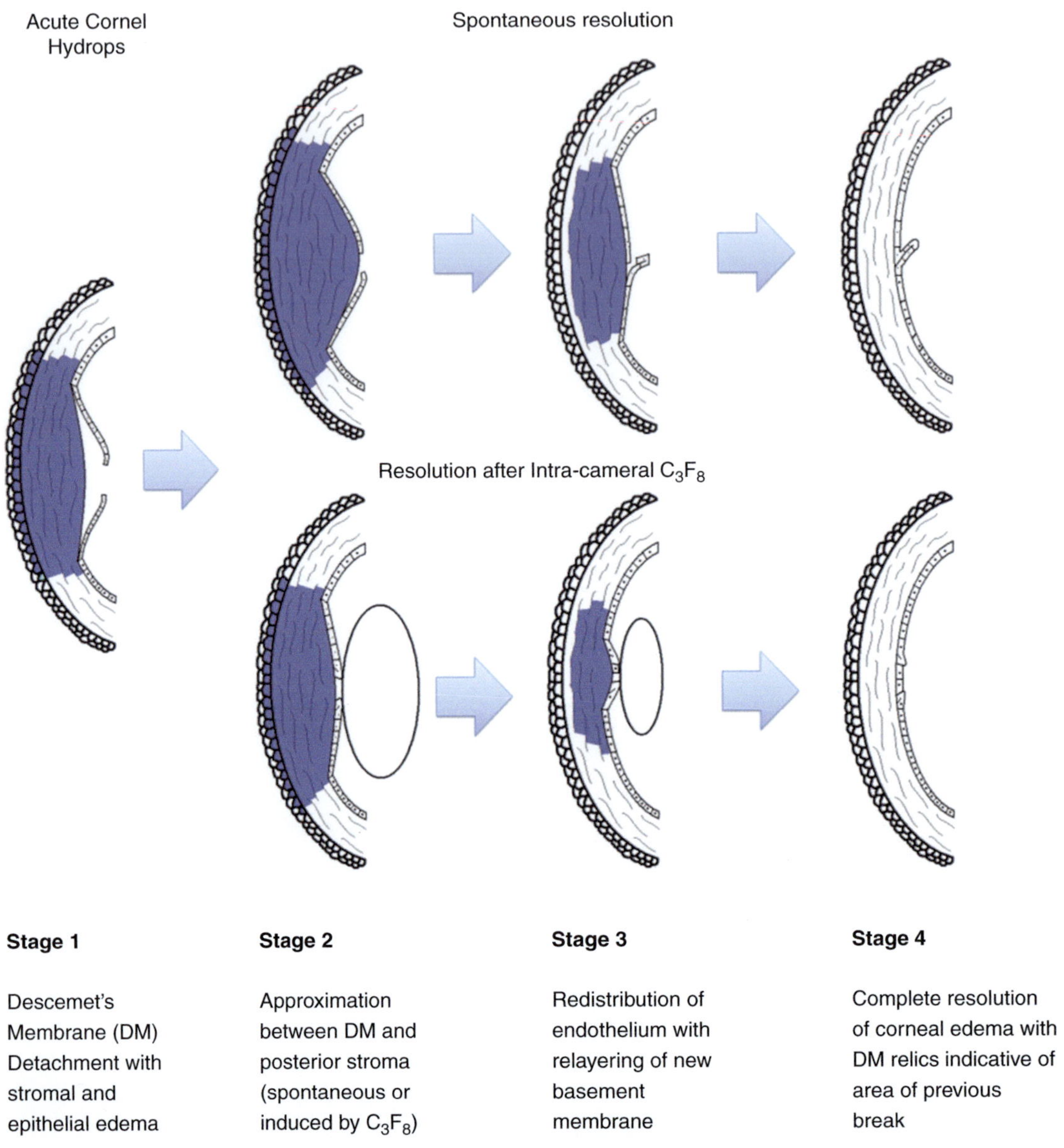

Fig. 12.10 A schematic diagram depicting the comparison of spontaneous resolution of acute hydrops versus rapid resolution following intracameral gas injection. Stage 1: Descemet's membrane detachment with stromal and epithelial edema. Stage 2: approximation between DM and posterior stroma (spontaneous or induced by C_3F_8). Stage 3: redistribution of the endothelium with relayering of new basement membrane. Stage 4: complete resolution of corneal edema with DM relics indicative of area of previous break

rence of secondary glaucoma is more common in cases wherein gas has been injected and depends on the amount of air/gas injected [5]. C_3F_8 persists in the anterior chamber for a longer period compared with SF_6; hence, the chances of developing secondary glaucoma are higher. A peripheral iridectomy may be done in cases wherein C_3F_8 is used, or the pupil should be dilated postoperatively till the gas bubble is less than half the volume of the anterior chamber [5]. Microbial keratitis and cataract formation may also occur postoperatively [59].

12.7.2.3 Compression Sutures with Intracameral Gas Injection

The injection of intracameral gas alone may not suffice in severe hydrops cases with large DM tears as it may lead to intrastromal migration of air, causing delayed resolution of edema which may incite inflammation and neovascularization [44, 61]. Rajaraman et al. proposed the use of compression corneal sutures in addition to intracameral perfluoropropane in the treatment of acute hydrops in a retrospective case series of 17 patients (16 keratoconus and 1 PMCD) [62]. The patients received either 0.2 mL of iso-expansile mixture of 14% C_3F_8 alone or with compression sutures. The decision to introduce compression sutures was only made after injection of the gas if (a) a stromal cleft was noted after gas tamponade or (b) a tracking of gas through the stroma was noted during gas injection. Corneal edema resolved faster in eyes with C_3F_8 and compression sutures than eyes with pneumopexy alone (8.9 ± 4.9 days and 27.5 days, respectively); however, the sample size was too small to be conclusive. Application of compressive sutures along with gas injection brings the gaping edges closer and prevents intrastromal migration of the gas which hastens the resolution of the edema. Two to five full-thickness sutures with 10–0 nylon is applied perpendicular to the tear, starting from 1 to 2 mm from its edges after the introduction of the gas. Suture removal is done 2–6 weeks later.

12.7.2.4 Amniotic Membrane Transplantation with Cauterization

There is a higher prevalence of acute hydrops in the differently abled (Down syndrome) patients which is attributed to the habit of vigorous eye rubbing. Another probable reason for this condition is that keratoplasty is less frequently performed on these patients, which leads to the progression of their disease for a longer period [63]. Medical treatment of hydrops remains the mainstay of therapy in these patients, but severe cases might need surgical intervention such as thermocauterization or penetration keratoplasty (associated with higher rejection rates) [1]. In such cases, cauterization coupled with stromal puncture allows the excess fluid from the stroma to evaporate and leaves a thermally injured epithelium and stroma. When combined with amniotic membrane transplantation, it strongly reduces inflammation, vascularization, and scarring and improves the corneal clarity without intense scarring [64].

12.7.2.5 Penetrating Keratoplasty (PK)

Traditionally, PK has been employed for patients with persistent corneal opacification, suboptimal visual recovery, or contact lens intolerance following resolution of corneal hydrops for visual rehabilitation [45, 46]. It is rarely indicated in cases of acute corneal hydrops unless in exceptional situations like perforation [65]. Although keratoconus has shown best outcomes for PK [66, 67], the endothelial rejection episodes were greater in eyes with longer duration of corneal hydrops and coexistent ocular allergy [45, 46]. Notwithstanding these risks, the long-term graft survival and visual outcomes after PK in eyes with keratoconus are excellent, irrespective of previous corneal hydrops [46].

12.7.2.6 Deep Anterior Lamellar Keratoplasty (DALK)

Because of the greater risk of endothelial graft rejection and reduced success of long-term graft survival noted following PK in earlier studies and the development of hydrops in younger age group, in the recent years, DALK has gained popularity wherever feasible for post-hydrops keratoconus patients [67, 68]. DALK poses technical challenges over those posed by PK, largely due to the depth and density of scarring in severe cases and the significant risk of deep perforation at the site of the DM rupture. Therefore, many of the techniques described for lamellar dissection are contraindicated. Modified dissection techniques have been described in all published case series of DALK following hydrops, most suggesting careful manual dissection down to near DM [67, 68]. Jacob et al. have proposed pre-Descemetic DALK (pDALK) as primary treatment modality for acute hydrops. Their technique modifications included creating tissue emphysema as a guide for dissection, using small aliquots of air directed away from break, manual deeper dissection using a blunt dissector, centripetal dissection leaving the area of DM break for last, retention of minimal stroma above DM tear, and tamponade of DM tear with air in the anterior chamber [69].

Primary pDALK thus avoids the need for a second surgical procedure. It addresses multiple pathologies associated with acute hydrops by closure of the DM break, providing anatomical correction for ectasia and thinning in these patients with severe keratoconus and providing optical correction by improving corneal topography, regaining corneal structure and transparency, and avoiding healing by scarring while also retaining host DM and the endothelium. It allows early and rapid visual and anatomical rehabilitation, and comorbidities and costs associated with a second surgical procedure can be avoided [69].

12.7.2.7 Endothelial Keratoplasty (EK)

Tu was the first to perform DMEK in a patient with chronic edema (7 months) after an episode of acute corneal hydrops in patient with keratoconus [70]. Bachman et al. published a small case series advocating the role of mini-DSAEK in rapid deswelling of the cornea, early visual rehabilitation along with reduced likelihood of scar formation [71]. Although the role of EK in the management of acute corneal hydrops needs further validation, this approach addresses the problem of loss of DM and endothelial barrier directly.

12.8 Visual Rehabilitation Post-Corneal Hydrops

Literature on contact lens strategies for post-hydrops visual rehabilitation is particularly scarce. Studies on the outcome of scleral lenses in moderate to severe keratoconus typically do not include post-corneal hydrops cases [72–74]. Kreps et al. have shown the value of scleral lenses in post-corneal hydrops visual rehabilitation where they were able to achieve a satisfactory visual acuity of 20/40 in 68.8% of the eyes post-hydrops with scleral lenses (diameter 16.5–17.5 mm) [75]. The average comfortable wearing time of these lenses was about 10 hours per day [76, 77]. Mini-scleral lenses with a diameter of 16.5–17.5 mm have several advantages over full scleral lenses (diameter of 18 mm and more): they are thinner, weigh less, require lower clearance, and are easier to handle [78]. However, larger scleral lenses are desired to achieve a higher vault or distribute the lens weight better.

Keratoplasty (PK or DALK) is indicated for those cases of resolved corneal hydrops that are not amenable to further visual impairment with contact lenses [45, 46, 66]. To lower the risk of endothelial rejection with PK, some authors advocate modified deep anterior lamellar keratoplasty (DALK) techniques, whereby careful manual dissection is performed down to near DM [68]. Overall, the visual outcome of DALK versus PK in keratoconus has not been proven to be superior [79, 80]. Moreover, in post-hydrops patients, scarring at the level of the posterior stroma and DM after hydrops may limit postoperative visual acuity. Risks of complications associated with keratoplasty, such as high corneal astigmatism, graft rejection, infection, cataract, and glaucoma, remain applicable to both techniques and should be considered when advising patients on therapeutic options after the resolution of acute corneal hydrops [66]. The evolution of a wide range of scleral lenses as an effective and safe alternative to keratoplasty has definitely led to a lesser need for keratoplasty overall in post-corneal hydrops eyes [75].

12.9 Summary and Conclusion

Acute corneal hydrops is a rare complication of progressive corneal ectasia most commonly seen in keratoconus, although it can occur in any form of primary or secondary keratectasia. The natural history of the disease suggests that it is a self-limiting condition and that the corneal edema resolves almost completely with time. This happens because of the partial reattachment of the detached and broken ends of the DM and the endothelial redistribution of the intervening posterior surface of the corneal stroma. The healing process can take several weeks to months and results in significant visual morbidity in the interim. Recent advances in corneal imaging and surgery have resulted in several promising innovations in the diagnosis and treatment of acute corneal hydrops. While intracameral C_3F_8 gas injection and use of compression sutures reduce the duration of corneal edema, lamellar corneal grafting in the form of pDALK and EK can rapidly reduce edema resulting in improved corneal clarity and vision. With increasing awareness and screening for corneal ectasia using corneal topography and Scheimpflug imaging in recent years, combined with the increasing use of specially designed contact lenses and collagen cross-linking for keratectasia, the incidence of acute corneal hydrops has probably significantly reduced. This preventive aspect is an equally critical component in the overall context of keratoconus and other corneal ectasias and must be emphasized. Challenges still remain in young children with severe allergy and eye rubbing, especially those with Down syndrome.

References

1. Tuft SJ, Gregory WM, Buckley RJ. Acute corneal hydrops in keratoconus. Ophthalmology. 1994;101(10):1738–44.
2. McClellan KA, Billson FA. Acute hydrops in keratoglobus. Arch Ophthalmol. 1987;105(10):1432–3.
3. Carter JB, Jones DB, Wilhelmus KR. Acute hydrops in pellucid marginal corneal degeneration. Am J Ophthalmol. 1989;107(2):167–70.
4. Ashenhurst M, Slomovic A. Corneal hydrops in Terrien's marginal degeneration: an unusual complication. Can J Ophthalmol. 1987;22(6):328–30.
5. Basu S, Vaddavalli PK, Ramappa M, Shah S, Murthy SI, Sangwan VS. Intracameral perfluoropropane gas in the treatment of acute corneal hydrops. Ophthalmology. 2011;118(5):934–9.
6. Grewal S, Laibson PR, Cohen EJ, Rapuano CJ. Acute hydrops in the corneal ectasias: associated factors and outcomes. Trans Am Ophthalmol Soc. 1999;97:187–98. discussion: 198-203
7. Sridhar MS, Mahesh S, Bansal AK, Nutheti R, Rao GN. Pellucid marginal corneal degeneration. Ophthalmology. 2004;111(6):1102–7.
8. Sharma R, Titiyal JS, Prakash G, Sharma N, Tandon R, Vajpayee RB. Clinical profile and risk factors for keratoplasty and development of hydrops in north Indian patients with keratoconus. Cornea. 2009;28(4):367–70.
9. Akova YA, Dabil H, Kavalcioglu O, Duman S. Clinical features and keratoplasty results in keratoconus complicated by acute hydrops. Ocul Immunol Inflamm. 2000;8(2):101–9.
10. Stoiber J, Muss W, Ruckhofer J, Grabner G. Acute keratoconus with perforation in a patient with Down's syndrome. Br J Ophthalmol. 2003;87(1):120.
11. Jhanji V, Sharma N, Vajpayee RB. Management of keratoconus: current scenario. Br J Ophthalmol. 2011;95(8):1044–50.
12. Mandal AK. Acute corneal hydrops in children with primary infantile glaucoma: a report of 31 cases over 23 years at the LVPEI. PLoS One. 2016;11(6):e0156108.
13. Diaz-Aljaro P, Monés-Liivina A, Romanic-Bubalo N, Castillo Capponi F, Sabala-Llopart A. Management of Descemet membrane detachment secondary to forceps assisted delivery in a newborn. Arch Soc Esp Oftalmol (Engl Ed). 2020;95(9):447–50.
14. Chen CL, Tai MC, Chen JT, Chen CH, Chang CJ, Lu DW. Acute corneal hydrops with perforation after LASIK-associated keratectasia. Clin Exp Ophthalmol. 2007;35(1):62–5.
15. Sharma N, Sachdev R, Jindal A, Titiyal JS. Acute hydrops in keratectasia after radial keratotomy. Eye Contact Lens. 2010;36(3):185–7.
16. Javadi MA, Feizi S, Kanavi MR, Faramarzi A, Hashemian J, Mirbabaee F. Acute hydrops after deep anterior lamellar keratoplasty in a patient with keratoconus. Cornea. 2011;30(5):591–4.
17. Ezra DG, Mehta JS, Allan BD. Late corneal hydrops after penetrating keratoplasty for keratoconus. Cornea. 2007;26(5):639–40.
18. Oshida T, Fushimi N, Sakimoto T, Sawa M. Acute hydrops in a host cornea after penetrating keratoplasty for keratoconus. Jpn J Ophthalmol. 2011;55(4):418–9.
19. Said DG, Faraj L, Elalfy MS, Miri A, Maharajan SV, Dua HS. Atypical hydrops in keratoconus. Int Ophthalmol. 2014;34(4):951–5.
20. Goldberg MA, Lubniewski AJ, Williams JM, Smith ME, Pepose JS. Cystic hydrops and spontaneous perforation in Fuchs' superficial marginal keratitis. Am J Ophthalmol. 1996;121(1):91–3.
21. Fuentes E, Sandali O, El Sanharawi M, Basli E, Hamiche T, Goemaere I, Borderie V, Bouheraoua N, Laroche L. Anatomic predictive factors of acute corneal hydrops in keratoconus: an optical coherence tomography study. Ophthalmology. 2015;122(8):1653–9.
22. Sandali O, El Sanharawi M, Temstet C, Hamiche T, Galan A, Ghouali W, Goemaere I, Basli E, Borderie V, Laroche L. Fourier-domain optical coherence tomography imaging in keratoconus: a corneal structural classification. Ophthalmology. 2013;120(12):2403–12.
23. Seiler T, Quurke AW. Iatrogenic keratectasia after LASIK in a case of forme fruste keratoconus. J Cataract Refract Surg. 1998;24(7):1007–9.

24. Seiler T, Koufala K, Richter G. Iatrogenic keratectasia after laser in situ keratomileusis. J Refract Surg. 1998;14(3):312–7.
25. Spadea L, Cantera E, Cortes M, Conocchia NE, Stewart CW. Corneal ectasia after myopic laser in situ keratomileusis: a long-term study. Clin Ophthalmol. 2012;6:1801–13.
26. Meyer CH, Mennel S, Schmidt JC. Acute keratoconus-like hydrops after laser in situ keratomileusis. J Ophthalmol. 2009;2009:363482.
27. Holland SP, Srivannaboon S, Reinstein DZ. Avoiding serious corneal complications of laser assisted in situ keratomileusis and photorefractive keratectomy. Ophthalmology. 2000;107(4):640–52.
28. Seitz B, Rozsíval P, Feuermannova A, Langenbucher A, Naumann GO. Penetrating keratoplasty for iatrogenic keratoconus after repeat myopic laser in situ keratomileusis: histologic findings and literature review. J Cataract Refract Surg. 2003;29(11):2217–24.
29. Chung SH, Im CY, Lee ES, Choi SY, Kwon YA, Kim EK. Clinical manifestation and pathologic finding of unilateral acute hydrops after bilateral laser in situ keratomileusis. J Cataract Refract Surg. 2005;31(6):1244–8.
30. Cooke MD, Koenig SB. Spontaneous resolution of acute corneal hydrops in a patient with post-LASIK ectasia. Cornea. 2015;34(7):835–7.
31. Gupta C, Tanaka TS, Elner VM, Soong HK. Acute hydrops with corneal perforation in post-LASIK ectasia. Cornea. 2015;34(1):99–100.
32. Cason JB, Yiu SC. Acute hydrops in the donor cornea graft in non-keratoconus patients. Middle East Afr J Ophthalmol. 2013;20(3):265–7.
33. Bechrakis N, Blom ML, Stark WJ, Green WR. Recurrent keratoconus. Cornea. 1994;13(1):73–7.
34. Bourges JL, Savoldelli M, Dighiero P, Assouline M, Pouliquen Y, BenEzra D, Renard G, Behar-Cohen F. Recurrence of keratoconus characteristics: a clinical and histologic follow-up analysis of donor grafts. Ophthalmology. 2003;110(10):1920–5.
35. Karseras AG, Ruben M. Aetiology of keratoconus. Br J Ophthalmol. 1976;60(7):522–5.
36. Wickremasinghe SS, Smith GT, Pullum KW, Buckley RJ. Acute hydrops in keratoconus masquerading as acute corneal transplant rejection. Cornea. 2006;25(6):739–41.
37. Dursun D, Fernandez V, Dubovy S, Trentacosta J, Alfonso EC. Hydrops in a corneal graft. Cornea. 2002;21(5):535.
38. Pramanik S, Musch DC, Sutphin JE, Farjo AA. Extended long-term outcomes of penetrating keratoplasty for keratoconus. Ophthalmology. 2006;113(9):1633–8.
39. Jafarinasab MR, Rahmati-Kamel M, Kanavi MR, Feizi S. Dissection plane in deep anterior lamellar keratoplasty using the big-bubble technique. Cornea. 2010;29(4):388–91.
40. Nakagawa T, Maeda N, Okazaki N, Hori Y, Nishida K, Tano Y. Ultrasound biomicroscopic examination of acute hydrops in patients with keratoconus. Am J Ophthalmol. 2006;141(6):1134–6.
41. Cameron JA, Al-Rajhi AA, Badr IA. Corneal ectasia in vernal keratoconjunctivitis. Ophthalmology. 1989;96(11):1615–23.
42. Basu S, Vaddavalli PK, Vemuganti GK, Ali MH, Murthy SI. Anterior segment optical coherence tomography features of acute corneal hydrops. Cornea. 2012;31(5):479–85.
43. Stone DL, Kenyon KR, Stark WJ. Ultrastructure of keratoconus with healed hydrops. Am J Ophthalmol. 1976;82(3):450–8.
44. Rowson NJ, Dart JK, Buckley RJ. Corneal neovascularisation in acute hydrops. Eye (Lond). 1992;6(Pt-4):404–6.
45. Meyer JJ, Gokul A, Crawford AZ, McGhee CNJ. Penetrating keratoplasty for keratoconus with and without resolved corneal hydrops: long-term results. Am J Ophthalmol. 2016;169:282–9.
46. Basu S, Reddy JC, Vaddavalli PK, Vemuganti GK, Sangwan VS. Long-term outcomes of penetrating keratoplasty for keratoconus with resolved corneal hydrops. Cornea. 2012;31(6):615–20.
47. Thota S, Miller WL, Bergmanson JP. Acute corneal hydrops: a case report including confocal and histopathological considerations. Cont Lens Anterior Eye. 2006;29(2):69–73.
48. Feder RS, Wilhelmus KR, Vold SD, O'Grady RB. Intrastromal clefts in keratoconus patients with hydrops. Am J Ophthalmol. 1998;126(1):9–16.
49. Chi HH, Katzin HM, Teng CC. Histopathology of keratoconus. Am J Ophthalmol. 1956;42(6):847–60.
50. Sharma N, Mannan R, Jhanji V, Agarwal T, Pruthi A, Titiyal JS, Vajpayee RB. Ultrasound biomicroscopy-guided assessment of acute corneal hydrops. Ophthalmology. 2011;118(11):2166–71.
51. Basu S, Mukhopadhyay S. Acute corneal hydrops. Ophthalmology. 2012;119(10):2197-2197.e1. author reply: 2198
52. Aurich H, Pham DT, Wirbelauer C. Biometric evaluation of keratoconic eyes with slit lamp-adapted optical coherence tomography. Cornea. 2011;30(1):56–9.
53. Lockington D, Fan Gaskin JC, McGhee CN, Patel DV. A prospective study of acute corneal hydrops by in vivo confocal microscopy in a New Zealand population with keratoconus. Br J Ophthalmol. 2014;98(9):1296–302.
54. Donnenfeld ED, Schrier A, Perry HD, Ingraham HJ, Lasonde R, Epstein A, Farber B. Infectious keratitis with corneal perforation associated with corneal hydrops and contact lens wear in keratoconus. Br J Ophthalmol. 1996;80(5):409–12.

55. Leibowitz HM, Morello S. Keratoconus and noninflammatory thinning disorders. In: Leibowitz HM, Waring GO, editors. Corneal disorders: clinical diagnosis and management. 2nd ed. Philadelphia: WB Saunders Company; 1998. p. 349–74.
56. Krachmer JH, Mannis MJ, Holland EJ. Non-inflammatory ectatic disorders. In: Krachmer JH, Mannis MJ, Holland EJ, editors. Cornea fundamentals, diagnosis and management. 2nd ed. St. Louis: Elsevier Mosby; 2005. p. 955–74.
57. Aquavella JV, Buxton JN, Shaw EL. Thermokeratoplasty in the treatment of persistent corneal hydrops. Arch Ophthalmol. 1977;95(1):81–4.
58. Miyata K, Tsuji H, Tanabe T, Mimura Y, Amano S, Oshika T. Intracameral air injection for acute hydrops in keratoconus. Am J Ophthalmol. 2002;133(6):750–2.
59. Panda A, Aggarwal A, Madhavi P, Wagh VB, Dada T, Kumar A, Mohan S. Management of acute corneal hydrops secondary to keratoconus with intracameral injection of sulfur hexafluoride (SF6). Cornea. 2007;26(9):1067–9.
60. Green K, Cheeks L, Stewart DA, Norman BC. Intraocular gas effects on corneal endothelial permeability. Lens Eye Toxic Res. 1992;9(2):85–91.
61. Sharma N, Mannan R, Titiyal JS. Nonresolution of acute hydrops because of intrastromal migration of perfluoropropane gas. Cornea. 2010;29(8):944–6.
62. Rajaraman R, Singh S, Raghavan A, Karkhanis A. Efficacy and safety of intracameral perfluoropropane (C3F8) tamponade and compression sutures for the management of acute corneal hydrops. Cornea. 2009;28(3):317–20.
63. Sugar J. Stromal corneal dystrophies and ectasias. In: Yanoff M, Duker JS, editors. Ophthalmology. Philadelphia: Mosby; 1999. p. 5.1–10.
64. Wylegala E, Tarnawska D. Amniotic membrane transplantation with cauterization for keratoconus complicated by persistent hydrops in mentally retarded patients. Ophthalmology. 2006;113(4):561–4.
65. Aldave AJ, Mabon M, Hollander DA, McLeod SD, Spencer WH, Abbott RL. Spontaneous corneal hydrops and perforation in keratoconus and pellucid marginal degeneration. Cornea. 2003;22(2):169–74.
66. De Lavalette JG, De Lavalette AR, Van Rij G, et al. Long-term results of corneal transplantations in keratoconus patients. Doc Ophthalmol. 1985;59(1):93–7.
67. Nanavaty MA, Daya SM. Outcomes of deep anterior lamellar keratoplasty in keratoconic eyes with previous hydrops. Br J Ophthalmol. 2012;96(10):1304–9.
68. Anwar HM, Anwar M. Predescemetic dissection for healed hydrops—judicious use of air and fluid. Cornea. 2011;30(12):1502–9.
69. Jacob S, Narasimhan S, Agarwal A, Sambath J, Umamaheshwari G, Saijimol AI. Primary modified predescemetic deep anterior lamellar keratoplasty in acute corneal hydrops. Cornea. 2018;37(10):1328–33.
70. Tu EY. Descemet membrane endothelial keratoplasty patch for persistent corneal hydrops. Cornea. 2017;36(12):1559–61.
71. Bachmann B, Händel A, Siebelmann S, Matthaei M, Cursiefen C. Mini-descemet membrane endothelial keratoplasty for the early treatment of acute corneal hydrops in keratoconus. Cornea. 2019;38(8):1043–8.
72. Koppen C, Kreps EO, Anthonissen L, Van Hoey M, Dhubhghaill SN, Vermeulen L. Scleral lenses reduce the need for corneal transplants in severe keratoconus. Am J Ophthalmol. 2018;185:43–7.
73. DeLoss KS, Fatteh NH, Hood CT. Prosthetic replacement of the ocular surface ecosystem (PROSE) scleral device compared to keratoplasty for the treatment of corneal ectasia. Am J Ophthalmol. 2014;158(5):974–82.
74. Barnett M, Mannis MJ. Contact lenses in the management of keratoconus. Cornea. 2011;30(12):1510–6.
75. Kreps EO, Claerhout I, Koppen C. The outcome of scleral lens fitting for keratoconus with resolved corneal hydrops. Cornea. 2019;38(7):855–8.
76. Schornack MM. Scleral lenses: a literature review. Eye Contact Lens. 2015;41(1):3–11.
77. Fan Gaskin JC, Patel DV, McGhee CN. Acute corneal hydrops in keratoconus—new perspectives. Am J Ophthalmol. 2014;157(5):921–8.
78. Fadel D. Modern scleral lenses: mini versus large. Cont Lens Anterior Eye. 2017;40(4):200–7.
79. Ramamurthi S, Ramaesh K. Surgical management of healed hydrops: a novel modification of deep anterior lamellar keratoplasty. Cornea. 2011;30(2):180–3.
80. Keane M, Coster D, Ziaei M, Williams K. Deep anterior lamellar keratoplasty versus penetrating keratoplasty for treating keratoconus. Cochrane Database Syst Rev. 2014;7:CD009700.
81. Ting DS, Srinivasan S. Pneumodescemetopexy with perfluoroethane (C2F6) for the treatment of acute hydrops secondary to keratoconus. Eye (Lond). 2014;28(7):847–51.
82. Yahia Chérif H, Gueudry J, Afriat M, Delcampe A, Attal P, Gross H, Muraine M. Efficacy and safety of pre-Descemet's membrane sutures for the management of acute corneal hydrops in keratoconus. Br J Ophthalmol. 2015;99(6):773–7.
83. Vajpayee RB, Maharana PK, Kaweri L, Sharma N, Jhanji V. Intrastromal fluid drainage with air tamponade: anterior segment optical coherence tomography guided technique for the management of acute corneal hydrops. Br J Ophthalmol. 2013;97(7):834–6.

Contact Lenses for Keratoconus

13

Varsha M. Rathi, Somasheila I. Murthy, Vishwa Sanghavi, Subhajit Chatterjee, and Rubykala Praskasam

13.1 Introduction

Keratoconus is a bilateral progressive ectatic thinning disorder of the cornea. Poor vision in keratoconus is due to irregular astigmatism [1]. The ectasia occurs at the point or area of thinning. Early stages of keratoconus are benefited with spectacles when myopia or astigmatism is low. However, with increasing severity of keratoconus, the curvature becomes steeper and irregular astigmatism is produced when spectacles do not correct the irregular astigmatism, and contact lenses are prescribed to improve vision. Variety of contact lenses are available for a contact lens practitioner to choose. The first lens is selected based on the severity of the disease though rigid gas permeable (RGP) contact lenses are the preferred lenses. The other parameters considered in selection of the lenses include associated ocular and systemic conditions [2–5]. Fitting a contact lens in a patient having keratoconus is challenging—this chapter will help in getting acceptable fitting of the right lens with proper selection of lenses (soft lenses such as spherical and toric, rigid gas permeable lenses such as corneal, corneo-scleral, mini-scleral and scleral, piggy-back lenses, hybrid lenses) so that keratoplasty can be obviated in patients of keratoconus [2, 3]. We will also discuss about role of the ocular imaging devices such as corneal topography and anterior segment optical coherence tomography (AS-OCT) that assist in contact lens fitting. Special situations such as after collagen cross-linking and after corneal intracorneal ring segment for contact lens fitting are discussed.

V. M. Rathi (✉)
Allen Foster Community Eye Health Research Centre, Gullapalli Pratibha Rao International Centre for Advancement of Rural Eye Care, L V Prasad Eye Institute, Hyderabad, Telangana, India

Indian Health Outcomes, Public Health and Economics (IHOPE) Research Centre, L V Prasad Eye Institute, Hyderabad, Telangana, India

The Cornea Institute, L V Prasad Eye Institute, Hyderabad, Telangana, India
e-mail: varsharathi@lvpei.org

S. I. Murthy
The Cornea Institute, L V Prasad Eye Institute, Hyderabad, Telangana, India
e-mail: smurthy@lvpei.org

V. Sanghavi · S. Chatterjee
Bausch & Lomb Contact Lens Centre, L V Prasad Eye Institute, Hyderabad, Telangana, India
e-mail: vishwa@lvpei.org; subhajit@lvpei.org

R. Praskasam
Standard Chartered LVPEI Academy for Eye Care Education, L V Prasad Eye Institute, Hyderabad, Telangana, India
e-mail: ruby@lvpei.org

13.2 Prerequisite for Fitting

13.2.1 Clinical Examination

A good slit-lamp examination is must to know the severity of keratoconus with its signs such as Vogt's striae, scar, or healed hydrops. One must

S. Das (ed.), *Keratoconus*, https://doi.org/10.1007/978-981-19-4262-4_13

rule out active allergic conjunctivitis or vernal keratoconjunctivitis. Presence of dry eyes also should be ruled out. The presence of any active disease may result in drop out of patients from contact lens wearing. Therefore, management of ocular surface issues and allergies is must before we start fitting contact lenses in such patients. Excessive watering in a patient may result in poor assessment of contact lens fitting.

13.3 Investigations

13.3.1 Corneal Topography

Corneal topography and tomography are very useful and are used in fitting contact lenses [4, 5]. Corneal topography has three major roles in keratoconus: (a) to aid in the diagnosis of early keratoconus, (b) to know the type and severity of cone of keratoconus that will aid in contact lens fitting, and (c) to assess the progression of the disease.

Though scissor's reflex or split reflex on retinoscopy will make one suspect keratoconus, corneal topography is a must for fitting contact lenses and will help the practitioner in educating the patients on progression and help in choosing either glasses or soft lenses in the initial stages of keratoconus. There are various classifications of keratoconus. Based on the topography values, the keratoconus has been classified into mild, moderate, severe, and advanced. If corneal topography is not available, one may do keratometry in the center and inferior cornea to know the difference in the center and inferior dioptric power of cornea. However, it is preferred to have corneal topography done in all patients of keratoconus, before initiating the fitting process. Based on the keratometry values, keratoconus is classified as mild (<45.00 D), moderate (45.00 D to <52.00 D), advanced (52.00 D to <62 D), and severe if >62.00 D [6]. In addition to this, the keratoconus is classified based on the shape of the cone as round or oval cone [7].

The dioptric power that can be measured with keratometry ranges between 36D and 52D. This can be increased to 61D with the use of +1.25 D spherical lens in front of the objective of keratometers. The topography machines have contact lens fitting software. One such software is Fitscan technology. Mandathara et al. have reported that selection of the base curve of the initial trial lens should be 0.22 mm steeper than the FITSCAN calculated base curve, so that chair time of the patients can be reduced [8]. AS-OCT is useful in assessing the relationship of the lens to the corneal surface, the vault of the lens, and the relationship of lens edge and central area in RGP fitting [9, 10].

13.4 Selection of a Lens

There are various types of lenses available for fitting keratoconus patients for vision improvement and selection of the lens is dependent on many factors. Based on the shape of cone, keratoconus is divided into three types: (a) nipple cone which is usually central within 5 mm of diameter and is very steep and observed in 50% of patients; (b) oval cones are between 5 and 7.5 mm in diameter and are located inferotemporally or inferonasally; (c) more than 75% of cornea are involved in globus type of cones (Fig. 13.1). It is important to know the shape of the cone for a practitioner because lens can be selected accordingly, viz. small central nipple cone—smaller diameter, and as the size of the cone increases, one selects larger diameter lenses for fitting.

To begin with, for lower refractive errors, or milder form of keratoconus, one may choose soft contact lens and as the astigmatism increases with improvement in vision, one may go in for various lenses based on the keratometry values as sometimes it may not be possible to get a proper refraction in advanced cases.

13.4.1 Soft Lenses

Spherical soft lenses have a limited role in improving vision in keratoconus though these lenses can be prescribed in early stages [11–13]. Soft spherical contact lenses can be prescribed with cylindrical lenses in the spectacles if required. These spherical soft lenses are also pre-

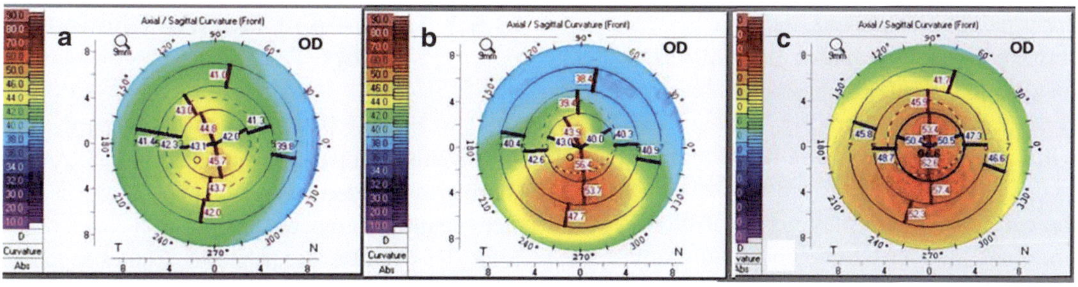

Fig. 13.1 Showing the various shapes of keratoconus on corneal topography: (**a**) nipple cone, which is small central—will need smaller size of RGP lenses; (**b**) oval cone, inferior cone—will need larger diameter of RGP lenses; (**c**) globus cone, involves more than 75% of cornea and will need larger diameter of lenses or other varieties of lenses

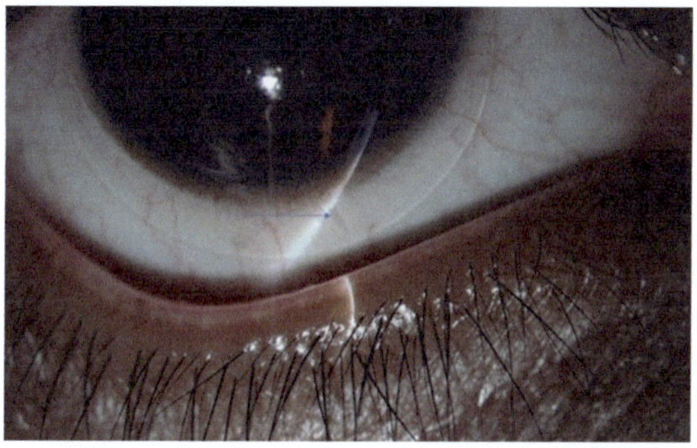

Fig. 13.2 Kerasoft lens (soft toric lens) on eye in a patient with mild keratoconus with laser mark (arrow)

scribed as a base for piggyback lenses when wearing RGP lenses associated with discomfort for the patients. Thicker lenses, larger in size which cause less movement and neutralize astigmatism, may be tried. Smaller lenses may result in poor visual acuity due to decentrations of the lens on the eye [14]. The higher-order aberrations also can be reduced with soft toric lenses [14–16].

Customized toric lenses are available in the market which can be used in keratoconus [17]. Lenses with steeper base curves are available [17–19]. Figure 13.2 shows the Kerasoft lens on the eye. These are available as conventional hydrogel or silicone hydrogel lenses and have front surface aspheric design and quadrant-specific changes can be done while fitting. These are similar to soft toric lenses with a single laser marking at the 6-o' clock position to assess the rotation and eye rotation should be minimal although movement of 1–2 mm of the lens is considered to be acceptable. The lens may take time to settle. It is better to assess the fitting of these lenses after 30 min, as the lens may become steeper on the eye and cause discomfort later to the patients if not assessed over time. With these lenses, improvement in vision and comfort goes hand in hand and can be prescribed. These lenses are also prescribed in patients who had intracorneal ring segments implanted in the eye [12]. One may use the locally made customized soft toric lenses, provided these are comfortable and improve vision in patients of keratoconus. Quite often the soft toric lenses may not be able to improve vision in advanced or severe keratoconus or keratoconus with scars and one may have to use the gold standard—rigid gas permeable lens for improvement in vision.

13.4.2 Rigid Gas Permeable Lenses

RGP lens is the lens of choice. These are smaller diameter lenses which rest on the cornea. The other RGP lenses available are Corneo-Scleral: 12.9–13.5 mm, Semi-Scleral: 13.6–14.9 mm, Mini-Scleral: 15.0–18.0 mm, and Full Scleral: 18.1–24 mm [19, 20].

Selection of RGP lens is dependent on the shape and the dioptric power of the cone, RGP being a stiffer lens, compared to soft, does not drape the cornea the way soft lens does, it usually rests on the cone. Flexure of RGP lens may cause reduction in vision and discomfort and so it is not preferred. In keratoconus, the cone is steeper and surrounding area is flatter. In milder cones, one may be able to fit a bicurve RGP lens but as the cone becomes steeper (Fig. 13.1), RGP lenses with tricurve or multicurve are required. Special trial sets are required for fitting keratoconus. In the early stage, one may get ideal fit but sometimes one may have to accept a compromised fit.

13.5 Fitting Philosophies

Korb et al. have reported scarring in patients having apical bearing and no scarring in patients with apical clearance [21]. Leung et al. too have described these fitting philosophies for keratoconus [22]. Table 13.1 describes various fitting philosophies. These are apical clearance, apical bearing or three-point touch.

13.5.1 Apical Clearance

As the name suggests, it has no touch in the center part of the cornea and with no touch or bearing, the central cornea is devoid of touch with reduced risk of scar. The lens bearing is however directed toward periphery. This may result in lesser tear exchange [22]. This is usually with smaller diameter steeper lenses which are centered over the cone.

13.5.2 Apical Bearing

As the name suggests, there is a touch or bearing on the apex of the cone that results in good visual acuity. However, sometimes the bearing may become heavy due to flatter fitting of these lenses on the eye, resulting in corneal scarring, and intolerance later.

Table 13.1 Fitting philosophies

◆	Apical clearance
◆	Apical bearing
◆	Three-point touch

13.5.3 Three-Point Touch or Divided Support

The lens bearing is divided into three parts, central and the midperiphery of the cornea. As the bearing is divided, tear exchange happens and there is minimal risk of scarring at the apex of the cone. This is also described as feather touch of the lens to the eye (RoseK). This fitting pattern gives good comfort with prolonged wearing time and provides good vision. Figure 13.3 shows the fluorescein pattern of these fitting philosophies.

13.5.4 Fitting RGP Lenses

Once a trial lens is chosen, the lens should be inserted in the eye and a waiting for 20–30 minutes should be allowed so that the patient becomes comfortable and there should not be any watering in the eye. The fitting should be assessed for both—dynamic fitting of the lens on the eye, in relation to the movement of the eye and static fitting of the lens on the eye—after fluorescein instillation. Table 13.2 shows the details to be seen during these assessments.

An ideal fit would be a central feather touch with a peripheral edge lift of 0.5–0.7 mm [17]. However, with advanced cone, the edges may stand off with more pooling of fluorescein. In such scenarios, the edges can be steepened in those meridians—certain companies do allow these meridional changes.

13.6 Lens Designs

Keratoconic corneas have steeper curvature in the area of cone and surrounding curvature is flatter. Most of the designs have central steep base curve and then the base curve flattens in the periphery with multiple radii of curvatures. The lenses can be tricurve or multicurve. Appropriate trial sets are important to have so that one can modify the various curves or optic zones as needed, in consultation with the company. With advanced kera-

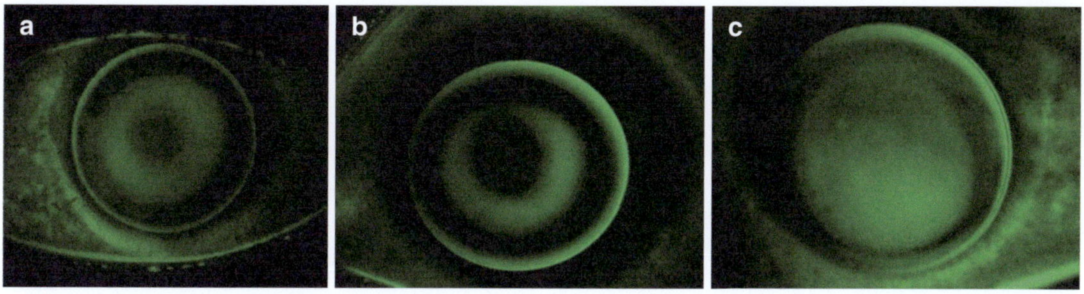

Fig. 13.3 The three fitting philosophies in fitting contact lenses: (**a**) three-point touch with very light fluorescein in the center; (**b**) apical bearing—with more bearing of lens in the center of the cornea compared to (**a**), darker in appearance; (**c**) apical clearance—more fluorescein in the center

Table 13.2 Assessment of dynamic and static fitting

♦	Dynamic fitting
	• Preferable under the lid fit or interpalpebral fit
	• Adequately centered after blink, no decentration
	• Movements 1 mm or so
	• Does not cross the limbus in all gazes of eye movement
	• Patient should be comfortable
♦	Static fitting
	• This is done in the interpalpebral area. Instill fluorescein and then assess the fit in relation to the corneal surface using cobalt blue light with the use of Wratten filter (if not available, one can use a yellow gelatin paper)

toconus, when refraction is not possible, one needs to select a steeper base curve with high power of the lens.

13.6.1 Rose K Lenses

Rose K lenses (Menicon Co, Ltd., Nagoya, Japan) are multicurve lenses with six curves and have a small optic zone that results in a feather touch fluorescein pattern, especially in nipple type of cones. About 90–100% of patients can be fitted successfully with Rose K lens [23–25]. These lenses can be the first lens of choice for fitting keratoconus patients as these lenses are more comfortable compared to regular RGP lenses [26].

An optimal fitting is possible with the small, central nipple cone. Rose K lens can be fitted in any type of keratoconus and 95% of fittings may need a minimum of three lenses [23]. A variety of Rose K lenses are available Rose K2, RoseK2 NC (Nipple Cone), IC, (for Advanced Cones), PG (Post Graft), and XL for larger cones or after keratoplasty. The diameter of the lenses varies, and lens may be selected based on the morphology and severity of cone.

For mild to moderate keratoconus, the lens selected is 0.2 mm steeper than the average keratometry values, for advanced keratoconus—same as the average keratometry values, and for the advanced keratoconus, 0.3 mm flatter than average keratometry values. Mandathara et al. had shown that selecting the initial trial lens base curve based on the 5-mm average *k* values obtained with corneal topography (Orbscan 11z), reduces the number of trials and thereby reduces the chair time [23].

Based on the location, smaller central cone, smaller diameter and steeper base curve, and for large cones, larger diameter lenses are chosen. The advantages of using Rose K lenses are flexible peripheral fit is possible with its toric peripheral curves. It uses asymmetric corneal technology and may be able to steepen the lens curves in particular meridian.

13.6.2 Assessment of Fitting

As discussed earlier in Table 13.2, similar to the other RGP lenses, Rose K lens fitting is assessed. Ideally a feather touch (three-point touch or divided support) should be obtained. This is more so with smaller cones with Rose K NC. With oval cone, as in Fig. 13.1, an ideal touch is seen. With oval and globus cones, larger diameter lenses are needed, and the fitting may appear as superior alignment.

13.6.3 Intralimbal Lenses

These are larger in diameter (10.4–12.0 mm) and the preferred contact lens fitting is under the upper lid [27]. These are usually fitted when the lenses are not stable on the surface or for advanced cases, inferior cones or ectasias other than keratoconus such as pellucid marginal degeneration. The comfort with these lenses is more compared to smaller diameter lenses. The fitting principle is like RGP lenses. Once an optimal fit is achieved, the over-refraction on these lenses is done with loose spherical lens in the trial frame to order new lens with added power.

13.6.4 Piggybacking Lenses

One lens rides over the other on the eye—RGP over SCL (Fig. 13.4). Soft contact gives for comfort and RGP lens improves vision. Here soft contact lens and RGP lenses are used together—one above the other. These lenses are indicated when a patient is intolerant to RGP lenses, unstable RGP lens, 3- and 9-o' clock staining or thin edge clearance. However, it is very difficult to maintain the two lens cleaning solutions, and these are very rarely used nowadays. RGP lens selection is same as above and the soft lens to be used is of low power to give comfort. Corneal topography is done on the silicone hydrogel soft contact lens placed on the eye and then RGP trial is performed using the dioptric values obtained.

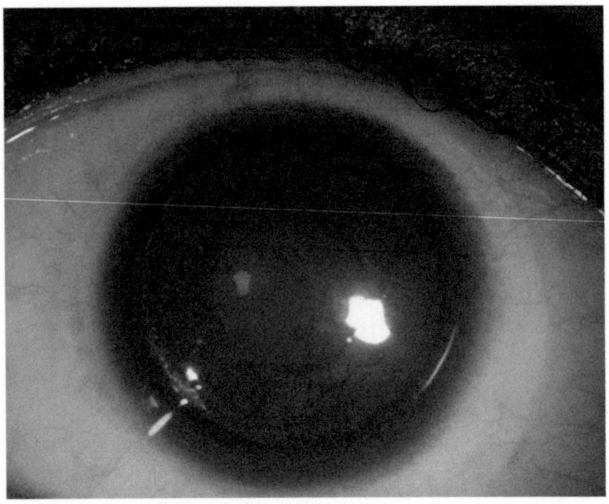

Fig. 13.4 Piggyback contact lens—the arrows show the edges of soft lens and the rigid gas permeable lens. RGP lens over the SCL

The fitting of both lenses is independent of each other and should be assessed individually. Once an optimal fit is achieved, over-refraction is done and then the power is added to the RGP lens. Romero-Jimenez et al. have shown that negative-powered soft contact lenses provide a flatter anterior surface in comparison to positive-powered lenses and should be preferred [28]. High-Dk lenses or hyper-Dk lenses are preferred for piggyback lens system [29–31]. These lenses are also used in patients having intracorneal ring segments [30].

Custom piggyback lenses, though rarely used, are lathe-cut lenses wherein presence of a circular groove in soft contact lens allows RGP lens in it so that there is little interaction of RGP with lids and comfort is improved. The thickness also is reduced so that hypoxia-related complications are reduced. Disadvantages are hypoxia-related changes, papillary conjunctivitis, and difficulty in handling two cleaning regimens of soft and RGP lenses [19, 32, 33].

13.6.5 Hybrid Lenses

As the name says, it has got both soft and rigid lens combined, RGP in the center to give vision and soft contact lens in periphery for achieving optimal fit and providing comfort (Fig. 13.5). Examples of these lenses are Saturn lens, Soft perm lens, SynergEyes lens (SynergEyes, Inc., Carlsbad, CA) [34–37], Eyebrid lenses (LCS Laboratories, Caen, France), AirFlex lenses [38], and UltraHealth lenses.

These lenses are indicated when patient is unable to tolerate RGP lenses or the fitting with RGP lens is suboptimal. There is minimal or no apical touch and lens movement is minimal (0.25 mm) on blink. Sometimes, even less movement is acceptable as these are made up of high-Dk material. To avoid refitting which was reported earlier, a flatter lens is selected nowadays so that even when lens settles, it does not become tight on the eye [36]. The disadvantages of using these lenses are corneal clouding, hypoxia-related changes, frequent tear in the soft skirt, and poor vision sometimes [39–41]. Dropouts were more in sagging cones in one study [38].

Corneo-scleral lenses are of 13.0–15.5 mm in diameter and rest at cornea, limbus, and on sclera and show movement—Rose K2 XL semi-scleral contact lens (Menicon Co. Ltd., Nagoya, Japan).

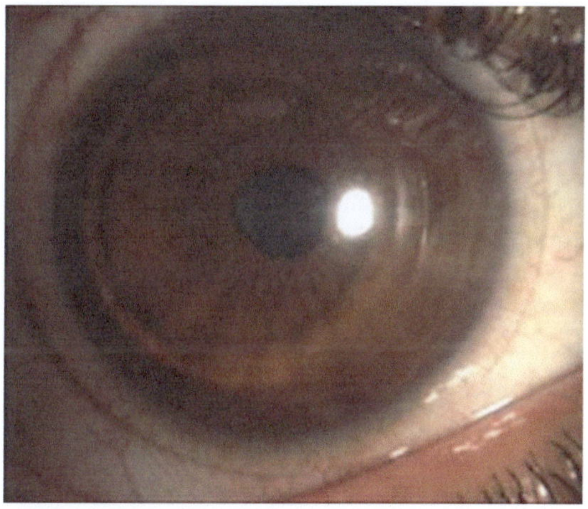

Fig. 13.5 Hybrid lens with central rigid material and peripheral soft skirt

13.6.6 Scleral Lenses

Pullum et al. have brought scleral lenses into practice [42]. Rosenthal is the first one to use CADCAM software and computerized lathe machine and high-Dk material for manufacturing scleral lenses [43]. Various studies have reported the usefulness of scleral lenses in improving vision [44–46]. A true ones rest on sclera and do not touch the cornea [19]. There is a space between scleral lens and the cornea which is termed as vault (Fig. 13.6a, b). These lenses are filled with saline (unisol or normal saline) and then placed on the eye. Technological advances in the last few decades have seen the resurgence of the scleral lenses. This is due to the availability of high-Dk material, advanced techniques in manufacturing and designs [47–49]. These lenses are indicated when all other modalities fail, though some contact lens fitters start with these lenses in advanced keratoconus [50]. The indications are when all other contact lens modalities fail either to improve vision or improve comfort, RGP intolerance, popping out of RGP lenses, and hypoxia-related changes. These lenses are also used for improvement in vision before a patient undergoes keratoplasty as sometimes these lenses can delay or obviate the need for keratoplasty [3, 51]. For example, PROSE (Prosthetic Replacement of the Ocular Surface Ecosystem), BostonSight Scleral lens, MSD (Blanchard Contact Lens Inc., Manchester, UK; 15.8 mm),

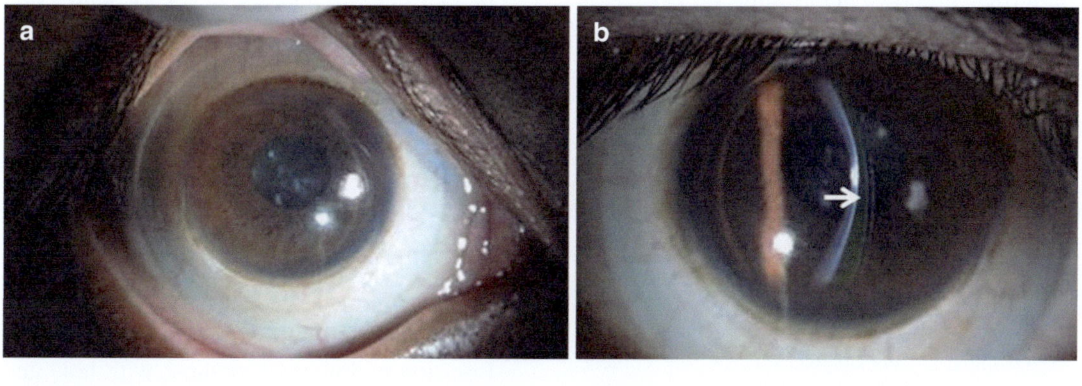

Fig. 13.6 True scleral lens of 19 mm diameter: (**a**) shows the diffuse fitting of the lens on the sclera, no conjunctival crowding or compression of conjunctival blood vessels seen; (**b**) shows the fluorescein level (ununiform – arrow) between the back surface of the lens and the front surface of the cornea

Europa and Jupiter lens (Visionary Optics, 15.0–18.2 mm), Boston mini-scleral (Boston Foundation for Sight, Needham Heights, MA, USA; any diameter 15 mm or more), Tru-scleral (Tru-Form Optics Inc., San Antonio, TX, USA; 16.0–20.0 mm), and Innovative sclerals (15.0–23.0 mm). EyePrintPRO (Advanced Vision Technologies, Lakewood, Colo.) scleral lens is fitted with 3D printing using lathe machine on the posterior surface of the impression mold taken from the eye [48].

These lenses may be fenestrated or nonfenestrated and may have channels for tear exchange. Scleral lens is divided into haptic and optic with a transition zone between them. These need to be evaluated separately while fitting the lenses. Principle of fitting mostly is the same, but the changes are done as per the company's guidelines. We describe fitting of PROSE lens which is a customized lathe-cut lens manufactured using a computerized software program. For keratoconus, usually a true scleral lens of >18 mm diameter or a lens with 18 mm diameter is preferred. Once the lens is placed on the eye, the first thing is to check comfort of the patient and then for presence of air bubble in the saline reservoir. If found, then the lens should be removed, refilled with normal saline, and reinserted in the eye. Once no air bubble is noted, the lens fit is examined immediately, and then after half an hour. The final lenses are ordered after assessing the lens fit on eye after 4–6 h of wear as the lens settles on the eye [9]. Parameters to be checked during fitting are shown in the Table 13.3.

Table 13.3 Assessing scleral lens fit

◆	Subjective—comfort	
◆	Slit-lamp biomicroscopy	
	• Vault	– For presence of air bubbles, debris, and the amount of vault
	• Haptic	– For blanching of conjunctival blood vessels
	• Optic	– Usually, as it is large, it covers the pupil
	• Limbal area	– For conjunctival crowding, corneal edema
	• Edges	– Apposition of the lens to the scleral surface, whether tight (digging in the conjunctiva, or lift—Allowing air bubble or debris seeping in)

13.7 Assessment of Fitting

The lens should not move on eye [52]. A corneal clearance is must. On slit-lamp examination, one can compare this with the thickness of cornea (either peripheral or central or even known thickness of the scleral lens). Objective methods of assessment include ASOCT measurements. OCT should be done immediately and then after 4–6 h of lens wear as lens may settle, more so in keratoconus [9].

As per Table 13.3, assessment should be done. It is continued even when scleral lens is removed. Suction felt while removing the scleral lens indicates that the lens is tight and haptic of the scleral lens should be flattened.

Fluorescein staining of the conjunctiva is done immediately after the lens is removed. Presence of staining of conjunctiva indicates that the lens is too tight, and the edges are digging on the conjunctiva. This is most common with toric sclera and based on the presence of conjunctival staining, one may have to add toricity to the lens.

Figure 13.7 shows the globus cone of keratoconus that is fitted with scleral lens—Vault is visible with fluorescein staining of the postlens tear film or fluid reservoir of scleral contact lens showing adequate vault. The edges of the scleral lens are apposed to sclera. As any other lens, once the fit is optimized, over-refraction is done with loose spherical lens and the power is added to the scleral lens power.

In addition to the basics of fitting, with some of the lenses such as PROSE or BostonSight Sclerals, it is possible to change the curvature of the front surface with change in asphericity values. Front surface eccentricity (FSE) 0.6 is preferred and based on the improvement of vision, presence of ghosting of images, one may change it to other FSE [53]. The FSE values can change/reduce the aberrations of the eye. Similarly, the wavefront-optimized scleral lenses are available that can reduce the aberrations [54–56].

Insertion is done with plunger with hole and removal is done with a small diameter plunger which does not have a hole. Plunger is placed in the center of the fenestrated lenses for removal. The nonfenestrated lenses are removed by

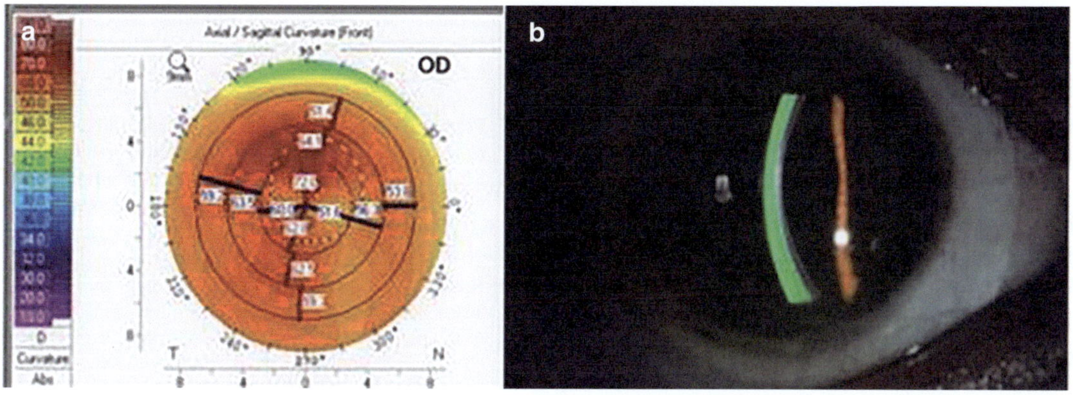

Fig. 13.7 Globus cone of keratoconus: (**a**) fitted with scleral lens—the normal saline is stained with fluorescein; and (**b**) the irregularity of vault is visible

applying the plunger at the limbus, i.e., at the junction of the optic and the haptic.

The most preferred advantage of scleral lenses is improved comfort and vision and delays or obviates the need for keratoplasty. However, the disadvantages include difficulty in initial stages of lens insertion and removal, plungers are used for insertion and removal, and saline bottles or unims needed for filling the lenses.

13.8 Contact Lenses in Special Scenarios

13.8.1 Keratoconus with Vernal Keratoconjunctivitis or Allergic Conjunctivitis

Usually, a scleral lens is preferred as these are more comfortable, do not touch the cornea and rest on sclera. There is no movement of the lens on the eye and so no irritation in these patients [57]. The other lenses which can be considered are Hybrid lenses or customized soft lenses.

13.8.2 After Collagen Cross-Linking

Usually, the patients can start wearing their lenses after a month or so. Mandathara et al. have shown that 62.5% (n = 20 eyes) were prescribed new rigid gas permeable lenses and 37.5% (n = 12 eyes) continued using their own lenses after cross-linking [58].

13.8.3 After Intracorneal Ring Segment Surgeries

Soft lenses, scleral lenses, and RGP lenses can be fitted over intracorneal ring segments (ICRSs) [30, 59–61].

13.8.4 Keratoconus with Stevens-Johnson Syndrome

Scleral lens is preferred in these patients as it improves comfort and vision [62, 63].

13.8.5 Warpage or Progression after RGP Fitting

The contact lens warpage is a reversible condition and appears as smile on the colored map of topography. This reversible change is usually seen in a week or two. Maximum changes in the keratometry occur within first week of discontinuation of lenses [64]. However, the preferred practice is to wait for 2 weeks to note the changes. Based on this, one can differentiate warpage from progression of keratoconus.

13.9 Conclusion

To summarize, use of contact lenses in keratoconus improves vision and delays or avoids surgery such as corneal transplants. RGP lens is the first choice though the selection of a contact lens is based on the morphology or shape of the cone. A high minus lens is selected when refraction is not possible in a keratoconic patient. Soft contact lenses are prescribed in early cases and toric or customized toric lenses may be prescribed when keratoconus is mild or patient is intolerant to RGP contact lenses. As the cone progresses, the lens type changes. RGP is the lens of choice for visual improvement, and one may use any trial lens set available with them or Rose K lenses. Piggyback contact lenses or hybrid lenses may be prescribed when patient is unable to use RGP lenses. Mini-scleral and Scleral lenses improve comfort and vision. Scleral lenses are used as last resort when it is not possible to achieve optimal fitting with improved vision. Use of anterior segment OCT in fitting scleral lenses is useful in keratoconus as based on the vault one may predict the settling of the lenses over time and order lenses accordingly.

Acknowledgments We thank Ms. Sabera Banu, the librarian, for the entire network of L V Prasad Eye Institute, Hyderabad, Telangana, 5000034, India.

Funding Support Hyderabad Eye Research Foundation, Hyderabad, Telangana, 5,000,034, India (for all the authors).

References

1. Rabinowitz YS. Keratoconus. Surv Ophthalmol. 1998;42(4):297–319.
2. Smiddy WE, Hamburg TR, Kracher GP, Stark WJ. Keratoconus. Contact lens or keratoplasty? Ophthalmology. 1988;95(4):487–92.
3. Koppen C, Kreps EO, Anthonissen L, Van Hoey M, Dhubhghaill SN, Vermeulen L. Scleral lenses reduce the need for corneal transplants in severe keratoconus. Am J Ophthalmol. 2018;185:43–7.
4. Rabinowitz YS, Garbus JJ, Garbus C, McDonnell PJ. Contact lens selection for keratoconus using a computer-assisted videophotokeratoscope. CLAO J. 1991;17(2):88–93.
5. Ramdas WD, Vervaet CJ, Bleyen I. Corneal topography for pancorneal toric edge rigid gas-permeable contact lens fitting in patients with keratoconus, and differences in age and gender. Cont Lens Anterior Eye. 2014;37(1):20–5.
6. Buxton JN, Buxton DF, Dias AK, Scorsetti DH. Keratoconus basic and clinical features. In: The CLAO guide to basic science and clinical practice, vol. 3. 3rd ed. Iowa: Kendall/Hunt; 1995. p. 101–22.
7. Perry HD, Buxton JN, Fine BS. Round and oval cones in keratoconus. Ophthalmology. 1980;87(9):905–9.
8. Mandathara PS, Fatima M, Taureen S, Dumpati S, Ali MH, Rathi V. RGP contact lens fitting in keratoconus using FITSCAN technology. Cont Lens Anterior Eye. 2013;36(3):126–9.
9. Rathi VM, Mandathara PS, Dumpati S, Sangwan VS. Change in vault during scleral lens trials assessed with anterior segment optical coherence tomography. Cont Lens Anterior Eye. 2017;40(3):157–61.
10. Elbendary AM, Abou SW. Evaluation of rigid gas permeable lens fitting in keratoconic patients with optical coherence tomography. Graefes Arch Clin Exp Ophthalmol. 2013;251(6):1565–70.
11. Fernandez-Velazquez FJ. Kerasoft IC compared to Rose-K in the management of corneal ectasias. Cont Lens Anterior Eye. 2012;35(4):175–9.
12. Nicula C, Nicula D, Suciu C. Results in keratoconus correction with Kerasoft 3 contact lenses. Rom J Ophthalmol. 2020;64(2):122–7.
13. Su S, Johns L, Rah MJ, Ryan R, Barr J. Clinical performance of KeraSoft(®) IC in irregular corneas. Clin Ophthalmol. 2015;9:1953–64.
14. Jinabhai A, O'Donnell C, Tromans C, Radhakrishnan H. Optical quality and visual performance with customised soft contact lenses for keratoconus. Ophthalmic Physiol Opt. 2014;34(5):528–39.
15. Jinabhai A, Radhakrishnan H, Tromans C, O'Donnell C. Visual performance and optical quality with soft lenses in keratoconus patients. Ophthalmic Physiol Opt. 2012;32(2):100–16.
16. Katsoulos C, Karageorgiadis L, Vasileiou N, Mousafeiropoulos T, Asimellis G. Customized hydrogel contact lenses for keratoconus incorporating correction for vertical coma aberration. Ophthalmic Physiol Opt. 2009;29(3):321–9.
17. Rathi VM, Mandathara PS, Dumpati S. Contact lens in keratoconus. Indian J Ophthalmol. 2013;61(8):410–5.
18. González-Méijome JM, Jorge J, de Almeida JB, Parafita MA. Soft contact lenses for keratoconus: case report. Eye Contact Lens. 2006;32(3):143–7.
19. Barnett M, Mannis MJ. Contact lenses in the management of keratoconus. Cornea. 2011;30(12):1510–6.
20. Niechwiej-Szwedo E, Kennedy SA, Colpa L, Chandrakumar M, Goltz HC, Wong AM. Effects of induced monocular blur versus anisometropic amblyopia on saccades, reaching, and eye-hand coordination. Invest Ophthalmol Vis Sci. 2012;53(8):4354–62.
21. Korb DR, Finnemore VM, Herman JP. Apical changes and scarring in keratoconus as related to contact lens fitting techniques. J Am Optom Assoc. 1982;53(3):199–205.
22. Leung KK. RGP fitting philosophies for keratoconus. Clin Exp Optom. 1999;82(6):230–5.

23. Mandathara Sudharman P, Rathi V, Dumapati S. Rose K lenses for keratoconus—an Indian experience. Eye Contact Lens. 2010;36(4):220–2.
24. Ozkurt YB, Sengor T, Kurna S, Evciman T, Acikgoz S, Haboğlu M, Aki S. Rose K contact lens fitting for keratoconus. Int Ophthalmol. 2008;28(6):395–8.
25. Jain AK, Sukhija J. Rose-K contact lens for keratoconus. Indian J Ophthalmol. 2007;55(2):121–5.
26. Betts AM, Mitchell GL, Zadnik K. Visual performance and comfort with the rose K lens for keratoconus. Optom Vis Sci. 2002;79(8):493–501.
27. Ozbek Z, Cohen EJ. Use of intralimbal rigid gas-permeable lenses for pellucid marginal degeneration, keratoconus, and after penetrating keratoplasty. Eye Contact Lens. 2006;32(1):33–6.
28. Romero-Jiménez M, Santodomingo-Rubido J, Flores-Rodríguez P, González-Méijome JM. Which soft contact lens power is better for piggyback fitting in keratoconus? Cont Lens Anterior Eye. 2013;36(1):45–8.
29. Sengor T, Kurna SA, Aki S, Ozkurt Y. High-Dk piggyback contact lens system for contact lens-intolerant keratoconus patients. Clin Ophthalmol. 2011;5:331–5.
30. Smith KA, Carrell JD. High-Dk piggyback contact lenses over Intacs for keratoconus: a case report. Eye Contact Lens. 2008;34(4):238–41.
31. O'Donnell C, Maldonado-Codina C. A hyper-Dk piggyback contact lens system for keratoconus. Eye Contact Lens. 2004;30(1):44–8.
32. Moschos MM, Nitoda E, Georgoudis P, Balidis M, Karageorgiadis E, Kozeis N. Contact lenses for keratoconus—current practice. Open Ophthalmol J. 2017;11:241–51.
33. Kok JH, van Mil C. Piggyback lenses in keratoconus. Cornea. 1993;12(1):60–4.
34. Maguen E, Caroline P, Rosner IR, Macy JI, Nesburn AB. The use of the SoftPerm lens for the correction of irregular astigmatism. CLAO J. 1992;18(3):173–6.
35. Maguen E, Martinez M, Rosner IR, Caroline P, Macy J, Nesburn AB. The use of Saturn II lenses in keratoconus. CLAO J. 1991;17(1):41–3.
36. Abdalla YF, Elsahn AF, Hammersmith KM, Cohen EJ. SynergEyes lenses for keratoconus. Cornea. 2010;29(1):5–8.
37. Hashemi H, Shaygan N, Asgari S, Rezvan F, Asgari S. ClearKone-Synergeyes or rigid gas-permeable contact lens in keratoconic patients: a clinical decision. Eye Contact Lens. 2014;40(2):95–8.
38. Kloeck D, Koppen C, Kreps EO. Clinical outcome of hybrid contact lenses in keratoconus. Eye Contact Lens. 2021;47(5):283–7.
39. Harbiyeli II, Erdem E, Isik P, Yagmur M, Ersoz R. Use of new-generation hybrid contact lenses for managing challenging corneas. Eur J Ophthalmol. 2021;31(4):1802–8.
40. Carracedo G, González-Méijome JM, Lopes-Ferreira D, Carballo J, Batres L. Clinical performance of a new hybrid contact lens for keratoconus. Eye Contact Lens. 2014;40(1):2–6.
41. Fernandez-Velazquez FJ. Severe epithelial edema in Clearkone SynergEyes contact lens wear for keratoconus. Eye Contact Lens. 2011;37(6):381–5.
42. Pullum KW, Whiting MA, Buckley RJ. Scleral contact lenses: the expanding role. Cornea. 2005;24(3):269–77.
43. Rosenthal P. The Boston lens and the management of keratoconus. Int Ophthalmol Clin. 1986;26(1):101–9.
44. Visser ES, Visser R, van Lier HJ, Otten HM. Modern scleral lenses part I: clinical features. Eye Contact Lens. 2007;33(1):13–20.
45. van der Worp E, Bornman D, Ferreira DL, Faria-Ribeiro M, Garcia-Porta N, González-Meijome JM. Modern scleral contact lenses: a review. Cont Lens Anterior Eye. 2014;37(4):240–50.
46. Barnett M, Courey C, Fadel D, Lee K, Michaud L, Montani G, van der Worp E, Vincent SJ, Walker M, Bilkhu P, Morgan PB. CLEAR—Scleral lenses. Cont Lens Anterior Eye. 2021;44(2):270–88.
47. Schein OD, Rosenthal P, Ducharme C. A gas-permeable scleral contact lens for visual rehabilitation. Am J Ophthalmol. 1990;109(3):318–22.
48. Nguyen MTB, Thakrar V, Chan CC. EyePrintPRO therapeutic scleral contact lens: indications and outcomes. Can J Ophthalmol. 2018;53(1):66–70.
49. Rathi VM, Mandathara PS, Taneja M, Dumpati S, Sangwan VS. Scleral lens for keratoconus: technology update. Clin Ophthalmol. 2015;9:2013–8.
50. Segal O, Barkana Y, Hourovitz D, Behrman S, Kamun Y, Avni I, Zadok D. Scleral contact lenses may help where other modalities fail. Cornea. 2003;22(4):308–10.
51. Ling JJ, Mian SI, Stein JD, Rahman M, Poliskey J, Woodward MA. Impact of scleral contact lens use on the rate of corneal transplantation for keratoconus. Cornea. 2021;40(1):39–42.
52. Jacobs DS, Rosenthal P. Boston scleral lens prosthetic device for treatment of severe dry eye in chronic graft-versus-host disease. Cornea. 2007;26(10):1195–9.
53. Hussoin T, Le HG, Carrasquillo KG, Johns L, Rosenthal P, Jacobs DS. The effect of optic asphericity on visual rehabilitation of corneal ectasia with a prosthetic device. Eye Contact Lens. 2012;38(5):300–5.
54. Hastings GD, Applegate RA, Nguyen LC, Kauffman MJ, Hemmati RT, Marsack JD. Comparison of wavefront-guided and best conventional scleral lenses after habituation in eyes with corneal ectasia. Optom Vis Sci. 2019;96(4):238–47.
55. Sabesan R, Johns L, Tomashevskaya O, Jacobs DS, Rosenthal P, Yoon G. Wavefront-guided scleral lens prosthetic device for keratoconus. Optom Vis Sci. 2013;90(4):314–23.
56. Marsack JD, Ravikumar A, Nguyen C, Ticak A, Koenig DE, Elswick JD, Applegate RA. Wavefront-guided scleral lens correction in keratoconus. Optom Vis Sci. 2014;91(10):1221–30.
57. Rathi VM, Mandathara PS, Vaddavalli PK, Srikanth D, Sangwan VS. Fluid-filled scleral contact lens in pediatric patients: challenges and outcome. Cont Lens Anterior Eye. 2012;35(4):189–92.

58. Mandathara PS, Kalaiselvan P, Rathi VM, Murthy SI, Taneja M, Sangwan VS. Contact lens fitting after corneal collagen cross-linking. Oman J Ophthalmol. 2019;12(3):177–80.
59. Carballo-Alvarez J, Puell MC, Cuiña R, Diaz-Valle D, Vazquez JM, Benitez-Del-Castillo JM. Soft contact lens fitting after intrastromal corneal ring segment implantation to treat keratoconus. Cont Lens Anterior Eye. 2014;37(5):377–81.
60. Rathi VM, Mandathara PS, Dumpati S, Sangwan VS. Scleral lens after intracorneal ring segments in patients with keratoconus. Cont Lens Anterior Eye. 2018;41(2):234–7.
61. Dalton K, Sorbara L. Fitting an MSD (mini scleral design) rigid contact lens in advanced keratoconus with INTACS. Cont Lens Anterior Eye. 2011;34(6):274–81.
62. Rathi VM, Taneja M, Dumpati S, Mandathara PS, Sangwan VS. Role of scleral contact lenses in Management of Coexisting Keratoconus and Stevens-Johnson Syndrome. Cornea. 2017;36(10):1267–9.
63. Saeed HN, Kohanim S, Le HG, Chodosh J, Jacobs DS. Stevens-Johnson syndrome and corneal ectasia: management and a case for association. Am J Ophthalmol. 2016;169:276–81.
64. Kumar P, Ali MH, Reddy JC, Vaddavalli PK. Short-term changes in topometric indices after discontinuation of rigid gas permeable lens wear in keratoconic eyes. Indian J Ophthalmol. 2020;68(12):2911–7.

Corneal Cross-Linking in Keratoconus

14

Farhad Hafezi and Mark Hillen

14.1 Introduction

First used over 20 years ago for the treatment of the corneal ectasia, keratoconus, corneal cross-linking (CXL) is a procedure that has evolved over this period into one that is able to not only treat several different ectasia types, but be used as an infectious keratitis therapy too.

CXL involves saturating the corneal stroma with riboflavin, followed by a period of ultraviolet (UV)-A irradiation (Fig. 14.1) [1]. Riboflavin absorbs the UV-A energy, generating riboflavin radicals and reactive oxygen species (ROS), which go on to have multiple effects. The intended effect in CXL for ectasia is the covalent binding together of stromal molecules (mostly collagen), which makes the cornea stiffer and stronger [2]. Corneal ectasias like keratoconus tend to develop a cone-like shape, as weakened corneas are less able to resist the distending forces of intraocular pressure. CXL has a side benefit of making the cornea more resistant to this distension and helps flatten it (although the extent of flattening is hard to predict). The covalent binding together of stromal molecules also reduces the number of available metalloproteinase cleavage sites – an effect called steric hindrance – making the cornea less susceptible to enzymatic digestion [3, 4]. ROS can also directly damage the cell membranes and nucleic acids of any pathogens present. UV-A irradiation can also kill pathogens by its damaging effect on nucleic acids, but adding riboflavin to UV-A irradiation results in a ten-fold increase in cytotoxicity compared with UV-A irradiation alone [5]. This is exactly the same mechanism of action exploited when photoactivated riboflavin is used to reduce the pathogen load in not only blood and blood products [6–9], but also drinking water, in a process called Solar Disinfection (SODIS) [8]. It has been postulated that CXL has anti-inflammatory and antinociceptive effects, through the inhibition of the synthesis of inflammatory cytokines substances like TNF-, IL-1, IL-6, and interferon [10, 11]. Importantly, these effects mean that the cornea is rendered sterile after CXL is performed [12–14], and represents an attractive treatment

F. Hafezi (✉)
Ocular Cell Biology Group, Center for Applied Biotechnology and Molecular Medicine, University of Zurich, Zurich, Switzerland

ELZA Institute AG, Dietikon, Switzerland

Department of Ophthalmology, Keck School of Medicine, University of Southern California, Los Angeles, CA, USA

Faculty of Medicine, University of Geneva, Geneva, Switzerland

Department of Ophthalmology, Wenzhou Medical University, Wenzhou, China
e-mail: farhad@hafezi.ch

M. Hillen
ELZA Institute AG, Dietikon, Switzerland
e-mail: mhillen@elza-institute.com

S. Das (ed.), *Keratoconus*, https://doi.org/10.1007/978-981-19-4262-4_14

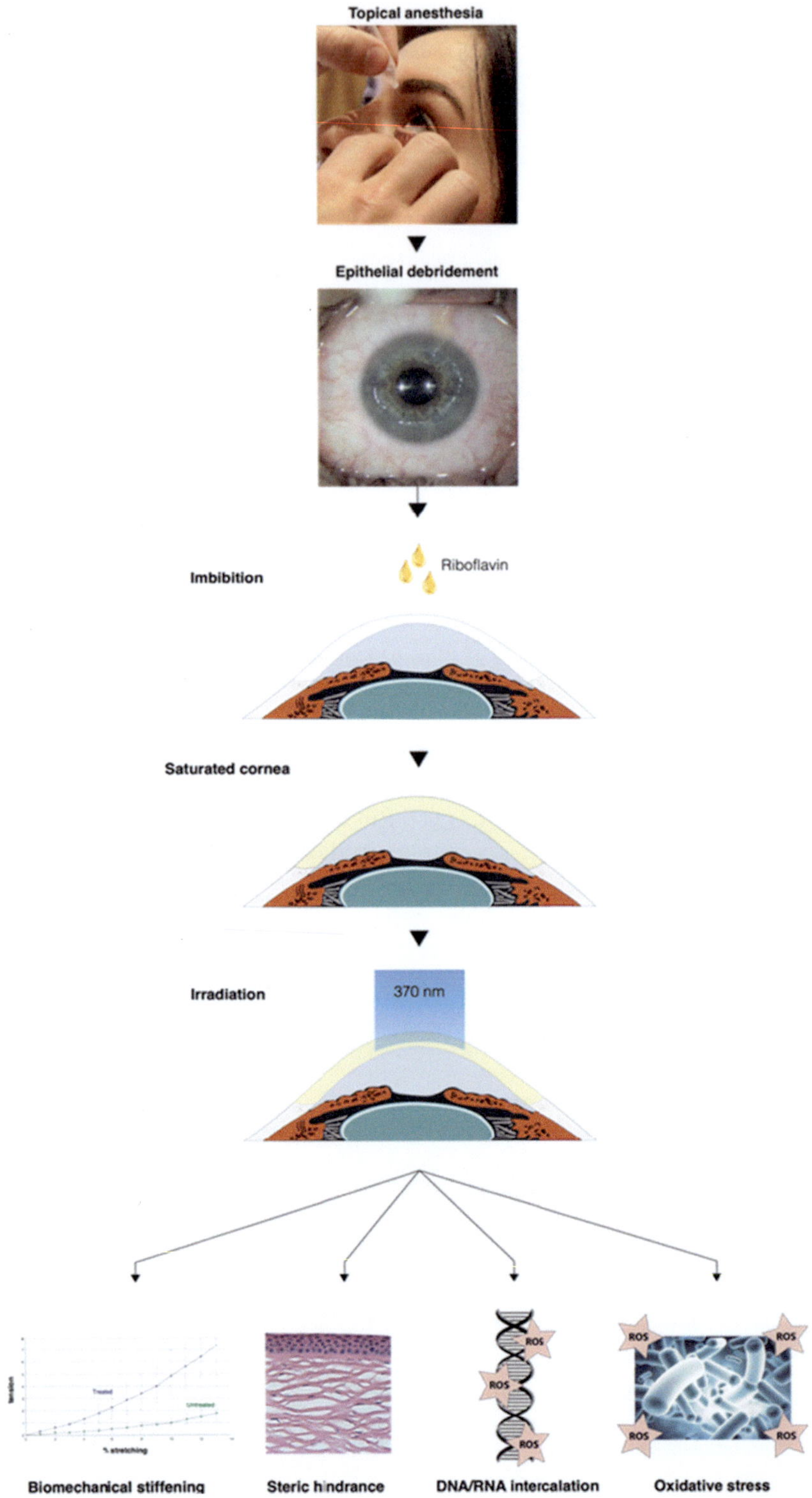

Fig. 14.1 Illustration of a classic epithelium-off corneal cross-linking (CXL) procedure and the effects the photoactivated riboflavin has on the cornea. Dresden protocol CXL dictates that the UV-A irradiation is 30 min of 3 mW/cm^2 UV irradiance to deliver a fluence of 5.4 J/cm^2

option for infectious keratitis, where it is termed photoactivated chromophore for keratitis-corneal cross-linking (PACK-CXL) [15].

14.2 CXL to Arresting Keratoconus Progression

The prototype CXL-for-ectasia protocol, developed 20 years ago, is called the "Dresden protocol", after the city in which it was first developed [16]. This protocol requires around an 8-mm diameter of the corneal epithelium to be removed as a first step after anesthesia and is referred to as an epithelium off ("epi-off") procedure [16]. The reason for this is that riboflavin does not ordinarily penetrate the tight junction between these cells [17], which function to protect the cornea from the outside world. The riboflavin needs to reach the collagen-rich stroma directly underneath to exert its effects. Fortunately, the corneal epithelium is repopulated after the procedure, but the process of epithelial regrowth can take over a week, and topical antimicrobial medication, analgesia, and bandage contact lenses are required for approximately two weeks after the procedure, in order to manage pain and the increased infection risk of an open cornea. Dresden protocol CXL also requires a 30-min period of saturating the stroma with riboflavin drops, before a 30-min period of UV-A irradiation (365–370 nm) is commenced, with riboflavin drops being applied to the cornea every 5 min during this process.

Dresden protocol CXL is considered to be the gold standard method of performing the procedure, as it has been shown to be the most effective method of halting the progression of keratectasia in general, as has been demonstrated in multiple short- and long-term studies [18–20]. Using this method, the keratoconus progression can successfully be arrested, with sustained improvements in clinical outcomes demonstrated for up to 10 years of follow-up [21]. However, several attempts have been made since the introduction of the Dresden protocol to work around several of its drawbacks, with mixed success.

14.3 Epi-on *Versus* Epi-off CXL

In an ideal world, a CXL procedure that did not require epithelial removal for riboflavin to penetrate the stroma (an "epi-on" procedure) would be preferable, and many groups have strived to achieve this. However, the efficacy of these epi-on approaches has, historically, been less effective at achieving the principal clinical endpoint: cessation of ectasia progression. One randomized-controlled trial reported evidence of keratoconus progression in 23% of eyes that underwent epi-on CXL, whereas progression was halted in all epi-off-treated eyes [22].

Several molecules that increase the permeability of tight intraepithelial junctions to riboflavin have been evaluated, and include tetracaine, benzalkonium chloride, ethylenediaminetetraacetic acid (EDTA), and trometamol, all of which are toxic to the corneal epithelium. While a meta-analysis has shown that epi-on CXL protocols that employed pretreatment with penetration enhancers certainly reduce the corneal curvature as effectively as eyes treated with standard epithelium-off protocol; [23] it is clear that historically, epi-on protocols with chemical enhancers alone are less effective than epi-off protocols at halting keratoconus progression [24].

Another approach to enable riboflavin to penetrate the epithelium is iontophoresis, in which an electric field is created to increase the diffusion of negatively charged riboflavin through the epithelium and into the stroma. A meta-analysis of 455 eyes with keratoconus by Wen *et al.* found that after 1 year of follow-up, standard epi-off CXL was associated with significantly greater reductions ($p = 0.03$) in mean K values than epi-on protocols, but a subgroup analysis found that standard epi-off CXL had a similar effect in reducing mean K values as epi-on CXL protocols that utilized chemical penetration enhancers, but had a much greater effect at reducing mean K values than transepeithelial epi-on CXL protocols ($p = 0.01$) although there were no statistically significant differences between the groups in terms of the other outcomes measured (uncorrected distance visual acuity, maximum keratometry, corrected distance visual acuity, mean refractive spherical equivalent, central corneal thickness, endothelial cell density and the occurrence of adverse events) [23].

14.4 Accelerated CXL Protocols

The Dresden protocol requires 30 min of 3 mW/cm^2 UV-A irradiation of the stroma to deliver a total UV-A dose (or "fluence") of 5.4 J/cm^2. Ideally, this period would be shorter, as decreasing the procedure time benefits both patients and doctors [25]. Twenty years ago, technological limitations defined and constrained the irradiation parameters, as more powerful UV light sources were not available back then. However, since the advent of UV-A emitting LEDs over a decade ago, higher-intensity UV-A light sources have become readily available. Photochemical reactions can be described by the Bunsen-Roscoe Law of reciprocity, which states that if all the reaction reagents (riboflavin and UV-A light) are in excess, the amount of photochemical reaction that occurs is determined by the fluence, regardless of whether the 5.4 J/cm^2 fluence is delivered as 3 mW/cm^2 for 30 min, or 30 mW/cm^2 for 3 min. This was the rationale for developing accelerated CXL protocols.

Unfortunately, Bunsen-Roscoe does not apply to the stiffening effect of CXL. Accelerated protocols that delivered 5.4 J/cm^2 fluence with a greater intensity over a shorter period all resulted in a lower biomechanical stiffening effect [25–27]. The reason for this was that there was an additional and essential reaction component that was not accounted for: oxygen. In accelerated protocols, once UV irradiation is commenced, stromal oxygen is consumed and depleted at a faster rate than it can be replenished by diffusion. In other words, oxygen diffusion into the cornea is the rate-limiting step [24]. Almost every epi-on CXL procedure tried has therefore failed to deliver Dresden protocol levels of corneal strengthening, although a consensus has formed around a 9 mW/cm^2 for 10-min protocol as an acceptable trade-off between speeding the procedure time while still retaining acceptable levels of corneal strengthening [28].

14.5 Attempts to Overcome the Rate-Limiting Effects of Oxygen

Several approaches have been taken to work around this oxygen availability limitation, principally pulsed UV-A irradiation, and the use of supplemental oxygen. Pulsed fractionation of UV-A energy delivery appears to increase the depth of the cross-linking effect when performed clinically [29, 30], but laboratory assessments show that this approach does not substantially improve corneal biomechanical strength [31]. Another pulsed UV-A approach, this time using an epi-on iontophoresis approach to deliver riboflavin, while delivering an enhanced UV-A fluence of 18 mW/cm^2 for 6.38 min, has been performed, with 3-year follow-up data showing mean visual acuity being greater and mean maximum keratometry readings being lower than preoperative values, and demarcation line depth that is close to that of one created by the standard epithelium-off cross-linking [32].

Supplemental oxygen combined with a pulsed UV-A irradiation applied to the corneal surface, can increase the depth and strengthening effect of corneal cross-linking, as has been demonstrated in laboratory studies [33, 34]. Clinical studies are underway to determine this protocol's real-world effectiveness.

14.6 CXL in Thin Corneas

While the epithelial cells on the surface of the cornea can be damaged and debrided, and will grow back over the course of a week or so, the same does not apply to the endothelial cells at the base of the cornea. Further, there is a threshold level of UV-A irradiation that can start to cause epithelial cell apoptosis. However, riboflavin acts as a shield against UV-A energy penetrating into the cornea too deeply – although this is a shield that is consumed by the UV energy, from the top down. The Dresden protocol specified that for CXL to be performed safely, corneas should have a minimum corneal

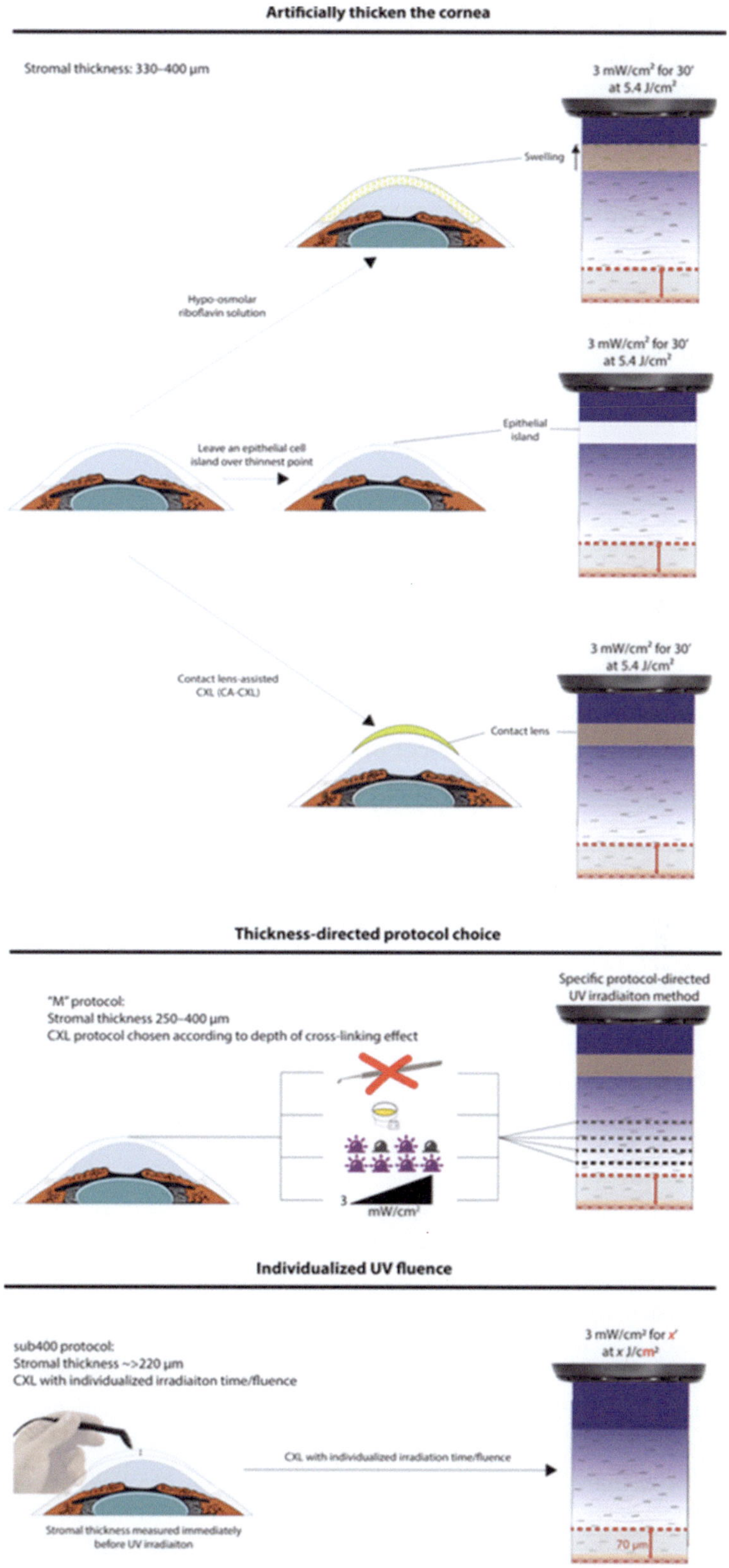

Fig. 14.2 Methods of cross-linking corneas thinner than 400 µm

thickness of 400 μm after epithelial debridement [17]. In a 400-μm-thick cornea, the Dresden protocol cross-links the superficial ~330 μm of the stroma, leaving ~70 μm of unreacted riboflavin in the basal stroma, as a safety margin to protect the corneal endothelium (Fig. 14.2). This safety margin distance was calculated based on riboflavin concentration estimates and the total fluence delivered to the cornea, to keep the endothelial cell UV-A exposure below damage threshold levels. However, the consequence of this is that the 400-μm corneal thickness limitation excludes many corneas with corneal ectatic disease that would benefit from CXL, many of whom will eventually otherwise require keratoplasty.

14.6.1 Artificial Thickening Approaches

Over the years, several modifications have been made to the Dresden protocol to overcome the 400 μm limit, most of which artificially thicken the cornea. However, these approaches are associated with drawbacks that may result in unpredictable outcomes, and consequently can reduce the subsequent efficacy of cross-linking [35–37].

The first approach was developed by Hafezi *et al.* in 2009 [35], which involved the preoperative swelling of the cornea with hypo-osmolaric riboflavin. Of the 20 eyes treated, keratectasia remained stable in all eyes after 6 months of follow-up, with no cases of endothelial cell loss being observed. However, the swelling effect using the same riboflavin soaking regime can be highly variable between corneas [38]. Jacob *et al.* took a contact lens-assisted CXL (CA-CXL) approach, which used an iso-osmolaric riboflavin-soaked contact lens to artificially "thicken" the cornea [36]. This approach achieved the minimum 400-μm corneal thickness before irradiation, but had the disadvantage that oxygen diffusion into the stroma was hindered by the contact lens [39]. This method was associated with a ~ 30% reduction in cross-linking efficacy compared with Dresden protocol CXL, as measured by Brillouin microscopy thermal shrinkage tests and biomechanical stress–strain measurements [40, 41]. Repurposed small-incision lenticule extraction (SMILE) lenticules have also been used in a similar manner [42].

Mazzotta [37] *et al.* offered "epithelial island cross-linking," where epithelial cells over the thinnest point of the cornea are not debrided, leaving an additional 40–50 μm of tissue above the stroma, with any riboflavin accumulating in the epithelial cells helping to attenuate the UV-A energy over these regions. However, there are some conceptual concerns with this approach: the epithelium would have a shielding effect not only in terms of UV energy, but also oxygen diffusion, and there are concerns that epithelial island edges might refract UV-A energy into the intermediate stroma, making the cross-linking effect more difficult to predict. In reality, this approach has resulted in an unequal demarcation line between epithelialized and de-epithelialized areas [40], and in addition to attenuating the UV dose received in the stroma, this additional restriction on oxygen diffusion results in a shallower cross-linking effect: areas under the epithelium-intact region had 150 μm of corneal cross-linked, whereas this was 250 μm in the epithelium-debrided regions [43–45].

14.6.2 Choosing a Protocol that Delivers the Desired Cross-Linking Depth

The "M" protocol is one approach that exploits the fact that non-Dresden protocol cross-linking methods are less effective than the original and cross-link less deeply [46] The M protocol cross-references the depth of cross-linking achieved by existing CXL methods that employ different technical settings (e.g., pulsed and continuous light, iontophoresis, different UV intensities, etc.) and pairs the known depth of effect from each method with the thickness of the thin cornea needing cross-linked. The drawback of this approach is that it requires surgeons to have access to a range of cross-linking technologies to be able to treat all thin corneas of a thickness between 250 and 400 μm.

14.6.3 Individualizing Fluence to each Patient's Corneal Thickness

A logical alternative approach is to individualize the UV-A fluence delivered to each patient based on their corneal thickness, which can be achieved by simply reducing the irradiation time. Recently, the "sub400" protocol has been developed that uses an algorithm that accounts for UV intensity, oxygen and stromal riboflavin levels during the cross-linking procedure to predict the extent of biomechanical stiffening achieved after CXL, and the duration of UV irradiation required to cross-link the stroma to the same safety threshold/distance from the corneal epithelial cells [24, 31]. Clinical validation of the sub400 algorithm was recently published [47], in which 39 patients with progressive keratoconus and stromal thicknesses ranging from 214 to 398 μm were treated with an epi-off approach. After epithelial cell debridement, patients' corneas were soaked with 0.1% hypotonic riboflavin solution for 20 min to saturate the stroma. UV irradiation was then performed at an intensity of 3 mW/cm^2 with the duration (and therefore the total fluence) adapted to the intraoperative stromal thickness of each eye under treatment. After 1 year of follow-up, individualized sub400 protocol CXL successfully prevented keratoconus progression in these ultra-thin keratoconic corneas in 90% of cases, and not a single cornea showed clinical signs of endothelial decompensation. There was a significant correlation between demarcation line depth and irradiation time, but no significant correlation between the depth of the demarcation line and change in *K*max.

14.6.4 Cross-Linking Corneal Infections

As mentioned earlier, the ROS produced during the UV-riboflavin interaction can disrupt the cell membranes of pathogens and intercalate with pathogen nucleic acids, resulting in a pathogen-killing effect. Furthermore, covalently cross-linking together molecules in the stroma, through steric hindrance, reduces the number of binding sites available for pathogen-produced proteases to act on. For these reasons, PACK-CXL has been actively investigated as an alternative to antimicrobial therapy for the treatment of infectious keratitis, with the greatest evidence for its efficacy being for the treatment of bacterial, fungal, or mixed bacterial/fungal keratitis.

The first instance of cross-linking being used to treat corneal infections was in 2008, when Iseli et al. used Dresden protocol CXL (5.4 J/cm^2 fluence) to treat five patients with advanced corneal melts of an infectious origin (two patients had fungal keratitis, three had *Mycobacterium* spp infection) unresponsive to maximal topical and systemic antimicrobial therapy [48].

Recently, Ting *et al.* performed a systematic review and meta-analysis of the PACK-CXL literature, assessing the efficacy of adjuvant PACK-CXL (i.e., PACK-CXL plus the standard-of-care antimicrobial therapy) as infectious keratitis therapy [49]. They identified 46 studies, including four randomized controlled trials, that included a total of 435 patients. They found that compared with standard-of-care antimicrobial treatment alone, adjuvant PACK-CXL resulted in a shorter mean time to complete corneal healing (−7.44 days; 95% CI, −10.71 to −4.16) and quicker infiltrate resolution at 7 days (−5.49 mm^2; 95% CI, −7.44 to −3.54) and at 14–30 days (−5.27 mm^2; 95% CI, −9.12 to −1.41), with no significant differences between groups being observed in terms of epithelial defect size, corrected distance visual acuity (CDVA), and adverse event risk.

Makdoumi [50] *et al.* revealed the potential of PACK-CXL to be used as a first-line monotherapy for bacterial keratitis in a pilot study that involved 16 patients who initially presented with a corneal ulcer. Initially, all patients responded to CXL, with only two patients needing adjunctive treatment with systemic and topical antibiotics.

More recently, Torres-Netto [51] *et al.* reported on the results of an international open-label prospective randomized controlled multicenter phase III trial of PACK-CXL for the treatment of infectious keratitis. The trial randomized 42 eyes (42 patients) with infiltrates and early ulcers <4 mm in diameter and <300 μm in depth of either bacterial or fungal origin, to either standard of care antimicrobial treatment [52] ($n = 23$) or PACK-CXL ($n = 19$) with a total fluence of either 5.4 or 7.2 J/cm^2, with the time to corneal re-epithelialization being the primary efficacy endpoint. The researchers observed no significant differences in re-epithelialization time between the medication and PACK-CXL-only treatment groups (respectively, 15.5 ± 15.0 vs. 10.7 ± 7.7 days, $p = 0.791$). Despite a (nonsignificant, 5-day) longer time to healing, 89% of patients in the PACK-CXL treatment group healed without the use of antimicrobial therapy, which compares with a 93% successful treatment rate in the antimicrobial treatment group. It became clear during the execution of this trial that the bacteria-killing efficacy of PACK-CXL is greatly improved when a total fluence of 7.2 J/cm^2 is applied [53], and this observation informed Torres-Netto *et al*'s decision to start applying a 7.2 J/cm^2 total fluence in their trial [51].

There is increasing and promising evidence that high UV fluences [54] and even the use of an alternative chromophore (rose bengal instead of riboflavin) with visible light at a wavelength of 532 nm (instead of 365–370 nm) could be potentially effective strategies for treating infections of the cornea of bacterial, fungal, and parasitic origin, but further investigation and optimization are required before wider clinical deployment can start [55–58].

14.6.5 The Future of CXL

There is a global unmet need, particularly in low-to-middle income countries (LMICs), for CXL technology to be made available to more patients who would benefit from the procedure. In both developed and LMICs, there is intense pressure to reduce costs and resource usage in healthcare systems. In terms of CXL (and PACK-CXL), one of the largest cost drivers is the fact that most CXL procedures are performed in operating theaters. Given the fact that CXL renders a cornea essentially sterile at the end of the procedure, the main advantage of an operating theater setting, sterility, no longer applies. The availability of portable, slit lamp-mountable cross-linking UV light sources has brought CXL and PACK-CXL out of the operating room and out to any location one might find a slit lamp such as a procedure room or a doctor's office should bring cost savings in any setting, but from the perspective of an LMIC, this move has further benefits. Operating theaters exist only in hospitals, which tend to exist in large population centers, which in LMICs, make this a location (and therefore the procedure) that is not only physically out of the reach of much of the rural dwelling population, but thanks to the costs associated with running an operating theater, out of financial reach too. Transitioning toward an office-based setting has the potential to bring a valuable and effective sight-saving treatment to many more people who need it, who might otherwise never receive it, be it CXL for keratoconus, or PACK-CXL for infectious keratitis.

References

1. Randleman JB, Khandelwal SS, Hafezi F. Corneal cross-linking. Surv Ophthalmol. 2015;60(6):509–23.
2. Wollensak G, Spoerl E, Seiler T. Riboflavin/ultraviolet-a-induced collagen crosslinking for the treatment of keratoconus. Am J Ophthalmol. 2003;135(5):620–7.
3. Berman MB. Collagenase inhibitors: rationale for their use in treating corneal ulceration. Int Ophthalmol Clin. 1975;15(4):49–66.
4. Spoerl E, Wollensak G, Seiler T. Increased resistance of crosslinked cornea against enzymatic digestion. Curr Eye Res. 2004;29(1):35–40.
5. Wollensak G, Spoerl E, Reber F, Seiler T. Keratocyte cytotoxicity of riboflavin/UVA-treatment in vitro. Eye (Lond). 2004;18(7):718–22.
6. Ruane PH, Edrich R, Gampp D, Keil SD, Leonard RL, Goodrich RP. Photochemical inactivation of selected viruses and bacteria in platelet concentrates using riboflavin and light. Transfusion. 2004;44(6):877–85.
7. Reddy HL, Dayan AD, Cavagnaro J, Gad S, Li J, Goodrich RP. Toxicity testing of a novel riboflavin-based technology for pathogen reduction and white blood cell inactivation. Transfus Med Rev. 2008;22(2):133–53.
8. Heaselgrave W, Kilvington S. Antimicrobial activity of simulated solar disinfection against bacterial, fungal, and protozoan pathogens and its enhancement by riboflavin. Appl Environ Microbiol. 2010;76(17):6010–2.
9. Goodrich RP. The use of riboflavin for the inactivation of pathogens in blood products. Vox Sang. 2000;78(Suppl-2):211–5.
10. Bertollo CM, Oliveira AC, Rocha LT, Costa KA, Nascimento EB Jr, Coelho MM. Characterization of the antinociceptive and anti-inflammatory activities

of riboflavin in different experimental models. Eur J Pharmacol. 2006;547(1–3):184–91.
11. Toyosawa T, Suzuki M, Kodama K, Araki S. Effects of intravenous infusion of highly purified vitamin B2 on lipopolysaccharide-induced shock and bacterial infection in mice. Eur J Pharmacol. 2004;492(2–3):273–80.
12. Kumar V, Lockerbie O, Keil SD, Ruane PH, Platz MS, Martin CB, Ravanat JL, Cadet J, Goodrich RP. Riboflavin and UV light-based pathogen reduction: extent and consequence of DNA damage at the molecular level. Photochem Photobiol. 2004;80:15–21.
13. Naseem I, Ahmad M, Hadi SM. Effect of alkylated and intercalated DNA on the generation of superoxide anion by riboflavin. Biosci Rep. 1988;8(5):485–92.
14. Tsugita A, Okada Y, Uehara K. Photosensitized inactivation of ribonucleic acids in the presence of riboflavin. Biochim Biophys Acta. 1965;103(2):360–3.
15. Hafezi F, Randleman JB. PACK-CXL: defining CXL for infectious keratitis. J Refract Surg. 2014;30(7):438–9.
16. Gore DM, O'Brart DP, French P, Dunsby C, Allan BD. A comparison of different corneal iontophoresis protocols for promoting transepithelial riboflavin penetration. Invest Ophthalmol Vis Sci. 2015;56(13):7908–14.
17. Wollensak G, Sporl E, Seiler T. Treatment of keratoconus by collagen cross linking. Ophthalmologe. 2003;100(1):44–9.
18. Wittig-Silva C, Chan E, Islam FM, Wu T, Whiting M, Snibson GR. A randomized, controlled trial of corneal collagen cross-linking in progressive keratoconus: three-year results. Ophthalmology. 2014;121(4):812–21.
19. Seyedian MA, Aliakbari S, Miraftab M, Hashemi H, Asgari S, Khabazkhoob M. Corneal collagen cross-linking in the treatment of progressive keratoconus: a randomized controlled contralateral eye study. Middle East Afr J Ophthalmol. 2015;22(3):340–5.
20. Tasci YY, Taslipinar G, Eyidogan D, Sarac O, Cagil N. Five-year long-term results of standard collagen cross-linking therapy in patients with keratoconus. Turk J Ophthalmol. 2020;50(4):200–5.
21. Raiskup F, Theuring A, Pillunat LE, Spoerl E. Corneal collagen crosslinking with riboflavin and ultraviolet-a light in progressive keratoconus: ten-year results. J Cataract Refract Surg. 2015;41(1):41–6.
22. Soeters N, Wisse RP, Godefrooij DA, Imhof SM, Tahzib NG. Transepithelial versus epithelium-off corneal cross-linking for the treatment of progressive keratoconus: a randomized controlled trial. Am J Ophthalmol. 2015;159(5):821–828.e3.
23. Wen D, Song B, Li Q, Tu R, Huang Y, Wang Q, McAlinden C, O'Brart D, Huang J. Comparison of epithelium-off versus transepithelial corneal collagen cross-linking for keratoconus: a systematic review and meta-analysis. Cornea. 2018;37(8):1018–24.
24. Richoz O, Hammer A, Tabibian D, Gatzioufas Z, Hafezi F. The biomechanical effect of corneal collagen cross-linking (CXL) with riboflavin and UV-A is oxygen dependent. Transl Vis Sci Technol. 2013;2(7):6.
25. Wernli J, Schumacher S, Spoerl E, Mrochen M. The efficacy of corneal cross-linking shows a sudden decrease with very high-intensity UV light and short treatment time. Invest Ophthalmol Vis Sci. 2013;54(2):1176–80.
26. Hammer A, Richoz O, Mosquera S, Tabibian D, Hoogewoud F, Hafezi F. Corneal biomechanical properties at different corneal collagen cross-linking (CXL) irradiances. Invest Ophthalmol Vis Sci. 2014;55(5):2881–4.
27. Webb JN, Su JP, Scarcelli G. Mechanical outcome of accelerated corneal crosslinking evaluated by Brillouin microscopy. J Cataract Refract Surg. 2017;43(11):1458–63.
28. Mazzotta C, Raiskup F, Hafezi F, Torres-Netto EA, Armia Balamoun A, Giannaccare G, Bagaglia SA. Long-term results of accelerated 9 mW corneal crosslinking for early progressive keratoconus: the Siena eye-cross study 2. Eye Vis (Lond). 2021;8(1):16.
29. Moramarco A, Iovieno A, Sartori A, Fontana L. Corneal stromal demarcation line after accelerated crosslinking using continuous and pulsed light. J Cataract Refract Surg. 2015;41(11):2546–51.
30. Peyman A, Nouralishahi A, Hafezi F, Kling S, Peyman M. Stromal demarcation line in pulsed versus continuous light accelerated corneal cross-linking for keratoconus. J Refract Surg. 2016;32(3):206–8.
31. Kling S, Richoz O, Hammer A, Tabibian D, Jacob S, Agarwal A, Hafezi F. Increased biomechanical efficacy of corneal cross-linking in thin corneas due to higher oxygen availability. J Refract Surg. 2015;31(12):840–6.
32. Mazzotta C, Bagaglia SA, Sgheri A, Di Maggio A, Fruschelli M, Romani A, Vinciguerra R, Vinciguerra P, Tosi GM. Iontophoresis corneal cross-linking with enhanced fluence and pulsed UV-A light: 3-year clinical results. J Refract Surg. 2020;36(5):286–92.
33. Seiler TG, Komninou MA, Nambiar MH, Schuerch K, Frueh BE, Buchler P. Oxygen kinetics during corneal cross-linking with and without supplementary oxygen. Am J Ophthalmol. 2021;223:368–76.
34. Hill J, Liu C, Deardorff P, Tavakol B, Eddington W, Thompson V, Gore D, Raizman M, Adler DC. Optimization of oxygen dynamics, UV-A delivery, and drug formulation for accelerated epi-on corneal crosslinking. Curr Eye Res. 2020;45(4):450–8.
35. Hafezi F, Mrochen M, Iseli HP, Seiler T. Collagen crosslinking with ultraviolet-a and hypoosmolar riboflavin solution in thin corneas. J Cataract Refract Surg. 2009;35(4):621–4.
36. Jacob S, Kumar DA, Agarwal A, Basu S, Sinha P, Agarwal A. Contact lens-assisted collagen cross-linking (CACXL): a new technique for cross-linking thin corneas. J Refract Surg. 2014;30(6):366–72.
37. Mazzotta C, Ramovecchi V. Customized epithelial debridement for thin ectatic corneas undergoing corneal cross-linking: epithelial island cross-linking technique. Clin Ophthalmol. 2014;8:1337–43.

38. Wollensak G, Sporl E. Biomechanical efficacy of corneal cross-linking using hypoosmolar riboflavin solution. Eur J Ophthalmol. 2019;29(5):474–81.
39. Kling S, Hafezi F. An algorithm to predict the biomechanical stiffening effect in corneal cross-linking. J Refract Surg. 2017;33(2):128–36.
40. Wollensak G, Sporl E, Herbst H. Biomechanical efficacy of contact lens-assisted collagen cross-linking in porcine eyes. Acta Ophthalmol. 2019;97(1):e84–90.
41. Zhang H, Roozbahani M, Piccinini AL, Golan O, Hafezi F, Scarcelli G, Randleman JB. Depth-dependent reduction of biomechanical efficacy of contact lens-assisted corneal cross-linking analyzed by Brillouin microscopy. J Refract Surg. 2019;35(11):721–8.
42. Sachdev MS, Gupta D, Sachdev G, Sachdev R. Tailored stromal expansion with a refractive lenticule for crosslinking the ultrathin cornea. J Cataract Refract Surg. 2015;41(5):918–23.
43. Deshmukh R, Hafezi F, Kymionis GD, Kling S, Shah R, Padmanabhan P, Sachdev MS. Current concepts in crosslinking thin corneas. Indian J Ophthalmol. 2019;67(1):8–15.
44. Kaya V, Utine CA, Yilmaz OF. Efficacy of corneal collagen cross-linking using a custom epithelial debridement technique in thin corneas: a confocal microscopy study. J Refract Surg. 2011;27(6):444–50.
45. Torres-Netto EA, Kling S, Hafezi N, Vinciguerra P, Randleman JB, Hafezi F. Oxygen diffusion may limit the biomechanical effectiveness of iontophoresis-assisted transepithelial corneal cross-linking. J Refract Surg. 2018;34(11):768–74.
46. Mazzotta C, Romani A, Burroni A. Pachymetry-based accelerated crosslinking: the "M nomogram" for standardized treatment of all-thickness progressive Ectatic corneas. Int J Kerat Ect Cor Dis. 2018;7(2):137–44.
47. Hafezi F, Kling S, Gilardoni F, Hafezi N, Hillen M, Abrishamchi R, Gomes JAP, Mazzotta C, Randleman JB, Torres-Netto EA. Individualized corneal cross-linking with riboflavin and UV-A in ultrathin corneas: the Sub400 protocol. Am J Ophthalmol. 2021;224:133–42.
48. Iseli HP, Thiel MA, Hafezi F, Kampmeier J, Seiler T. Ultraviolet a/riboflavin corneal cross-linking for infectious keratitis associated with corneal melts. Cornea. 2008;27(5):590–4.
49. Ting DSJ, Henein C, Said DG, Dua HS. Photoactivated chromophore for infectious keratitis - corneal cross-linking (PACK-CXL): a systematic review and meta-analysis. Ocul Surf. 2019;17(4):624–34.
50. Makdoumi K, Mortensen J, Sorkhabi O, Malmvall BE, Crafoord S. UVA-riboflavin photochemical therapy of bacterial keratitis: a pilot study. Graefes Arch Clin Exp Ophthalmol. 2012;250(1):95–102.
51. Torres-Netto E, Shetty R, Knyazer B, Chen S, Hosny M, Gilardoni F, Hafezi F. Corneal cross-linking for treating infectious keratitis: final results of the prospective randomized controlled multicenter trial. Poster Presentation, 38th Congress of the ESCRS, Virtual Meeting, Oct 2020.
52. Lin A, Rhee MK, Akpek EK, Amescua G, Farid M, Garcia-Ferrer FJ, Varu DM, Musch DC, Dunn SP, Mah FS. American Academy of ophthalmology preferred practice pattern cornea and external disease panel. Bacterial keratitis preferred practice pattern®. Ophthalmology. 2019;126(1):P1–P55.
53. Kling S, Hufschmid FS, Torres-Netto EA, Randleman JB, Willcox M, Zbinden R, Hafezi F. High fluence increases the antibacterial efficacy of PACK cross-linking. Cornea. 2020;39(8):1020–6.
54. Nateghi Pettersson M, Lagali N, Mortensen J, Jofre V, Fagerholm P. High fluence PACK-CXL as adjuvant treatment for advanced acanthamoeba keratitis. Am J Ophthalmol Case Rep. 2019;15:100499.
55. Amescua G, Arboleda A, Nikpoor N, Durkee H, Relhan N, Aguilar MC, Flynn HW, Miller D, Parel JM. Rose Bengal photodynamic antimicrobial therapy: a novel treatment for resistant fusarium keratitis. Cornea. 2017;36(9):1141–4.
56. Cherfan D, Verter EE, Melki S, Gisel TE, Doyle FJ Jr, Scarcelli G, Yun SH, Redmond RW, Kochevar IE. Collagen cross-linking using rose bengal and green light to increase corneal stiffness. Invest Ophthalmol Vis Sci. 2013;54(5):3426–33.
57. Naranjo A, Arboleda A, Martinez JD, Durkee H, Aguilar MC, Relhan N, Nikpoor N, Galor A, Dubovy SR, Leblanc R, Flynn HW Jr, Miller D, Parel JM, Amescua G. Rose Bengal photodynamic antimicrobial therapy for patients with progressive infectious keratitis: a pilot clinical study. Am J Ophthalmol. 2019;208:387–96.
58. Zarei-Ghanavati M. Rose Bengal-green light for collagen cross-linking. J Ophthalmic Vis Res. 2017;12(2):241–2.

15 Penetrating Keratoplasty in Keratoconus

Ankit Anil Harwani and Prema Padmanabhan

15.1 History of Keratoplasty in Keratoconus

In 1888, corneal transplantation was described as a lamellar procedure only to be replaced by penetrating keratoplasty (PK) in 1905, when the first successful penetrating keratoplasty was performed by Edward Zinn [1]. For keratoconus per se, the first penetrating keratoplasty was recorded to have been performed in 1936 by Ramon Castroviejo Briones. The report submitted by Castroviejo involved more than 200 cases with an excellent visual outcome and graft survival, making it a landmark study for successful penetrating keratoplasty in keratoconus [2].

Penetrating keratoplasty dominated the scene for almost eight decades thereafter, becoming the treatment of choice for keratoconus. Over the years, the surgical procedure has been refined with improvements in suture material and advancements in microsurgical instruments and the ophthalmic microscope allowing greater surgical precision.

A. A. Harwani · P. Padmanabhan (✉)
Medical Research Foundation, Sankara Nethralaya, Chennai, Tamil Nadu, India
e-mail: drpp@snmail.org

15.2 Long-Term Results of Penetrating Keratoplasty in Keratoconus

Of all the indications for corneal transplants, keratoconus offers one of the best prognoses, and the available long-term data from the literature show excellent results both in terms of functional outcome and graft survival [3–7].

The visual results are excellent with an average best-corrected visual acuity of more than 20/40 in 72% to 97% of cases after a mean follow-up ranging from 3 to 11 years [3, 4, 6–9]. The visual outcome can get affected due to the variable refractive error developing after the PK with a mean spherical equivalent ranging from −1 to −4 D, including the mean refractive cylinder ranging from 2.8 to 5.6 D requiring spectacles, contact lens wear or other measures for improvement [4, 8–10]. A significantly improved functional visual acuity was achieved in 30–67% of patients with spectacles alone [3, 8, 11]. However, around 26–47% of cases required contact lenses for visual rehabilitation after penetrating keratoplasty [3, 8]. As noted, the postoperative visual outcome largely depends upon astigmatism, while cataract, glaucoma, and trauma can also result in less than expected visual improvement. The graft remained clear in more than 90% of cases in the long-term studies with the mean follow-up ranging from 3 to 11 years [3, 4, 6–9, 12].

S. Das (ed.), *Keratoconus*, https://doi.org/10.1007/978-981-19-4262-4_15

In the last few decades, however, the indications for surgery in general, and PK in particular, for keratoconus have vastly reduced. The introduction of collagen cross-linking to slacken or even prevent the progression of the disease, the visual improvement offered by scleral contact lenses, and the gaining popularity of Deep Anterior Lamellar Keratoplasty (DALK) have all been responsible for the shift in approach in the management of keratoconus.

15.3 Indications for PK in the Era of DALK

Recently, DALK has been increasingly replacing PK for the treatment of advanced keratoconus. However, there are still a few conditions where PK continues to be the preferred procedure. These conditions include acute keratoconus or hydrops, prior hydrops, maximum keratometry >60 D, macroperforations in Descemet's membrane (DM) during DALK, large and deep stromal scars, and regrafting after initial penetrating keratoplasty done for keratoconus [13, 14].

15.4 Surgical Steps of PK

The steps of PK in keratoconus are similar to those of keratoplasty for any other indication. Few modifications which need to be kept in mind are elaborated here wherever necessary. The surgery can be done under regional anesthesia; however, if the patient is a child or apprehensive or has an associated systemic disease with mental growth abnormality like Down's syndrome, then general anesthesia may be preferred.

The donor tissue to be used should be of good quality, especially in terms of endothelial cell density (ECD), to provide for long-term survival of the graft as the PK is performed at a relatively younger age in keratoconus. The variables which influence the donor ECD most include the donor age and the preservation time [15]. Although young donor tissue would be expected to have a good cell count, some studies do report an associated higher incidence of graft rejection [16, 17]. On the contrary, Feizi et al. studied the outcome of PK in keratoconus patients with respect to donor characteristics and found no significant correlation of the donor variables with the long-term graft survival, as long as the minimum ECD of the donor tissue was>2000 cells/mm^2 [18].

Preoperatively, a miotic can be used to prevent damage to the crystalline lens unless a concurrent cataract surgery is planned. Scleral ring or Flieringa ring can be used to stabilize the globe especially in younger patients and in patients with connective tissue disorders with an associated thin sclera.

While trephining the host cornea, the center of the pupil or the corneal apex is used as a guide for centration of the trephine. The size of the trephine is determined by the extent of the cone and should ideally encompass the ectasia [19]. However, if the cone is decentered, the trephination can also be decentered taking care that the edge of the trephine does not overlap the pupillary area. In keratoconus, the trephination of the ectatic steep cornea, having a naturally deep anterior chamber, leaves an elongated and steep recipient rim which can cause postoperative myopia and astigmatism after keratoplasty.

The donor cornea can be trephined from the epithelial or the endothelial side. Trephination from the endothelial side generally creates a 0.2-mm smaller graft than when trephination is performed from the epithelial side [20, 21]. Surgeons have mixed opinions about the ideal graft-host size disparity in keratoconus. A donor graft 0.25 mm smaller than the recipient bed causes a significant and consistent reduction in myopia compared to a same-size graft [22–25]. Apart from the flattening of the cornea with the same-size trephine (smaller graft), the reduction in axial length by an average of 0.46 mm also contributes to the decrease in myopia postoperatively [23, 26]. Although undersized grafts could be expected to be associated with problems in wound healing, difficulty in suturing, postoperative glaucoma, excessive hyperopia, and contact lens fitting issues, no significant difficulties were reported in studies [23, 25]. It is thus a popular practice to use the same-size trephine, to cut the recipient cornea from the epithelial side and the donor cornea from the endothelial side (giving a 0.2-mm smaller graft) in keratoconus cases.

While trephining, care should be exercised in keeping the cut edges vertical and smooth, avoiding tilting of trephine, and avoiding uneven pressure or side to side movements to reduce postoperative astigmatism [27].

As with any PK, suturing techniques include interrupted, single running, double running, and combined interrupted and running, the choice ultimately resting with the surgeon.

15.5 Femto-Assisted PK

A vertical edge-to-edge graft-host junction typically requires tighter sutures for maintaining a secure wound and risks wound dehiscence after suture removal. After Busin [28] introduced the concept of a stepped lamellar wound to improve graft-host apposition, Farid et al. [29] used the precision provided by the femtosecond laser to include the "mushroom", "top hat", "zig-zag", and "Christmas tree" (Fig. 15.1a–d). The interlocking edges of these shaped profiles confer greater wound stability with less scope for sliding or torque within the wound. The improved wound alignment facilitates faster and better wound healing and quicker visual rehabilitation. However, the cost and equipment for the procedure preclude its widespread use.

15.6 Deep Anterior Lamellar Keratoplasty (DALK) Versus PK

Comparisons between PK and DALK have examined different aspects of their outcomes, and understanding the nuances of each procedure will help the surgeon make a judicious choice for a given patient. The differences in the procedures will be discussed with respect to the different aspects as below.

15.6.1 Learning Curve

The surgical learning curve is allegedly longer and steeper, for a novice, to learn DALK as compared to PK [30]. While this may affect the outcome of the DALK during the learning phase, the results, in experienced hands, are comparable to those of a PK.

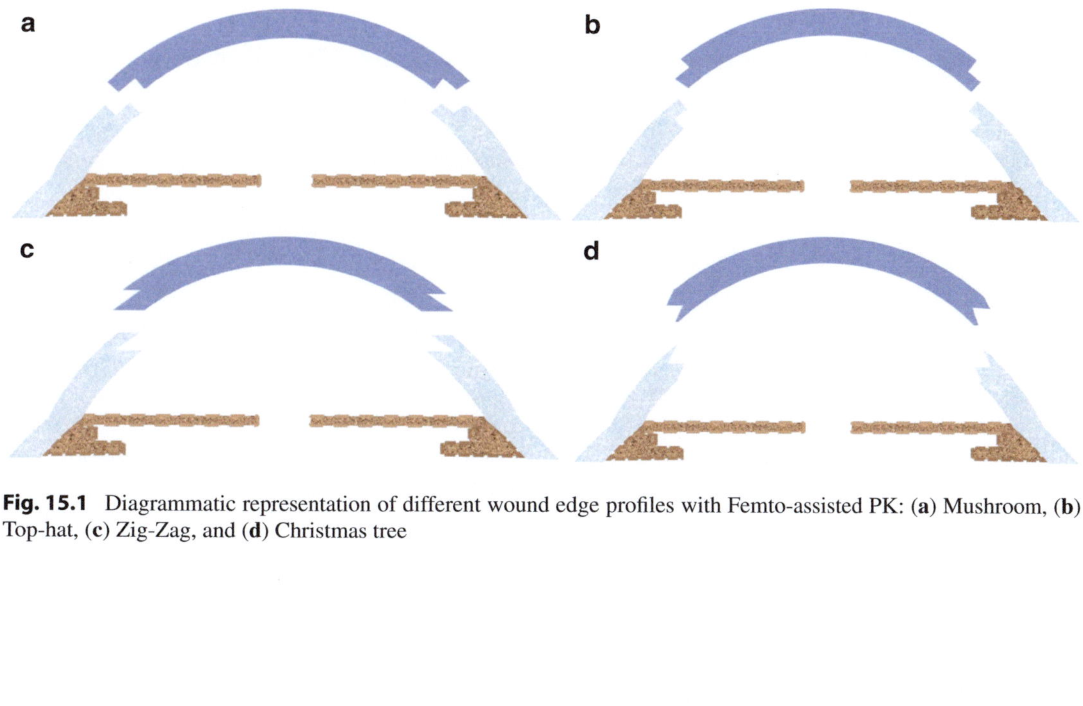

Fig. 15.1 Diagrammatic representation of different wound edge profiles with Femto-assisted PK: (**a**) Mushroom, (**b**) Top-hat, (**c**) Zig-Zag, and (**d**) Christmas tree

15.6.2 Visual Acuity

The varied and heterogeneous data in reported literature make it difficult to conclusively establish the superiority of one procedure over the other with respect to the visual outcome. Most of the studies, including meta-analyses, have shown no significant difference in the visual outcome between DALK and PK [14, 31–33]. Occasional differences among reported outcomes could be attributed to the surgeons' experience and to the depth till which the stroma had been dissected during the DALK procedure. A residual stromal bed of more than 60 μ to 80 μ in the recipient has been proposed to be associated with poor outcomes in DALK [10, 34]. This issue got addressed in 2002 when Anwar reported the "big bubble technique", where he used air to achieve a dissection plane by injecting a big air bubble between the DM and the stroma creating a deep and smooth interface for transplantation [35]. The Anwar Big bubble technique in DALK provided a better achievement rate of best spectacle-corrected visual acuity ≥6/12, if not equal to reported results with PK. These advancements in technique and instrumentation, lead to a better visual outcome and graft survival in DALK comparable to PK and have made DALK a preferred choice, where possible, among most surgeons.

15.6.3 Refractive Astigmatism

Meta-analyses and various other individual reports have found no significant difference in the postoperative refractive astigmatism between DALK and PK [14, 31, 33]. The mean astigmatism was found to range from 2.2 to 7.3 D for DALK and 2.8 to 7.9 D for PK [13].

15.6.4 Topographic or Keratometric Astigmatism

The factors that influence the keratometric and refractive astigmatism after a PK or a DALK include donor-recipient size disparity and the amount of preoperative ametropia [10, 25]. Accordingly, analogous to refractive astigmatism, various studies and meta-analysis of randomized control trials reveal no significant difference in the keratometric or topographic astigmatism between DALK and PK [10, 13, 14].

15.6.5 Spherical Equivalent

There is no difference in the overall spherical equivalent between the two procedures as concluded in various studies and meta-analyses [10, 31]. There are a few studies that have found the spherical equivalent to be greater post-DALK, although this may have more to do with axial length of the keratoconic eyes than with the type of surgery.

15.6.6 Q Value

The asphericity of the cornea is denoted by the Q value. A normal cornea has a prolate shape with a larger radius of curvature in the periphery than the center and a Q value ranging from −0.26 to −0.42. After keratoplasty, whether DALK or PK, almost all corneas develop a highly oblate shape with a mean Q value of 11.6 [14].

15.6.7 Corneal Densitometry

Corneal densitometry is a measure of corneal transparency and light scattering, which can be measured quantitatively with Pentacam HR (Oculus, Wetzlar, Germany). Some patients post-keratoplasty perceive glare and photophobia in spite of a clear graft, which can be attributed to the changes in the corneal densitometry resulting in backward light scattering and affecting visual acuity. Changes in corneal densitometry occur due to extracellular tissue remodeling and keratocyte repopulation, some of which transform into myofibroblasts giving rise to the post-DALK interface haze. This haze is more pronounced when stromal dissection is carried out manually rather with an air bubble and is responsible for the higher densitometry values reported after DALK than after PK [36].

15.6.8 Contrast Sensitivity

Apart from the visual acuity, the quality of vision can be assessed with other parameters like contrast sensitivity. The contrast sensitivity is found to be comparable between DALK and PK; provided the recipient stroma is dissected till the DM, as achieved by the big bubble technique. Other techniques that result in stromal interface scarring or irregularities can result in a reduced contrast sensitivity in DALK cases [37].

15.6.9 Endothelial Cell Loss

Long-term follow-up data of up to 5 years suggest that annual endothelial cell loss rate in PK is 14%, while in DALK it is 5.8%, both of which are far more than the normal cell loss rates, i.e., 0.6% per year. However, there has been no significant difference reported in the late endothelial failure between both procedures [14, 38].

15.6.10 Graft Survival

A systematic review of graft survival revealed no significant difference between procedures, but conclusions are unreliable when the follow-up duration in the reviewed studies was only 12 months [10]. However, in a long-term study, the median predicted survival of the PK graft was 17 years while that of the DALK graft was 49 years [39].

15.6.11 Graft Rejections

Graft rejections are more common in PK as the amount of antigenic load is more and transplanted corneal endothelial cells are more vulnerable to host inflammatory and immune response. Patients with PK have been found to have a 2.69 times greater risk of developing graft rejections than patients with DALK [13].

15.6.12 Corneal Biomechanics

Corneal hysteresis and corneal resistance factor are the two parameters measured by the Ocular Response Analyzer to describe the viscoelastic properties of the cornea.

Although the difference between DALK and PK for these parameters was not found to be statistically significant, the corneal biomechanical properties post-DALK were reported to resemble those of a normal cornea more closely, possibly due to the retention of the host DM and endothelium, providing better tissue strength. However, studies that compare the biomechanical properties of transplanted corneas by both procedures are inconclusive due to differences in the dissection techniques used in DALK and in the assessment being done at disparate follow-up periods [40].

15.6.13 Miscellaneous

Suture removal in DALK can be done at 6–12 months, while in PK it is usually done at around 18–24 months [30].

15.6.14 Complications

Systematic review and meta-analysis have suggested that the incidence of complications is more with PK than with DALK, 44% and 10% respectively. The nature of reported complications is different between the two techniques, but the most common ones after either procedure are high refractive error and immune graft rejection [13, 14, 30].

The risk of intraocular pressure elevation is ten times more with PK (26%) as compared to DALK (2.6%), which can, in part be attributed to long-term use of steroids after PK. Endothelial rejections with PK have been reported to occur in 8–13% of cases, while stromal and epithelial rejections after DALK are rare [14]. Cataract was also found to be more common after PK, which can be attributed to the intraocular nature of the surgery and prolonged use of steroids [41].

Complications peculiar to DALK include perforation of DM and double anterior chamber. The DM perforation rate during DALK has been found to be 4–39%, of which large DM tears needing conversion into PK were relatively low, 2.3% to 27% [14].

15.6.15 Conclusion

Based on available evidence, it can be concluded that both procedures, PK and DALK, enjoy comparable outcomes in terms of major aspects such as BCVA, astigmatism, and graft survival. DALK has the advantage of reduced overall complications rate, particularly of endothelial rejection, which makes it a favorable option especially in places where good-quality donor tissue is scarce.

15.7 Complications of PK in Keratoconus (KC)

Most of the intraoperative and postoperative complications of PK stem from the fact that it is an intraocular surgery, with a 360° wound requiring 360° suturing. Complications like endophthalmitis, choroidal hemorrhage, secondary glaucoma, postoperative astigmatism, secondary cataract, etc. are common to all PKs whatever be the indication for which it was done, so will not be dealt with in this section. Here, we confine ourselves to complications with specific reference to keratoconus.

15.8 Graft-Host Misalignment

The most obvious aspect of keratoplasty performed on keratoconic cornea with spatially varying corneal thickness is the wound mismatch with the donor cornea resulting in graft-host malposition. While alignment of the epithelial surface can be directly visualized under a surgical microscope, the misalignments of the internal graft-host interface are common and often ignored. Although oversized grafts are believed to be more likely to be associated with internal wound alignment errors due to the curled shape of the internal surface of the larger graft [42], they could also occur with isometric grafts [43]. The introduction of the anterior segment optical coherence tomography (AS-OCT) has allowed better analysis of the internal wound. Kaiserman et al. reported internal graft-host malappositions in 78.4% in keratoconic eyes as compared to 50% in those that received corneal transplantation for other corneal diseases [44]. Postkeratoplasty alignment patterns have been classified into four basic types: regular, step, protrusion, and gape. Graft step and host step are subtypes of step, while hill and tag are subtypes of protrusion (Fig. 15.2a–f) [44, 45]. Kaiserman et al. used AS-OCT to study the internal corneal wound of 13 post-PK keratoconic eyes and reported 34.6% with step, 22.1% with gape, and 22.1% with protrusion patterns of misalignment, although these patterns would depend on the grade of keratoconus, size of the graft, suturing technique and could vary along the circumference of the wound [44]. Steeper grafts were shown to correlate with thinner, less stable graft-host touch. Graft-host misalignments may result in weaker unstable wounds, irregular astigmatism, and optical aberrations following keratoplasty.

15.9 Wound Healing in Keratoconus

The reparative process to injury has been shown to be altered in keratoconus. An aberrant cytokine expression profile, keratocyte apoptosis, and an abnormal extracellular matrix, which characterize keratoconic corneas, would be expected to alter the wound healing and remodeling process needed after penetrating keratoplasty [46].

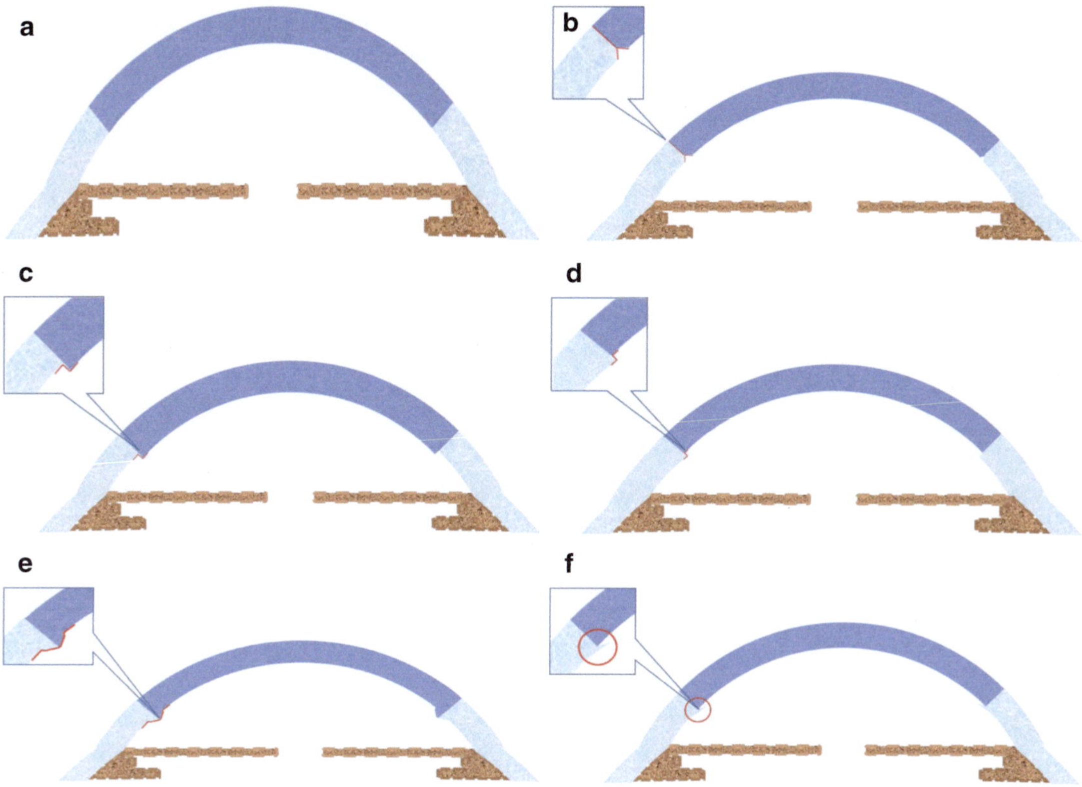

Fig. 15.2 Diagrammatic representation of different patterns of inner wound appositions: (**a**) Normal, (**b**) Gape, (**c**) Graft step, (**d**) Host step, (**e**) Hill protrusion, and (**f**) Tag protrusion

15.10 Post-PK Refractive Errors

The main challenge of PK in a keratoconic eye is to reduce, rather than compound the refractive state of an eye that already has a highly aberrated optical system. Oversized grafts using donor buttons 0.5 mm larger than the recipient bed are usually preferred in conventional PK to avoid irido-corneal compression and secondary glaucoma. However, in keratoconic eyes, which usually have a deep anterior chamber, most surgeons prefer a same-size graft. Oversized grafts in keratoconus have been associated with an increased postoperative myopic shift in refraction.

15.11 Post-PK Astigmatism

Post-PK astigmatism, as with any PK depends on the graft size, trephination, and technique. Additionally, in keratoconic eyes, it is also influenced by the severity of the disease, being more unpredictable and irregular in advanced keratoconus [47].

The outcomes of penetrating keratoplasty in terms of visual acuity have greatly improved over the years. However, high astigmatism after PK is encountered in 10–20% cases and can be a reason for impaired visual acuity, despite a clear graft [4]. The factors contributing to post-PK astigmatism may be host-related, donor-related, surgery-related, or a combination of these. The donor-related factors include diameter, edge profile, and intrinsic astigmatism. The host-related factors include edge thinning due to keratoconus itself, scleral thinning or ectasia, scarring, and edge profile. The surgical factors include mainly suture-related (depth, tension, technique, radiality, timing of removal), trephine tilt, and scleral ring placement. To correct the post-PK astigmatism, optical methods like spectacles and contact lenses are first attempted before surgical options are sought. The surgical options can be individualized to each patient and consist of suture removal or adjustment, incisional procedures, wedge resection, toric intraocular lens (IOL), and intrastromal ring segments [48]. Before deciding upon the option of treatment for astigmatism, it is important to evaluate the patient on a slit lamp and assess astigmatism with corneal topography.

15.11.1 Spectacles and Contact Lenses

Spectacles should be the initial choice of treatment for mild to moderate postkeratoplasty astigmatism. However, it is not uncommon for spectacle use to cause aniseikonia if the difference in the power between the two eyes is more than 3 diopters. This can be dealt with using contact lenses, which also increase the binocularity. As the surface after PK is irregular, rigid gas permeable (RGP) lenses are most commonly used for the correction of the refractive error. The contact lenses can be used after 3–4 months of surgery. Recent addition to the armamentarium of the contact lenses has been the prosthetic replacement of the ocular surface ecosystem (PROSE) lenses. These are large scleral lenses resting on the sclera while creating a vault hoarding fluid over the cornea. The RGP lenses may sometimes fit poorly or cause discomfort after a PK having a highly irregular surface, in such cases PROSE lenses resting over the sclera would be preferable. However, the cost of the lens and of its maintenance precludes its conventional usage in post-PK astigmatism. Contact lens usage is often associated with suture-related problems like infiltrates, punctate erosions and corneal vascularization, and increased chances of graft rejection. These associations often preclude contact lens use postpenetrating keratoplasty. Surgical techniques are resorted to when optical measures fail to correct astigmatism.

15.11.2 Suture Removal or Adjustments

Suture adjustments can be done intraoperatively, to have better stability and early visual rehabilitation [49]. If the astigmatism is <3D and the patient is comfortable with the visual acuity and if there are no obvious suture-related problems, sutures can be left in situ. If continuous with interrupted sutures are placed, the interrupted ones can be removed at 2–3 weeks, and if only interrupted sutures are placed, they can be removed at around 12 weeks or when the wound appears adequately stable [48].

Depending on the topographic pattern, the steepest meridian is determined, and one or two sutures removed in the area or 180 degrees apart if symmetric pattern is seen. The results of suture removal are unpredictable and are also dependent on the topographic pattern. Nonetheless, the results from the various study show final astigmatism of <3D in nearly 70% of cases after suture removal [48, 50–52].

Suture adjustments are done for a single continuous suture. The suture is loosened in the area of steep meridian by tightening it in the flat meridian. Repeat adjustments can be done if significant astigmatism persists after 3 weeks. Suture adjustments should be done carefully to avoid breakage, loose loops, and wound gape. Single continuous suture causes astigmatism of around 6D which can be reduced to <3D with 1 or 2 suture adjustments [48, 53].

15.11.3 Relaxing Incisions

Relaxing incision is a partial depth (70–80%) incision in the steep meridian, at the graft-host interface, causing flattening of the steep meridian and steepening of the flat meridian. It can reduce astigmatism by 40%, to even 70% when combined with compression sutures at the flat meridian which offers the added advantage of allowing some degree of postoperative adjustment [54]. Although the results are extremely variable and there are chances of inadvertent perforation, it is a relatively easy procedure, can correct a large range of astigmatism (0–15 D), and has a short stabilization period. The incisions can be given in pairs 180 degrees apart, or a single incision if there is a focal steepening, or as a sequentially paired incision if there is a significant skewing of the steep axis [48]. The refractive stability after relaxing incisions with or without compression sutures occurs at around 2–4 months [55]. Relaxing incisions have a better effect than astigmatic keratotomy and hence should be the initial incisional procedure of choice to correct astigmatism.

15.11.4 Astigmatic Keratotomy

A transverse or arcuate partial incision on the donor cornea, placed at 6–7 mm optical zone, centered on the visual axis irrespective of the graft position, can reduce the astigmatism by an average of 60%. Various nomograms are available to determine the length, depth, and site of the incisions, but the results are, by and large, unpredictable. Surgeons can modify the nomograms based on their own individual experiences [48].

15.11.5 Wedge Resection

A wedge of corneal tissue 90% in depth is excised from the flat meridian, resulting in steepening of that meridian and flattening of the steep meridian. For each 0.1-mm wedge of tissue excised, there is a 1–2 D correction of astigmatism. Sutures are placed to close the wound and to mildly overcorrect astigmatism, allowing titration of astigmatism after 2–4 weeks by suture removal if necessary. Though the results are very unpredictable, it can correct 10–20 D of astigmatism and thus is reserved for extremely high astigmatism of >8 D [48].

15.11.6 Intraocular Lens

As keratoconus patients requiring transplants are usually young, prolonged use of steroids after keratoplasty can predispose these cases to the development of cataract. Astigmatism can be addressed during the cataract removal by using a toric IOL. Toric IOLs are contraindicated in irregular astigmatisms, which is usually the case after penetrating keratoplasty. In a study, with fairly regular post-PK astigmatism, 75% achieved manifest astigmatism ≤1D after toric IOL implantation [56]. Other options, such aphakic IOLs and Piggyback IOLs have also been tried.

15.11.7 Intrastromal Ring Segments

Intrastromal ring segments have been tried to reduce post-PK astigmatism with good results sometimes achieving a reduction of about 3–5 D [57]. Thus, management of the postkeratoplasty astigmatism should begin intraoperatively by taking appropriate precautions during donor and recipient trephination and suturing. Postoperatively, if optical methods and suture-related methods fail to correct astigmatism, incisional or surgical procedures should be sought.

15.12 Recurrence/Progression of Keratoconus Following PK

Although the long-term prognosis of PK for keratoconus is acknowledged to be excellent, there have been a few reports of a recurrence of ectasia decades after PK [58, 59]. A progressive increase in postoperative astigmatism several years after postsuture removal refractive stability, was seen in 70% of patients [19]. A 20-year post-PK probability of recurrence in 10% of cases, with a mean time to recurrence of 17.9–21.9 years has been reported [1]. The paucity of literature on this subject makes it difficult to determine whether it is the host cornea or the graft that develops keratoconus. Yoshida et al., using multivariate regression analysis, showed that smaller grafts carried a higher risk of showing progression [60].

15.13 Rejection

The clear avascular cornea in keratoconus represents a situation that is least vulnerable to immune rejection compared to any other. Allogenic graft rejection could still occur and has been variously reported in 10–35% [3, 4, 6–9]. Most of the rejections episodes are observed within the first year of penetrating keratoplasty, although the contralateral eye corneal transplantation appears to put the first graft at risk of developing a rejection episode even years later [3, 4, 7]. The rejections are less likely to cause graft failure after PK in keratoconus cases, accounting for about 2.4% of grafts. Large grafts, decentered grafts that encroach the corneal limbus, conditions that predispose to localized vascularization like loose sutures, corneal infections, or regrafts for previously failed grafts, could increase the risk of immune rejection [5].

Even though there has been a paradigm shift in the approach to the treatment of keratoconus in recent years, PK retains an important role in appropriately selected situations and as a bail-out procedure in others.

References

1. Arnalich-Montiel F, Alió Del Barrio JL, Alió JL. Corneal surgery in keratoconus: which type, which technique, which outcomes? Eye Vis (Lond). 2016;3:2.
2. Castroviejo R. Keratoplasty for the treatment of keratoconus. Trans Am Ophthalmol Soc. 1948;46:127–53.
3. Sharif KW, Casey TA. Penetrating keratoplasty for keratoconus: complications and long-term success. Br J Ophthalmol. 1991;75(3):142–6.
4. Kirkness CM, Ficker LA, Steele AD, Rice NS. The success of penetrating keratoplasty for keratoconus. Eye (Lond). 1990;4(Pt 5):673–88.
5. Epstein RJ, Seedor JA, Dreizen NG, Stulting RD, Waring GO 3rd, Wilson LA, Cavanagh HD. Penetrating keratoplasty for herpes simplex keratitis and keratoconus. Allograft rejection and survival. Ophthalmology. 1987;94(8):935–44.
6. Ehlers N, Olsen T. Long-term results of corneal grafting in keratoconus. Acta Ophthalmol. 1983;61(5):918–26.
7. Paglen PG, Fine M, Abbott RL, Webster RG Jr. The prognosis for keratoplasty in keratoconus. Ophthalmology. 1982;89(6):651–4.
8. Brierly SC, Izquierdo L Jr, Mannis MJ. Penetrating keratoplasty for keratoconus. Cornea. 2000;19(3):329–32.
9. Troutman RC, Lawless MA. Penetrating keratoplasty for keratoconus. Cornea. 1987;6(4):298–305.
10. Henein C, Nanavaty MA. Systematic review comparing penetrating keratoplasty and deep anterior lamellar keratoplasty for management of keratoconus. Cont Lens Anterior Eye. 2017;40(1):3–14.
11. Lim L, Pesudovs K, Coster DJ. Penetrating keratoplasty for keratoconus: visual outcome and success. Ophthalmology. 2000;107(6):1125–31.
12. Chandler JW, Kaufman HE. Graft reactions after keratoplasty for keratoconus. Am J Ophthalmol. 1974;77(4):543–7.
13. Song Y, Zhang J, Pan Z. Systematic review and meta-analysis of clinical outcomes of penetrating keratoplasty versus deep anterior lamellar keratoplasty for keratoconus. Exp Clin Transplant. 2020;18(4):417–28.
14. Yüksel B, Kandemir B, Uzunel UD, Çelik O, Ceylan S, Küsbeci T. Comparison of visual and topographic outcomes of deep-anterior lamellar keratoplasty and penetrating keratoplasty in keratoconus. Int J Ophthalmol. 2017;10(3):385–90.
15. Armitage WJ, Jones MN, Zambrano I, Carley F, Tole DM, NHSBT Ocular Tissue Advisory Group and Contributing Ophthalmologists OTAG Audit Study 12. The suitability of corneas stored by organ culture for penetrating keratoplasty and influence of donor and recipient factors on 5-year graft survival. Invest Ophthalmol Vis Sci. 2014;55(2):784–91.
16. Palay DA, Kangas TA, Stulting RD, Winchester K, Litoff D, Krachmer JH. The effects of donor age on the outcome of penetrating keratoplasty in adults. Ophthalmology. 1997;104(10):1576–9.
17. Inoue K, Amano S, Oshika T, Tsuru T. Risk factors for corneal graft failure and rejection in penetrating keratoplasty. Acta Ophthalmol Scand. 2001;79(3):251–5.
18. Feizi S, Javadi MA, Ghasemi H, Javadi F. Effect of donor graft quality on clinical outcomes after penetrating keratoplasty for keratoconus. J Ophthalmic Vis Res. 2015;10(4):364–9.
19. de Toledo JA, de la Paz MF, Barraquer RI, Barraquer J. Long-term progression of astigmatism after penetrating keratoplasty for keratoconus: evidence of late recurrence. Cornea. 2003;22(4):317–23.
20. Troutman RC. Astigmatic considerations in corneal graft. Ophthalmic Surg. 1979;10(5):21–6.

21. Olson RJ. Variation in corneal graft size related to trephine technique. Arch Ophthalmol. 1979;97(7):1323–5.
22. Girard LJ, Eguez I, Esnaola N, Barnett L, Maghraby A. Effect of penetrating keratoplasty using grafts of various sizes on keratoconic myopia and astigmatism. J Cataract Refract Surg. 1988;14(5):541–7.
23. Girard LJ, Esnaola N, Rao R, Barnett L, Rand WJ. Use of grafts smaller than the opening for keratoconic myopia and astigmatism. A prospective study. J Cataract Refract Surg. 1992;18(4):380–4.
24. Perry HD, Foulks GN. Oversize donor buttons in corneal transplantation surgery for keratoconus. Ophthalmic Surg. 1987;18(10):751–2.
25. Wilson SE, Bourne WM. Effect of recipient-donor trephine size disparity on refractive error in keratoconus. Ophthalmology. 1989;96(3):299–305.
26. Lanier JD, Bullington RH Jr, Prager TC. Axial length in keratoconus. Cornea. 1992;11(3):250–4.
27. van Rij G, Waring GO 3rd. Configuration of corneal trephine opening using five different trephines in human donor eyes. Arch Ophthalmol. 1988;106(9):1228–33.
28. Busin M. A new lamellar wound configuration for penetrating keratoplasty surgery. Arch Ophthalmol. 2003;121(2):260–5.
29. Farid M, Kim M, Steinert RF. Results of penetrating keratoplasty performed with a femtosecond laser zigzag incision initial report. Ophthalmology. 2007;114(12):2208–12.
30. Watson SL, Ramsay A, Dart JK, Bunce C, Craig E. Comparison of deep lamellar keratoplasty and penetrating keratoplasty in patients with keratoconus. Ophthalmology. 2004;111(9):1676–82.
31. Keane M, Coster D, Ziaei M, Williams K. Deep anterior lamellar keratoplasty versus penetrating keratoplasty for treating keratoconus. Cochrane Database Syst Rev. 2014;7:CD009700.
32. Reinhart WJ, Musch DC, Jacobs DS, Lee WB, Kaufman SC, Shtein RM. Deep anterior lamellar keratoplasty as an alternative to penetrating keratoplasty—a report by the american academy of ophthalmology. Ophthalmology. 2011;118(1):209–18.
33. Pedrotti E, Passilongo M, Fasolo A, Ficial S, Ferrari S, Marchini G. Refractive outcomes of penetrating keratoplasty and deep anterior lamellar keratoplasty in fellow eyes for keratoconus. Int Ophthalmol. 2017;37(4):911–9.
34. Han DC, Mehta JS, Por YM, Htoon HM, Tan DT. Comparison of outcomes of lamellar keratoplasty and penetrating keratoplasty in keratoconus. Am J Ophthalmol. 2009;148(5):744-751.e1.
35. Anwar M, Teichmann KD. Big-bubble technique to bare Descemet's membrane in anterior lamellar keratoplasty. J Cataract Refract Surg. 2002;28(3):398–403.
36. Alzahrani K, Dardin SF, Carley F, Brahma A, Morley D, Hillarby MC. Corneal clarity measurements in patients with keratoconus undergoing either penetrating or deep anterior lamellar keratoplasty. Clin Ophthalmol. 2018;12:577–85.
37. Fontana L, Parente G, Sincich A, Tassinari G. Influence of graft-host interface on the quality of vision after deep anterior lamellar keratoplasty in patients with keratoconus. Cornea. 2011;30(5):497–502.
38. Kubaloglu A, Koytak A, Sari ES, Akyol S, Kurnaz E, Ozerturk Y. Corneal endothelium after deep anterior lamellar keratoplasty and penetrating keratoplasty for keratoconus: a four-year comparative study. Indian J Ophthalmol. 2012;60(1):35–40.
39. Borderie VM, Sandali O, Bullet J, Gaujoux T, Touzeau O, Laroche L. Long-term results of deep anterior lamellar versus penetrating keratoplasty. Ophthalmology. 2012;119(2):249–55.
40. Ziaei M, Vellara HR, Gokul A, Ali NQ, McGhee CNJ, Patel DV. Comparison of corneal biomechanical properties following penetrating keratoplasty and deep anterior lamellar keratoplasty for keratoconus. Clin Exp Ophthalmol. 2020;48(2):174–82.
41. Khattak A, Nakhli FR, Al-Arfaj KM, Cheema AA. Comparison of outcomes and complications of deep anterior lamellar keratoplasty and penetrating keratoplasty performed in a large group of patients with keratoconus. Int Ophthalmol. 2018;38(3):985–92.
42. Jhanji V, Constantinou M, Beltz J, Vajpayee RB. Evaluation of posterior wound profile after penetrating keratoplasty using anterior segment optical coherence tomography. Cornea. 2011;30(3):277–80.
43. Zhao Y, Zhuang H, Hong J, Tian L, Xu J. Malapposition of graft-host interface after penetrating keratoplasty (PK) and deep anterior lamellar keratoplasty (DALK): an optical coherence tomography study. BMC Ophthalmol. 2020;20(1):41.
44. Kaiserman I, Bahar I, Rootman DS. Corneal wound malapposition after penetrating keratoplasty: an optical coherence tomography study. Br J Ophthalmol. 2008;92(8):1103–7.
45. Sung MS, Yoon KC. Evaluation of graft-host interface after penetrating keratoplasty using anterior segment optical coherence tomography. Jpn J Ophthalmol. 2014;58(3):282–9.
46. Cheung IM, McGhee CNJ, Sherwin T. Deficient repair regulatory response to injury in keratoconic stromal cells. Clin Exp Optom. 2014;97(3):234–9.
47. Choi JA, Lee MA, Kim MS. Long-term outcomes of penetrating keratoplasty in keratoconus: analysis of the factors associated with final visual acuities. Int J Ophthalmol. 2014;7(3):517–21.
48. Riddle HK Jr, Parker DA, Price FW Jr. Management of postkeratoplasty astigmatism. Curr Opin Ophthalmol. 1998;9(4):15–28.
49. Serdarevic ON, Renard GJ, Pouliquen Y. Randomized clinical trial of penetrating keratoplasty. Before and after suture removal comparison of intraoperative and postoperative suture adjustment. Ophthalmology. 1995;102(10):1497–503.
50. Burk LL, Waring GO 3rd, Radjee B, Stulting RD. The effect of selective suture removal on astigmatism fol-

lowing penetrating keratoplasty. Ophthalmic Surg. 1988;19(12):849–54.
51. Binder PS. Selective suture removal can reduce postkeratoplasty astigmatism. Ophthalmology. 1985;92(10):1412–6.
52. Harris DJ Jr, Waring GO 3rd, Burk LL. Keratography as a guide to selective suture removal for the reduction of astigmatism after penetrating keratoplasty. Ophthalmology. 1989;96(11):1597–607.
53. Lin DT, Wilson SE, Reidy JJ, Klyce SD, McDonald MB, Kaufman HE, McNeill JI. An adjustable single running suture technique to reduce postkeratoplasty astigmatism. A preliminary report. Ophthalmology. 1990;97(7):934–8.
54. Mandel MR, Shapiro MB, Krachmer JH. Relaxing incisions with augmentation sutures for the correction of postkeratoplasty astigmatism. Am J Ophthalmol. 1987;103(3 Pt 2):441–7.
55. Fronterrè A, Portesani GP. Relaxing incisions for postkeratoplasty astigmatism. Cornea. 1991;10(4):305–11.
56. Wade M, Steinert RF, Garg S, Farid M, Gaster R. Results of toric intraocular lenses for post-penetrating keratoplasty astigmatism. Ophthalmology. 2014;121(3):771–7.
57. Coscarelli S, Ferrara G, Alfonso JF, Ferrara P, Merayo-Lloves J, Araújo LP, Machado AP, Lyra JM, Torquetti L. Intrastromal corneal ring segment implantation to correct astigmatism after penetrating keratoplasty. J Cataract Refract Surg. 2012;38(6):1006–13.
58. Yoshida J, Murata H, Miyai T, Shirakawa R, Toyono T, Yamagami S, Usui T. Characteristics and risk factors of recurrent keratoconus over the long-term after penetrating keratoplasty. Graefes Arch Clin Exp Ophthalmol. 2018;256(12):2377–83.
59. Fujita A, Yoshida J, Toyono T, Usui T, Miyai T. Severity assessment of acute hydrops due to recurrent keratoconus after penetrating keratoplasty using anterior segment optical coherence tomography. Curr Eye Res. 2019;44(11):1189–94.
60. Yoshida J, Toyono T, Shirakawa R, Miyai T, Usui T. Risk factors and evaluation of keratoconus progression after penetrating keratoplasty with anterior segment optical coherence tomography. Sci Rep. 2020;10(1):18594.

16 Lamellar Keratoplasty in Keratoconus

Jagadesh C. Reddy, Zarin Modiwala, and Maggie Mathew

16.1 Introduction

As discussed in the earlier chapter, replacement of ectatic cornea with a healthy donor cornea has been the last resort in the visual rehabilitation of patients with advanced keratoconus. Full-thickness penetrating keratoplasty (PKP) has been the preferred choice for keratoconus with good visual outcomes and graft survival [1]. The major complications leading to a short fall of PKP were higher endothelial graft rejection, secondary glaucoma, and graft dehiscence needing wound re-suturing [2, 3]. The advent of anterior lamellar keratoplasty (ALKP) has revolutionized the keratoplasty care for patients with keratoconus. This has decreased the graft failures because of endothelial rejection, long-term endothelial cell loss, and thus improved the graft survival rates [1, 2]. In the current scenario, PKP could be reserved for cases where keratoconus eyes are associated with endothelial dysfunction or when deep corneal scarring involving the visual axis up to the Descemet membrane (DM) level [4]. In some instances with residual scarring, safety of ALKP can outperform the better visual acuity achieved with PK [5].

Indications for ALK in patients with keratoconus:

- Any case of keratoconus with healthy endothelium.
- Patients with advanced keratoconus and intolerant to contact lenses or intra corneal ring segments (ICRS).
- Patients with previous hydrops who have poor vision with contact lenses.
- Keratoconus in a case of Downs syndrome wherein ALKP can provide better tectonic stability than PKP and minimize graft dehiscence secondary to trauma.
- Patients with atopy with a high risk of graft rejection and failure.
- The other eye of the patient had repeated graft rejections.
- Monocular patient with an increased risk of trauma.
- Patients suspected to have poor compliance with follow-ups and treatment.

The initial ALKP was not very successful compared to PKP because of poor visual outcomes. According to the depth of dissection, ALKP techniques are of two categories (Fig. 16.1): (a) superficial anterior lamellar

J. C. Reddy (✉)
Cataract and Refractive Services, Pristine Eye Hospitals, Madhapur, Hyderabad, Telangana, India

Z. Modiwala
Cataract and Refractive Services, Pristine Eye Hospitals, Madhapur, Hyderabad, Telangana, India

The Cornea Institute, L V Prasad Eye Institute, Hyderabad, India

M. Mathew
Birmingham Midland Eye Center, Birmingham City Hospital, Birmingham, UK

S. Das (ed.), *Keratoconus*, https://doi.org/10.1007/978-981-19-4262-4_16

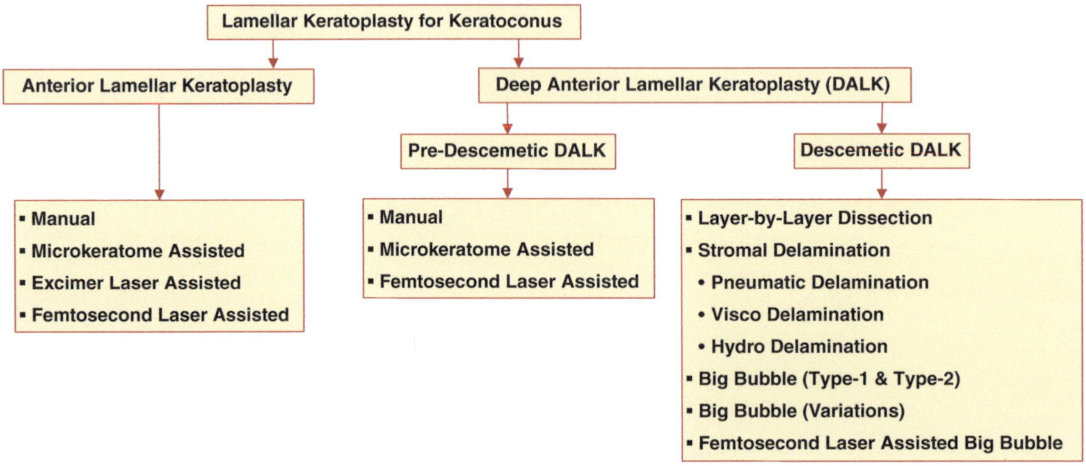

Fig. 16.1 A flow diagram showing different nomenclature for lamellar keratoplasty, and techniques used for a successful procedure. Black color represents recipient cornea, and the red color represents donor cornea

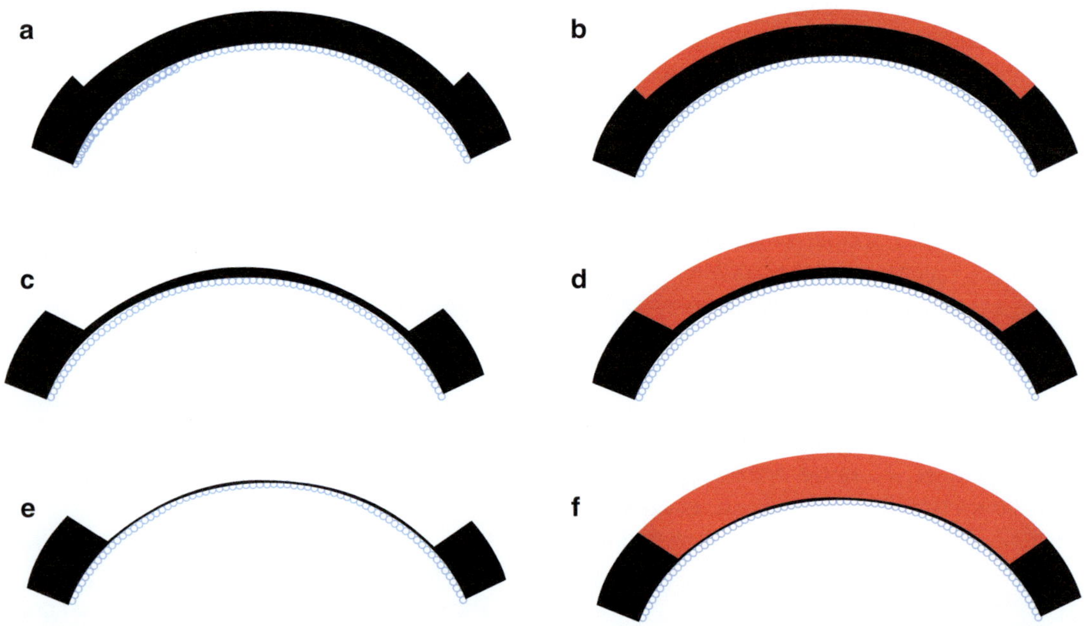

Fig. 16.2 (**a**) Diagrammatic representation of anterior lamellar keratoplasty technique, (**b**) Anterior one-third of cornea with disease is removed and replaced with donor cornea of similar size, (**c**) Larger amount of recipient cornea removed without baring Descemet membrane (DM), (**d**) Donor cornea of similar size is transplanted, (**e**) Recipient cornea up to DM has been removed, and (**f**) Donor cornea without DM replaced. (**a, b**) Anterior lamellar keratoplasty, (**c, d**) Predescemet membrane deep anterior lamellar keratoplasty (DALK), and (**e, f**) Descemetic DALK

keratoplasty (ALK) wherein the residual stromal tissue of 25% or more is left behind, and (b) deep anterior lamellar keratoplasty (DALK) wherein the residual stroma left behind is less than 25% of central corneal thickness. DALK is further classified into (a) predescemet membrane DALK (pd-DALK) wherein less than 25% of stroma are left intact over the Descemet membrane (DM) at the end of dissection, and (b) Descemetic DALK (d-DALK) procedure wherein complete excision of stroma baring the DM is accomplished (Fig. 16.2) [6–8].

16.2 Anterior Lamellar Keratoplasty

The ALKP procedure is preferred in situations where there is a higher risk of DM perforations thus affecting the overall success of the graft. The potential disadvantages with this technique would be a possible irregular stromal bed leading to interface haze, irregular astigmatism, and recurrence of ectasia [9]. This technique can be facilitated by layer-by-layer manual dissection, microkeratome, excimer laser or femtosecond laser-assisted ALK [10].

16.2.1 Manual ALKP

This technique is performed by partial trephination of desired diameter encompassing the entire cone. The stromal tissue is dissected layer by layer. It is difficult to judge the residual stromal thickness unless an intraoperative optical coherence tomography (OCT) is used. But a fair idea can be achieved by closely observing the orientation of the stromal fibers. Once the stromal dissection is done, the donor cornea fashioned with approximately similar thickness is secured in place with the help of sutures [11]. The major disadvantage of this procedure is the possibility of irregular stromal dissection leading to interface haze and irregular astigmatism.

16.2.2 Automated ALKP/ Microkeratome-Assisted ALKP (MALKP)/Automated Lamellar Therapeutic Keratoplasty (ALTK)

To avoid the possibility of irregular stromal bed, microkeratome is used to allow safe and relatively safe reproducible stromal dissection [12]. Microkeratome-assisted LKP is aimed at not only removing the central ectatic corneal tissue but also reshaping the cornea by suturing under tension a lamellar button which is thicker and smaller than the recipient bed. The microkeratome is used to prepare both the recipient and the donor. The ALTK system consists of microkeratome with interchangeable heads and an artificial anterior chamber.

16.2.3 Procedure

16.2.3.1 Recipient Preparation

Using gentian violet, 16 radial marks are placed over the cornea. A suction ring is placed on the recipient and the intraocular pressure is increased to facilitate a smoother dissection. Microkeratome (automated/hand-driven) is advanced in the sliver provided for sliding until the anterior corneal lamellar cap is free. A special nomogram is used for ectatic corneas to facilitate the use of appropriate ring size to achieve a desired diameter of dissection. Usually a 250-micron microkeratome is used for preparation of recipient tissue.

16.2.3.2 Donor Preparation

A donor cornea is mounted on an artificial anterior chamber. The same microkeratome with a 350-micron head is used for preparation of donor lamellar tissues of a diameter of 8.5 mm. The lamellar donor graft is sutured to the recipient bed using 16 interrupted 10–0 nylon sutures [13].

The drawbacks of this procedure have been a high percentage of patients having significant astigmatism, expensive procedure, unpredictability in matching of donor- recipient thickness and/ or size, recurrence of keratoconus because of progressive nature of the disease, and poor suitability of the procedure for advanced keratoconus with thin cornea. Complications like buttonhole, double anterior chamber, and persistent central folds were reported [14]. Busin et al. have reported good outcomes with modified microkeratome-assisted lamellar keratoplasty (MALK) for keratoconus [14]. At 12 months, the spectacle-corrected distance visual acuity was 20/25 in about 69% of patients.

16.2.4 Excimer Laser-Assisted LKP (ELLKP)

To overcome the deficiencies in sizing of the recipient and donor cornea using the manual or microkeratome-assisted procedures, excimer laser is used as it has been shown to have micron level precision [15]. A plano excimer laser ablation is done on the donor and the recipient of desired thickness and diameter. After de-epithelialization, a stainless-steel mask is used over to the cornea to achieve vertical and regular edge of ablation. Studies have shown predictable nature of the procedure and good visual outcomes. The outcomes achieved by this technique were comparable to those achieved with PKP [16–18]. The drawbacks of this technique have been expensive nature, and residual ectatic tissue leading to recurrence of ectasia [18, 19].

16.2.5 Femtosecond Laser-Assisted ALK (FALK)

The precision of the corneal tissue dissection has improved with the introduction of femtosecond laser. Based on the predictability of the lasers in keratorefractive surgery, performing keratoplasty has been an extended indication as a smoother surface can be achieved. FALK is performed with or without sutures based on thickness of stromal removal. The precision of the depth of dissection decreases with severity of keratoconus. In advanced keratoconus, there is a higher tendency of DM perforation [20, 21].

16.3 DALK Surgical Techniques

DALK based on the depth of dissection can be pd-DALK or d-DALK. There are several reports studying the effect of residual stroma on the final visual outcomes. Marchini et al. showed comparable visual outcomes with up to 50 microns of residual stroma with complete dissection [22]. Ardjomand et al. demonstrated that eyes with a residual stromal bed thickness of less than 20 μm had visual acuity comparable to eyes with a PK, whereas those with a residual stromal bed thickness of greater than 80 μm had a significantly reduced visual acuity [23]. This could be explained by the fact that the residual bed thickness can determine the stiffness and corresponding resistance against the compressive forces of the donor graft. So, it is been hypothesized that thick residual recipient bed, together with a steep preoperative cornea and greater axial length, contributes to postoperative myopia in DALK. These results are consistent with several clinical studies available in literature comparing the visual outcome of d-DALK and pd-DALK [24–26]. Various methods have been adopted to achieve a deeper dissection.

16.3.1 Layer-by-Layer Manual Dissection

It is the oldest technique of lamellar keratoplasty. This technique is preferred in situations with very advanced thinning with deep stromal scar, previous corneal hydrops, or in cases where survival of the graft is more important than the visual acuity achieved. In this technique, partial trephination (60–70%) of the desired diameter is done and this is followed by dissection using a spatula or crescent knife to reach deep stromal plane. Multiple layers of stromal dissection are done. When a deep and regular stromal plane is achieved, a full-thickness donor cornea is then sutured. The major limitations of this procedure are interface haze, poor visual acuity, and recurrence of ectasia due to residual stroma (Fig. 16.3) [27–29].

Sugita and Kondo showed that there are no differences in visual acuity using a manual dissection technique that leaves a small amount of stroma, in place of the complete stromal dissection [11].

Rama et al. used a manual dissection technique guided by a calibrated knife incision based on ultrasonic pachymetry values and treated 288 eyes [30]. Both Rama et al. and Ardjomand et al. showed that eyes with lower values of recipient residual thickness are associated with better visual acuity [23, 30].

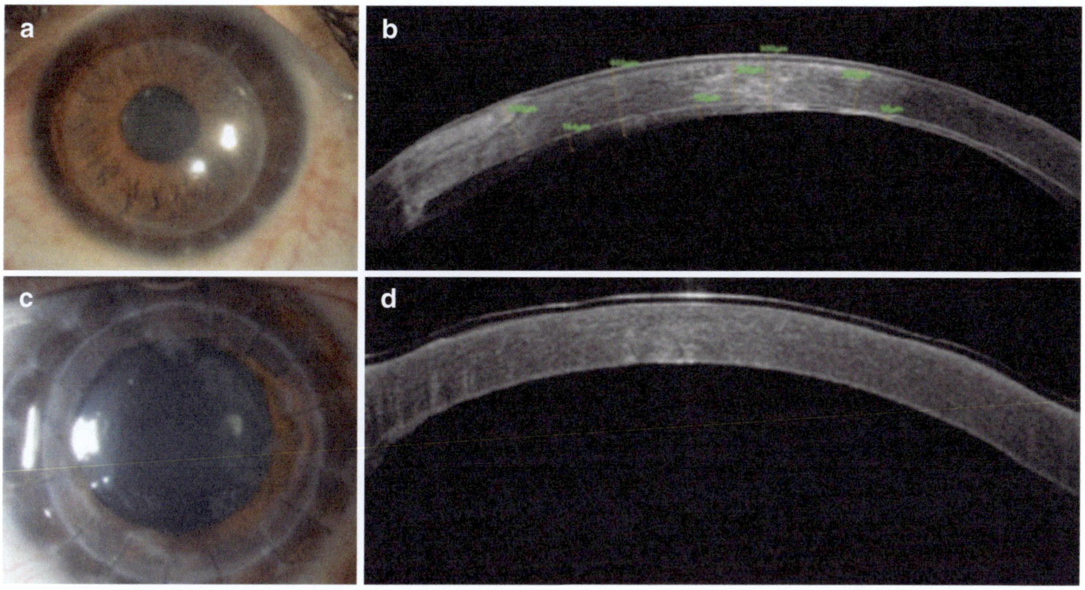

Fig. 16.3 DALK over ALK: (**a**) diffuse slit-lamp image of a patient with a clear graft and trace central haze causing poor visual acuity, (**b**) optical coherence tomography (OCT) showing residual stroma, (**c**) diffuse slit-lamp image showing a clear graft on the first postoperative day after big bubble DALK, and (**d**) OCT showing a compact graft with a well-attached DM with no residual stroma

16.3.2 Visco-Delamination

The technique of visco-delamination is performed by use of viscoelastic to achieve the cleavage cleaning between DM and stroma. This technique is preferred in patients with a previous episode of hydrops or those who had a near full-thickness corneal scar or a healed keratitis. In this procedure, anterior keratectomy is performed after partial corneal trephination. Then to visualize the depth of corneal incision and lamellar dissection, anterior chamber is filled with air through a paracentesis, so that creation of an air to endothelium interface behaves as a convex mirror. To inject viscoelastic through a cannula, a golf blade is used to create a deep incision. A dark band which is nonreflective can be seen between the tip of the blade and the light reflex representing the nonincised corneal tissue between the blade and air to endothelium interface. As you advance into deep stromal layers, the thickness of the dark band reduces and the depth at which the blade is in the stroma can be judged. The air is removed from the anterior chamber followed by injecting viscoelastic in stroma to create a visco-bubble. The progression of viscoelastic between the two layers is outlined by a typical golden ring reflex. The anterior corneal stroma is removed by trephination or dissection. This is followed by suturing of the full-thickness donor cornea [31, 32]. Though this technique showed a good outcome in a few studies, there were studies showing poor visual outcomes because of the residual stromal bed that was left over after dissection [33].

16.3.3 Hydro-Delamination

This technique involves achieving a cleavage plane between the DM and the stroma using balance salt solution (BSS). Initially, partial trephination of desired depth is done followed by injection of BSS using a blunt needle into the posterior stroma to reach the plane between the DM and the posterior stroma. The BSS passes between the collagen lamellae leading to swelling of the cornea which facilitates the easy dissection of stroma to reach DM. This technique has not become very popular because of the technical difficulty, and the possibilities of reaching the DM without leaving the posterior stroma are difficult [34].

16.3.4 Pneumo-Delamination

This technique involves injection of air into the posterior corneal stroma to achieve a plane of dissection between DM and stroma. This technique was described several years ago by Archila but became popular only after a successful modification of a big bubble technique, by Anwar and Teichmann in 2002 [35, 36]. The big bubble techniques remain a very popular and the most widely used technique of DALK.

The big bubble technique involves a partial thickness corneal trephination of up to 60–80% depth using vacuum trephine (Barron Radial Vacuum Trephine, Katena, USA). A 27- or 30-gauge needle attached to an air-filled syringe is inserted deep into paracentral stroma through the bottom of trephination groove and advanced with the bevel parallel to DM, facing downward. The approach to the center of the cornea is avoided as the cornea may be thinner in this location in patients with keratoconus. As the air is injected into the stroma, the bubbles seep into the space between corneal lamellae and based on the type of bubble the pattern changes. In situation of achieving a big bubble, disk-shaped semi-opaque circular changes are seen suggestive of a big bubble formation between the DM and corneal stroma. This is followed by creation of a small opening at the center of the anterior wall of the bubble to gain access into the space above the DM. This leads to collapse of the air bubble. The remaining stromal layers are lifted with a blunt spatula, severed with a blade, and excised with scissors.

Based on pattern of spread of air in the cornea, three types of bubbles can be achieved facilitating baring of DM. In majority of instances (80%–85%), Type-1 bubble is achieved followed by Type-2 or mixed bubbles. The Type-1 big bubble is formed when the air separates predescemet's layer (PDL) from the deep stroma creating a large central single bubble of around 8–9 mm in diameter (Fig. 16.4a). The posterior lamellae retained consist of PDL, DM, and endothelial cells. The Type-2 big bubble is formed when the air creates a cleavage between the PDL and DM. The retained lamellae consist of only the DM and endothelial cells thus making it susceptible to perforation (Fig. 16.4b). The mixed big bubble pattern is seen when the above two coexist. The Type-1 big bubble arises from the center and is smaller than the Type-2 bubble which

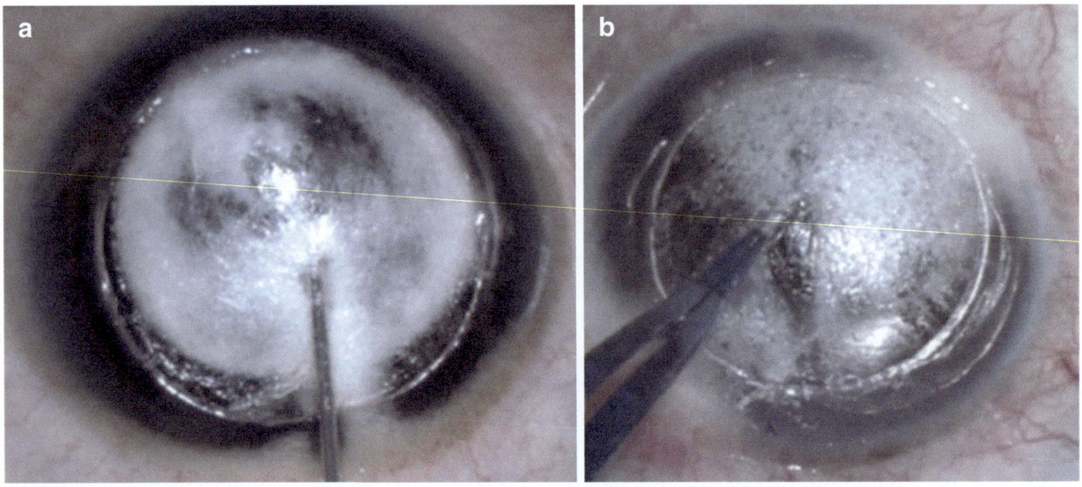

Fig. 16.4 Snapshot form surgical video showing: (**a**) Type-1 Big bubble, (**b**) Type-2 Big bubble

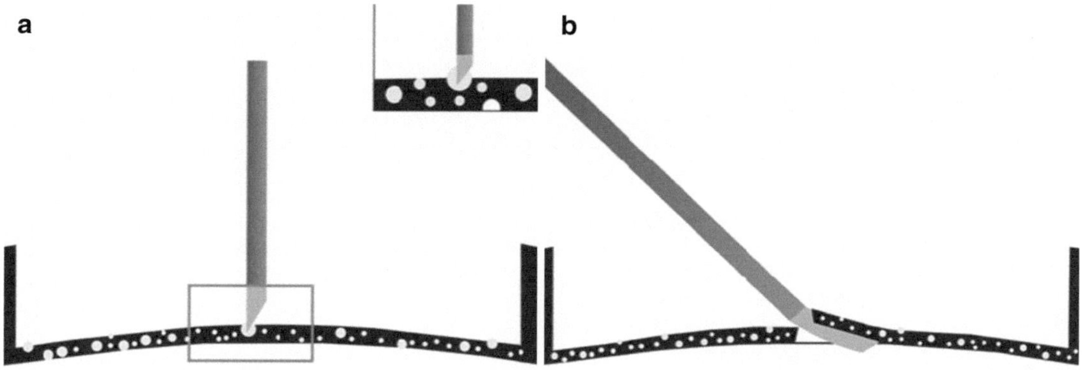

Fig. 16.5 Schematic diagram showing small air bubbles in the posterior stroma: (**a**) sharp needle used to rupture the anterior wall, (**b**) through the opening made access to the predescemet layer can be achieved

arises from the periphery and extends to the center [37–39].

16.3.5 Modifications of Big Bubble Technique

16.3.5.1 Small Bubble-Guided Big Bubble Technique

This technique involves completing a partial dissection as discussed earlier. This is followed by making a paracentesis and injecting multiple small bubbles into the anterior chamber. When air is injected into the posterior stroma and Type-1 big bubble is achieved, the convex bowing of DM into the AC will displace the small bubbles to the periphery. In situations of multiple attempts to achieve a big bubble may lead to opaque cornea with the air. In such situations, the small bubble-guided techniques aid in confirming the achievement of a big bubble. Baring the DM once big bubble is achieved will be similar to the method described above [40].

16.3.5.2 Microbubble-Assisted Baring of DM

In certain situations when the injection of air is more anterior or mid stroma wherein the collagen lamellae are more compact than the posterior stroma, can lead to diffuse emphysema of the corneal stroma with no big bubble. In order to bare DM, manual dissection has to be done until posterior stroma is reached. Manual dissection at the level of DM can lead to perforation. By rupturing the small bubbles, the space between the posterior stroma and the PDL can be safely reached (Fig. 16.5) [41].

16.3.5.3 Femtosecond Laser-Assisted DALK (FS-DALK)

The precision of femtosecond laser paved for deeper stromal dissection. The trephination done using femtosecond laser assisted in achieving BB in majority of the times. There is lower rate of perforation and conversion to PKP with FS-DALK. The use of FS-DALK in conjunction with intraoperative optical coherence tomography has improved the rate of achieving BB. Recently, the creation of intrastromal pockets to guide injection of air at appropriate depth and achieve a big bubble has been successful. The rate of achieving was about 90–100%. The added advantage of use of femtosecond laser has been customization of the donor and recipient trephination.

16.3.5.4 DALK after ICRS

ICRS have been popular in improving visual acuity in mild-moderate keratoconus by flattening the central cornea and thus making the cornea regular. Patients with complications like extrusion, or dissatisfaction due to poor visual improvement, glare, and holes may require PKP or DALK [42–44]. The procedure of DALK will be like what has been discussed above but the likelihood of achieving BB will be high if air is injected into the

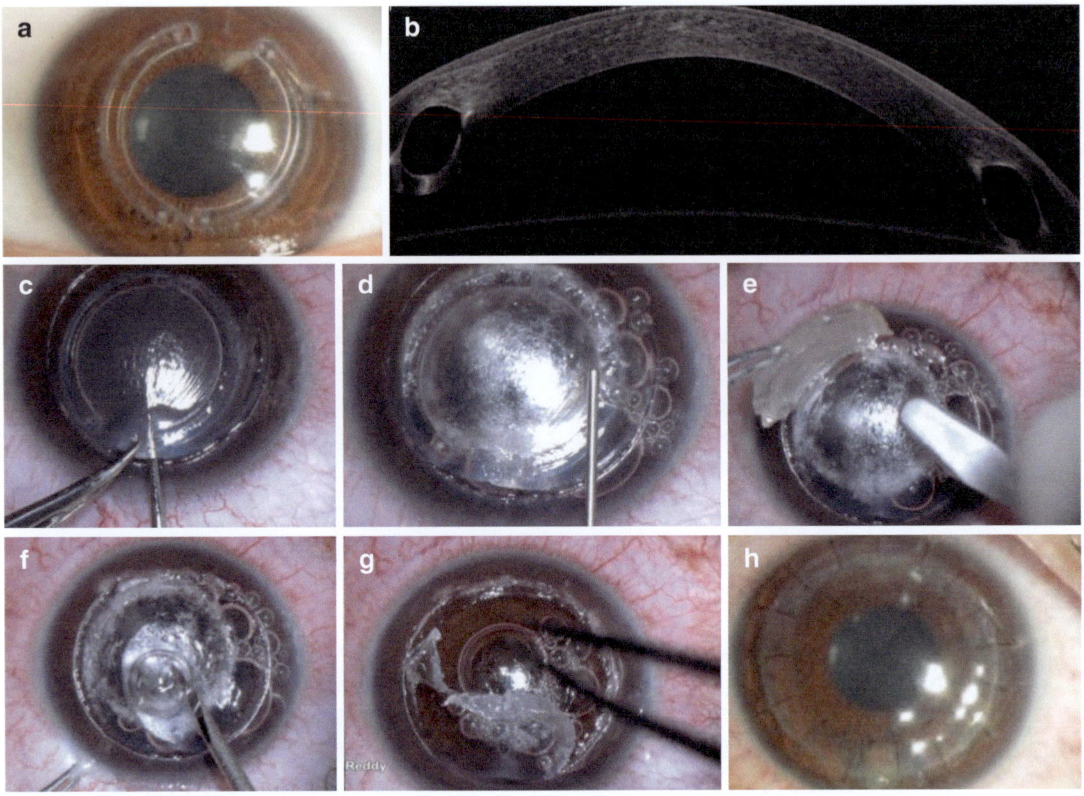

Fig. 16.6 DALK after intracorneal ring segment implantation (ICRS): (**a**) diffuse slit-lamp picture showing a clear cornea and ICRS, (**b**) optical coherence tomography (OCT)showing the ICRS in the posterior stroma, (**c**) after partial trephination, a pointed dissector is inserted under the ICRS to create a canal for the cannula to inject air, (**d**) Type-1 big bubble achieved after air injection, (**e**) excision of the anterior-midstroma along with ICRS complex, (**f**) brave slash to rupture the anterior wall of the big bubble, (**g**) removal of the posterior stroma to bare DM, and (**h**) postoperative slit-lamp picture with a clear graft and intact sutures

stroma under the ICRS prior to their removal (Fig. 16.6). Though rare complications like segment exposure, extrusion, corneal infection, and vascularization can occur [43]. The visual and refractive outcomes after ICRS explantation and DALK have been good with improved spectacle-corrected distance visual acuity (CDVA) and lower astigmatism levels [45, 46].

16.3.5.5 DALK after Resolved Hydrops

Acute corneal hydrops is a result of progressive keratoconus leading to gross corneal edema. The edema would resolve in 2–4 months but would result in corneal scarring. Removal of scarred tissue and achieving DM baring DALK are technically difficult and hence majority of times a PKP is considered. The DM perforation rate with an attempted DALK ranges from 0% to 100% [47]. The rate of corneal graft rejection was higher and graft survival at 5 years was lower in patients after PKP for resolved hydrops compared to those without hydrops [48].

To achieve a successful DALK, manual dissection is preferred over BB technique to avoid perforation. Initially intrastromal air is injected into the stroma followed by layer-layer dissection with or without baring the DM. The visual outcomes were good despite leaving a thin layer of posterior stroma in situations where there is a higher chance of developing a macroperforation (Fig. 16.7) [47, 49]. Goweida et al. have described a technique of peripheral pneumatic dissection followed by peeling to complete DALK [49].

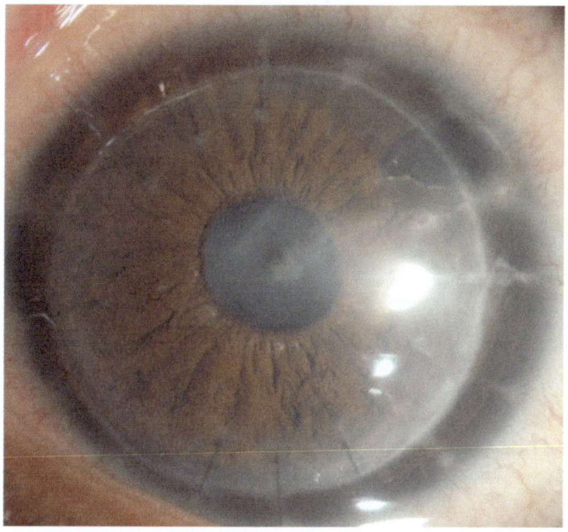

Fig. 16.7 Diffuse slit-lamp picture of a patient after predescemet membrane for resolved hydrops. A trace scar can be seen in the posterior stroma because of the residual stroma

Majority of studies reported CDVA of 20/40 or better after DALK for resolved hydrops [49].

16.3.6 Outcomes

16.3.6.1 Visual Refractive and Graft Success

Several studies have compared the outcomes of DALK and PK in keratoconus patients.

16.3.6.2 CDVA

Most of the studies have shown a comparable CDVA between DALK and PKP at 6 and 12 months [3, 50–53]. Javadi et al. and Sari et al. have shown a favorable outcome with PKP comparable to DALK [1, 54]. The mean difference in the percentage of patients who achieved CDVA better than 0 LogMAR by 12 months was seen in patients after PKP than DALK [3, 50, 51, 53, 55–57]. This needs further validation with RCTs.

16.3.6.3 Spherical Equivalent (SE)

Several studies have shown a comparable refractive SE at 12 months between patients who underwent DALK versus PKP. Though the suture removal timing may have been different, the SE was comparable. The mean ranged from −1.0 to −7.73 D and − 1.0 to −4.17 D after DALK and PKP, respectively [1, 2, 51–55, 58].

16.3.6.4 Astigmatism

The refractive astigmatism in several studies has shown to be lower in patients after DALK compared to PKP at 12 months. The mean ranged from −2.2 to −4.0 D and − 2.8 to −5.83 D after DALK to PKP, respectively [2, 3, 51, 54–58]. The keratometry astigmatism at 12 months was shown to be comparable between PKP and DALK [1, 2, 52, 58, 59].

16.3.6.5 Endothelial Cell Density (ECD)

At 12 months, the postoperative ECD was higher in patients after DALK compared to PKP. However, it was not statistically different between DALK and PKP. The rate of loss of ECD over long-term follow-up was higher after PKP compared to DALK [33, 58, 60, 61].

16.3.6.6 Graft Rejection Episodes

The superiority of DALK over PK has been with retaining host endothelial cells thus avoiding endothelial cell rejection which is the most common form of rejection after keratoplasty. Stromal rejection was the most common form of rejection noted after DALK. DALK was favored over PKP in the number of graft rejection episodes and outcomes of graft rejection [1–3, 33, 50, 53–58].

16.3.6.7 Graft Survival

In a recent meta-analysis, Henein et al. have shown a comparable graft survival rate between PKP and DALK [58]. Both RCTs and comparative studies have shown a similar trend [1–3, 50, 51, 53–58].

16.3.6.8 Complications

Both PKP and DALK have complications in common and which are unique to each procedure as shown in Table 16.1.

Table 16.1 Complications of DALK and PK

The complications unique to DALK	Complications common to PKP and DALK
• Microperforation of DM • Macroperforation of DM • Large lamellar splits in DM • DM perforation while suturing • Pseudo anterior chamber (AC)/double AC • Endothelial cell loss secondary to air/synthetic gas, perforation of DM • Interface haze • Interface vascularization, epithelial ingrowth, microbial keratitis • Wrinkles of DM • Urrets-Zavalia syndrome (fixed dilated pupil) • Re-epithelialization problems	• Ocular surface disease • Donor-to-host transmission of infection • Ametropias, high/irregular astigmatism • Suture-related issues (sterile inflammation, microbial keratitis, premature loosening) • Graft rejection: Epithelial and stromal rejection • Recurrence of keratoconus • Globe rupture

DALK Deep anterior lamellar keratoplasty, *DM* Descemet membrane, *PKP* Penetrating keratoplasty

16.4 Perforation of DM

Descemet's membrane perforation or rupture is the most common intraoperative complication of DALK procedure. The incidence of rupture ranges from 4% to 39% [62, 63]. DALK for keratoconus is shown to have higher rate of DM perforation compared to other indications [29]. The rate of perforation also depends on the techniques used to bare the DM with the lowest for BB technique [26]. The rupture of DM can occur at different stages of the procedure like partial trephination, air bubble injection, brave slash, removal of stroma, and while suturing [26, 29]. Based on size, perforations have been classified as micro- or macroperforations. The management of these perforations is discussed in Table 16.2. In cases of perforations of a smaller size, the use of fibrin glue or augmentation with small stromal tissue can aid in successfully completing the procedure (Fig. 16.8) [64–66]. There has been a greater loss of endothelial cells after DM perforation compared to those with no perforation [62]. Majority of the times it is difficult to salvage macroperforation which may necessitate conversion to PKP. The rate of conversion to PKP ranges from 0 to 100% [67].

16.4.1 Double Anterior Chamber (AC)/Pseudo AC

In case of DM, perforation during the DALK procedure can lead to double AC or pseudo AC (Fig. 16.9) [29, 67, 68]. The risk of double AC is high in keratoconus patients with corneal scar, intraoperative perforation, and Type-2 bubble formation [68]. At times, this can also happen without a noticeable perforation because of the buckling of donor cornea over the stretched host DM. The double AC can resolve spontaneously or may require injection of air or gases like C_3F_8/sulfur hexafluoride (SF_6) gas into the anterior chamber postoperatively [29, 67]. But in situation of residual recipient, stroma over the DM may lead to persistent detachment and needs a PKP.

16.4.2 Pupillary Block and Fixed Dilated Pupil (Urrets-Zavalia Syndrome)

Permanent pupillary mydriasis can result from injecting air into the anterior chamber at the end of surgery or for detached DM. This could be due to iris ischemia, immobile iris, and glaucomflecken/anterior subcapsular cataract because of anterior lens epithelial cell infarcts [69, 70]. Timely diagnosis of the pupillary block and management with pupil dilation or paracentesis to reduce the size of the gas bubble, deepen the anterior chamber, and eliminating the pupillary block will often prevent these complications [29, 69, 70].

Table 16.2 DALK: DM perforation; timing of perforation, their management, and prevention are discussed

Timing of perforation	Management	Prevention
Partial trephination	• If the perforation <1/third of the circumference of trephination: To place a full-thickness suture and then continue dissection from a different location. • If the perforation >1/third of the circumference of trephination: To convert of PKP.	• To be aware of corneal thickness in the zone of trephination. • To use a predictable vacuum trephine.
Air bubble injection	• Usually, perforation would be in the central cornea. To consider stromal removal till the size of the perforation is identified. If there is a microperforation—Can consider leaving some residual stroma around the perforation or applying fibrin glue. Air bubble should be placed in the anterior chamber throughout the procedure. • If the perforation is large to convert to PKP.	• To avoid sudden gush of air into the stroma. • To avoid big bubble in the presence of posterior stromal scar like in hydrops. • To check the patency of the canula prior to injection of air.
Brave slash	• To consider stromal removal till the size of the perforation is identified. In many instances there would be a microperforation—Can consider leaving some residual stroma around the perforation or applying fibrin glue. Air bubble should be placed in the anterior chamber throughout the procedure. • If the perforation is large to convert to PKP.	• To place a blog of viscoelastic to avoid sudden egress of air. • To consider performing the manoeuvre with the MVR blade at an angle and not perpendicular.
Stromal removal	• Perforation usually happens while dissecting the peripheral stroma. If there is a microperforation—Can consider leaving some residual stroma around the perforation or applying fibrin glue. Air bubble should be placed in the anterior chamber throughout the procedure. • If the perforation is large to convert to PKP.	• To separate adhesions between the posterior stroma and the PDL before excising. • To avoid excessive stretch posterior stroma perpendicular to the DM. • To avoid use of sharp instruments.
Suturing	• In case of DM perforation, there is egress of aqueous while passing the needle through the recipient to donor. • Majority of times the perforation is small and by air tamponade we can avoid detachment of DM.	• To visualize the passing of needle always can avoid a perforation.

PKP Penetrating keratoplasty, *PDL* Predescemetic layer, *DM* Descemet membrane

16.4.3 Graft Rejection

DALK procedure trades better than PK by avoiding endothelial rejection. In about 3–14% of patients, subepithelial and stromal rejections have been reported [71]. The episodes of rejection are reported more in patients associated with ocular allergy and young age (Fig. 16.10) [72, 73]. These rejections are very much reversible with intense topical steroids. If untreated can lead to graft failure [29].

16.4.4 Interface Complications

An interface is created in DALK between the recipient DM and the donor posterior stroma. This potential space can be source of vascularization and for lodging microbes. In patients with uncontrolled allergy can lead to vascularization in the interface. This could lead to acute graft rejection or interface bleeding [72]. One of the most common organisms retrieved from interface is Candida. The common cause has been transplanting a contaminant donor.

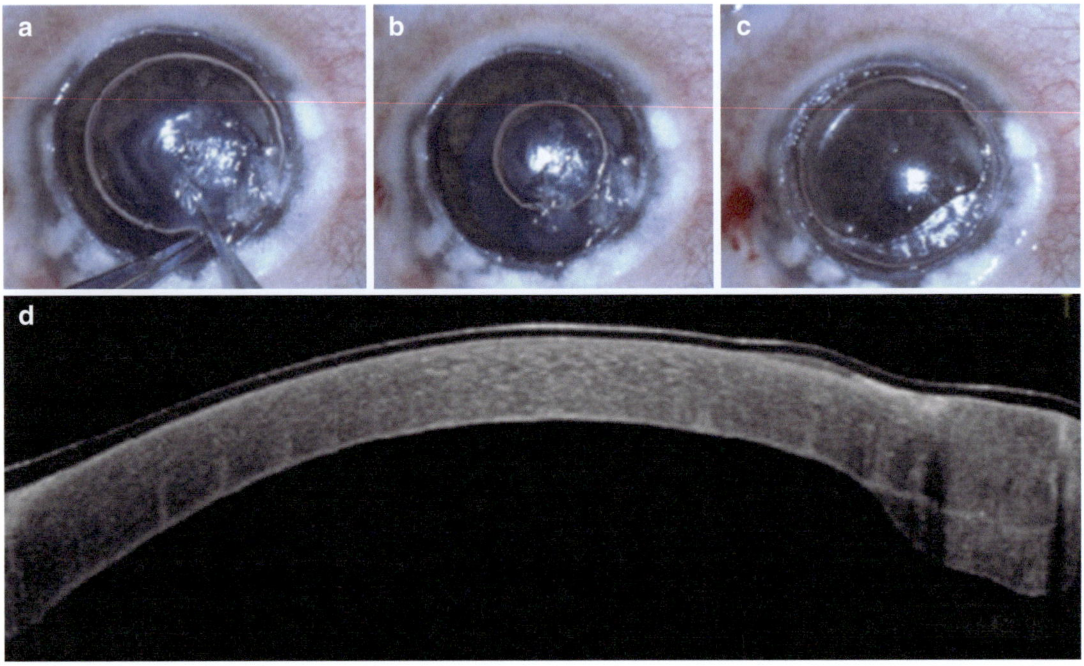

Fig. 16.8 Snapshot form surgical video after anterior keratectomy and no big bubble: (**a**) microbubble-assisted DALK is planned with a MVR knife, small bubbles are being punctured, (**b**) there is escape of air from anterior chamber and escape of aqueous because of microperforation, (**c**) the posterior stroma was successfully removed manually but residual stroma was left behind in the area of perforation, and (**d**) OCT showing a well-placed graft with residual stroma in the periphery

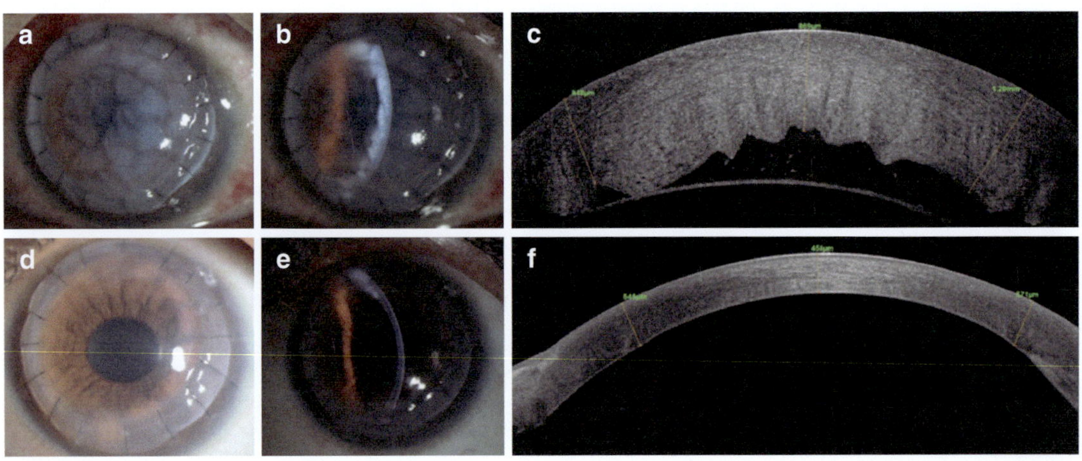

Fig. 16.9 Double anterior chamber (AC) after DALK: (**a**) slit-lamp diffuse image with severe graft edema, (**b**) slit image showing detached DM and a double AC, (**c**) OCT showing a thick, edematous graft with a detached DM, (**d**) slit-lamp diffuse image showing a clear graft after rebubbling with air, (**e**) slit image showing a well-attached DM, and (**f**) OCT showing a well-attached DM and a compact cornea

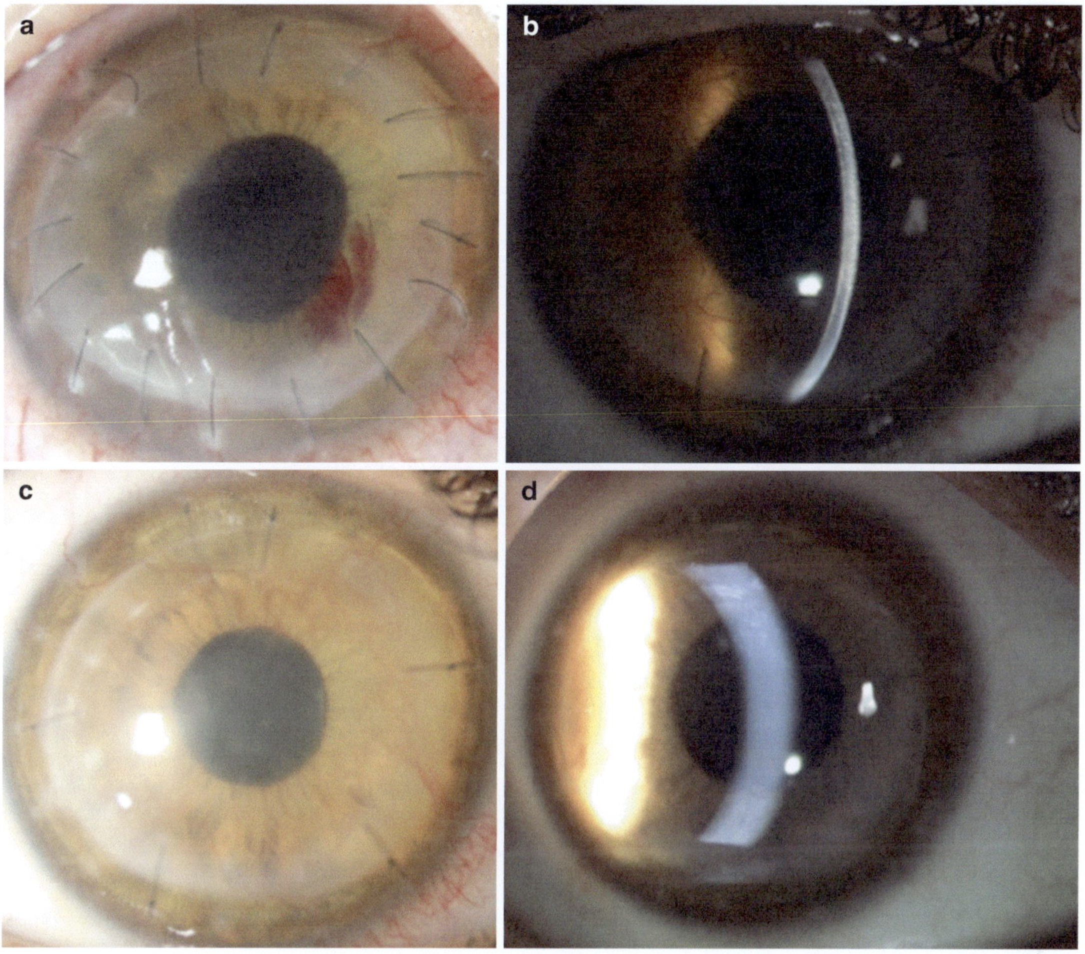

Fig. 16.10 (**a**) 17-year-old male who had a history of ocular allergy and keratoconus underwent DALK: (**b**) diffuse slit image showing a graft edema, interface vascularization, bleeding suggestive of acute stromal rejection, (**c**) 6 weeks later with intense steroids showing a decrease in graft edema, and (**d**) 6 months after rejection showing clear graft and ghost vessels

The presence of the recipient DM delays the spread of infection intraocularly. Because of the location, it is difficult to treat and gain access to the material for microbiological evaluation. Often these cases may end up having PKP [29, 74].

16.5 Conclusion

Modifications of keratoplasty techniques for patients with keratoconus have been done over the years. Lamellar keratoplasty has evolved to the present DALK technique which appears as a very promising alternative to PKP in most of the keratoconus patients with healthy endothelial cells. However, there is still some scope for future research to explore alternatives to donor cornea and thus improve long-term outcomes of DALK for keratoconus.

References

1. Javadi MA, Feizi S, Yazdani S, Mirbabaee F. Deep anterior lamellar keratoplasty versus penetrating keratoplasty for keratoconus: a clinical trial. Cornea. 2010;29(4):365–71.
2. Song Y, Zhang J, Pan Z. Systematic review and meta-analysis of clinical outcomes of penetrating

keratoplasty versus deep anterior lamellar keratoplasty for keratoconus. Exp Clin Transplant. 2020;18(4):417–28.
3. MacIntyre R, Chow SP, Chan E, Poon A. Long-term outcomes of deep anterior lamellar keratoplasty versus penetrating keratoplasty in Australian keratoconus patients. Cornea. 2014;33(1):6–9.
4. El-Agha MS, El Sayed YM, Harhara RM, Essam HM. Correlation of corneal endothelial changes with different stages of keratoconus. Cornea. 2014;33(7):707–11.
5. Parker JS, van Dijk K, Melles GR. Treatment options for advanced keratoconus: a review. Surv Ophthalmol. 2015;60(5):459–80.
6. Tan DT, Dart JK, Holland EJ, Kinoshita S. Corneal transplantation. Lancet. 2012;379(9827):1749–61.
7. Baradaran-Rafii A, Eslani M, Sadoughi MM, Esfandiari H, Karimian F. Anwar versus Melles deep anterior lamellar keratoplasty for keratoconus: a prospective randomized clinical trial. Ophthalmology. 2013;120(2):252–9.
8. Singh NP, Said DG, Dua HS. Lamellar keratoplasty techniques. Indian J Ophthalmol. 2018;66(9):1239–50.
9. Richard JM, Paton D, Gasset AR. A comparison of penetrating keratoplasty and lamellar keratoplasty in the surgical management of keratoconus. Am J Ophthalmol. 1978;86(6):807–11.
10. Patil M, Mehta JS. Lamellar keratoplasty for advanced keratoconus. Asia Pac J Ophthalmol (Phila). 2020;9(6):580–8.
11. Sugita J, Kondo J. Deep lamellar keratoplasty with complete removal of pathological stroma for vision improvement. Br J Ophthalmol. 1997;81(3):184–8.
12. Springs CL, Joseph MA, Odom JV, Wiley LA. Predictability of donor lamellar graft diameter and thickness in an artificial anterior chamber system. Cornea. 2002;21(7):696–9.
13. Busin M, Zambianchi L, Arffa RC. Microkeratome-assisted lamellar keratoplasty for the surgical treatment of keratoconus. Ophthalmology. 2005;112(6):987–97.
14. Busin M, Scorcia V, Zambianchi L, Ponzin D. Outcomes from a modified microkeratome-assisted lamellar keratoplasty for keratoconus. Arch Ophthalmol. 2012;130(6):776–82.
15. Spadea L, De Rosa V. Current techniques of lamellar keratoplasty for keratoconus. Saudi Med J. 2016;37(2):127–36.
16. Kubota T, Seitz B, Tetsumoto K, Naumann GO. Lamellar excimer laser keratoplasty: reproducible photoablation of corneal tissue. A laboratory study. Doc Ophthalmol. 1992;82(3):193–200.
17. Bilgihan K, Ozdek SC, Sari A, Hasanreisoğlu B. Excimer laser-assisted anterior lamellar keratoplasty for keratoconus, corneal problems after laser in situ keratomileusis, and corneal stromal opacities. J Cataract Refract Surg. 2006;32(8):1264–9.
18. Buratto L, Belloni S, Valeri R. Excimer laser lamellar keratoplasty of augmented thickness for keratoconus. J Refract Surg. 1998;14(5):517–25.
19. Serdarevic ON, Hanna K, Gribomont AC, Savoldelli M, Renard G, Pouliquen Y. Excimer laser trephination in penetrating keratoplasty. Morphologic features and wound healing. Ophthalmology. 1988;95(4):493–505.
20. Alio JL, Abdelghany AA, Barraquer R, Hammouda LM, Sabry AM. Femtosecond laser-assisted deep anterior lamellar keratoplasty outcomes and healing patterns compared to manual technique. Biomed Res Int. 2015;2015:397891.
21. Chan CC, Ritenour RJ, Kumar NL, Sansanayudh W, Rootman DS. Femtosecond laser-assisted mushroom configuration deep anterior lamellar keratoplasty. Cornea. 2010;29(3):290–5.
22. Marchini G, Mastropasqua L, Pedrotti E, Nubile M, Ciancaglini M, Sbabo A. Deep lamellar keratoplasty by intracorneal dissection: a prospective clinical and confocal microscopic study. Ophthalmology. 2006;113(8):1289–300.
23. Ardjomand N, Hau S, McAlister JC, Bunce C, Galaretta D, Tuft SJ, Larkin DF. Quality of vision and graft thickness in deep anterior lamellar and penetrating corneal allografts. Am J Ophthalmol. 2007;143(2):228–35.
24. Schiano-Lomoriello D, Colabelli-Gisoldi RA, Nubile M, Oddone F, Ducoli G, Villani CM, Mastropasqua L, Pocobelli A. Descemetic and predescemetic DALK in keratoconus patients: a clinical and confocal perspective study. Biomed Res Int. 2014;2014:123156.
25. Fontana L, Parente G, Sincich A, Tassinari G. Influence of graft-host interface on the quality of vision after deep anterior lamellar keratoplasty in patients with keratoconus. Cornea. 2011;30(5):497–502.
26. Sarnicola V, Toro P, Gentile D, Hannush SB. Descemetic DALK and predescemetic DALK: outcomes in 236 cases of keratoconus. Cornea. 2010;29(1):53–9.
27. Shimazaki J, Shimmura S, Ishioka M, Tsubota K. Randomized clinical trial of deep lamellar keratoplasty vs penetrating keratoplasty. Am J Ophthalmol. 2002;134(2):159–65.
28. Reinhart WJ, Musch DC, Jacobs DS, Lee WB, Kaufman SC, Shtein RM. Deep anterior lamellar keratoplasty as an alternative to penetrating keratoplasty a report by the american academy of ophthalmology. Ophthalmology. 2011;118(1):209–18.
29. Karimian F, Feizi S. Deep anterior lamellar keratoplasty: indications, surgical techniques and complications. Middle East Afr J Ophthalmol. 2010;17(1):28–37.
30. Rama P, Knutsson KA, Razzoli G, Matuska S, Viganò M, Paganoni G. Deep anterior lamellar keratoplasty using an original manual technique. Br J Ophthalmol. 2013;97(1):23–7.
31. Melles GR, Remeijer L, Geerards AJ, Beekhuis WH. A quick surgical technique for deep, anterior lamellar keratoplasty using visco-dissection. Cornea. 2000;19(4):427–32.
32. Manche EE, Holland GN, Maloney RK. Deep lamellar keratoplasty using viscoelastic dissection. Arch Ophthalmol. 1999;117(11):1561–5.

33. Bahar I, Kaiserman I, Srinivasan S, Ya-Ping J, Slomovic AR, Rootman DS. Comparison of three different techniques of corneal transplantation for keratoconus. Am J Ophthalmol. 2008;146(6):905–912.e1.
34. Panda A, Singh R. Intralamellar dissection techniques in lamellar keratoplasty. Cornea. 2000;19(1):22–5.
35. Archila EA. Deep lamellar keratoplasty dissection of host tissue with intrastromal air injection. Cornea. 1984–1985;3(3):217–8.
36. Anwar M, Teichmann KD. Big-bubble technique to bare Descemet's membrane in anterior lamellar keratoplasty. J Cataract Refract Surg. 2002;28(3):398–403.
37. Dua HS, Katamish T, Said DG, Faraj LA. Differentiating type 1 from type 2 big bubbles in deep anterior lamellar keratoplasty. Clin Ophthalmol. 2015;9:1155–7.
38. Dua HS, Faraj LA, Said DG, Gray T, Lowe J. Human corneal anatomy redefined: a novel pre-Descemet's layer (Dua's layer). Ophthalmology. 2013;120(9):1778–85.
39. Anwar DS, Kruger MM, Mootha VV. Blunt scissors stromal dissection technique for deep anterior lamellar keratoplasty. Clin Ophthalmol. 2014;8:1849–54.
40. Parthasarathy A, Por YM, Tan DT. Use of a "small-bubble technique" to increase the success of Anwar's "big-bubble technique" for deep lamellar keratoplasty with complete baring of Descemet's membrane. Br J Ophthalmol. 2007;91(10):1369–73.
41. Riss S, Heindl LM, Bachmann BO, Kruse FE, Cursiefen C. Microbubble incision as a new rescue technique for big-bubble deep anterior lamellar keratoplasty with failed bubble formation. Cornea. 2013;32(2):125–9.
42. Samimi S, Leger F, Touboul D, Colin J. Histopathological findings after intracorneal ring segment implantation in keratoconic human corneas. J Cataract Refract Surg. 2007;33(2):247–53.
43. Colin J, Malet FJ. Intacs for the correction of keratoconus: two-year follow-up. J Cataract Refract Surg. 2007;33(1):69–74.
44. Kymionis GD, Siganos CS, Tsiklis NS, Anastasakis A, Yoo SH, Pallikaris AI, Astyrakakis N, Pallikaris IG. Long-term follow-up of Intacs in keratoconus. Am J Ophthalmol. 2007;143(2):236–44.
45. Fontana L, Parente G, Sincich A, Tassinari G. Deep anterior lamellar keratoplasty after Intacs implantation in patients with keratoconus. Cornea. 2009;28(1):32–5.
46. Titiyal JS, Chawla B, Sharma N. Deep anterior lamellar keratoplasty with Intacs explantation in keratoconus. Eur J Ophthalmol. 2010;20(5):874–8.
47. Chew AC, Mehta JS, Tan DT. Deep lamellar keratoplasty after resolution of hydrops in keratoconus. Cornea. 2011;30(4):454–9.
48. Basu S, Reddy JC, Vaddavalli PK, Vemuganti GK, Sangwan VS. Long-term outcomes of penetrating keratoplasty for keratoconus with resolved corneal hydrops. Cornea. 2012;31(6):615–20.
49. Goweida MB, Sobhy M, Seifelnasr M, Liu C. Peripheral pneumatic dissection and scar peeling to complete deep anterior lamellar keratoplasty in eyes with healed hydrops. Cornea. 2019;38(4):504–8.
50. Han DC, Mehta JS, Por YM, Htoon HM, Tan DT. Comparison of outcomes of lamellar keratoplasty and penetrating keratoplasty in keratoconus. Am J Ophthalmol. 2009;148(5):744–751.e1.
51. Amayem AF, Hamdi IM, Hamdi MM. Refractive and visual outcomes of penetrating keratoplasty versus deep anterior lamellar keratoplasty with hydrodissection for treatment of keratoconus. Cornea. 2013;32(4):e2–5.
52. Jafarinasab MR, Feizi S, Javadi MA, Hashemloo A. Graft biomechanical properties after penetrating keratoplasty versus deep anterior lamellar keratoplasty. Curr Eye Res. 2011;36(5):417–21.
53. Jones MN, Armitage WJ, Ayliffe W, Larkin DF, Kaye SB, NHSBT Ocular Tissue Advisory Group and Contributing Ophthalmologists (OTAG Audit Study 5). Penetrating and deep anterior lamellar keratoplasty for keratoconus: a comparison of graft outcomes in the United Kingdom. Invest Ophthalmol Vis Sci. 2009;50(12):5625–9.
54. Söğütlü Sari E, Kubaloğlu A, Ünal M, Piñero Llorens D, Koytak A, Ofluoglu AN, Özertürk Y. Penetrating keratoplasty versus deep anterior lamellar keratoplasty: comparison of optical and visual quality outcomes. Br J Ophthalmol. 2012;96(8):1063–7.
55. Zhang YM, Wu SQ, Yao YF. Long-term comparison of full-bed deep anterior lamellar keratoplasty and penetrating keratoplasty in treating keratoconus. J Zhejiang Univ Sci B. 2013;14(5):438–50.
56. Funnell CL, Ball J, Noble BA. Comparative cohort study of the outcomes of deep lamellar keratoplasty and penetrating keratoplasty for keratoconus. Eye (Lond). 2006;20(5):527–32.
57. Watson SL, Ramsay A, Dart JK, Bunce C, Craig E. Comparison of deep lamellar keratoplasty and penetrating keratoplasty in patients with keratoconus. Ophthalmology. 2004;111(9):1676–82.
58. Henein C, Nanavaty MA. Systematic review comparing penetrating keratoplasty and deep anterior lamellar keratoplasty for management of keratoconus. Cont Lens Anterior Eye. 2017;40(1):3–14.
59. Kim MH, Chung TY, Chung ES. A retrospective contralateral study comparing deep anterior lamellar keratoplasty with penetrating keratoplasty. Cornea. 2013;32(4):385–9.
60. Oh BL, Kim MK, Wee WR. Comparison of clinical outcomes of same-size grafting between deep anterior lamellar keratoplasty and penetrating keratoplasty for keratoconus. Korean J Ophthalmol. 2013;27(5):322–30.
61. Kubaloglu A, Koytak A, Sari ES, Akyol S, Kurnaz E, Ozerturk Y. Corneal endothelium after deep anterior lamellar keratoplasty and penetrating keratoplasty for keratoconus: a four-year comparative study. Indian J Ophthalmol. 2012;60(1):35–40.
62. Leccisotti A. Descemet's membrane perforation during deep anterior lamellar keratoplasty: prognosis. J Cataract Refract Surg. 2007;33(5):825–9.

63. Den S, Shimmura S, Tsubota K, Shimazaki J. Impact of the descemet membrane perforation on surgical outcomes after deep lamellar keratoplasty. Am J Ophthalmol. 2007;143(5):750–4.
64. Alharbi SS, Alameer A. Use of fibrin glue in the management of descemet membrane perforation during deep anterior lamellar keratoplasty. Middle East Afr J Ophthalmol. 2019;26(3):168–71.
65. Nasr Hashem A, Tolees SS, Samir A. Novel technique for the management of macroperforation during deep anterior lamellar keratoplasty. Clin Ophthalmol. 2019;13:2075–80.
66. Srirampur A, Katta KR. Closure of microperforation during deep anterior lamellar keratoplasty with a corneal tissue fragment. Oman J Ophthalmol. 2019;12(2):138–40.
67. Goweida MB, Mahmoud S, Sobhy M, Liu C. Deep anterior lamellar keratoplasty with large Descemet's membrane perforation: should we stop conversion to penetrating keratoplasty? J Curr Ophthalmol. 2021;33(2):171–6.
68. Myerscough J, Bovone C, Mimouni M, Elkadim M, Rimondi E, Busin M. Factors predictive of double anterior chamber formation following deep anterior lamellar keratoplasty. Am J Ophthalmol. 2019;205:11–6.
69. UrretsZavalia A Jr. Fixed, dilated pupil, iris atrophy and secondary glaucoma. Am J Ophthalmol. 1963;56:257–65.
70. Maurino V, Allan BD, Stevens JD, Tuft SJ. Fixed dilated pupil (Urrets-Zavalia syndrome) after air/gas injection after deep lamellar keratoplasty for keratoconus. Am J Ophthalmol. 2002;133(2):266–8.
71. Al-Torbak AA, Al-Motowa S, Al-Assiri A, Al-Kharashi S, Al-Shahwan S, Al-Mezaine H, Teichmann K. Deep anterior lamellar keratoplasty for keratoconus. Cornea. 2006;25(4):408–12.
72. Williams KA, Lowe M, Bartlett C, Kelly TL, Coster DJ, Contributors A. Risk factors for human corneal graft failure within the Australian corneal graft registry. Transplantation. 2008;86(12):1720–4.
73. Watson SL, Tuft SJ, Dart JK. Patterns of rejection after deep lamellar keratoplasty. Ophthalmology. 2006;113(4):556–60.
74. Kanavi MR, Foroutan AR, Kamel MR, Afsar N, Javadi MA. Candida interface keratitis after deep anterior lamellar keratoplasty: clinical, microbiologic, histopathologic, and confocal microscopic reports. Cornea. 2007;26(8):913–6.

17 Intracorneal Ring Segments in Keratoconus

Andreas Katsimpris and George Kymionis

17.1 Introduction

ICRS are small circular devices made of poly (methyl methacrylate) (PMMA) which are implanted in the mid-peripheral corneal stroma aiming to reshape the geometry of corneal tissue, alter its refractive power, and improve patient's visual acuity. In contrast to other treatments, like contact lenses, which aim to correct refractive errors by changing the anterior corneal curvature, ICRS are a long-term intervention, which aim to improve the shape of the cornea and halt the progression of the cone.

Before the development of the modern ICRS, other intracorneal devices and surgical methodologies, like keratophakia, were used for the correction of refractive errors without promising clinical outcomes [1]. This led to a better understanding of the corneal physiology and the development of new materials and devices to reduce refractive errors. Among the newly developed intracorneal devices, ICRS were utilized principally in the reduction of refractive errors, mainly because of the various advantages compared to other surgical treatment options. Some of the main benefits of ICRS are the rapid improvement of visual acuity, adjustment of refractive correction by implant manipulation, preservation of an intact central cornea, and possibility of implant removal in case of complications [2].

The study of Blavatskaya in 1966 was the first to report the use intralamellar transplant rings in rabbit eyes to assess the effects on corneal curvature [3]. However, the first utilization of ICRS started in 1987 by Fleming et al. [4], where the insertion of an intracorneal device through a single peripheral corneal incision was found to diminish refractive errors in rabbit eyes by mechanically constricting or expanding the ring and as a result increasing or decreasing, respectively, the central corneal curvature. Later animal and human studies [5] contributed to the evolution of the ICRS from the initial 360-degree ring implants to C-shaped rings and ultimately, to incomplete ring segments, which were renamed to ICRS. The main reasons for remodeling the initial 360-degree rings were to facilitate an easier implementation and to eliminate incision-related complications [2]. KeraVision (Fremont, CA) Intacs ICRS underwent Food and Drug Administration (FDA)-regulated clinical trials [6] and in 1999 they were approved by the FDA for the treatment of myopia.

Despite the extensive research on ICRS and the proven safety, efficacy, and predictability of ICRS in the treatment of low and moderate myopia, this technology was overtaken by the success of the corneal excimer laser surgery, which has shown to have excellent refractive outcomes. However, due to the ability of ICRS to alter the

A. Katsimpris (✉) · G. Kymionis
First Department of Ophthalmology, National and Kapodistrian University of Athens, General Hospital "G. Gennimatas", Athens, Greece
e-mail: a.katsimpris@gna-gennimatas.gr; kymionis@med.uoc.gr

S. Das (ed.), *Keratoconus*, https://doi.org/10.1007/978-981-19-4262-4_17

corneal shape, the technology of ICRS was used as a potential interesting surgical alternative to avoid penetrating keratoplasty in patients with ectatic corneal disease. Thus, in 2000, Colin et al. were the first to report refractive outcomes of keratoconic patients without corneal scarring and with contact lens intolerance after ICRS implantation [7]. They found that ICRS implantation could reduce astigmatism and spherical correction and increase topographical regularity and visual acuity in keratoconic eyes. Since then, several studies have shown the positive clinical outcomes, with regard to refractive and visual acuity changes, occurring after ICRS implantation in eyes with keratoconus [8–11].

Nowadays, ICRS insertion constitutes a minimally invasive surgical option, which is also reversible, for treatment of keratoconus in patients with clear central cornea and contact-lens intolerance (stages II and III in standard Amsler-Krumeich classification [12]), but also of other types of ectatic corneal diseases, such as pellucid marginal degeneration and post-LASIK ectasia [13, 14]. The main aim of ICRS insertion is to improve contact lens tolerance and improve patients' visual acuity with spectacles, in order to delay or eliminate the need for penetrating keratoplasty or deep anterior lamellar keratoplasty.

17.2 Mechanism of Action of the Intracorneal Ring Segments and Effects on the Cornea

ICRS produce their refractive effects by acting as spacer elements between the corneal collagen lamellae and, thus, producing an arc-shortening effect of the corneal geometry [2]. The effects of ICRS insertion on corneal deformation have been assessed by analytical, finite-element, numerical, and empirical regression models [15–18] with consistent results and the refractive changes are exerted mainly through changing the curvature of the posterior and corneal surface and corneal apex position.

First, the arc-shortening effect of the ICRS on the corneal tissue results in flattening of the central cornea. Normal human corneas are aspheric with a gradual increase in thickness from central to peripheral cornea [19]. ICRS insertion flattens the pericentral portion of the cornea more than the central and thus, maintaining the prolate shape of the cornea and improving contact lens tolerance. In contrast, incisional and ablative surgical options produce more oblate corneas which are associated with spherical aberrations [20]. Second, it has been also shown that ICRS implantation increases corneal thickness up to several months postoperatively [21]. This effect has been hypothesized to be induced from corneal edema probably due to changes in endothelial cell function, especially in the area under the ICRS [22]. Another theory that could explain corneal thickening is that of collagen crowding and stromal infolding due to collagen remodeling; ICRS will compact corneal tissue postoperatively and, thus, increasing corneal thickness [22]. Third, in keratoconic eyes there has been observed a corneal axial apex shift up to 1 mm after ICRS implantation, which to a lesser extent contributes to the refractive changes seen postoperatively by decreasing anterior chamber depth [18]. Finally, apart from the effects of ICRS on corneal shape, ICRS implantation may act as a second limbus by adding mechanical support, relieving stress and improving the biomechanical properties of keratoconic corneas [23].

In general, the degree of corneal flattening after ICRS implantation is directly proportional to ICRS thickness and inversely proportional to ICRS diameter [24]; incremental increases in ICRS thickness and reductions in ring diameter sizes result in increased corneal flattening. However, the biomechanical, structural, and optical properties of keratoconic eyes are different than normal eyes and as a result the effects of ICRS on keratoconic eyes can be unpredictable. For example, it has been found that in keratoconic eyes the activity of proteolytic enzymes is increased [25], there is a lower number of collagen-producing keratocytes [26], corneal proteoglycan content is increased [27], orthogonal arrangement of collagen lamellae is lost and mean fibril diameter and spacing between collagen lamellae is decreased [27]. These structural alterations result in changes of corneal biomechanical integrity which may explain the unpredictability of clinical outcomes after ICRS placement in the mechanically weakened keratoconic eyes [28].

Most studies to date have extensively focused on the visual, refractive, and topographic outcomes post-ICRS insertion without taking into consideration the wound-healing corneal response. On the contrary, corneal histopathological changes have been assessed to a lesser extent, usually by utilizing optical coherence tomography, ultrasound, confocal or specular microscopy on human or animal corneas [29–31]. Outcomes from these studies have shown an increased production of extracellular and intracellular production of lipids [31] and deposition of apoptotic keratocytes in the anterior corneal stroma [32], which are directly proportional with ICRS thickness and the duration of ICRS implantation. The density of keratocytes has been found to be either decreased [29] or increased [31] in the corneal stroma adjacent to the ICRS.

Finally, several studies have demonstrated that the aforementioned biomechanical, topographical, and histological effects of ICRS are reversible [29, 33]. In general, ICRS are easily removed and after explantation, corneas can return to their original state, which is one of the main advantages of this treatment.

17.2.1 Types of Intracorneal Ring Segments

Currently there is a variety of ICRS models which are available for keratoconus treatment. All of them are made of PMMA and the main characteristics which vary among different types ICRS are arc length, cross section, thickness, optical zone size, inner and outer diameter (Table 17.1).

Intacs (Lombard, Illinois, USA) (Fig. 17.1) is the only commercially available ICRS in the USA, consisting of either two semicircular implants of 150° arc length or a single 210° implant, with a hexagonal cross-section shape. Intacs thickness ranges from 150 to 210 μm with higher thickness inducing higher refractive effects. In contrast, Intacs segment design (SK) has an oval transverse shape with a smaller inner diameter of 6 mm and are used in keratoconic eyes with high refractive errors, since they induce a higher corneal flattening effect.

Ferrara (Ferrara Ophthalmics, Belo Horizonte, Brazil) and Keraring (Mediphacos, Belo Horizonte, Brazil) (Fig. 17.2) are ICRS with triangular cross-section shapes, which share similar design characteristics (Table 17.1). The aim of the triangular shape in ICRS is to produce a prismatic effect and, thus, to diminish optical abbera-

Table 17.1 Main design characteristics of different ICRS models

Characteristics	Bisantis	Intacs	Intacs SK	Ferrara	Keraring	Keraring AS	Myoring
Arc length (degrees)	80	150–210	90–150	90–320	90–355	160–320	360
Cross-section	Oval	Hexagonal	Oval	Triangular	Triangular	Triangular	Triangular
Optical zone (mm)	3.5–4.5	7	6	5–6	5–6	5	5–8
Thickness (μm)	150	210–450	210–500	150–350	150–350	150–300[a]	200–320
Inner diameter (mm)	No data	6.77	6	4.4	5	5	5–8
Outer diameter (mm)	No data	8.1	7	5.6	6	6	5–8
FDA—approval	No	Yes	Yes	No	No	No	No
CE—marking	No data	Yes	Yes	Yes	Yes	Yes	Yes

FDA Food and Drug Administration
CE Communauté Européenne
[a]Keraring AS has progressive thickness profiles of 150–250 mm or 200–300 mm within the same implant

tions, especially in low light conditions [34]. In contrast to other ICRS, which have a constant ring thickness, Keraring Asymmetric (AS) (Mediphacos, Belo, Horizonte, Brazil) is the only one with progressively thickness profiles (from 150 to 250 mm or from 200 to 300 mm) within the same implant. The thinnest part of the ring is located near the corneal incision and progressively increases till the distal end of the ring, which has the highest thickness. The progression of ring thickness can be either clockwise or counterclockwise. This type of ICRS is indicated for keratoconic patients with asymmetric corneal topographic features, like in the Duck and or Snowman phenotypes [35].

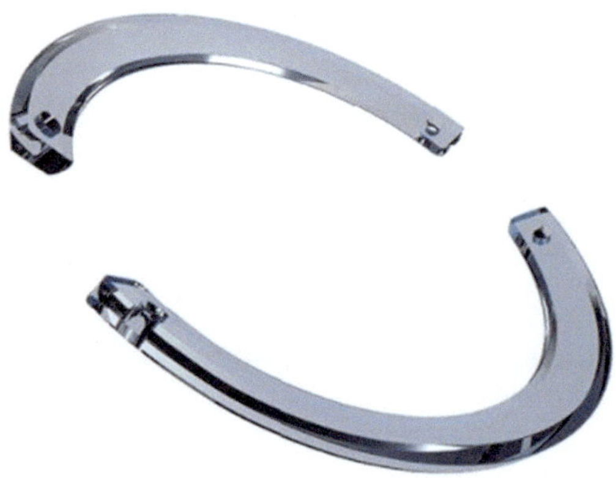

Fig. 17.1 Intacs intrastromal corneal ring segments

Bisantis (Optikon 2000 SpA and Soleko SpA, Rome, Italy) are intrastromal segmented perioptic implants of 80° arc length, with a vertical and horizontal diameter of 200 μm and 250 μm, respectively, and an oval cross-section. The degree of ring curvature is the only modifiable characteristic of these implants, which produces a range of optical zone sizes from 3.5 mm to 4.0 mm and, as a result, a range of applanation effects on the cornea [36]. Bisantis ICRS are no longer commercially available.

Myoring (Dioptex, Linz, Austria) is the only ICRS with a 360° arc length. Its anterior and posterior surfaces are convex and concave, respectively, and they are implanted into a corneal stromal pocket via a corneal incision tunnel after being folded [36]. Because of their full ring design, they produce higher biomechanical stability compared to the interrupted ring designs (<360°), and therefore have a greater capacity of corneal flattening. They also have the ability to significantly strengthen the cornea, eliminating the necessity of adding corneal cross-linking to the treatment [37]. However, they usually cannot eliminate high astigmatism and, thus, are indicated for keratoconic patients with high myopic refractive errors.

Selecting keratoconic patients who will benefit most from ICRS implantation is of great importance, with different types of ICRS usually

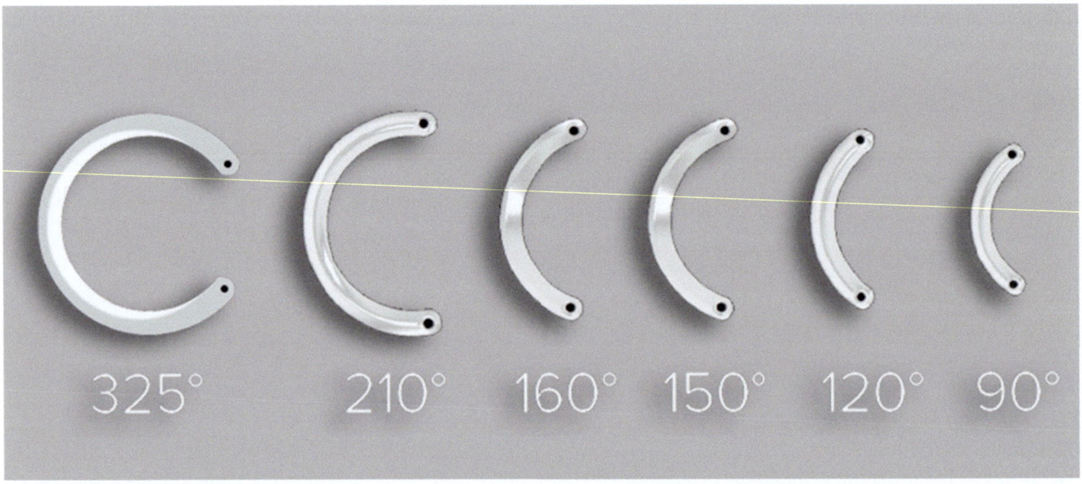

Fig. 17.2 Different options of Keraring intrastromal corneal ring segments

having different indications. This poses a great challenge, since several parameters should be taken into account in order to achieve the best possible refractive results for the patient. Mild and moderate stage keratoconus without central corneal scarring in patients with contact lens intolerance and/or not significant improvement in visual acuity with contact lenses or spectacles are considered the main indications for ICRS implantation [38]. Moreover, corneal thickness should be >400 μm at the location of the incision and corrected distance visual acuity >0.9 [39].

17.3 Nomograms for Intracorneal Ring Segments Implantation

ICRS implantation requires several parameters to be determined, like arc length, thickness, and location of incision and for this reason, the surgeon should utilize implementation nomograms. Nomograms are surgical and clinical guidelines which can help the clinician achieve the best possible refractive correction with ICRS. In addition to the several published nomograms in the literature [10, 40, 41], each manufacture provides their own nomograms [42], which are the ones that are mostly used in clinical practice.

In most nomograms, the parameters that need to be specified are the spherical equivalent, the location of the cone, and the keratometric axes. Moreover, depending on the nomograms chosen and the clinical and topographical parameters mentioned above, usually two symmetrical rings, two asymmetrical rings or one ring are implanted. For example, for Intacs ICRS, two symmetric implants are used when the location of the cone on the posterior float is in the central 3–5 mm corneal zone and the spherical power is greater than the cylindrical power in manifest refraction notated in positive cylinder, while two asymmetrical implants are used when these requirements are not met. There are also some studies that have reported similar or better clinical results with the implantation of a single rather than two ring segments [43–45]. Regarding the incision placement, most authors recommend the incision to be made either on the steepest axis [46, 47], with the aim to reduce astigmatism, or temporally [48, 49].

Despite the fact that most of the nomograms have been based in anecdotic clinical data and the experience of the surgeon and that a consensus on ICRS implantation guidelines does not exist, most surgeons have achieved good visual and refractive results after ICRS implantation [50]. Lastly, patients should undergo a complete ocular examination including slit lamp examination, fundus examination, corneal topography, pachymetry, uncorrected and best spectacle-corrected visual acuity before any nomogram implementation. Lastly, future research is needed for the development of more accurate mathematical models to predict the ICRS effects. Given that keratoconic eyes have different biomechanical characteristics compared to normal eyes, these models should take into consideration the ectatic corneal features so as to optimize their predictions and produce valid outcomes.

17.4 Surgical Techniques for Intracorneal Ring Segments Implantation

For the successful implantation of ICRS, we need to create corneal stromal tunnels, where the ICRS will be inserted. There are two ways to create these tunnels, either mechanically or with a femtosecond laser, both performed under topical anesthesia.

The mechanical technique was the first method reported in the literature for ICRS insertion. At first, a reference point should be created, which will be the center of the ICRS and will also be used as a guide for the corneal incisions. The pupil center is used as the reference point, usually identified with a 11-mm zone marker, and it is marked with a Sinskey hook. Then, a radial corneal incision of 1.2–1.8 mm is made with a calibrated diamond knife. The depth of the incision is made at a depth of 70% to 80% of the corneal thickness on the desired location, which is measured intraoperatively or preoperatively by ultrasonic corneal pachymetry. After this, pocket hooks are used to create corneal pockets on each side of the bottom of the incision and a suction ring is placed around the corneal limbus, initially operating at low vacuum pressure and later at higher pressures. Finally, two semicircular dissectors (Fig. 17.3) are gradually advanced into the corneal pockets, in a clockwise and counterclockwise manner, and two semicircular stromal tunnels with specific diameters are created [51].

Separation of corneal collagen layers for the creation of corneal stromal tunnels can also be done with a femtosecond laser-assisted technique via photodisruption, where initially a disposable suction ring is placed centered at the pupillary center in order to avoid decentration. Then, corneal flattening is achieved with the use of an applanation cone, facilitating fixation of the eye and precise focusing of the laser beam on corneal tissue. Similar to the manual procedure, the center of the pupil is marked as a reference point, corneal pachymetry is performed to assess corneal thickness at the incision point, and the corneal tunnels are created at a depth of 70–80% of the measured corneal thickness [51]. In both techniques, creation of the stromal tunnels is followed by the ICRS implantation.

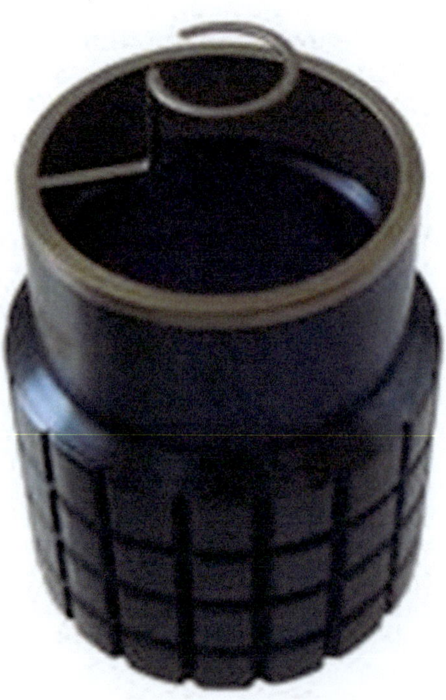

Fig. 17.3 Intrastromal tunnels dissector

17.5 Efficacy and Complications of Intracorneal Ring Segments Implantation

Since the advent of ICRS for keratoconus treatment, several studies have been conducted to assess the postoperative visual, keratometric, and refractive outcomes of this surgical technique. The majority of them have found ICRS to be an effective technique, with a recent systematic review and meta-analysis on the efficacy of ICRS in keratoconus reporting an overall improvement on all clinical postoperative parameters assessed [50]. In general, the parameters of interest which are usually evaluated postoperatively are uncorrected and corrected distance visual acuity (UDVA and CDVA), maximal and minimal keratometry (Kmax and Kmin), spherical equivalent, and cylinder.

According to the systematic review and meta-analysis of Benoist d'Azy et al. [50], the spherical equivalent after ICRS implantation has been shown to decrease, with a pooled effect size (ES) of −1.09 (95% confidence interval [95% CI]: −0.98 to −0.94) including 46 studies. Similarly, ICRS insertion permitted a reduction of cylinder (pooled ES: −0.99, 95% CI: −1.25 to −0.73, n = 54 studies), while the UDVA and CDVA showed improvement, with an increase of pooled ES of 1.25 (95% CI: 1.07 to 1.44, n = 58 studies) and 0.76 (95% CI: 0.64 to 0.87, n = 54 studies), respectively. Regarding the effect of ICRS surgery on topographic parameters, corneal flattening is exerted with an decrease of Kmax and Kmin [pooled ES of 0.85 (95% CI: 0.69 to 1.01, n = 46 studies) and 0.84 (95% CI: 0.69 to 0.98, n = 57 studies), respectively]. It is also important to take into account that ICRS surgery can be combined with other therapeutic procedures, like photorefractive keratectomy (PRK), corneal collagen cross-linking (CXL), and intraocular lenses (IOLs) insertion. These therapeutic combinations have been utilized by many surgeons in order to produce better clinical outcomes than performing ICRS insertion alone. The same systematic review and meta-analysis have reported on better visual, topographical, and refractive outcomes after combining surgical procedures, compared to ICRS implantation alone [50]. Combining ICRS with IOLs exerted the best outcomes, however these results need to be interpreted with caution mainly because of the relatively low number of studies that have been focused on these associations [50].

Moreover, systematically reviewed published evidence on the safety of ICRS implantation in keratoconic patients has indicated minimal complications [52]. Intraoperative complications include incomplete stromal tunnel creation and perforation of anterior corneal surface or anterior chamber, which occur more commonly with the mechanical dissection than the femtosecond laser-assisted technique [53, 54]. Moreover, the postoperative complications that account for almost all the ICRS removal are segment migration, ring extrusion, corneal thinning, corneal melting, and infectious keratitis. In conclusion, although ICRS is considered an effective and safe surgical procedure in the management of keratoconus, adequate patient selection and surgery planning should always be implemented in order to minimize adverse events.

References

1. Barraquer JI. Modification of refraction by means of intracorneal inclusions. Int Ophthalmol Clin. 1966;6(1):53–78.
2. Burris TE. Intrastromal corneal ring technology: results and indications. Curr Opin Ophthalmol. 1998;9(4):9–14.
3. Blavatskaia DE. The use of intralamellar homoplasty in order to reduce refraction of the eye. Uberstzt Aus Oftalmol Zh. 1966;7:530–7.
4. Fleming JF, Reynolds AE, Kilmer L, Burris TE, Abbott RL, Schanzlin DJ. The intrastromal corneal ring: two cases in rabbits. J Refract Surg. 1987;3(6):227–32.
5. Burris TE, Baker PC, Ayer CT, Loomas BE, Mathis ML, Silvestrini TA. Flattening of central corneal curvature with intrastromal corneal rings of increasing thickness: an eye-bank eye study. J Cataract Refract Surg. 1993;19(Suppl):182–7.
6. Twa MD, Karpecki PM, King BJ, Linn SH, Durrie DS, Schanzlin DJ. One-year results from the phase III investigation of the KeraVision Intacs. J Am Optom Assoc. 1999;70(8):515–24.
7. Colin J, Cochener B, Savary G, Malet F. Correcting keratoconus with intracorneal rings. J Cataract Refract Surg. 2000;26(8):1117–22.
8. Alió JL, Shabayek MH, Artola A. Intracorneal ring segments for keratoconus correction: long-term follow-up. J Cataract Refract Surg. 2006;32(6):978–85.
9. Alió JL, Shabayek MH, Belda JI, Correas P, Feijoo ED. Analysis of results related to good and bad outcomes of Intacs implantation for keratoconus correction. J Cataract Refract Surg. 2006;32(5):756–61.
10. Kymionis GD, Siganos CS, Tsiklis NS, Anastasakis A, Yoo SH, Pallikaris AI, Astyrakakis N, Pallikaris IG. Long-term follow-up of Intacs in keratoconus. Am J Ophthalmol. 2007;143(2):236–44.
11. Zare MA, Hashemi H, Salari MR. Intracorneal ring segment implantation for the management of keratoconus: safety and efficacy. J Cataract Refract Surg. 2007;33(11):1886–91.
12. Krumeich JH, Daniel J. Lebend-Epikeratophakie und Tiefe Lamelläre Keratoplastik zur Stadiengerechten chirurgischen Behandlung des Keratokonus (KK) I-III [live epikeratophakia and deep lamellar keratoplasty for I-III stage-specific surgical treatment of keratoconus]. Klin Monatsbl Augenheilkd. 1997;211(2):94–100.
13. Ertan A, Bahadir M. Management of superior pellucid marginal degeneration with a single intracorneal ring segment using femtosecond laser. J Refract Surg. 2007;23(2):205–8.
14. Kymionis GD, Tsiklis NS, Pallikaris AI, Kounis G, Diakonis VF, Astyrakakis N, Siganos CS. Long-term follow-up of Intacs for post-LASIK corneal ectasia. Ophthalmology. 2006;113(11):1909–17.
15. Djotyan GP, Kurtz RM, Fernández DC, Juhasz T. An analytically solvable model for biomechanical response of the cornea to refractive surgery. J Biomech Eng. 2001;123(5):440–5.
16. Fleming JF, Wan WL, Schanzlin DJ. The theory of corneal curvature change with the intrastromal corneal ring. CLAO J. 1989;15(2):146–50.
17. Patel S, Marshall J, Fitzke FW 3rd. Model for deriving the optical performance of the myopic eye corrected with an intracorneal ring. J Refract Surg. 1995;11(4):248–52.
18. Kling S, Marcos S. Finite-element modeling of intrastromal ring segment implantation into a hyperelastic cornea. Invest Ophthalmol Vis Sci. 2013;54(1):881–9.
19. Fares U, Otri AM, Al-Aqaba MA, Dua HS. Correlation of central and peripheral corneal thickness in healthy corneas. Cont Lens Anterior Eye. 2012;35(1):39–45.
20. Burris TE, Holmes-Higgin DK, Silvestrini TA, Scholl JA, Proudfoot RA, Baker PC. Corneal asphericity in eye bank eyes implanted with the intrastromal corneal ring. J Refract Surg. 1997;13(6):556–67.

21. Torquetti L, Cunha P, Luz A, Kwitko S, Carrion M, Rocha G, Signorelli A, Coscarelli S, Ferrara G, Bicalho F, Neves R, Ferrara P. Clinical outcomes after implantation of 320°-arc length intrastromal corneal ring segments in keratoconus. Cornea. 2018;37(10):1299–305.
22. Zare MA, Mehrjardi HZ, Afarideh M, Bahrmandy H, Mohammadi SF. Visual, Keratometric and corneal biomechanical changes after Intacs SK implantation for moderate to severe keratoconus. J Ophthalmic Vis Res. 2016;11(1):17–25.
23. Roberts CJ. Biomechanics in Keratoconus. In: Barbara A, editor. Textbook on Keratoconus: new insights. Jaypee Brothers Medical Publishers (P) Ltd.; 2012. p. 29–32.
24. Burris TE, Ayer CT, Evensen DA, Davenport JM. Effects of intrastromal corneal ring size and thickness on corneal flattening in human eyes. Refract Corneal Surg. 1991;7(1):46–50.
25. Cristina Kenney M, Brown DJ. The cascade hypothesis of keratoconus. Cont Lens Anterior Eye. 2003;26(3):139–46.
26. Ku JY, Niederer RL, Patel DV, Sherwin T, McGhee CN. Laser scanning in vivo confocal analysis of keratocyte density in keratoconus. Ophthalmology. 2008;115(5):845–50.
27. Akhtar S, Bron AJ, Salvi SM, Hawksworth NR, Tuft SJ, Meek KM. Ultrastructural analysis of collagen fibrils and proteoglycans in keratoconus. Acta Ophthalmol. 2008;86(7):764–72.
28. Daxer A, Fratzl P. Collagen fibril orientation in the human corneal stroma and its implication in keratoconus. Invest Ophthalmol Vis Sci. 1997;38(1):121–9.
29. Samimi S, Leger F, Touboul D, Colin J. Histopathological findings after intracorneal ring segment implantation in keratoconic human corneas. J Cataract Refract Surg. 2007;33(2):247–53.
30. Ruckhofer J, Böhnke M, Alzner E, Grabner G. Confocal microscopy after implantation of intrastromal corneal ring segments. Ophthalmology. 2000;107(12):2144–51.
31. Twa MD, Ruckhofer J, Kash RL, Costello M, Schanzlin DJ. Histologic evaluation of corneal stroma in rabbits after intrastromal corneal ring implantation. Cornea. 2003;22(2):146–52.
32. Kim WJ, Rabinowitz YS, Meisler DM, Wilson SE. Keratocyte apoptosis associated with keratoconus. Exp Eye Res. 1999;69(5):475–81.
33. Alió JL, Artola A, Ruiz-Moreno JM, Hassanein A, Galal A, Awadalla MA. Changes in keratoconic corneas after intracorneal ring segment explantation and reimplantation. Ophthalmology. 2004;111(4):747–51.
34. Siganos D, Ferrara P, Chatzinikolas K, Bessis N, Papastergiou G. Ferrara intrastromal corneal rings for the correction of keratoconus. J Cataract Refract Surg. 2002;28(11):1947–51.
35. Prisant O, Pottier E, Guedj T, Hoang XT. Clinical outcomes of an asymmetric model of intrastromal corneal ring segments for the correction of keratoconus. Cornea. 2020;39(2):155–60.
36. Ertan A, Colin J. Intracorneal rings for keratoconus and keratectasia. J Cataract Refract Surg. 2007;33(7):1303–14.
37. Daxer A. Biomechanics of corneal ring implants. Cornea. 2015;34(11):1493–8.
38. Kymionis GD. Actual indications for intracorneal ring segment implantation in keratoconus. In: Güell JL, editor. Cornea, ESASO Course Series, vol. 6. Basel: Karger; 2015. p. 66–73.
39. Vega-Estrada A, Alio JL. The use of intracorneal ring segments in keratoconus. Eye Vis (Lond). 2016;3:8.
40. Ertan A, Kamburoğlu G. Intacs implantation using a femtosecond laser for management of keratoconus: comparison of 306 cases in different stages. J Cataract Refract Surg. 2008;34(9):1521–6.
41. Shetty R, D'Souza S, Ramachandran S, Kurian M, Nuijts RM. Decision making nomogram for intrastromal corneal ring segments in keratoconus. Indian J Ophthalmol. 2014;62(1):23–8.
42. Rocha G, Silva LNP, Chaves LFOB, Bertino P, Torquetti L, de Sousa LB. Intracorneal ring segments implantation outcomes using two different Manufacturers' nomograms for keratoconus surgery. J Refract Surg. 2019;35(10):673–83.
43. Sharma M, Boxer Wachler BS. Comparison of single-segment and double-segment Intacs for keratoconus and post-LASIK ectasia. Am J Ophthalmol. 2006;141(5):891–5.
44. Alió JL, Artola A, Hassanein A, Haroun H, Galal A. One or 2 Intacs segments for the correction of keratoconus. J Cataract Refract Surg. 2005;31(5):943–53.
45. Rabinowitz YS. INTACS for keratoconus. Int Ophthalmol Clin. 2006;46(3):91–103.
46. Ibrahim TA. After 5-years follow-up: do Intacs help in keratoconus. J Cataract Refract Surg. 2006;1:45–8.
47. Shetty R, Kurian M, Anand D, Mhaske P, Narayana KM, Shetty BK. Intacs in advanced keratoconus. Cornea. 2008;27(9):1022–9.
48. Hellstedt T, Mäkelä J, Uusitalo R, Emre S, Uusitalo R. Treating keratoconus with intacs corneal ring segments. J Refract Surg. 2005;21(3):236–46.
49. Colin J, Cochener B, Savary G, Malet F, Holmes-Higgin D. INTACS inserts for treating keratoconus: one-year results. Ophthalmology. 2001;108(8):1409–14.
50. Benoist d'Azy C, Pereira B, Chiambaretta F, Dutheil F. Efficacy of different procedures of intra-corneal ring segment implantation in keratoconus: a systematic review and meta-analysis. Transl Vis Sci Technol. 2019;8(3):38.
51. Piñero DP, Alio JL. Intracorneal ring segments in ectatic corneal disease - a review. Clin Exp Ophthalmol. 2010;38(2):154–67.
52. Bautista-Llamas MJ, Sánchez-González MC, López-Izquierdo I, López-Muñoz A, Gargallo-Martínez B, De-Hita-Cantalejo C, Sánchez-González JM. Complications and Explantation reasons in

Intracorneal ring segments (ICRS) implantation: a systematic review. J Refract Surg. 2019;35(11):740–7.
53. Rabinowitz YS, Li X, Ignacio TS, Maguen E. INTACS inserts using the femtosecond laser compared to the mechanical spreader in the treatment of keratoconus. J Refract Surg. 2006;22(8):764–71.
54. Kubaloglu A, Sari ES, Cinar Y, Cingu K, Koytak A, Coşkun E, Ozertürk Y. Comparison of mechanical and femtosecond laser tunnel creation for intrastromal corneal ring segment implantation in keratoconus: prospective randomized clinical trial. J Cataract Refract Surg. 2010;36(9):1556–61.

18 Intraocular Lens (IOL) Implantation in Kertaoconus

Seyed Javad Hashemian

18.1 Introduction

Corneal ectasia included primary corneal ectasia (keratoconous, pellucid marginal corneal degeneration (PMD), and keratoglobus) and secondary corneal ectasia (Postlaser vision correction corneal ectasia, postcorneal trauma). Keratoconous is a bilateral progressive corneal disease with an incidence rate of 50–230 per 100,000 of the general population [1, 2]. Mostly, it could result in unavoidable conical protrusion, irregular astigmatism, and decreased visual acuity and quality [3]. Pellucid marginal corneal degeneration (PMD) is less common than keratoconus. It usually affects the inferior peripheral, rather than para-central, cornea in about 85% of cases and the superior peripheral cornea in 15%. It occurs in a crescentic fashion typically between the 5- and 7-o'clock positions [4, 5]. Keratectasia after refractive surgery is a rare but often visually devastating complication. It was first described after Laser in situ keratomileusis (LASIK) by Seiler in 1998 [6]. Its reported incidence ranges from 0.04 to 0.6% of post-LASIK cases [7, 8].

In early stages, visual symptoms of keratoconous could be managed with spectacles and contact lenses. However, as keratoconous progresses to severe stages, surgical intervention will be warranted to gain appropriate vision [9]. Most patients seek treatment for keratoconous for cessation of ectasia and improvement of refractive errors and aberrations. However, correction of corneal irregularity and reduction of higher-order and lower-order aberrations seem to be a very challenging aim to achieve in the cornea with irregular astigmatism [10].

Due to risk of induced keratectasia, keratoconous was considered as a contraindication for excimer laser refractive surgeries in previous decades. However, advancements in laser technology convince physicians to utilize these methods to lessen the refractive errors and aberrations in keratoconous patients [11]. On the other hand, it has been proven that accelerated corneal cross-linking (CXL) procedure is effective to stabilize the progression of keratoconous with a significant reduction in topographic keratometry values [12].

The multiple alternative options for patients with contact lens intolerance but with good contact lens-corrected vision have evolved and include stabilizing the cornea with corneal collagen cross-linking (CXL) [13], regularizing the cornea with intracorneal ring segment (ICRS) implantation [14–16] and performing topography-guided excimer laser ablation [17], and treating myopic astigmatism with toric phakic intraocular lens (pIOL) [18, 19]. Also for refractive management of keratoconus, PMD and postlaser vision correction corneal ectasia multiple procedures suggested to improve visual and refractive status

S. J. Hashemian (✉)
Eye Research Center and Department, The Five Senses Health Institute, School of Medicine, Iran University of Medical Sciences, Tehran, Iran

S. Das (ed.), *Keratoconus*, https://doi.org/10.1007/978-981-19-4262-4_18

and stabilizing corneal structure together comprise of CXL plus intracorneal ring segments implantation (ICRS); CXL plus phakic intraocular lens implantation (pIOL); CXL plus photorefractive keratectomy (PRK); and CXL plus ICRS plus pIOLs implantation [17, 18, 20, 21].

18.2 Phakic Intraocular Lens Implantation (pIOLs)

Phakic IOLs are important tools in refractive surgery; they can be used to accurately and stably correct high ametropias because they are not associated with wound healing, and they preserve the natural accommodation of the eye. pIOLs have the advantage of treating a much larger range of myopic and hyperopic refractive errors than can be safely and effectively treated with corneal refractive surgery. It is removable; therefore, the refractive effect should theoretically be reversible. The pIOL has the advantage of preserving natural accommodation and may have a lower risk of postoperative retinal detachment because of the preservation of the crystalline lens and minimal vitreous destabilization. Its nodal points are nearer the pupil and enhance the quality of the retinal image. The pIOLs result is highly predictable, easily adjustable with complementary fine tuning corneal surgeries, and immediately will be stable. According to their location inside the eye, phakic IOLs can be divided into three groups:

(a) Anterior chamber angle-supported phakic IOLs (e.g., AcrySof Cachet; Alcon).
(b) Anterior chamber iris-supported phakic IOLs (e.g., Artisan and Artiflex [both by Ophtec BV]; also marketed as the Verisyse and Veriflex by Abbott Medical Optics Inc.)
(c) Posterior chamber phakic IOLs (e.g., Visian ICL; STAAR Surgical).

18.2.1 Anterior Chamber pIOLs

18.2.1.1 Acrysof Cachet

The hydrophobic acrylic AcrySof Cachet (Alcon Inc., USA) is a single-piece, foldable, soft acrylic lens and is intended for implantation in the anterior chamber angle (Fig. 18.1). It has a 6.00 mm optic and four haptics to ensure angle fixation. It is available only for myopia correction (−6.00 to −16.50D) and comes in four sizes (12.5 mm, 13.0 mm, 13.5 mm, and 14.0 mm) [22].

18.2.1.2 Artisan/Verisyse

The Artisan lens (Fig. 18.2) is made of PMMA. The optic is 5.00 or 6 mm, convex–concave, and the two haptics are shaped like claws to grasp the mid-peripheral iris tissue. The 5.00-mm Artisan is available for correction of myopia (−2.00 to −23.00D), hyperopia (2.00 to 12.00D), and astigmatism (both myopic and hyperopic up to 7.50D). The 6.00 mm lens is available only for myopia correction (−2.00 to −14.50D). The

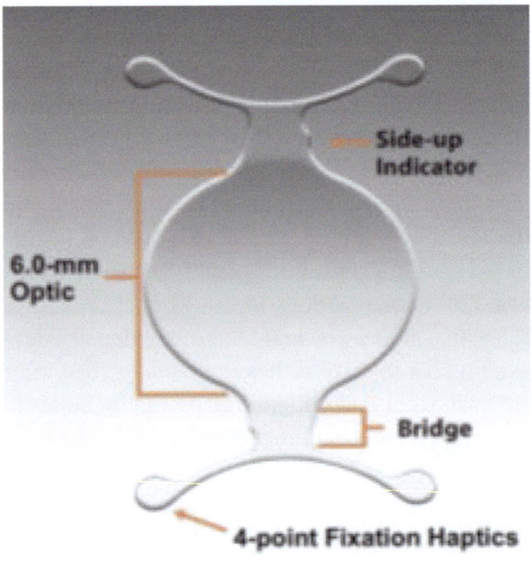

Fig. 18.1 AcrySof phakic angle-supported IOL

Fig. 18.2 Artisan/Verisyse pIOL (Abbott Medical Optics, Santa Ana, California, USA)

overall length of the Artisan is 8.5 mm; because the lens is iris-fixated, there is no need for different sizes [23]. The optic vaults approximately 0.87 mm anterior to the iris, providing good clearance from both the anterior lens capsule and the corneal endothelium.

18.2.1.3 Artiflex/Veriflex

The Artiflex is a foldable lens (Fig. 18.3) with a design similar to the Artisan. It has a 6.00 mm silicone optic and two PMMA haptics. The overall length is 8.5 mm. The Artiflex is available for the correction of myopia (−2.00 to −14.50D) and astigmatism (myopic up −5.00D, provided that the sphere plus cylinder does not exceed −14.50D) [23].

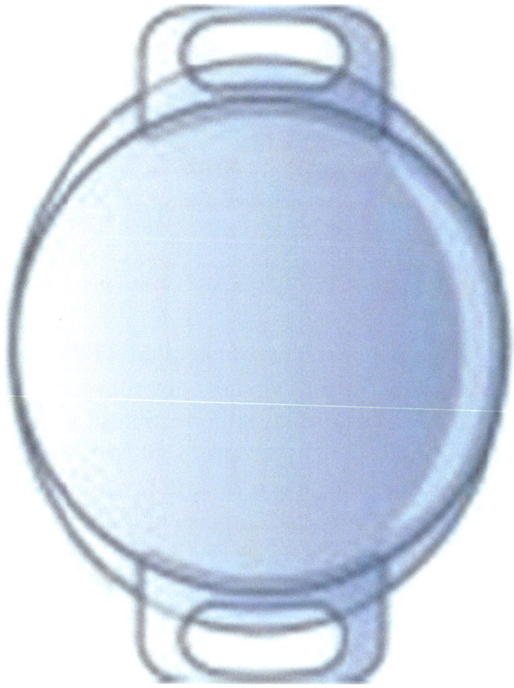

Fig. 18.3 Artiflex/Veriflex pIOL (Abbott Medical Optics, Santa Ana, California, USA)

18.2.2 Posterior Chamber pIOLs

Currently, two posterior chamber pIOLs are available, the Implantable Collamer Lens (ICL) (Staar Surgical Co.) and the Phakic Refractive Lens (PRL) (Carl Zeiss Meditec).

18.2.2.1 Visian ICL

The Visian ICL is designed to fit in the ciliary sulcus. It features a plate-haptic with central convex/concave optical zone design made of the proprietary material Collamer, a proprietary hydroxyethyl methacrylate/porcine-collagen-based biocompatible polymer material and an ultraviolet-absorbing chromophore. It has a refractive index of 1.442 at room temperature in balanced salt solution, with an optic diameter of 4.65 to 5.50 mm (myopia, according to power) or 5.50 mm (hyperopia). The basic design change of the ICL V4 addresses the vaulting. This model has an additional 0.13 to 0.21 mm anterior vault

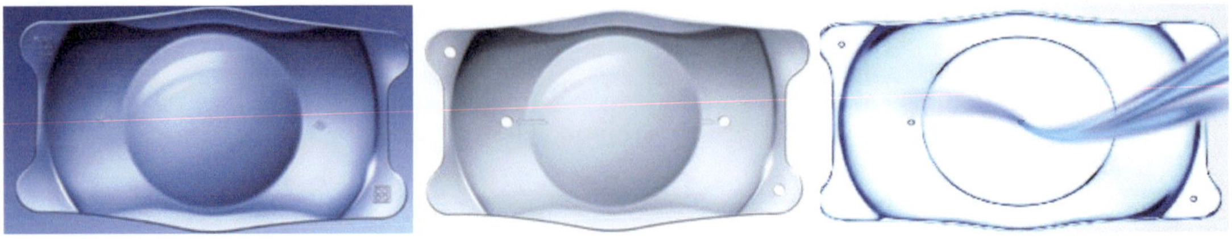

Fig. 18.4 Visian ICL; V4, V4b, V4c. Visian ICL V4c with Centra Flow™

due to the steeper radius of curvature of the base curve, which depends on the dioptric power. The Visian ICL is available for correction of myopia (−3.0 to −20.00D), hyperopia (+3.00 to +10.0D), and, with the brand name Toric ICL, astigmatism (1.00 to 4.00D). The ICL comes in four sizes for myopia and astigmatism (12.1, 12.6, 13.2, and 13.7 mm) and four for hyperopia (11.6, 12.1, 12.6, and 13.2 mm). The most recent version, the V4c, has a hole in the middle of the optic for improved aqueous humor flow (Fig. 18.4) [24].

The EVO ICL Model V5 is the latest release of the Implantable Collamer Lens. This pIOL has an optic diameter up to 6.10 mm depending on the power of the IOL, and it is larger than the previous model (V4c). Patients with larger pupils may benefit from these new pIOLs with larger optic diameters and good optical quality.

The V4c and V5 models have a central hole with a diameter of 0.36 mm to increase aqueous humor perfusion and reduce the risk for secondary cataract formation [25, 26].

- The V4c is the same design as the V4b with the addition of a central port. This port is the same size as the perioptic ports (360 microns).
- V4c model available for the myopic spheric and myopic toric lens versions.

18.2.3 Phakic Intraocular Lens Implantation (pIOLs) in Keratoconus

pIOLs can be used to correct myopia and compound myopic astigmatism in eyes with keratoconus (KCN), which has been stable at least for 2 years. It may be especially indicated for the management of high ametropia [27], and Toric pIOL implantation is beneficial according to measures of safety, efficacy, predictability and stability for KCN. The refractive stability suggests viability of the procedure as a surgical option [19, 28, 29].

18.3 Patient Selection

The most critical factor for the insertion of toric or nontoric phakic IOLs in keratoconus patients is the presence of stable, nonprogressive, and regular ectasia. The corneal shape in keratoconus, plays a role in refraction. The more irregular the cornea, the poorer the best spectacle-corrected distance visual acuity (BSCVA) and the more central the cone, the poorer the BSCVA as well. We can count on good results with toric or nontoric phakic IOLs in keratoconic eyes if the patient experiences good vision with glasses. Therefore, typically patients who do well with glasses preoperatively are the ones who will do well with the implantable lens postoperatively. Refractive correction with phakic IOLs should be limited to cases with good spectacles-corrected refraction, stable ectasia, and also to those who have repeatable and verifiable subjective refraction. A repeatable subjective refraction is the best guide. Also, the targeted postoperative refraction slightly myopic is planned, as a hyperopic end result is usually poorly tolerated. Patients should always be informed that reduced spectacle dependence is the target, not spectacle independence. The best candidates are patients with BSCVA of 20/40 or better, or UDVA to BSCVA with at least three lines of improvement. Generally, the visual rehabilitation for keratoconic corneas requires addressing three concerns: halting the ectatic process, improving corneal shape, and minimizing the residual refractive error. The treatment would depend on each of these concerns and its influence on the disease and quality of vision of the patient.

Progression of keratoconus leading to refraction change is a concern after implantation. Ideally, pIOL implantation should not be performed until refraction and keratometry are stabilized. To have a good result for pIOL implantation in patient with keratoconus, we should determine that, it is progressing or not, the cornea shape is irregular with high level of HOAs and poor CDVA or not, and finally the degree of associated ametropia. Generally recommended inclusion criteria for pIOL implantation: [30, 31]

- Age >21 years.
- Stable refraction at least 1 year.
- Ametropia not correctable with excimer laser surgery.
- Unsatisfactory vision with/intolerance of contact lenses or spectacles.
- Iridocorneal angle >30°.
- Anterior chamber depth (ACD) from the corneal endothelium to the anterior plane of the crystalline lens had to be at least 2.8 mm with a maximal clear lens rise of 600 μm.
- ECC >2500 cells/mm [2]: (>2800 cells/mm^2 if >21 years old, >2000 if >40 years old).
- No anomaly of iris or pupil function.
- Mesopic pupil size <5.0–6.0 mm.
- White to white value (W to W) of more than 11.0 mm.

Special recommended inclusion criteria for pIOL implantation in keratoconus:

- KCN with low irregularity and aberrations which stable at least for 2 years.
- Forme Fruste KCN.
- Clear central cornea.
- BSCVA >20/50.
- Mean keratometric values <52.00D.
- Keratoconus stage 1 to 2 (Amsler–Krumeich).
- Stable nonprogressive PMD.
- Postkeratoplasty with high ametropia or astigmatism (at least 1 year after suture removal).

Generally recommended exclusion criteria for pIOL implantation:

- Background of active disease in the anterior segment.
- Recurrent or chronic uveitis.
- Any form of clinically significant cataract.
- Previous corneal or intraocular surgery (to be evaluated).
- IOP >21 mm Hg or glaucoma.
- Pre-existing macular degeneration or macular pathology.
- Abnormal retinal condition.
- Systemic diseases (e.g., autoimmune disorder, connective tissue disease, atopy, diabetes mellitus).
- Pregnancy.

18.3.1 Preoperative Evaluations and Considerations

All patients should have a baseline ophthalmic examination which included the measurement of best spectacle corrected visual acuity (BSCVA) at a vertex distance of 12 mm, uncorrected visual acuity (UCVA), cycloplegic and manifest subjective refractions, slit-lamp examination, fundoscopy with dilated pupil and Goldmann tonometry.

Additional ancillary tests are necessary when using pIOLs in KCN such as specular microscopy or confocal microscopy to evaluate endothelial cell count (ECC) and morphology looking for polymegethism and pleomorphism, anterior chamber depth (ACD) measurement can be done by ultrasound, anterior segment optical coherence tomography (AS-OCT), optical biometry, slit-beam topography, or Scheimpflug imaging [32–34], White-to-White (WTW) diameter is mandatory for selection of the pIOL diameter. Corneal White-to-White (WTW) diameter can be measured by caliper at a slit-lamp or by scanning-slit topography system (Orbscan IIZ; Bausch and Lomb, Rochester, New York, USA). Corneal and ocular aberrometry and mesopic pupil size measurement should be done to determine the amount of corneal irregularity and higher-order aberrations (HOAs) and high-frequency ultrasound biomicroscopy (UBM) to directly measure the sulcus-to-sulcus distance, as a preferred method. In addition, surgeons should record axial length in these patients before surgery to prevent an IOL power error at cataract surgery time due to imprecise keratometry.

18.4 pIOL Sizing and Power Calculations

Historically, concerns related to pIOL safety have included sizing methodology because of the relationship of excessive or insufficient vault to adverse events such as lens exchange or explanation, pupillary block, endothelial cell loss, pigment dispersion, elevated intraocular pressure (IOP), and cataract. Sizing represents the methodology by which the appropriate overall lens diameter is selected for implantation to achieve a safe level of vault, which is the axial distance between the pIOL and the crystalline lens. Currently, there are three methods for pIOL sizing, especially for posterior chamber pIOLs:

(a) The most used method of sizing, which is based on the horizontal corneal white-to-white (WTW) distance and the anterior chamber depth (ACD), as recommended by manufacturers of lenses.
(b) Sulcus-to-sulcus-based sizing method includes the use of ultrasound biomicroscopy to measure the sulcus-to-sulcus (STS) distance.
(c) Anterior segment optical coherence tomography (AS-OCT)-based sizing formula; Anterior chamber width (ACW); and Crystalline lens rise (CLR).

18.4.1 WTW Distance and the Anterior Chamber Depth (ACD)-Based Sizing Formula

WTW can be measured by callipers or a variety of imaging devices such as Orbscan (Bausch & Lomb, Rochester, NY, USA), IOL Master (Carl Zeiss Meditec, Jena, Germany), Pentacam (Oculus, Irvine, CA, USA), and Lenstar (Haag Streit, Koeniz, Switzerland) [35, 36]. Although automated measurement of WTW is convenient and repeatable, it is not necessarily more accurate than measurement with manual callipers. Validation with manual callipers can help surgeons avoid detection errors due to anomalies in the limbal area such as arcus senilis, pigmentation, pinguecula, and peripheral corneal vascularization. This methodology leads to approximately 20% of cases outside the accepted vault range (<250 μm and > 1000 μm) [37, 38].

Various lens-sizing formulas, based on STS measurement determined by high-frequency ultrasound biomicroscopy (UBM) with a wide scanning field, have been developed [39–41]. However, these UBM-based formulas have not been widely adopted by surgeons, because UBM measurement requires probe-sensor contact with the eye, is time-consuming, and requires examiner experience. Ghoreishi and Mohammadinia [42] prospectively compared vault based on randomization to sizing based on either WTW ("WTW value was entered into the ICL calculation formula which was proposed by the manufacturer") or STS ("ICL size was ordered based on horizontal sulcus-to-sulcus measurement") and concluded, STS measurement, by itself, did not improve the ICL sizing results. Reinstein [43] et al. found a larger lens may have been used in 6% of eyes based on the WTW diameter formula when comparing the postoperative vault with sizing based on STS distance to the theoretical vault that would have been achieved with WTW-based sizing. However, Packer [44] revealed there was no meaningful significant difference between the achieved vault using sizing methodologies based on WTW and STS distance.

AS-OCT (CASIA2; Tomey Corp, Nagoya, Japan) can acquire anterior segment tomographic images with a width of 16 mm and a depth of 11 mm, which facilitates corneal shape analysis, anterior chamber angle analysis, and observation of the intraocular lens within about 0.3 seconds. Its light source is a 1310-nm super-luminescent diode. The instrument performs 50,000 axial scans per second. Its axial and transverse resolutions are approximately 10 μm and 30 μm, respectively.

The parameters measured using AS-OCT were defined as follows. The angle-to-angle (ATA) diameter was defined as the distance between the angle recesses on the nasal and temporal sides. Anterior chamber width (ACW) was defined as the distance between the scleral spurs on the nasal and temporal sides [45], ACW has been described by Goldsmith [46] et al. as the distance from angle recess to angle recess, which is equal to the ATA diameter. Lens vault (LV) was defined as the perpendicular distance between the anterior crystalline lens surface and a horizontal line joining the two scleral spurs (Fig. 18.5) [47].

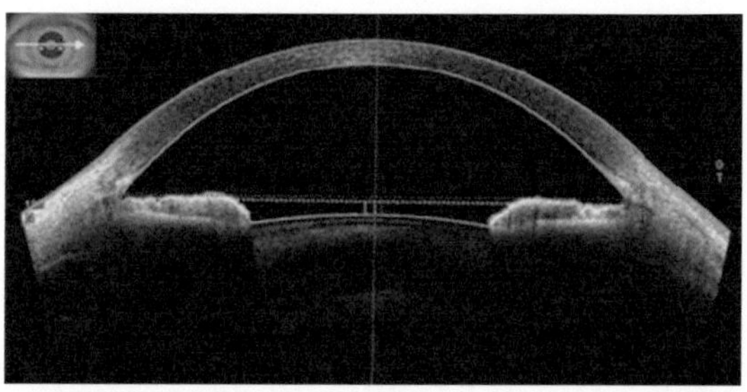

Fig. 18.5 Measurement of anterior segment parameters using the CASIA2; the software automatically finds the anterior and posterior corneal surfaces, the anterior iris surface, and the anterior crystalline lens surface and highlights each with green lines. ACW and ATA diameters are depicted with a dotted magenta line and a dotted yellow line, respectively. The software automatically specifies the position of the scleral spur and the angle recess and calculates the ACW distance and the ATA distance. Lens vault and crystalline lens rise are depicted with a solid magenta line and a solid yellow line, respectively (ACW = anterior chamber width; ATA = angle-to-angle)

Crystalline lens rise (CLR) was defined as the anteroposterior distance between the anterior crystalline lens surface and the angle recess to angle recess line [48]. The horizontal anterior chamber angle distance (ATA), measured using anterior segment optical coherence tomography (AS-OCT), is an alternative technique for assessing the transverse size of the eye and is proven to be well correlated to the STS [49–51].

Also, its assessment is more convenient for the patient and less operator-dependent compared to UBM. Recently, the AS-OCT has been used to assess the transverse size of the eye using the ATA, scleral-spur to scleral-spur distance, and applied to estimate the optimal ICL size [52, 53]. It has been demonstrated that patients presenting with a higher CLR (protruded crystalline anterior surfaces) tend to have lower vault [40, 53, 54]. Also, from the geometric design of the lens, the intrinsic sagittal depth of the ICL is regulated by its dioptric power and overall size, with more myopic ICL and larger diameter ICL presenting deeper sagittal depths [37].

Among the various preoperative anatomical and lens parameters measured, the multiple regression analysis identified the ATA, CLR, ICL size, ICL power, and age as relevant predictors of the vault, explaining 34% of the vault variance. This compares with the 37% found by Lee et al., 36% reported by Zheng et al., and more recently 41% [37, 52, 55].

18.4.2 NK-Formula Version 2 (NK-Formula V2)

NK formula was recently proposed that determines the optimal ICL size on the basis of anterior segment optical coherence tomography (AS-OCT) measurements [53].

Optimal ICL size (mm; in a balanced salt solution) = 4.575 + 0.688 × (ACW) (mm)+ 0.388 × (CLR) (mm).

NK-formula: Optimal ICL size (mm, in balanced salt solution) = 4.20 + 0.719 × (ACW) (mm) + 0.655 × (CLR) (mm).

In general, measurements of WTW, ATA, PTP, and STS do not correlate highly [41, 50, 56, 57],

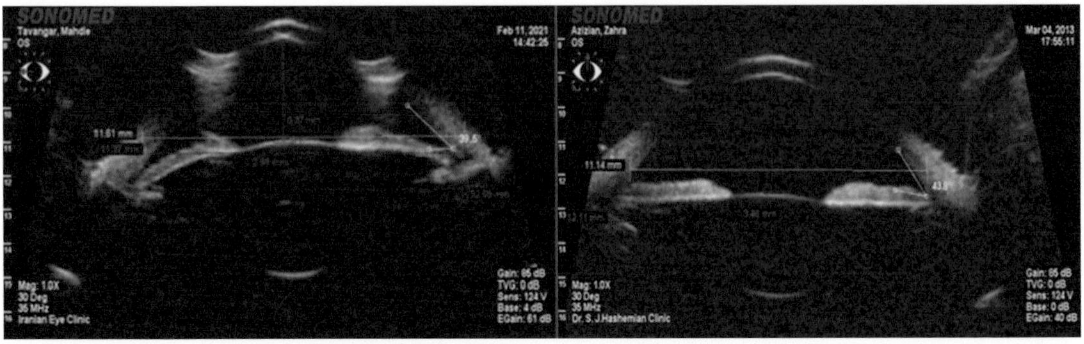

Fig. 18.6 Ultrasound biomicroscopy image showing the measurement of the sulcus-to-sulcus (STS) distance and the crystalline lens rise (CLR), angle-to-angle distance (ATA), and ciliary body position. The CLR was defined as the distance from the anterior pole of the lens to the STS plane. The patient had Intacs SK ring segment implantation (left picture)

although some authors have found varying degrees of correlation (Fig. 18.6) [58]. The degree of variation in vault is independent of sizing methodology and is related to the interaction of the lens implant with the anatomy and physiology of the posterior chamber. Neither clinically meaningful nor statistically significant difference in achieved vault differentiates, WTW- and STS-based sizing methodologies. The NK-formula shows higher accuracy for predicting vault than the STAAR nomogram.

In this issue especially for posterior chamber pIOLs implantation, I prefer to have an anterior segment OCT(ASOCT) analysis and measurement of sulcus-to-sulcus diameter and iris-ciliary angle by UBM. For power calculation, we follow the manufacturer software based on manifest subjective refraction and consider spherical correction according to push and plus refraction method.

The power calculation of the anterior chamber pIOLs (Artisan/Artiflex Toric pIOL) was performed by Ophtec BV (Groningen, The Netherlands) using the Van der Heijde formula [59, 60].

This formula uses the corneal curvature, adjusted ACD (ACD - 0.9), and the patient's subjective refraction to calculate the spherical and cylindrical power of the pIOL. Calculations were performed for 2-cylinder axes perpendicular to each other.

18.4.3 Safe Ranges of Vault

Authors have reported a range of values for the limits of safe vault, based on the likelihood that cataract or pupillary block may occur beyond that range. Data supported the conclusion that low vault, along with higher levels of myopia, constituted risk factors for anterior subcapsular cataract (ASC). Gonvers [61] et al. concluded that 150 μm should be regarded as a lower limit of safe vault. Zeng [62] et al. suggested a safe range of vault from 100 to 1000 μm. Dougherty [49] et al. suggested a safe range of vault from 90 to 1000 μm. Insufficient or excessive vault should be considered a risk factor, not a complication, and that only a percentage of eyes with vault beyond any predefined range experiences vault-related adverse events.

18.5 The Key Points for Successful pIOL Surgery in Keratoconus

- Careful selection of the patient and eye.
- Stable keratoconus with low irregularity.
- Careful preoperative examinations.
- Choosing the right IOL.
- Performing a good surgical operation.

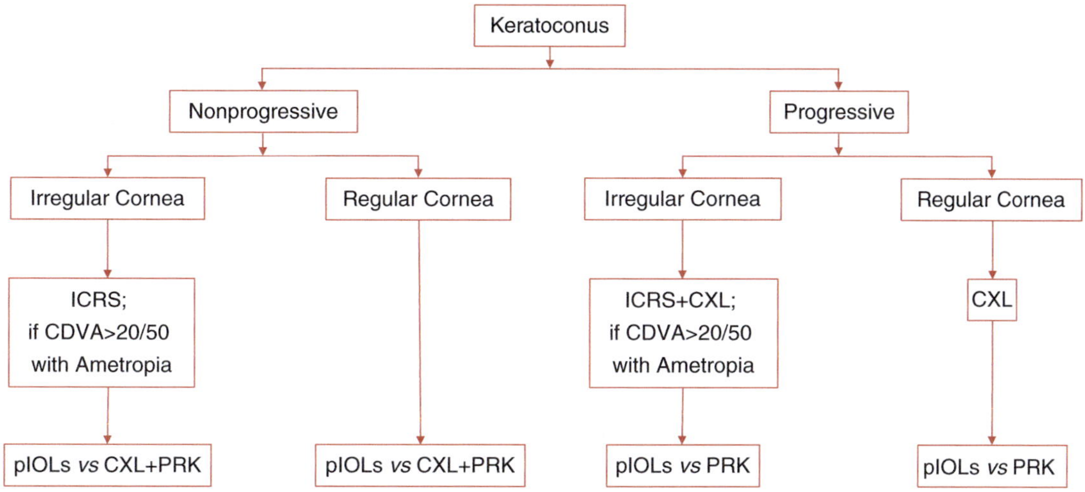

Fig. 18.7 Decision tree treatment considering the stability or progression, the corrected distance visual acuity (CDVA), and the refractive error. PRK = photorefractive keratectomy; pIOL = phakic intraocular lens; ICRS = intrastromal corneal ring segments; CXL = corneal collagen cross-linking

According to stability and regularity of cornea in patients with keratoconus, we have different treatment plans for pIOLs implantation (Fig. 18.7):

- Stable keratoconus with low irregularity.
- Unstable keratoconus with low irregularity.
- Stable keratoconus with high irregularity.
- Unstable keratoconus with high irregularity.

18.5.1 Stable Keratoconus (KC) with Low Irregularity

The best candidates are patients with stable and regular KC. Usually, these patients have BSCVA>20/50, relatively low HOAs, good MTF, and satisfied vision with glasses [19, 28, 29, 63].

Example 1

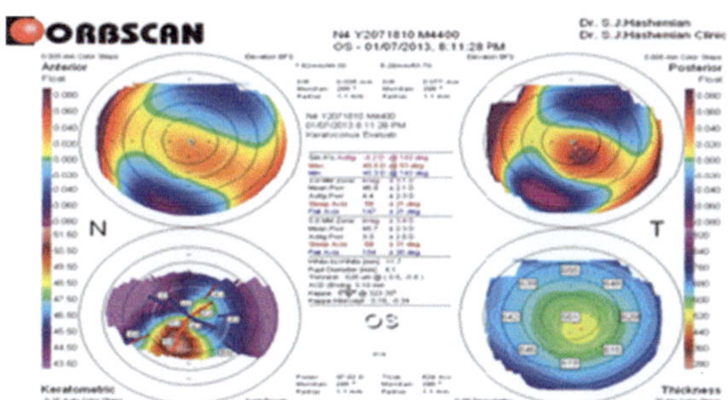

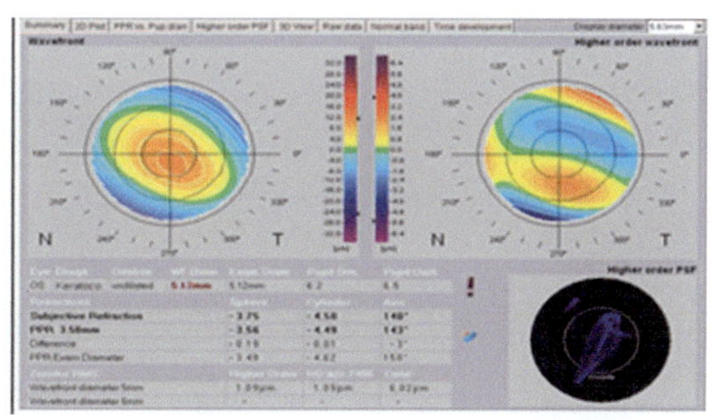

18.5.2 Unstable Keratoconus with Low Irregularity

The treatment goals of keratoconus management involve improved visual acuity and a reduction in or halting of disease progression. For contact lens – intolerant patients, the ideal sequence and staging of combined treatments, which may include CXL, toric pIOL implantation, remains to be fully elucidated. Corneal CXL is primarily a treatment to increase the biomechanical stability of the cornea. It has been shown to be effective in halting the progression of keratoconus over a period of years, and it could continue to induce longer-term corneal flattening with a resulting reduction in myopia [12, 13]. The pIOL selection should made a minimum of 6 months to 1 year after CXL treatment [64–66].

18.5.3 Stable Keratoconus with High Irregularity

For the irregular astigmatism component of reduced vision, corneal regularization can be achieved using ICRS implantation [14–16]. Fewer studies have reported on Visian TICL in the correction of myopia and irregular astigmatism associated with keratoconus and the safety and efficacy of TICL implantation after ICRS implantation [67–69]. The ICRS implantation improves corneal contour, making the cornea less irregular, flattening the cone, and making it more symmetric.

Example 2

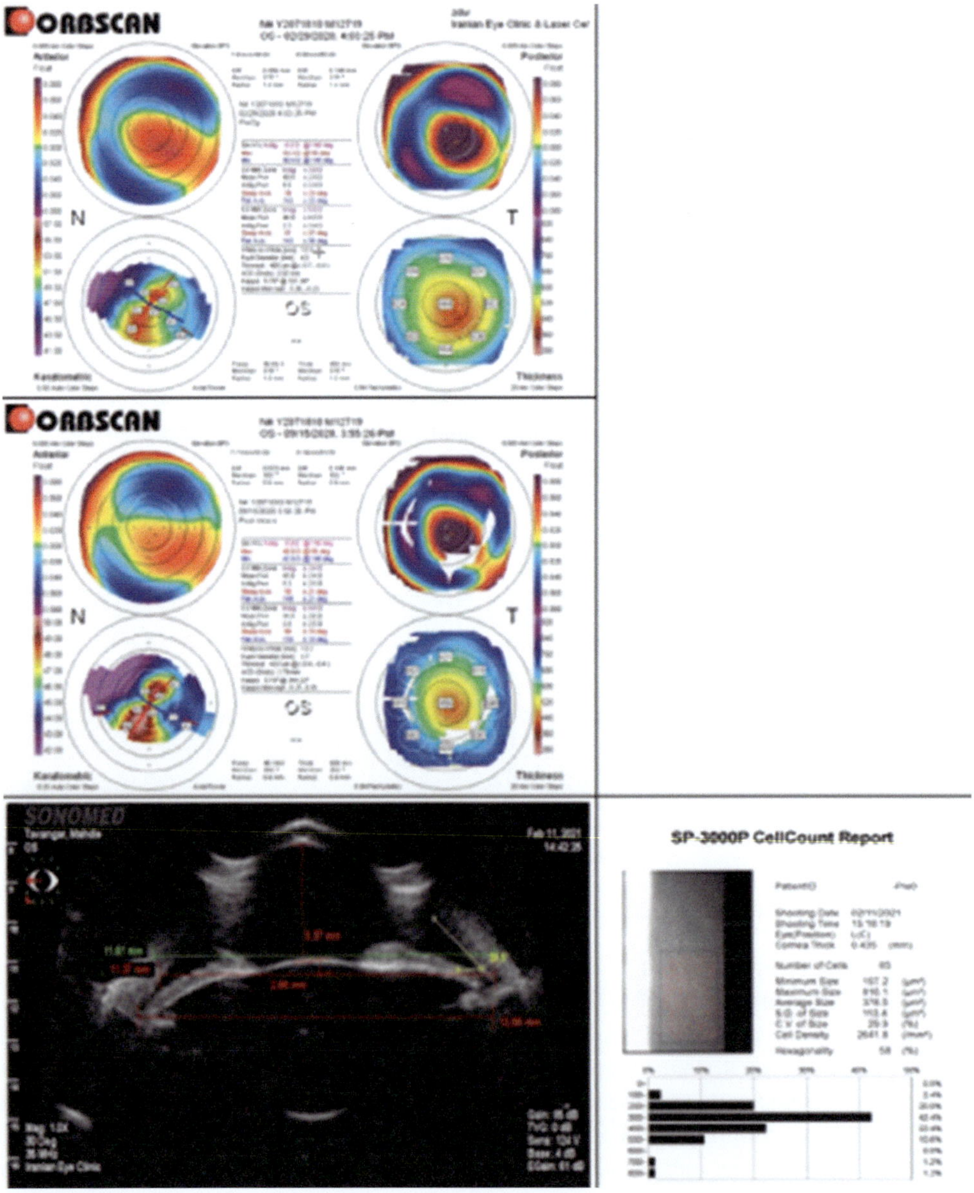

18.5.4 Unstable Keratoconus with High Irregularity

Combining cross-linking with therapeutic refractive procedures can enhance a patient's ability to wear soft contact lenses, improve visual acuity with glasses, or even improve uncorrected visual acuity. Therapeutic refractive options include intrastromal ring segment implantation and pIOLs.

Fewer investigation in which the Visian toric ICL was implanted for the treatment of residual refractive error 6 months after ICRS and CXL in stable keratoconus showed good safety and efficacy in patients with moderate to severe keratoconus [70]. The combination of three surgical modalities (ICRS, CXL, and toric pIOL) improved functional uncorrected vision in keratoconic eyes with a high refractive error and reduced keratoconus progression. This approach takes advantage of the benefits of each modality: ICRS to treat irregular astigmatism, CXL to reduce progression, and toric pIOL to treat the high-residual myopic astigmatism (Fig. 18.7) [71–73].

18.6 Surgical Technique

18.6.1 Artiflex/Veriflex

For Artiflex/Veriflex phakic IOL implantation, miosis can be achieved with topical pilocarpine 2% applied for 15 minutes before surgery or with intraoperative acetylcholine. Topical, peribulbar, or general anesthesia can be used, depending on patient and surgeon choice. The main surgical steps of implantation are:

- Create two 1.0-mm side port incisions at the 10- and 2-o'clock positions.
- Create the main incision (3.2 mm in clear cornea) at the 12-o'clock position.
- Fill the anterior chamber with cohesive OVD.
- Place the IOL in the spatula provided by Ophtec.
- Introduce the spatula with the IOL into the eye and, once the IOL is in the anterior chamber, press down on and remove the spatula.
- Rotate the Artiflex to the horizontal position.
- Fixate the IOL to the midperipheral iris. To perform this step, introduce the blunt needle provided by Ophtec through a side port incision and use forceps through the main incision to hold the haptic of the IOL. Then, with a bimanual technique, introduce a sufficient amount of iris tissue through the IOL haptics. This step is done in each haptic, and the amount of tissue grasped by the haptic must be at least 1.0 mm.
- Wash out all the OVD using I/A or passive irrigation.
- Perform iridectomy or iridotomy; this can alternatively be performed preoperatively with Nd:YAG laser.
- Close the wound with corneal hydration.

Postoperative medications include topical antibiotic (levofloxacin) four times daily for 1 weeks and steroids (prednisolone acetate) four times daily for 4 weeks.

18.6.2 Visian ICL

For Visian ICL implantation, mydriasis can be achieved with topical phenylephrine 1% and tropicamide 1%. Depending on patient and surgeon preference, topical, peribulbar, or general anesthesia can be used. The main surgical steps of implantation are:

- Create two 1.0 mm side port incisions at the 6- and 12-o'clock positions.
- Create the main incision (3.2 mm clear cornea) on the temporal side.
- Fill the anterior chamber with cohesive OVD.
- Introduce the IOL into the cartridge.
- Introduce the cartridge into the eye.
- Inject the IOL slowly into the anterior chamber, watching it unfold in the correct direction (note that the small mark on the leading haptic must be on the right and the mark on the trailing haptic on the left).

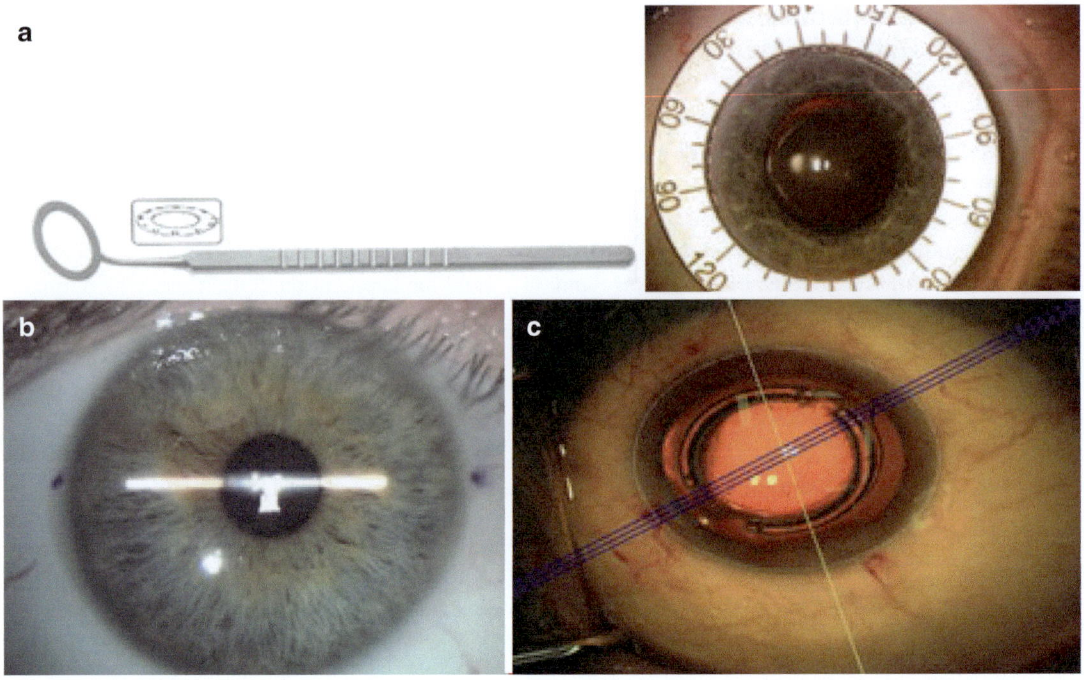

Fig. 18.8 Marking of toric pIOLs' axis: (**a**) Mendez, (**b**) Slit-lamp marking, (**c**) Callisto digital marking

- Introduce a soft-tip manipulator through the side port incisions and press down the tip of the haptics to move the ICL into the posterior chamber; never press on the optic.
- Wash out all OVD using I/A or passive irrigation.
- Perform iridectomy only if central hole is not present (hyperopia).
- Close the wound with corneal hydration.

Postoperatively, topical antibiotic four times daily for 1 weeks and steroid should be administered four times daily for 2–3 weeks. Cases of the Visian ICL being implanted upside-down have been described, but this is easily avoidable if one pays attention to the position of the haptic marks during unfolding.

The implantation of toric IOLs is similar to that of the spherical models, except that the axis of the IOL must be placed in the axis of astigmatism. The first step is to mark the axis of implantation in the patient's eye (Fig. 18.8a–c). This is commonly done at the slit lamp to avoid cyclotorsion, marking the limbus with a surgical pen or using digital marking system such as Callisto eye (Carl Zeiss Meditec; Fig. 18.8c) or the Verion Image-Guided System (Alcon). After implantation, the IOL should be aligned along the marked axis. With the Artisan and Artiflex lenses, the axis of the claws must be aligned with the limbus marks. The ICL is always implanted in the same axis (0° to 180°), as the cylinder is included in the lens design (Fig. 18.9).

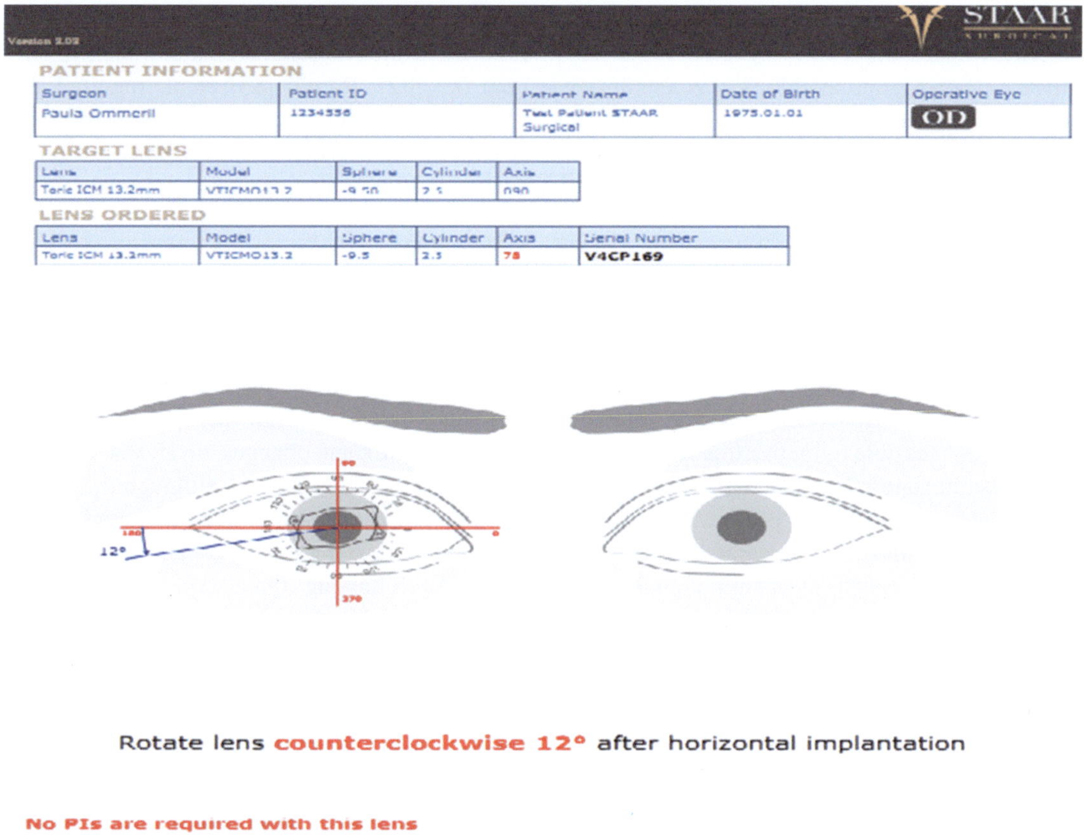

Fig. 18.9 Implantation orientation diagram

18.7 Results of pIOLs in KCN

18.7.1 Refractive Outcomes

18.7.1.1 Efficacy

The efficacy of this procedure was defined as the number and percentage of eyes achieving a UDVA of 20/40 or better. The efficacy index was defined as the ratio of mean postoperative UDVA to mean preoperative CDVA. The mean postoperative UDVA ranged between 0.01 ± 0.0635 and 0.3336 logMAR and 0.88 ± 0.1837 and 0.49 ± 0.2338 decimal. The percentage of eyes achieving a UDVA of 20/40 was reported to be 96.7% by Alfonso [63] et al., 93% by Kamiya [28] et al., 60% by Kurian [73] et al., 90.9% by Hashemian [19, 29] et al., and 100% by Doroodgar [74] et al. The efficacy index ranged between 0.72 and 1.75, indicating that postoperatively there was a gain in the UDVA compared to the preoperative CDVA. These results were comparable to those reported in the use of ICL implantation in nonkeratoconic eyes with myopic astigmatism [75, 76].

18.7.1.2 Predictability

Predictability is based on the number of eyes that achieved a postoperative spherical equivalent within ±0.50D of the targeted refraction. In these studies, the predictability for ±0.50D ranged widely between 18% [67] and 90% [63]. However, most studies reported a predictability between 70% and 85% [19, 74, 77–80]. The predictability for ±1.00D ranged between 50% and 100%, with most studies showing a predictability greater than 90% [18, 19, 74, 77–80].

18.7.1.3 Safety

Measures of safety include the safety index, the percentage of central corneal endothelial cell loss, and the rates of incidence for asymptomatic anterior subcapsular (ASC) opacity, visual significant cataract, pupillary block, pigment dispersion, and secondary surgical intervention. The safety index is the ratio of postoperative CDVA to preoperative CDVA. All studies reported a favorable safety ratio for the procedure between 0.72 and 2.2 (with maximum studies between 1 and 1.5). This implied that the postoperative CDVA was better than the preoperative values in most cases. None of the studies reported any significant change in the endothelial cell counts after surgery. Phakic iris-fixated anterior chamber lenses offer a feasible refractive treatment for stabilized keratoconus. Patients with lower preoperative astigmatism and pellucidal marginal degeneration (PMD)-like appearance of the keratoconus seem to benefit most from a phakic IOL implantation. The UDVA after pIOL implantation is equal or better than the preoperative CDVA in 71% and better in 34% in eyes with keratoconus. None of the patients lost two lines [81].

18.7.1.4 Stability

Stability outcomes are measured by clinically significant changes in the mean value of any component over the follow-up period. It was evaluated as loss of two or more lines of CDVA or gain of one or more line of CDVA during this period. The follow-up period ranged from 3 to 60 months. Kurian [73] et al. reported a stability of 90% because 10% of eyes showed a change of more than 0.50D between 1 and 6 months of follow-up. None of the studies reported a loss of two or more lines of CDVA in any patient during the follow-up period, thereby indicating that the results remained stable during the entire duration of follow-up [29].

18.7.2 Visual Quality Outcomes

18.7.2.1 HOAs

Several studies have shown that keratoconic eyes and eyes with other ectatic disorders have significantly greater HOAs than normal eyes [18, 82]. Various visual parameters correlated with good visual quality: modulation transfer function of greater than 30 cycles per degree (cpd), Strehl ratio of 1, and Objective Scatter Index of less than 0.5 [82]. Ramin [83] et al. reported that coma, trefoil, and tetrafoil were the dominant aberrations in a patient with keratoconus and a significant reduction in the internal trefoil occurred following TICL implantation ($p < 0.03$). Emerah [84] et al. reported that the surgery itself did not induce any new aberration, but the preexisting HOAs remained the same despite the correction of myopic astigmatism.

We reported that the ICL and TICL performed well in correcting high myopic astigmatism without significant changes in HOAs during a 6-month observation period, although the spherical aberration (Z400) increased significantly [85]. He et al. reported significant improvement in HOAs following three-step treatment with ICRS+CXL + ICL for keratoconus [72].

18.7.2.2 Glare

The reasons for glare and halo in patients after pIOLs implantation are peripheral iridotomy, large mesopic pupil size, IOL optic diameter, and central hole of V4c Visian ICL. It was reported in patients who underwent ICL implantation with peripheral iridotomy before ICL implantation [86]. With the introduction of the V4c model, iridotomy is no longer required, but glare was still reported to occur in 27% patients, possibly due to hole decentration [87, 88]. Camoriano et al. reported severe glare in one patient with PMD who underwent ICL implantation and subsequently required explantation [77]. This complaint decreased with the new model V5 or Evo plus ICL.

18.7.3 Corneal Biomechanical Effects of pIOLs Implantation

Studies showed that one advantage of foldable pIOLs implantation is this procedure does not affect corneal biomechanical properties such as corneal hysteresis and cornea-resistant factor. Li et al. studied the corneal biomechanics after V4c ICL implantation in subclinical keratoconus [89]. They used the Corvis ST (Oculus Optikgeräte

GmbH) to measure the Corvis Biomechanical Index and the Pentacam for the Tomographic and Biomechanical Index. They reported that all parameters returned to baseline levels at 3 months following surgery. Ali et al. used the Ocular Response Analyzer (Reichert Ophthalmic Instruments) and found no significant changes in corneal hysteresis or corneal resistance factor in both normal and keratoconic eyes following ICL implantation [90].

18.7.4 Complications of pIOLs in KCN

Most studies did not report any adverse outcomes after pIOLs implantation in eyes with corneal ectasia. Our study with the longest observational period so far (5 years) showed that the most complication in stable nonprogressive KCN subjects was lens rotation which treated with repositioning [29].

The most relevant potential complications of pIOLs include raised IOP, uveitis, traumatic pIOL dislocation, cataract formation, endothelial cell loss, endophthalmitis, and retinal detachment. The specific complications of pIOLs implantation in corneal ectasia include endothelial cell loss, asymptomatic anterior subcapsular (ASC) opacity, visual significant cataract, pupillary block, pigment dispersion, misalignment and lens rotation, keratoconus progression, and secondary surgical intervention.

18.8 ICL Replacement

Zeng [62] et al. adopted criteria for exchange as follows: vault less than 100 μm or direct contact between the ICL and the crystalline lens; or vault greater than 1000 μm and shallow anterior chamber with angle closure in any quadrant, or vault greater than 1000 μm without angle closure but pupil diameter larger than preoperative and unrelieved patient-reported glare. According to these criteria, 2.6% of eyes which ICLs sized according to WTW and ACD measurements should be replaced. In the US FDA in which sizing was also performed based on WTW and ACD, the ICL replacement for insufficient or excessive vault was 1.0% [91]. ICL exchange for insufficient or excessive vault in the absence of complications remains a matter of medical judgment. On the other hand, excessive vault in the presence of compromised anterior chamber angle function and insufficient vault in the presence of visually significant cataract are indications for surgical intervention.

18.8.1 Cataract

In a large retrospective study, Alfonso [92] et al. reported on 3420 eyes of 1898 patients who underwent implantation with the ICL V4, V4b, or V4c, Twenty-one eyes (0.61%) had explantation for anterior subcapsular cataract (ASC), and the mean time between ICL implantation and cataract surgery was 4.2 ± 1.8 years (range, 1–7 years). Schmidinger [93] et al. noted the association of insufficient vault with ASC cataract, and described a 17% rate of cataract surgery after 10 years of follow-up. Guber [94] et al. reported data from a cohort of 133 eyes of 78 patients, of which 75 eyes (56.4%) from 45 patients were examined 10 years after ICL implantation. The rate of lens opacity development was 40.9% (95% CI, 32.7%–48.8%) and 54.8% (95% CI, 44.7%–63.0%) at 5 and 10 years, respectively.

The incidence of ASC opacities ranges from 1.1% to 5.9%, and the incidence of ASC cataracts requiring surgery ranges from 0% to 1.8%. Higher myopia in Schmidinger [93] et al. and a relatively older population and higher myopia in Guber [94] et al. may help explain their higher rates of reported lens opacities and cataracts.

18.8.2 Pigment Dispersion Glaucoma

Guber [94] et al. noted normal vault (403 μm on a mean of 190–740 μm) among 16 cases of ocular hypertension controlled with IOP-lowering treatment, developing a mean of 7.3 years (range, 1.4–12 years) after implantation. In our study [[29]] with the longest observational period so far

(5 years), we have not seen cataract formation, pigment dispersion glaucoma, pupillary block, or any other vision-threatening complications at any time during the five-year period.

18.8.3 Endothelial Cell Loss

Corneal health has remained an important long-term safety concern for patients undergoing pIOLs implantation. Igarashi [95] reported 8-year follow-up on 41 eyes of 41 patients. They reported that the mean percentage of endothelial cell loss in posterior chamber pIOLs was 6.2 ± 8.6%, 8 years postoperatively, which was considerably lower than the findings in previous studies.

Five-year follow-up, reported by Alfonso [96] et al. demonstrated that the mean endothelial cell loss was 7.5%. In our study [29] we reported favorable safety outcomes, with endothelial cell loss of 7.88% at 5 years in stable nonprogressive KCN subjects. Park [96] et al. highlighted that exact calculation of the emmetropic ICL power is more difficult in patients with keratoconus than in other conditions with myopic astigmatism due to the difficulty in obtaining precise manifest refraction and keratometry readings.

The incidence of retinal detachment after posterior chamber pIOL insertion is very low. In a series of 418 eyes that underwent a posterior chamber PIOL procedure, rhegmatogenous retinal detachment developed in 3 eyes (0.7%) at a mean of 19.8 months postoperatively, a rate comparable to the expected natural history of detachment in eyes with similar degrees of myopia. Alió [97] et al. compared the outcomes of iris claw (Artiflex) and posterior chamber PIOL (ICL) in stable keratoconus. They did not find any statistically significant difference between the safety and stability of the two lenses.

18.9 Conclusion

According to review of the literature, use of non-toric and toric pIOLs in stable nonprogressive stable keratoconic patients (with low irregularity) with myopia and myopic astigmatism can be a safe and effective procedure with acceptable predictability and good stability. Ectatic disorders can progress after surgery, which would lead to unsatisfactory and fluctuating visual outcomes. Hence, only patients with ectasias that are stable with no progression should undergo ICL implantation [11].

In patients with PMD, the progression can occur at a later age than keratoconus; hence the age for surgery in this subgroup may be more than that of keratoconus. In the unexpected event of progression following surgery and a shift in the axis of astigmatism, the IOL can be replaced or repositioned, as reported by Camoriano [77] et al. in PMD. In patients with advanced disease presenting with highly irregular astigmatism or corneal scarring, keratoplasty remains the surgery of choice [98].

pIOLs implantation alone in patient with irregular or unstable KCN, may not provide an optimal refractive solution. Halting the progression of the disease and regularizing the corneal shape eventually lead to better visual outcomes. The treatment is to be tailored to suit the patient's requirements in combination with CXL, ICRS, or PRK, as indicated.

References

1. de Sanctis U, Loiacono C, Richiardi L, Turco D, Mutani B, Grignolo FM. Sensitivity and specificity of posterior corneal elevation measured by Pentacam in discriminating keratoconus/subclinical keratoconus. Ophthalmology. 2008;115(9):1534–9.
2. Piñero DP, Alió JL, Alesón A, Escaf Vergara M, Miranda M. Corneal volume, pachymetry, and correlation of anterior and posterior corneal shape in subclinical and different stages of clinical keratoconus. J Cataract Refract Surg. 2010;36(5):814–25.
3. Rabinowitz YS. Keratoconus. Surv Ophthalmol. 1998;42(4):297–319.
4. Jinabhai A, Radhakrishnan H, O'Donnell C. Pellucid corneal marginal degeneration: A review. Cont Lens Anterior Eye. 2011;34(2):56–63.
5. Sridhar MS, Mahesh S, Bansal AK, Nutheti R, Rao GN. Pellucid marginal corneal degeneration. Ophthalmology. 2004;111(6):1102–7.
6. Seiler T, Quurke AW. Iatrogenic keratectasia after LASIK in a case of forme fruste keratoconus. J Cataract Refract Surg. 1998;24(7):1007–9.

7. Randleman JB, Russell B, Ward MA, Thompson KP, Stulting RD. Risk factors and prognosis for corneal ectasia after LASIK. Ophthalmology. 2003;110(2):267–75.
8. Pallikaris IG, Kymionis GD, Astyrakakis NI. Corneal ectasia induced by laser in situ keratomileusis. J Cataract Refract Surg. 2001;27(11):1796–802.
9. Sakla H, Altroudi W, Muñoz G, Albarrán-Diego C. Simultaneous topography-guided partial photorefractive keratectomy and corneal collagen crosslinking for keratoconus. J Cataract Refract Surg. 2014;40(9):1430–8.
10. Lin DT, Holland S, Tan JC, Moloney G. Clinical results of topography-based customized ablations in highly aberrated eyes and keratoconus/ectasia with cross-linking. J Refract Surg. 2012;28(11 Suppl):S841–8.
11. Ormonde S. Refractive surgery for keratoconus. Clin Exp Optom. 2013;96(2):173–82.
12. Cınar Y, Cingü AK, Turkcu FM, Yüksel H, Sahin A, Yıldırım A, Caca I, Cınar T. Accelerated corneal collagen cross-linking for progressive keratoconus. Cutan Ocul Toxicol. 2014;33(2):168–71.
13. Wollensak G, Spoerl E, Seiler T. Riboflavin/ultraviolet-a-induced collagen crosslinking for the treatment of keratoconus. Am J Ophthalmol. 2003;135(5):620–7.
14. Coskunseven E, Kymionis GD, Tsiklis NS, Atun S, Arslan E, Jankov MR, Pallikaris IG. One-year results of intrastromal corneal ring segment implantation (KeraRing) using femtosecond laser in patients with keratoconus. Am J Ophthalmol. 2008;145(5):775–9.
15. Kymionis GD, Siganos CS, Tsiklis NS, Anastasakis A, Yoo SH, Pallikaris AI, Astyrakakis N, Pallikaris IG. Long-term follow-up of Intacs in keratoconus. Am J Ophthalmol. 2007;143(2):236–44.
16. Hashemian SJ, Farshchian N, Foroutam-Jazi A, Jafari ME, Hashemian MS, Hashemian SM. Visual and refractive outcomes and tomographic changes after femtosecond laser-assisted intrastromal corneal ring segment implantation in patients with keratoconus. J Ophthalmic Vis Res. 2018;13(4):376–82.
17. Kymionis GD, Kontadakis GA, Kounis GA, Portaliou DM, Karavitaki AE, Magarakis M, Yoo S, Pallikaris IG. Simultaneous topography-guided PRK followed by corneal collagen cross-linking for keratoconus. J Refract Surg. 2009;25(9):S807–11.
18. Coskunseven E, Onder M, Kymionis GD, Diakonis VF, Arslan E, Tsiklis N, Bouzoukis DI, Pallikaris I. Combined Intacs and posterior chamber toric implantable Collamer lens implantation for keratoconic patients with extreme myopia. Am J Ophthalmol. 2007;144(3):387–9.
19. Hashemian SJ, Soleimani M, Foroutan A, Joshaghani M, Ghaempanah J, Jafari ME. Toric implantable collamer lens for high myopic astigmatism in keratoconic patients after six months. Clin Exp Optom. 2013;96(2):225–32.
20. Andreanos KD, Hashemi K, Petrelli M, Droutsas K, Georgalas I, Kymionis GD. Keratoconus treatment algorithm. Ophthalmol Ther. 2017;6(2):245–62.
21. Fadlallah A, Dirani A, Chelala E, Antonios R, Cherfan G, Jarade E. Non-topography-guided PRK combined with CXL for the correction of refractive errors in patients with early stage keratoconus. J Refract Surg. 2014;30(10):688–93.
22. Knorz MC. The AcrySof cachet™ angle-supported Phakic IOL. In: Alio JL, Pérez-Santonja JJ, editors. Refractive surgery with Phakic IOLs: fundamentals and clinical practice. Jaypee Brothers Medical Publishers (P) Ltd; 2013. p. 86–95.
23. Budo CJR. Iris-fixated Phakic IOLs. In: Alio JL, Pérez-Santonja JJ, editors. Refractive surgery with Phakic IOLs: fundamentals and clinical practice. Jaypee Brothers Medical Publishers (P) Ltd; 2013. p. 64–76.
24. Lovisolo CF, Mazzolani F. ICL posterior chamber Phakic IOL. In: Alio JL, Pérez-Santonja JJ, editors. Refractive surgery with Phakic IOLs: fundamentals and clinical practice. Jaypee Brothers Medical Publishers (P) Ltd; 2013. p. 96–122.
25. Kawamorita T, Uozato H, Shimizu K. Fluid dynamics simulation of aqueous humour in a posterior-chamber phakic intraocular lens with a central perforation. Graefes Arch Clin Exp Ophthalmol. 2012;250(6):935–9.
26. Fujisawa K, Shimizu K, Uga S, Suzuki M, Nagano K, Murakami Y, Goseki H. Changes in the crystalline lens resulting from insertion of a phakic IOL (ICL) into the porcine eye. Graefes Arch Clin Exp Ophthalmol. 2007;245(1):114–22.
27. Alio JL, Sanz-Diez P. Phakic intraocular lenses in keratoconus. Int J Kerat Ect Cor Dis. 2015;4:103–6.
28. Kamiya K, Shimizu K, Kobashi H, Igarashi A, Komatsu M, Nakamura A, Kojima T, Nakamura T. Three-year follow-up of posterior chamber toric phakic intraocular lens implantation for the correction of high myopic astigmatism in eyes with keratoconus. Br J Ophthalmol. 2015;99(2):177–83.
29. Hashemian SJ, Saiepoor N, Ghiasian L, Aghai H, Jafari ME, Alemzadeh SP, Hashemian MS, Hashemian SM. Long-term outcomes of posterior chamber phakic intraocular lens implantation in keratoconus. Clin Exp Optom. 2018;101(5):652–8.
30. Güell JL, Morral M, Kook D, Kohnen T. Phakic intraocular lenses part 1: historical overview, current models, selection criteria, and surgical techniques. J Cataract Refract Surg. 2010;36(11):1976–93.
31. Aalders-Deenstra V, Bartels M, Beerthuizen J, et al. Consensus Refractie Chirurgie. 3rd ed. Nederlands Gezelschapvoor Refractie Chirurgie (NGRC); 2013.
32. Menezo JL, Peris-Martínez C, Cisneros AL, Martínez-Costa R. Phakic intraocular lenses to correct high myopia: Adatomed, Staar, and artisan. J Cataract Refract Surg. 2004;30(1):33–44.

33. Huang D, Schallhorn SC, Sugar A, Farjo AA, Majmudar PA, Trattler WB, Tanzer DJ. Phakic intraocular lens implantation for the correction of myopia: a report by the American Academy of ophthalmology. Ophthalmology. 2009;116(11):2244–58.
34. Doors M, Cals DW, Berendschot TT, de Brabander J, Hendrikse F, Webers CA, Nuijts RM. Influence of anterior chamber morphometrics on endothelial cell changes after phakic intraocular lens implantation. J Cataract Refract Surg. 2008;34(12):2110–8.
35. Salouti R, Nowroozzadeh MH, Zamani M, Ghoreyshi M, Khodaman AR. Comparison of horizontal corneal diameter measurements using the Orbscan IIz and Pentacam HR systems. Cornea. 2013;32(11):1460–4.
36. Sheng XL, Rong WN, Jia Q, Liu YN, Zhuang WJ, Gu Q, Sun Y, Pan B, Zhu DJ. Outcomes and possible risk factors associated with axis alignment and rotational stability after implantation of the Toric implantable collamer lens for high myopic astigmatism. Int J Ophthalmol. 2012;5(4):459–65.
37. Lee DH, Choi SH, Chung ES, Chung TY. Correlation between preoperative biometry and posterior chamber phakic Visian implantable Collamer lens vaulting. Ophthalmology. 2012;119(2):272–7.
38. Nam SW, Lim DH, Hyun J, Chung ES, Chung TY. Buffering zone of implantable Collamer lens sizing in V4c. BMC Ophthalmol. 2017;17(1):260.
39. Choi KH, Chung SE, Chung TY, Chung ES. Ultrasound biomicroscopy for determining visian implantable contact lens length in phakic IOL implantation. J Refract Surg. 2007;23(4):362–7.
40. Kojima T, Yokoyama S, Ito M, Horai R, Hara S, Nakamura T, Ichikawa K. Optimization of an implantable collamer lens sizing method using high-frequency ultrasound biomicroscopy. Am J Ophthalmol. 2012;153(4):632–7.
41. Hashemian SJ, Mohebbi M, Yaseri M, Jafari ME, Nabili S, Hashemian SM, Hashemian MS. Adjustment formulae to improve the correlation of white-to-white measurement with direct measurement of the ciliary sulcus diameter by ultrasound biomicroscopy. J Curr Ophthalmol. 2017;30(3):217–22.
42. Ghoreish M, Mohammadinia M. Correlation between preoperative sizing of implantable collamer lens (ICL) by white-to-white and sulcus-to-sulcus techniques, and postoperative vault size measured by sheimpflug imaging. J Clin Exp Ophthalmol. 2014;5(4):351.
43. Reinstein DZ, Lovisolo CF, Archer TJ, Gobbe M. Comparison of postoperative vault height predictability using white-to-white or sulcus diameter-based sizing for the visian implantable collamer lens. J Refract Surg. 2013;29(1):30–5.
44. Packer M. Meta-analysis and review: effectiveness, safety, and central port design of the intraocular collamer lens. Clin Ophthalmol. 2016;10:1059–77.
45. Moghimi S, Abdi F, Latifi G, Fakhraie G, Ramezani F, He M, Lin SC. Lens parameters as predictors of intraocular pressure changes after phacoemulsification. Eye (Lond). 2015;29(11):1469–76.
46. Goldsmith JA, Li Y, Chalita MR, Westphal V, Patil CA, Rollins AM, Izatt JA, Huang D. Anterior chamber width measurement by high-speed optical coherence tomography. Ophthalmology. 2005;112(2):238–44.
47. Nongpiur ME, He M, Amerasinghe N, Friedman DS, Tay WT, Baskaran M, Smith SD, Wong TY, Aung T. Lens vault, thickness, and position in Chinese subjects with angle closure. Ophthalmology. 2011;118(3):474–9.
48. Baïkoff G, Bourgeon G, Jodai HJ, Fontaine A, Lellis FV, Trinquet L. Pigment dispersion and artisan phakic intraocular lenses: crystalline lens rise as a safety criterion. J Cataract Refract Surg. 2005;31(4):674–80.
49. Dougherty PJ, Rivera RP, Schneider D, Lane SS, Brown D, Vukich J. Improving accuracy of phakic intraocular lens sizing using high-frequency ultrasound biomicroscopy. J Cataract Refract Surg. 2011;37(1):13–8.
50. Reinstein DZ, Archer TJ, Silverman RH, Rondeau MJ, Coleman DJ. Correlation of anterior chamber angle and ciliary sulcus diameters with white-to-white corneal diameter in high myopes using Artemis VHF digital ultrasound. J Refract Surg. 2009;25(2):185–94.
51. Kawamorita T, Uozato H, Kamiya K, Shimizu K. Relationship between ciliary sulcus diameter and anterior chamber diameter and corneal diameter. J Cataract Refract Surg. 2010;36(4):617–24.
52. Igarashi A, Shimizu K, Kato S, Kamiya K. Predictability of the vault after posterior chamber phakic intraocular lens implantation using anterior segment optical coherence tomography. J Cataract Refract Surg. 2019;45(8):1099–104.
53. Nakamura T, Isogai N, Kojima T, Yoshida Y, Sugiyama Y. Implantable Collamer lens sizing method based on swept-source anterior segment optical coherence tomography. Am J Ophthalmol. 2018;187:99–107.
54. Gonzalez-Lopez F, Bilbao-Calabuig R, Mompean B, Luezas J, Ortega-Usobiaga J, Druchkiv V. Determining the potential role of crystalline lens rise in vaulting in posterior chamber Phakic Collamer lens surgery for correction of myopia. J Refract Surg. 2019;35(3):177–83.
55. Zheng QY, Xu W, Liang GL, Wu J, Shi JT. Preoperative biometric parameters predict the vault after ICL implantation: a retrospective clinical study. Ophthalmic Res. 2016;56(4):215–21.
56. Oh J, Shin HH, Kim JH, Kim HM, Song JS. Direct measurement of the ciliary sulcus diameter by 35-megahertz ultrasound biomicroscopy. Ophthalmology. 2007;114(9):1685–8.
57. Werner L, Izak AM, Pandey SK, Apple DJ, Trivedi RH, Schmidbauer JM. Correlation between different measurements within the eye relative to phakic intraocular lens implantation. J Cataract Refract Surg. 2004;30(9):1982–8.
58. Piñero DP, Puche AB, Alió JL. Ciliary sulcus diameter and two anterior chamber parameters measured by optical coherence tomography and VHF ultrasound. J Refract Surg. 2009;25(11):1017–25.

59. Worst JG, van der Veen G, Los LI. Refractive surgery for high myopia. The Worst-Fechner biconcave iris claw lens. Doc Ophthalmol. 1990;75:335–41.
60. van der Heijde GL. Some optical aspects of implantation of an IOL in a myopic eye. Eur J Implant Refract Surg. 1989;1:245–8.
61. Gonvers M, Bornet C, Othenin-Girard P. Implantable contact lens for moderate to high myopia: relationship of vaulting to cataract formation. J Cataract Refract Surg. 2003;29(5):918–24.
62. Zeng QY, Xie XL, Chen Q. Prevention and management of collagen copolymer phakic intraocular lens exchange: causes and surgical techniques. J Cataract Refract Surg. 2015;41(3):576–84.
63. Alfonso JF, Fernández-Vega L, Lisa C, Fernandes P, González-Méijome JM, Montés-Micó R. Collagen copolymer toric posterior chamber phakic intraocular lens in eyes with keratoconus. J Cataract Refract Surg. 2010;36(6):906–16.
64. Kymionis GD, Grentzelos MA, Karavitaki AE, Zotta P, Yoo SH, Pallikaris IG. Combined corneal collagen cross-linking and posterior chamber toric implantable collamer lens implantation for keratoconus. Ophthalmic Surg Lasers Imaging. 2011;42 Online:e22–5.
65. Güell JL, Morral M, Malecaze F, Gris O, Elies D, Manero F. Collagen crosslinking and toric iris-claw phakic intraocular lens for myopic astigmatism in progressive mild to moderate keratoconus. J Cataract Refract Surg. 2012;38(3):475–84.
66. Fadlallah A, Dirani A, El Rami H, Cherfane G, Jarade E. Safety and visual outcome of Visian toric ICL implantation after corneal collagen cross-linking in keratoconus. J Refract Surg. 2013;29(2):84–9.
67. Navas A, Tapia-Herrera G, Jaimes M, Graue-Hernández EO, Gomez-Bastar A, Ramirez-Luquín T, Ramirez-Miranda A. Implantable collamer lenses after intracorneal ring segments for keratoconus. Int Ophthalmol. 2012;32(5):423–9.
68. Alfonso JF, Lisa C, Fernández-Vega L, Madrid-Costa D, Poo-López A, Montés-Micó R. Intrastromal corneal ring segments and posterior chamber phakic intraocular lens implantation for keratoconus correction. J Cataract Refract Surg. 2011;37(4):706–13.
69. Dirani A, Fadlallah A, Khoueir Z, Antoun J, Cherfan G, Jarade E. Visian toric ICL implantation after intracorneal ring segments implantation and corneal collagen crosslinking in keratoconus. Eur J Ophthalmol. 2014;24(3):338–44.
70. Coskunseven E, Sharma DP, Grentzelos MA, Sahin O, Kymionis GD, Pallikaris I. Four-stage procedure for keratoconus: ICRS implantation, corneal cross-linking, Toric Phakic intraocular lens implantation, and topography-guided photorefractive keratectomy. J Refract Surg. 2017;33(10):683–9.
71. Coşkunseven E, Sharma DP, Jankov MR 2nd, Kymionis GD, Richoz O, Hafezi F. Collagen copolymer toric phakic intraocular lens for residual myopic astigmatism after intrastromal corneal ring segment implantation and corneal collagen crosslinking in a 3-stage procedure for keratoconus. J Cataract Refract Surg. 2013;39(5):722–9.
72. He C, Joergensen JS, Knorz MC, McKay KN, Zhang F. Three-step treatment of keratoconus and post-LASIK ectasia: implantation of ICRS, corneal cross-linking, and implantation of Toric posterior chamber Phakic IOLs. J Refract Surg. 2020;36(2):104–9.
73. Kurian M, Nagappa S, Bhagali R, Shetty R, Shetty BK. Visual quality after posterior chamber phakic intraocular lens implantation in keratoconus. J Cataract Refract Surg. 2012;38(6):1050–7.
74. Doroodgar F, Niazi F, Sanginabadi A, Niazi S, Baradaran-Rafii A, Alinia C, Azargashb E, Ghoreishi M. Comparative analysis of the visual performance after implantation of the toric implantable collamer lens in stable keratoconus: a 4-year follow-up after sequential procedure (CXL+TICL implantation). BMJ Open Ophthalmol. 2017;2(1):e000090.
75. Nakamura T, Isogai N, Kojima T, Yoshida Y, Sugiyama Y. Posterior chamber Phakic intraocular lens implantation for the correction of myopia and myopic astigmatism: a retrospective 10-year follow-up study. Am J Ophthalmol. 2019;206:1–10.
76. Bhikoo R, Rayner S, Gray T. Toric implantable collamer lens for patients with moderate to severe myopic astigmatism: 12-month follow-up. Clin Exp Ophthalmol. 2010;38(5):467–74.
77. Camoriano GD, Aman-Ullah M, Purba MK, Sun J, Gimbel HV. Toric collagen copolymer phakic intraocular lens to correct myopic astigmatism in eyes with pellucid marginal degeneration. J Cataract Refract Surg. 2012;38(2):256–61.
78. Kamiya K, Shimizu K, Kobashi H, Komatsu M, Nakamura A, Nakamura T, Ichikawa K. Clinical outcomes of posterior chamber toric phakic intraocular lens implantation for the correction of high myopic astigmatism in eyes with keratoconus: 6-month follow-up. Graefes Arch Clin Exp Ophthalmol. 2011;249(7):1073–80.
79. Shuber HS. Implantable Collamer lens for correction of refractive errors in patients with keratoconus following collagen cross-linking: one year follow-up. Int J Kerat Ect Cor Dis. 2014;3(1):29–35.
80. Alfonso JF, Palacios A, Montés-Micó R. Myopic phakic STAAR collamer posterior chamber intraocular lenses for keratoconus. J Refract Surg. 2008;24(9):867–74.
81. Fischinger IR, Wendelstein J, Tetz K, Bolz M, Tetz MR. Toric phakic IOLs in keratoconus-evaluation of preoperative parameters on the outcome of phakic anterior chamber lens implantation in patients with keratoconus. Graefes Arch Clin Exp Ophthalmol. 2021;259(6):1643–9.
82. Miháltz K, Kovács I, Kránitz K, Erdei G, Németh J, Nagy ZZ. Mechanism of aberration balance and the effect on retinal image quality in keratoconus: optical and visual characteristics of keratoconus. J Cataract Refract Surg. 2011;37(5):914–22.
83. Ramin S, Sangin Abadi A, Doroodgar F, Esmaeili M, Niazi F, Niazi S, Alinia C, Golestani Y, Taj

AR. Comparison of visual, refractive and aberration measurements of INTACS versus Toric ICL lens implantation; a four-year follow-up. Med Hypothesis Discov Innov Ophthalmol. 2018;7(1):32–9.
84. Emerah SH, Sabry MM, Saad HA, Ghobashy WA. Visual and refractive outcomes of posterior chamber phakic IOL in stable keratoconus. Int J Ophthalmol. 2019;12(5):840–3.
85. Hashemian SJ, Farrokhi H, Foroutan A, Jafari ME, Hashemian SM, Alemzadeh SA, Hashemian MS. Ocular higher-order aberrations changes after implantable collamer lens implantation for high myopic astigmatism. J Curr Ophthalmol. 2017;30(2):136–41.
86. Tognetto D, De Giacinto C, Cirigliano G. Suture of symptomatic YAG laser peripheral Iridotomies following Phakic intraocular lens implantation. J Glaucoma. 2017;26(7):675–7.
87. Karandikar S, Bhandari V, Reddy J. Outcomes of implantable collamer lens V4 and V4c for correction of high myopia - a case series. Nepal J Ophthalmol. 2015;7(14):164–72.
88. Martínez-Plaza E, López-Miguel A, Fernández I, Blázquez-Arauzo F, Maldonado MJ. Effect of central hole location in phakic intraocular lenses on visual function under progressive headlight glare sources. J Cataract Refract Surg. 2019;45(11):1591–6.
89. Li K, Wang Z, Zhang D, Wang S, Song X, Li Y, Wang MX. Visual outcomes and corneal biomechanics after V4c implantable collamer lens implantation in subclinical keratoconus. J Cataract Refract Surg. 2020;46(10):1339–45.
90. Ali M, Kamiya K, Shimizu K, Igarashi A, Ishii R. Clinical evaluation of corneal biomechanical parameters after posterior chamber phakic intraocular lens implantation. Cornea. 2014;33(5):470–4.
91. Sanders DR, Vukich JA, Doney K, Gaston M. Implantable contact lens in treatment of myopia study group. U.S. Food and Drug Administration clinical trial of the implantable contact lens for moderate to high myopia. Ophthalmology. 2003;110(2):255–66.
92. Alfonso JF, Lisa C, Fernández-Vega L, Almanzar D, Pérez-Vives C, Montés-Micó R. Prevalence of cataract after collagen copolymer phakic intraocular lens implantation for myopia, hyperopia, and astigmatism. J Cataract Refract Surg. 2015;41(4):800–5.
93. Schmidinger G, Lackner B, Pieh S, Skorpik C. Long-term changes in posterior chamber phakic intraocular collamer lens vaulting in myopic patients. Ophthalmology. 2010;117(8):1506–11.
94. Guber I, Mouvet V, Bergin C, Perritaz S, Othenin-Girard P, Majo F. Clinical outcomes and cataract formation rates in eyes 10 years after posterior Phakic lens implantation for myopia. JAMA Ophthalmol. 2016;134(5):487–94.
95. Igarashi A, Shimizu K, Kamiya K. Eight-year follow-up of posterior chamber phakic intraocular lens implantation for moderate to high myopia. Am J Ophthalmol. 2014;157(3):532–9.
96. Park SW, Kim MK, Wee WR, Lee JH. Partial visual rehabilitation using a toric implantable collamer lens in a patient with keratoconus: a case report with 20 months of follow-up. Korean J Ophthalmol. 2013;27(3):211–4.
97. Alió JL, Peña-García P, Abdulla GF, Zein G, Abu-Mustafa SK. Comparison of iris-claw and posterior chamber collagen copolymer phakic intraocular lenses in keratoconus. J Cataract Refract Surg. 2014;40(3):383–94.
98. Vazirani J, Basu S. Keratoconus: current perspectives. Clin Ophthalmol. 2013;7:2019–30.

Stromal Augmentation Techniques for Keratoconus

19

Sunita Chaurasia

19.1 Introduction

Several novel treatment strategies have evolved in the last decade as alternatives to keratoplasty in keratoconus. The exact pathogenesis of keratoconus is not clearly understood, but it is well known that there is a biomechanical weakening of the corneal stroma leading to ectasia, which is progressive in a large majority of eyes [1]. Deep anterior lamellar keratoplasty (DALK) is the current standard, safe, and effective technique in the management of those advanced keratoconus and contact lens intolerance [2]. Penetrating keratoplasty (PK) is the conventional strategy of managing keratoconus that is now largely favored in eyes with hydrops in the past and those with failure of deep anterior lamellar keratoplasty (DALK) either intraoperatively or postoperatively [3, 4]. A quest for surgical options that are minimally invasive and have a potential to avoid sutures are gaining interest.

Historically, intrastromal additive techniques using synthetic inlays had been investigated in animal models and patients with ectasias. The introduction of femtosecond laser enabled feasibility of several stromal augmentation procedures in keratoconus.

This chapter discusses the various surgical options that are currently available as alternatives to standard technique of DALK and holds the promise of evolving into newer standards of management in keratoconus. Broadly, these include the Bowman's layer transplantation (BLT), stromal lenticule addition keratoplasty (SLAK), and intrastromal implantation of regenerated stromal lamina.

19.2 Corneal Stroma-Applied Surgical Anatomical Considerations

The cornea comprises epithelium, Bowman's layer (BL), stroma, fine Dua's layer, and Descemet membrane endothelium complex. The BL is the anterior limiting lamina that is acellular, ~12 microns thick, and composed of type I and III collagen fibrils and proteoglycans. The diameter of these collagen fibrils is ~20–30 nm [5]. The BL receives insertion from obliquely arranged anterior stromal collagen lamellae and contributes to the formation of anterior corneal mosaic [6]. This is believed to contribute to the shape and biomechanical strength of the anterior cornea [7]. The BL undergoes thinning with age and does not regenerate upon injury. The functional significance of absence of BL and its impact on corneal biomechanics is not clear.

S. Chaurasia (✉)
The Cornea Institute, LV Prasad Eye Institute, Hyderabad, Telangana, India

Ramayamma International Eye Bank, L V Prasad Eye Institute, Hyderabad, Telangana, India
e-mail: sunita@lvpei.org

S. Das (ed.), *Keratoconus*, https://doi.org/10.1007/978-981-19-4262-4_19

Many mammals do not have BL, and still there is no compromised corneal stability. Likewise, agenesis of BL is reported in normal corneas and the iatrogenic loss of BL as happens in photorefractive keratectomy (PRK) does not exhibit any increased risk of ectasia when compared to LASIK [8, 9]. In contrast to these observations, it is believed that BL may be the strongest biomechanical component of the cornea followed by anterior one-third of the cornea [10].

A notable feature of keratoconus is the fragmentation of BL and the proliferation of collagen tissue derived from anterior stroma beneath the rupture [11]. BL can be successfully isolated from the donor cornea, akin to Descemet's membrane, and this resulted in feasibility of its transplantation in keratoconus.

19.3 Bowman's Membrane Transplant (BLT)

The BLT was earlier used in treating subepithelial scarring after PRK. In 2014, van Dijk et al were the first to describe isolated BLT in the treatment of keratoconus with contact lens intolerance [12]. This surgical procedure is advocated in keratoconus based on the premise that replacement of ruptured BL with isolated BL harvested from donor cornea will provide additional strength to the weak cornea and flatten the anterior corneal surface and thereby improve visual acuity and arrest disease progression.

19.4 Surgical Technique

19.4.1 Graft Preparation

The technique of BL graft preparation was initially described in 2010 [13]. The BL graft is prepared either from whole globes or donor cornea is mounted on an artificial anterior chamber. The epithelium is debrided, and air is injected into the donor cornea beneath the BL. A 30-gauge needle is used to incise the BL, 360° just within the limbal region. The BL is lifted and grasped with a McPherson forceps and carefully peeled from the underlying stroma, obtaining a graft of ~9–11 mm in size. The BL graft tends to form a single or a double roll with epithelial border on the outside. The BL roll is rinsed with 70% alcohol for 30 s to remove remnant epithelial cells and stored in corneal preservation solution until the time of surgery.

Recently, femtosecond laser has been used for preparing donor BL graft. Initial analysis showed that the laser cuts had relatively smoother posterior cut edges but were significantly thicker than manually prepared grafts due to some amount of anterior stroma [14].

19.4.2 Surgery in the Recipient

The surgery is performed under a local anesthesia. A conjunctival peritomy is performed. A 5-mm partial-thickness scleral tunnel is made 1–2 mm outside the limbus and dissected into the clear cornea using a crescent knife. A paracentesis port is made to fill the anterior chamber with air. The mid-stromal pocket is dissected manually over 360° up to the limbus. The dissection plane is targeted at 50% depth that is gauged using the air-endothelial reflex to avoid inadvertent anterior and/or posterior perforations. Following this, the air is released from the anterior chamber. A surgical glide is placed in the lamellar pocket. The BL graft is rinsed thoroughly with balanced salt solution, stained with trypan blue, and introduced into the stromal pocket over the glide. The glide is removed, and the BL graft is unfolded and positioned within the stromal pocket (Fig. 19.1). The anterior chamber is irrigated with BSS to physiological intraocular pressure, conjunctiva is repositioned to cover the external incision, and the eye is patched.

19.4.3 Clinical Outcomes

BLT is a relatively newer surgical procedure, and hence, there is limited literature on its outcomes. Table 19.1 summarizes the results of BLT from the currently available studies [15–20]. The pro-

Fig. 19.1 Diagram illustrating the Bowman layer transplantation (inlay technique)

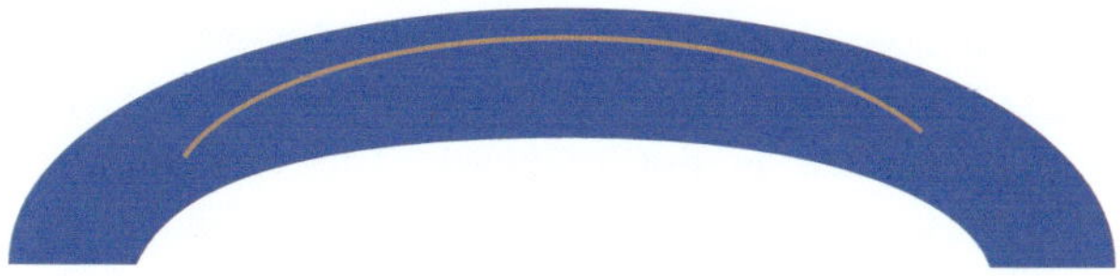

Table 19.1 Outcomes of BLT

Author	Number of eyes	Inclusion criteria	Observations and outcomes	Follow-up duration	Complications
van Dijk et al [12], 2014	10	Advanced KC with contact lens intolerance	Decreased mean Kmax from 74.5D to 68.3D at 6 months, stable till 12 months, improved contact lens tolerance	12 months	None
van Dijk et al [15], 2015	22	Advanced KC, Kmax ≥70D	Decreased K from 77.2 ± 6.2 to 69.2 ± 3.7D by 6 months, stable thereafter	21 ± 7 months	Intraoperative DM perforation (2 eyes)
Luceri et al [16], 2016	15	Advanced KC	Improved spectacle-corrected VA, reduction in corneal HOA	12 months	Increased corneal densitometry
Blasberg et al [17], 2017	1	Advanced, progressive KC	Corneal flattening, restoration of contact lens fit	–	None
van Dijk et al [18], 2018	20	Advanced KC	84% of eyes had stable disease and persistent flattened corneas	5 years	–
Garcia de Oteyza et al [19], 2019	2	KC	Femtolaser stromal pocket dissection was safe, with lower risk of inadvertent perforation	–	None
Tong et al [20], 2019	21	KC	Intraoperative OCT-assisted manual stromal dissection safe	–	Intraoperative perforation (2 eyes)

KC Keratoconus, *HOA* Higher-order aberrations, *OCT* Optical coherence tomography, *DM* Descemet membrane

cedure leads to a decrease in corneal curvatures, increased pachymetry, improved spectacle-corrected visual acuity, and better tolerance of contact lens. The short- and mid-term results show its efficacy in advanced keratoconus. The largest single-center clinical outcomes up to 7 years after the surgery are available from the innovators of BLT [21]. In the first clinical series, the operated eyes showed an average reduction in 8-9D in maximum keratometry values that remained stable thereafter [12]. The slit-lamp examination of the graft in the postoperative period is visible faintly as a thin white line. There was improvement in spectacle-corrected visual acuity, a decrease in spherical aberration, and improvement in contact lens tolerance. There was some increase in corneal backscatter up to 5 years after BLT, which was attributed to interface irregularities and differences in refractive indices between the BL graft and the recipient stroma. The clinical impact of increased backscatter was reportedly insignificant. In 3 eyes of 2 patients, who had a history of severe eye rubbing and atopy, hydrops occurred at 4.5, 6, and 6.5 years after BLT.

The advantages of BLT are that it is a sutureless procedure. There is a reduced risk of allograft rejection as the BL is acellular. The risk of other post-keratoplasty complications is steroid-related cataract and glaucoma, and infections are minimized. However, BLT is relatively tedious procedure and has a learning curve in graft preparation. The mid-stromal dissection in advanced keratoconus can be challenging with high risk of perforations and subsequent need for conventional surgical procedures. Nevertheless, the surgical procedure may be an alternative or can be a promising strategy to postpone the more invasive corneal surgery such as DALK or PK.

More recently, the Bowman layer onlay grafting [22] has been investigated, where the dissection of cornea is not required. The clinical outcomes seemed to be comparable to the inlay technique of BLT.

19.5 Stromal Lenticule Addition Keratoplasty (SLAK)

The procedure described by Mastropasqua et al [23] entails implanting a negative meniscus-shaped lenticule that is thinner in the center and thicker in the periphery. The surgery is based on the principle to augment the corneal thickness and achieve corneal flattening like the effect achieved after intrastromal corneal ring segments [24].

19.5.1 Surgical Technique

The surgery involves creation of a stromal pocket using femtosecond laser. The allogenic lenticule, 6.7 mm in diameter, is sculpted in the donor cornea with the exact shape, size, and geometry using femtolaser (VisuMax, Zeiss, Germany) and is extracted for implantation in the stromal pocket within the recipient's cornea.

19.5.1.1 Clinical Outcomes

The early outcomes of SLAK have been shown to improve the corneal shape and regularity in keratoconus [23]. There was a significant improvement in mean uncorrected and corrected distance visual acuity, which ranged between 1 and 3 lines. The allogenic meniscus-shaped lenticules induced a generalized flattening of the cone, with a reduction in anterior Km and increase in thickness of central and mid-peripheral corneal thickness. Confocal microscopy (HRT II Rostock Cornea Module, Germany) revealed the lenticule–host interfaces. The anterior and posterior lenticule interfaces showed a hyperreflectivity that decreased over time. There was no occurrence of stromal rejection in the follow-up period.

The advantage of the procedure is its relative ease due to the application of femtosecond laser in stromal pocket creation and lenticule preparation. The procedure is more suitable for less severe cases of keratoconus.

19.6 Cellular Therapy of the Corneal Stroma

Cellular therapy following corneal cell expansion and tissue engineering of the corneal stroma has gained interest over the last decade as a potential alternative to conventional keratoplasty [25–27]. The successful application of this modality has several challenges and is dependent on identifying an ideal cellular substitute that holds the promise of nearly similar structural and optical characteristics as that of corneal stroma. Autologous ocular stem cells have some disadvantages such as difficulties in isolation and limitations of availability in high density. On the contrary, autologous stem cells from extraocular sources as human adipose tissue have been shown to differentiate in vivo into adult human keratocytes and produced collagen within the host stroma. The mesenchymal stromal cells (MSCs) derived from human adipose tissue are an ideal source due to ease of access, high cell retrieval efficiency, and differentiation potential. The mesenchymal stem cells have immunomodulatory properties in syngenic, allogenic, and xenogenic models, thus making these lucrative for their use in corneal stroma regeneration therapies. Additionally, acellular corneal extracellular matrix has been shown to behave as an excellent scaffold for implantation in cornea. The growing interest in corneal cell expansion and regeneration using stem cells and collagen matrix has led to its potential application in restoring the abnormal stroma in keratoconus.

19.7 Autologous Adipose-Derived Adult Stem Cells (ADASCs) Isolation and Intrastromal Implantation Techniques

Standard liposuction is performed under local anesthesia, and ~ 250 ml of adipose tissue is obtained from the patient. The adipose tissue is then processed and cultured in Dulbecco's modified Eagle medium. Approximately three million cells are prepared in phosphate-buffered saline for direct transplantation [25]. In another technique, the cells were cultured on each surface of decellularized corneal stromal lamina prepared using the femtosecond laser and then inserted into the stromal pockets of the recipient, unfolded, and centered [26].

19.7.1 Clinical Outcomes

The authors have reported new collagen production at the level of stromal pocket [25]. Further, there was an increase in unaided and corrected distance visual acuity at 6, 12, and 36 months of follow-up. An increase in thickness of the thinnest point and central cornea was observed. There was a notable improvement in anterior Km and Kmax values and higher-order aberrations. No adverse events were noted during 3-year follow-up except in one patient, who had a mild early haze that was due to lenticular edema. Although this approach seems promising, the technique needs more scientific evidence to support its application in different severity of the disease.

19.8 Conclusion

The application of femtosecond lasers in ophthalmology has opened alternative avenues to perform corneal surgeries. Stromal augmentation techniques with/without femtosecond lasers are the newer evolving management strategies of keratoconus. Although the literature is limited to fewer cases and shorter follow-up periods, these can offer several advantages over the current standard techniques such as minimally invasive therapies, avoidance of sutures, and its complications.

References

1. Mas Tur V, MacGregor C, Jayaswal R, O'Brart D, Maycock N. A review of keratoconus: diagnosis, pathophysiology, and genetics. Surv Ophthalmol. 2017;62(6):770–83.
2. Gadhvi KA, Romano V, Fernández-Vega Cueto L, Aiello F, Day AC, Allan BD. Deep anterior lamellar Keratoplasty for keratoconus: multisurgeon results. Am J Ophthalmol. 2019;201:54–62.
3. Mohammadpour M, Heidari Z, Hashemi H. Updates on managements for keratoconus. J Curr Ophthalmol. 2017;30(2):110–24.
4. Parker JS, van Dijk K, Melles GR. Treatment options for advanced keratoconus: a review. Surv Ophthalmol. 2015;60(5):459–80.
5. Nishida T, Saika S, Morishige N. Cornea and sclera: anatomy and physiology. In: Mannis MJ, Holland EJ, editors. Cornea. New York: Elsevier Inc.; 2017. p. 1–22.
6. Bron AJ, Tripathi RC. The anterior corneal mosaic. Br J Physiol Opt. 1970;25(1):8–13.
7. Bron AJ, Tripathi RC, Tripathi BJ. Wolff's anatomy of the eye and orbit. 8th ed. London: Chapman & Hall Medical; 1997. p. 736.
8. Kasner L, Mietz H, Green WR. Agenesis of Bowman's layer. A histopathological study of four cases. Cornea. 1993;12(2):163–70.
9. Lagali N, Germundsson J, Fagerholm P. The role of Bowman's layer in corneal regeneration after phototherapeutic keratectomy: a prospective study using in vivo confocal microscopy. Invest Ophthalmol Vis Sci. 2009;50(9):4192–8.
10. Dragnea DC, Birbal RS, Ham L, Dapena I, Oellerich S, van Dijk K, Melles GRJ. Bowman layer transplantation in the treatment of keratoconus. Eye Vis (Lond). 2018;5:24.
11. Salomão MQ, Hofling-Lima AL, Gomes Esporcatte LP, Correa FF, Lopes B, Sena N Jr, Dawson DG, Ambrósio R Jr. Ectatic diseases. Exp Eye Res. 2021;202:108347.
12. van Dijk K, Parker J, Tong CM, Ham L, Lie JT, Groeneveld-van Beek EA, Melles GR. Midstromal isolated Bowman layer graft for reduction of advanced keratoconus: a technique to postpone penetrating or deep anterior lamellar keratoplasty. JAMA Ophthalmol. 2014;132(4):495–501.
13. Lie J, Droutsas K, Ham L, Dapena I, Ververs B, Otten H, van der Wees J, Melles GR. Isolated Bowman layer transplantation to manage persistent subepithelial haze after excimer laser surface ablation. J Cataract Refract Surg. 2010;36(6):1036–41.
14. Parker JS, Huls F, Cooper E, Graves P, Groeneveld-van Beek EA, Lie J, Melles GRJ. Technical feasibil-

ity of isolated Bowman layer graft preparation by femtosecond laser: a pilot study. Eur J Ophthalmol. 2017;27(6):675–7.
15. van Dijk K, Liarakos VS, Parker J, Ham L, Lie JT, Groeneveld-van Beek EA, Melles GR. Bowman layer transplantation to reduce and stabilize progressive, advanced keratoconus. Ophthalmology. 2015;122(5):909–17.
16. Luceri S, Parker J, Dapena I, Baydoun L, Oellerich S, van Dijk K, Melles GR. Corneal densitometry and higher order aberrations after Bowman layer transplantation: 1-year results. Cornea. 2016;35(7):959–66.
17. Blasberg C, Geerling G, Schrader S. Transplantation der Bowman-Lamelle bei progressivem Keratokonus – was bringt's? [Bowman layer transplantation in progressive keratoconus - what is it good for?]. Klin Monatsbl Augenheilkd. 2017;234(6):776–9.
18. van Dijk K, Parker JS, Baydoun L, Ilyas A, Dapena I, Groeneveld-van Beek EA, Melles GRJ. Bowman layer transplantation: 5-year results. Graefes Arch Clin Exp Ophthalmol. 2018;256(6):1151–8.
19. García de Oteyza G, González Dibildox LA, Vázquez-Romo KA, Tapia Vázquez A, Dávila Alquisiras JH, Martínez-Báez BE, García-Albisua AM, Ramírez M, Hernández-Quintela E. Bowman layer transplantation using a femtosecond laser. J Cataract Refract Surg. 2019;45(3):261–6.
20. Tong CM, Parker JS, Dockery PW, Birbal RS, Melles GRJ. Use of intraoperative anterior segment optical coherence tomography for Bowman layer transplantation. Acta Ophthalmol. 2019;97(7):e1031–2.
21. Zygoura V, Birbal RS, van Dijk K, Parker JS, Baydoun L, Dapena I, Melles GRJ. Validity of Bowman layer transplantation for keratoconus: visual performance at 5-7 years. Acta Ophthalmol. 2018;96(7):e901–2.
22. Dapena I, van der Star L, Groeneveld-van Beek EA, Quilendrino R, van Dijk K, Parker JS, Oellerich S, Melles GRJ. Bowman layer Onlay grafting: proof-of-concept of a new technique to flatten corneal curvature and reduce progression in keratoconus. Cornea. 2021;40(12):1561–6.
23. Mastropasqua L, Nubile M, Salgari N, Mastropasqua R. Femtosecond laser-assisted stromal Lenticule addition Keratoplasty for the treatment of advanced keratoconus: a preliminary study. J Refract Surg. 2018;34(1):36–44.
24. Fasolo A, Galzignato A, Pedrotti E, Chierego C, Cozzini T, Bonacci E, Marchini G. Femtosecond laser-assisted implantation of corneal stroma lenticule for keratoconus. Int Ophthalmol. 2021;41(5):1949–57.
25. Alió Del Barrio JL, El Zarif M, de Miguel MP, Azaar A, Makdissy N, Harb W, El Achkar I, Arnalich-Montiel F, Alió JL. Cellular therapy with human autologous adipose-derived adult stem cells for advanced keratoconus. Cornea. 2017;36(8):952–60.
26. El Zarif M, Alió JL, Alió Del Barrio JL, De Miguel MP, Abdul Jawad K, Makdissy N. Corneal stromal regeneration: a review of human clinical studies in keratoconus treatment. Front Med (Lausanne). 2021;8:650724.
27. El Zarif M, Alió JL, Alió Del Barrio JL, Abdul Jawad K, Palazón-Bru A, Abdul Jawad Z, De Miguel MP, Makdissy N. Corneal stromal regeneration therapy for advanced keratoconus: long-term outcomes at 3 years. Cornea. 2021;40(6):741–54.

Cataract Surgery in Keratoconus 20

Wassef Chanbour and Elias Jarade

20.1 Introduction

As the life expectancy is increasing worldwide [1], a higher number of keratoconus patients will be presenting for cataract surgery. In addition, it is well known that keratoconic eyes have higher chances of developing cataract at a younger age compared to the general population, and this might be due to the association with high myopia, atopy, and the frequent use of topical steroid medications [2, 3]. Thinning and cone shape protrusion of the cornea are the hallmark of keratoconus which lead to decrease in the best corrected visual acuity (BCVA) due to irregular astigmatism [4].

In the past, when rigid gas permeable (RGP) contact lens failed, penetrating keratoplasty with or without cataract extraction was the only treatment used to improve the visual acuity in patients with keratoconus. However, with the advent of corneal collagen crosslinking (CXL), which is the only proved treatment to halt the progression of keratoconus, a new era has emerged. In addition to the RGP contact lens, scleral contact lens, intrastromal corneal ring segments (ICRS) [5], phakic toric implantable collamer lenses (ICL) [6], and deep anterior lamellar keratoplasty are currently applied to provide this population with the best possible visual acuity. Ophthalmologists are facing new challenges when patients present for cataract surgery with prior abovementioned surgical procedure. Each patient requires a customized approach tailored to his previous surgical treatments, taking into consideration his corrected distance visual acuity (CDVA) prior to cataract development, current topography, the astigmatism axis (manifest and topographic axis), the accuracy of the recorded keratometry and axial length measurements. Different strategies and multiple surgeries may be applied to provide the patients with the best visual outcomes, to preserve the corneal stability and to increase independence from glasses or contact lens after cataract surgeries.

As keratoconus patients get older, a progressive decrease of visual acuity may be attributed to cataract. The most commonly identified type is nuclear sclerosis [7]. Also, it is well known that any surgical intervention involving corneal incisions in eyes with keratoconus can induce a progression of the corneal ectasia. Therefore, a complete preoperative assessment of the stability and the stage of the disease is necessary, to improve the surgical and refractive outcomes [8].

W. Chanbour
Ophthalmology Department, Lebanese University, Beirut, Lebanon

Ophthalmology Department, University of Minnesota, Minneapolis, MN, USA

E. Jarade (✉)
Ophthalmology Department, Lebanese University, Beirut, Lebanon

Cornea and Refractive Surgery Department, Beirut Eye and ENT Specialist Hospital, Beirut, Lebanon

Mediclinic, Dubai Mall, Dubai, UAE

S. Das (ed.), *Keratoconus*, https://doi.org/10.1007/978-981-19-4262-4_20

20.2 Preoperative Evaluation

Preoperative assessment for every keratoconus patient or those with high astigmatism and a suspicion of ectasia requires a careful review of the medical and ophthalmological history, a slit lamp exam followed by biometric and topographic measurements. Even though keratoconus is a progressive disease, it tends to stabilize in the after the age of 30. However, ectasia progression and corneal topographic changes have been documented beyond this age [9].

In patients previously diagnosed with keratoconus, the cataract surgery evaluation starts by identifying the history of the disease. A history of good, corrected distance visual acuity (CDVA) before the development of cataract improves the prognosis after cataract extraction, while a poor known CDVA can decrease patient's satisfaction after the surgery. Previous topographies should be reviewed looking for stability, especially in young patients diagnosed with cataract. Also of importance is comparing the magnitude and axis of manifest astigmatic (which can be retrieved from the patient's file or by measuring the patient's eyeglasses) before cataract development relative to the position and magnitude of the topographic astigmatism.

Medical history should be closely reviewed as many of the keratoconus patients have associated connective tissue diseases (Ehlers–Danlos syndrome, Marfan syndrome), allergies, obstructive sleep apnea, and genetic diseases (Down syndrome). These patients require a visit to the primary care practitioner and special intraoperative considerations for their anesthesia and positioning during the surgery.

Slit-lamp examination is next step in the surgical planning. Cornea should be evaluated for central haze, scarring, or thinning that may block to surgeon's intraoperative view and increase the risk of intraoperative complications and vitreous loss (cases of advanced keratoconus). Furthermore, in case of advanced corneal scarring and poor visual potential, the surgeon may elect to do a combined cataract extraction and keratoplasty.

Topography has become the standard of care for the preoperative screening in patients with high corneal astigmatism and especially when planning for toric intraocular lens (IOL) implantation. In countries with high prevalence of keratoconus (like the Middle East area), it is not uncommon to diagnose keratoconus in elderly patients presenting for cataract surgery. In addition, topography is the most important imaging modality in the decision making; it identifies the stage of keratoconus and the regularity of astigmatism. To the best of our knowledge, an algorithm for the management of keratoconus eyes with cataract is considered the latest guideline to plan cataract surgeries in keratoconus eyes [10]. Patients with a history of good CDVA and previous identical manifest and topographic axis of astigmatism were candidates for toric IOL, compared to those with different manifest and topographic axis of astigmatism, in which a monofocal IOL was preferred. Authors recommended an ICRS implantation before proceeding with cataract surgery in patients with moderate keratoconus and poor CDVA. And they also concluded that toric implantable Collamer lens (ICL) implantation after cataract surgery may be used in pseudophakic eyes to correct residual ametropia. Figure 20.1 represents an updated algorithm to be followed when planning a cataract surgery in this population.

Intraocular lens power calculation requires a biometry. Multiple studies have compared the reliability and reproducibility of optical devices versus ultrasound (US) biometry in normal eyes; it was reported that optical systems give more accurate and reliable results compared to the US biometry [11, 12]. Optical and US biometric measurements have been also compared in keratoconus. One study found that US and Lenstar (Haag-Streit AG, Koeniz, Switzerland) measurements were highly correlated [13]. US biometer was successful in every measurement, while the Lenstar could not measure at least one of the biometric properties in one eye and did not give the automatic corrected anterior chamber depth approximately in 2/3 of the studied population of 42 patients. In addition, the central corneal thickness (CCT), the lens thickness, and axial length were larger using US compared with the Lenstar in keratoconic eyes, and the difference in CCT between the devices increases with the increase

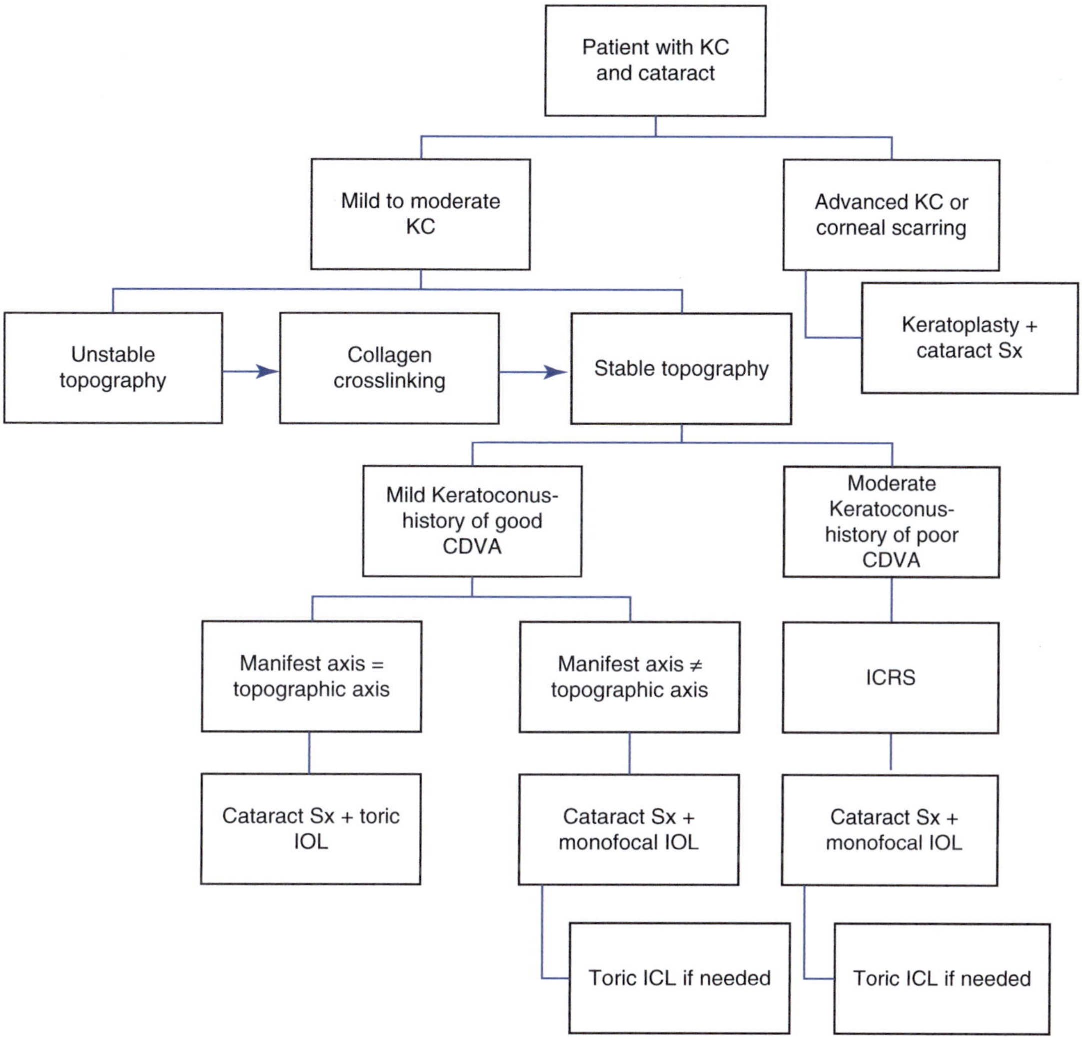

Fig. 20.1 Updated Dr. Jarade's algorithm for the management of keratoconus with cataract

in keratometry. The authors concluded that the reported differences were clinically acceptable. But the US and Lenstar measurements cannot be used interchangeably.

20.3 CXL and ICRS Prior to Cataract

Even though keratoconus is a disease of younger population, it may continue to progress beyond the fourth decade. Of 449 patients, less than 10% of eyes were found to progress beyond the age of 30, having increase in more than 1D of keratometry measurements (Kmax or Kmean) per year [9]. This has major implications for the consideration of CXL in older subjects planned for cataract surgery and considering toric IOL. CXL has been proved safe and effective in patients older than 35 years, and a comparative study found a complication rate of 3.9% of 103 eyes in patients <35 years, compared with 2.6% complication rate in 38 eye of patients >35 years. Corneal haze was the adverse event in the older patients [14]. In our practice, we recommend monitoring new keratoconus patient with cataract and with unknown medical history and younger than 50 years for corneal stability for at least 6 months before operating the cataract (unless it is a very dense cataract and the benefit of early cataract extraction overweight risk of waiting for stability increasing the likelihood of corneal endothelial injury). In case of a documented progression, we recommend waiting for at least 3–6 months after CXL and before proceeding with cataract surgery. Studies showed a corneal stability as early as 3 months post-CXL, and no significant difference in topographic values was reported between the 3-month and 12-month of follow-ups [15].

Patients with moderate keratoconus presenting with irregular corneas and history of poor CDVA present a challenge to ophthalmologists. These patients are less likely to benefit from a toric IOL or a regular monofocal IOLs with expected poor CDVA postoperatively and are at high risk for postoperative glare, decreased contrast sensitivity, and quality of vision. In these cases, ICRS is recommended at least 6 months before proceeding with cataract surgery. Currently, there are no comparative studies evaluating the cataract surgery outcomes with and without ICRS. However, a retrospective review including 70 patients with keratoconus showed statistically significant improvement of the mean uncorrected distance visual acuity (UDVA) and CDVA after each procedure (both ICRS and cataract surgery). Six months after monofocal IOL implantation, 9 eyes had no change in CDVA and 61 gained one or more lines [16]. Even though Ferrara ICRS were used in previously mentioned study, other types of ICRS (Intacs, Keraring) can be used according to the surgeon's preference as they were also proved effective in reshaping the cornea and improving CDVA in patients with keratoconus.

20.4 Intraocular Lens Power Calculation Formulas

The accuracy of keratometry readings and axial length measurements in keratoconus patients may present a challenge to ophthalmologists. Minor changes may affect the IOL power calculation since all the available formulas require these two parameters.

The keratometric power of the cornea may be overestimated for the following reasons. First, keratoconus patients have an abnormal tear film which may affect the topographic measurements. Second, corneal multifocality [17] and a displaced corneal visual axis can make fixation difficult during the measurement. Third, the disparity between the anterior and posterior corneal is greater than in normal eyes and may have an unpredictable impact on IOL power calculation formulas [18]. An overestimated steeper keratometric value in these eyes will result in the selection of a low-power IOL, hence leading to postoperative hyperopia. The concept of keratometry measurement requires a symmetrical corneal curvature around the measurement axis to obtain an accurate and reproducible reading. Such condition is hardly attained in asymmetric keratoconus corneas.

The repeatability of keratometry measurements using five different devices (Pentacam, EyeSys, Orbscan II, IOL Master, and Javal Manual Keratometer) was compared in 78 keratoconic eye; the results showed that eyes with K < 55D had good repeatability, being the highest with Pentacam (OCULUS Optikgeraete GmbH; Wetzlar, Germany) and the lowest in Orbscan II (Bausch & Lomb, Orbtek Inc., Salt Lake City, UT). In patients with advanced keratoconus and K > 55, all the devices had poor repeatability [19]. Another study compared the repeatability of Scheimpflug analyzer (Galilei DSA; Ziemer) and Nidek AL Scan (Nidek CO, Aichi, Japan) between keratoconus and normal eyes. Both devices had good repeatability in low stages of keratoconus, and Nidek AL scan had higher K readings compared to Galilei [20]. These aforementioned studies highlight the difficulty in obtaining reliable keratometry values in advanced keratoconus. One author reported the use of an intraoperative autorefractometer to determine the optimal power of the IOL to be implanted in these cases [21].

In more complicated scenarios where ICRS were previously implanted, K readings are even harder to predict. A subjective measurement technique was reported in a case series by Jarade et al. The technique consists of identifying an inner central effective optical zone that is subjectively determined according to the diameter of the ring segment inserted, pupil size, and the regularity of the central cornea. The surgeon averages the corneal curvature at 12 different circumferential corneal points between 2.7 to 3 mm diameter zone to obtain a K reading that will be used in the SRK/T formula [22]. In the same work, Jarade et al. described a method to obtain "near" accurate K reading in case of corneal ectasia after LASIK. Same method of averaging the central K reading is implemented, and the "real" value should be converted using the postrefractive surgery methods to obtain accurate K reading.

Furthermore, another reason for the inaccuracy in IOL power measurements is that keratoconus patients tend to have large axial lengths and deep anterior chambers, which makes the effective lens position less accurate compared to normal eyes [7, 23]. One study showed a higher correlation between axial length and postoperative spherical equivalence compared to keratometry [24].

In the latest review, published in 2020, summarizing the results of all the studies and case reports on IOL implantation in keratoconus [25], authors concluded that SRK/T formula yielded the best outcomes compared to the remaining third-generation (Hoffer Q and Holladay) and fourth-generation (Holladay 2, Haigis and Barrett Universal II) formulas used in the studies. Also, all the studies reported decrease in the accuracy of formulas in advance keratoconus with higher K readings.

Moreover, SRK/T formula was most accurate using topographic-guided keratometry, EyeSys(EyeSys, INC, Houston, TX) or Pentacam, for mild and moderate keratoconus, whereas both SRK/T and SRK II formulas were most reliable using either topography and manual keratometry for severe keratoconus [26].

Efforts are being made to improve the accuracy of IOL power calculations. The OCULUS Pentacam® AXL (OCULUS Optikgeraete GmbH; Wetzlar, Germany) is a new device which adds the axial length measurements and IOL power calculation for spherical and toric IOL to the usual tomography. The Optovue Cornea Advance (Optovue Inc., CA, USA) can measure directly both the anterior and the posterior corneal curvatures using an OCT technology. These advancements will make the choice of IOL power safer and more predictable in patients with keratoconus [27].

20.5 Intraocular Lens Choice

Monofocal IOL is the first choice in patients with advanced or progressive keratoconus. It is recommended to be implanted if a future keratoplasty is planned or if the patient is going to use RGP or scleral contact lens after cataract extraction. Placing a RGP lens, a scleral lens or performing a keratoplasty after a toric IOL implantation will make the toric degree manifest, resulting in increase in the cylindrical component and change in the refraction [28, 29]. Furthermore, monofocal IOL is recommended after ICRS implantation [10], a study evaluation of 70 eyes after sequential ICRS and monofocal IOL placement reported good visual outcomes [16].

In our new refractive surgery era, there is an increase demand on spectacle and contact lens independence after cataract surgeries. Multiple studies proved that toric IOL implantation during cataract surgery is effective in improving UDVA, CDVA, and spherical equivalence in keratoconus patients [8, 10, 24, 26, 30–36]. All these studies concluded that toric IOL is unpredictable in late stages and irregular corneal astigmatism and that it should be limited to stable, mild-to-moderate grade keratoconus and keep in mind, refractive manifest astigmatism before cataract development should coincide with the topographic astigmatism in order to proceed with toric IOL implantation [10].

In addition to the decreased outcome of toric IOL in case of irregular corneal astigmatism, there is an increased risk of postoperative IOL rotation. Postoperative change in the toric axis has been linked to high myopia and large capsular bag size. Since keratoconic eyes tend to be myopic with large axial lengths [23, 37]. It is assumed that they may have an enlarged capsular bag [38] leading to toric IOL rotation.

Toric multifocal/trifocal IOL was reported to be used in mild stable keratoconus, a case series of 10 eyes [30], and two case reports [39, 40] showed good near and distant visual acuity outcome. Another case series of 17 eyes reported good near and distance vision following sequential ICRS and an extended range of vision IOL implantation in patients with keratoconus and cataract [16]. Even though there is not enough evidence to recommend the use of these type of lenses, careful patient selection is advised before implanting one.

The IOL power calculation in case of planned triple procedure (phacoemulsification, IOL implantation and keratoplasty) is beyond the scope of this chapter. In summary, each case should be assessed for keratoconus severity and stability. The location of the cone and the regularity of the astigmatism should be well identified before making the appropriate IOL power selection, taking into consideration the patient's desire for distance vision, near vision, and independence from glasses or contact lens [41].

20.6 Surgical Technique

Modern phacoemulsification with smaller corneal incisions and new advancements in phacoemulsification machines has made the cataract extraction a safe and predictable surgery. Mild keratoconus cases can be managed as a normal cataract surgery. However, multiple challenges face the surgeons when operating on eyes with moderate to severe keratoconus.

First, corneal scarring and abnormal corneal collagen tissue increase the risk of wound leaking after clear corneal incisions. Second, an incision located on the steep corneal axis may destabilize the cornea by changing its shape in an unpredictable manner. Third, advanced keratoconus patients have unstable tear film and high irregular corneas which may distort the intraoperative surgeons view of the anterior chamber and increase the risk of complications [42].

Therefore, planning cataract surgical incision should be done preoperatively taking into consideration the topography and the pachymetry. In order to maintain the structural integrity of the cornea, it is recommended that the corneal incision is made as closer to the limbus as possible or using a scleral tunnel technique [23]. The main incision should be 90 degrees away from the steep corneal axis (supero-temporal in case of infero-temporal cone or temporal in very rare cases of superior cone). If a clear corneal incision is made, the surgeons should avoid operating through scarred tissue as wound may not bet self-sealing and they are advised to use 10–0 nylon so close the incision [42, 43]. A progression of ectasia has been reported to occur following cataract surgery [44], and one case report of a 38-year-old man whose cornea was stable following a cross-linking surgery had a rapid ectasia progression following cataract surgery [45].

In order to overcome an intraoperative image distortion in advanced cases of keratoconus, the surgeon may use the following maneuvers. Applying an ophthalmic viscosurgical device on the cornea may smoothen its surface and improve visibility, the drawback of this technique is that it is not sustainable due to surface exposure to active fluid flow from the instruments which will irrigate away the viscoelastic substance. Injecting trypan blue into the anterior chamber may improve the visibility of anterior capsule during capsulorrhexis. Intraoperative use of a regular RGP contact lens (9 mm) has been described before, and it was reported to improve the visibility and surgeon's depth of perception by overcoming the irregular astigmatism in advance corneal ectasia [46]. A larger modified RGP contact lens (12 mm) was recently reported to be used in case of optical distortion caused by keratoconus or corneal grafts (Fig. 20.2). It provided a wider view to the anterior chamber. Notches were drilled on the contact lens at the location of corneal incision, following the surgeon's preference, to improve its stability during ocular maneuvers [47].

An additional counseling is needed when a toric IOL insertion is planned. If the patient was found to have axial myopia (axial length>25 mm) with a large white to white measurements (>12.5 mm), a capsular tension ring placement may be considered to decrease the risk of IOL rotation postoperatively [41].

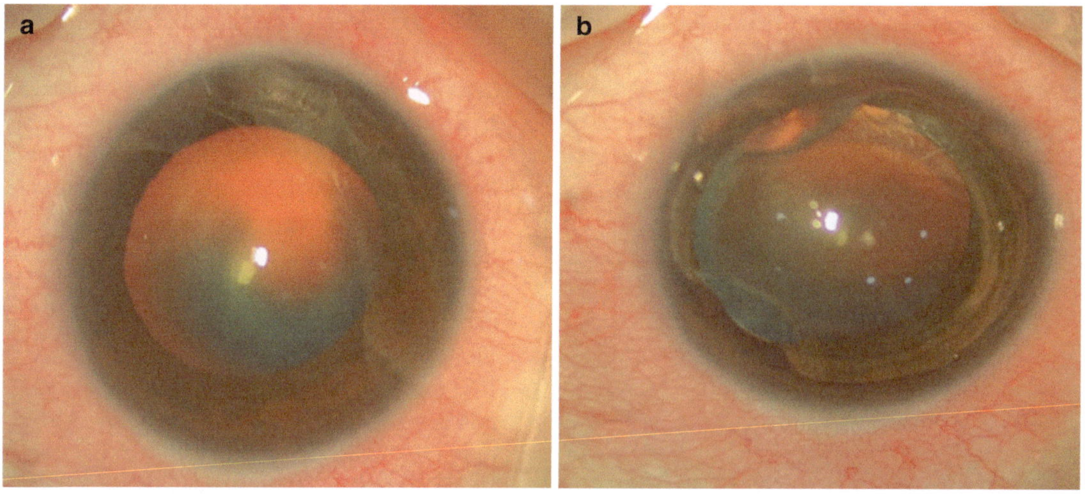

Fig. 20.2 Intraoperative view during cataract surgery showing: (**a**) microscope image distortion due to advance keratoconus and (**b**) clearer view to the anterior capsule when a notched RGP contact lens is placed over the cornea

20.7 Vision Recovery Following Cataract Surgery

Due to the unpredictability of IOL power calculation in keratoconus, especially in advanced disease, the surgeon may face refractive surprises after cataract surgery. Also, even if IOL calculation was accurate, the patient's vision may be suboptimal due to corneal irregularities, and they may require further interventions. The post-phacoemulsification visual rehabilitation may be surgical (lens-based or corneal-based) or nonsurgical (using contact lens or glasses).

20.7.1 Lens-Based Surgeries

In case of large refractive surprise after cataract surgery, the surgeon may elect to do an monofocal IOL exchange. in a study including 34 eyes with cataract and stage 1 and 2 keratoconus, 32% of the cases required an IOL exchange due to inaccurate IOL power calculation [21]. If the IOL was implanted more than 6 months ago, the capsular bag can be fibrosed, exchanging the IOL may pose additional risks to the patient, and therefore, piggyback IOL or phakic ICL implantation may be better choices. Recently, an article including 3 patients having toric ICL implantation following cataract surgery reported good outcomes in keratoconus [10].

20.7.2 Corneal-Based Surgeries

In case of minimal residual refractive errors after cataract surgery, corneal procedures may be considered. ICRS implantation after cataract surgery has never been attempted before. Due to the unpredictability of this surgery following IOL insertion, it is less likely to benefit these patients. However, topography-guided PRK has been proved safe and effective in keratoconus patients when performed simultaneously with CXL [48]. PRK may be attempted following noncomplicated cataract surgery in stable corneas previously treated with CXL. More studies need to be performed to prove the safety and long-term stability of this procedure.

20.7.3 Contact Lens

Contact lens use is cautiously considered safe and effective way to improve the BCVA following cataract surgery in keratoconus. It may avoid the risks related to the intraocular and the corneal surgeries previously mentioned but on the other hand, it -may impose a significant risk in the era of dry eyes, non-proper handling after cataract surgery in elderly people. RGP or scleral Lens may be required to achieve better refractive outcomes. The fitting of these contact lenses should be delayed until after the cataract surgery, because the corneal irregularity may change or worsen following corneal incisions [26, 44]. Furthermore, a bitoric RGP lens may be required to neutralize a new manifest astigmatism after a toric IOL malrotation.

20.8 Conclusion

Managing cataract and keratoconus require an extensive preoperative planning, good intraoperative execution, and careful postoperative rehabilitation. New devices are being evaluated for accurate biometric measurements in advanced keratoconus. Further studies are also needed to prove the accuracy of the newest fourth-generation formulas in calculating IOL power in all stages of keratoconus. Finally, we summarized below some useful tips that ophthalmologist can rely on when managing a keratoconus patient with cataract:

- Before proceeding with cataract surgery, ectasia stability should be documented, and the stage of keratoconus should be identified.
- If the ectasia was proved progressive, preoperative CXL is recommended at least 3 months prior to cataract surgery. However, if the topography was proved stable, reshaping the cornea with ICRS may be considered to optimize the outcomes of cataract surgery by improving the BCVA.
- Pentacam has the best repeatability in mild keratoconus, but other topographer has also good repeatability. All topographers and keratometers showed low accuracy when keratometry exceeded 55D.
- AL measurements are accurate using both optical and US biometers.
- SRK/T formula is currently the most accurate in calculating IOL power in mild keratoconus. All the formula's predictability is still debatable in advance stages of keratoconus.
- Using the smallest size incision, placing it 90 degrees away from the steep corneal axis and suturing the incision are ideal to preserve corneal stability.
- Toric IOL may be considered in mild stable keratoconus with a "relatively" less distorted corneal astigmatism, and the manifest astigmatic axis coincides with the topography astigmatic axis. If the axial length is >25 mm, capsular tension rings may be inserted for more stability.
- IOL exchange, piggyback IOL, ICL, and RGP contact lens can be considered in case of postoperative refractive error. More studies need to be performed before considering PRK as treatment of residual refractive error in stable corneas following CXL and cataract surgery.

References

1. Robine JM, Cubaynes S. Worldwide demography of centenarians. Mech Ageing Dev. 2017;165(Pt B):59–67.
2. Thebpatiphat N, Hammersmith KM, Rapuano CJ, Ayres BD, Cohen EJ. Cataract surgery in keratoconus. Eye Contact Lens. 2007;33(5):244–6.
3. Mehrjerdi MA, Hashemi H, Kalantari F, Rajabi MB, Tafti MR. Comparison of refractive outcomes of different intraocular lens power calculation formulas in keratoconic patients undergoing phacoemulsification. J Curr Ophthalmol. 2014;26(2):66.
4. Mas Tur V, MacGregor C, Jayaswal R, O'Brart D, Maycock N. A review of keratoconus: diagnosis, pathophysiology, and genetics. Surv Ophthalmol. 2017;62(6):770–83.
5. Lisa C, Fernández-Vega Cueto L, Poo-López A, Madrid-Costa D, Alfonso JF. Long-term follow-up of intrastromal corneal ring segments (210-degree arc length) in central keratoconus with high corneal Asphericity. Cornea. 2017;36(11):1325–30.
6. Antonios R, Dirani A, Fadlallah A, Chelala E, Hamade A, Cherfane C, Jarade E. Safety and visual outcome of Visian Toric ICL implantation after corneal collagen cross-linking in keratoconus: up to 2 years of follow-up. J Ophthalmol. 2015;2015:514834.
7. Bozorg S, Pineda R. Cataract and keratoconus: minimizing complications in intraocular lens calculations. Semin Ophthalmol. 2014;29(5–6):376–9.
8. Zvornicanin J, Cabric E, Jusufovic V, Musanovic Z, Zvornicanin E. Use of the toric intraocular lens for keratoconus treatment. Acta Inform Med. 2014;22(2):139–41.

9. Gokul A, Patel DV, Watters GA, McGhee CNJ. The natural history of corneal topographic progression of keratoconus after age 30 years in non-contact lens wearers. Br J Ophthalmol. 2017;101(6):839–44.
10. Arej N, Chanbour W, Zaarour K, Amro M, El-Rami H, Harb F, Jarade E. Management of cataract in keratoconus: early visual outcomes of different treatment modalities. Int J Ophthalmol. 2019;12(10):1654–8.
11. Goel S, Chua C, Butcher M, Jones CA, Bagga P, Kotta S. Laser vs ultrasound biometry--a study of intra- and interobserver variability. Eye (Lond). 2004;18(5):514–8.
12. Németh J, Fekete O, Pesztenlehrer N. Optical and ultrasound measurement of axial length and anterior chamber depth for intraocular lens power calculation. J Cataract Refract Surg. 2003;29(1):85–8.
13. Cınar Y, Cingü AK, Sahin M, Sahin A, Yüksel H, Türkcü FM, Cınar T, Caça I. Comparison of optical versus ultrasonic biometry in Keratoconic eyes. J Ophthalmol. 2013;2013:481238.
14. Baenninger PB, Bachmann LM, Wienecke L, Kaufmann C, Thiel MA. Effects and adverse events after CXL for keratoconus are independent of age: a 1-year follow-up study. Eye (Lond). 2014;28(6):691–5.
15. Tiveron MC Jr, Pena CRK, Hida RY, Moreira LB, Branco FRE, Kara-Junior N. Topographic outcomes after corneal collagen crosslinking in progressive keratoconus: 1-year follow-up. Arq Bras Oftalmol. 2017;80(2):93–6.
16. Alfonso JF, Lisa C, Fernández-Vega Cueto L, Poo-López A, Madrid-Costa D, Fernández-Vega L. Sequential intrastromal corneal ring segment and monofocal intraocular lens implantation for keratoconus and cataract: long-term follow-up. J Cataract Refract Surg. 2017;43(2):246–54.
17. Jarade EF, Abdelmassih Y, El-Khoury S. Reply. Am J Ophthalmol. 2017;181:183–4.
18. Piñero DP, Nieto JC, Lopez-Miguel A. Characterization of corneal structure in keratoconus. J Cataract Refract Surg. 2012;38(12):2167–83.
19. Hashemi H, Yekta A, Khabazkhoob M. Effect of keratoconus grades on repeatability of keratometry readings: comparison of 5 devices. J Cataract Refract Surg. 2015;41(5):1065–72.
20. Yağcı R, Kulak AE, Güler E, Tenlik A, Gürağaç FB, Hepşen İF. Comparison of anterior segment measurements with a dual Scheimpflug Placido corneal topographer and a new partial coherence interferometer in Keratoconic eyes. Cornea. 2015;34(9):1012–8.
21. Leccisotti A. Refractive lens exchange in keratoconus. J Cataract Refract Surg. 2006;32(5):742–6.
22. Jarade E, Dirani A, Fadlallah A, Chelala E, Fakhoury H, Cherfan G. Intraocular lens power calculation after intracorneal ring segment surgery for the treatment of post-LASIK ectasia. SM Opthalmol J. 2015;1(1):1005.
23. Ernst BJ, Hsu HY. Keratoconus association with axial myopia: a prospective biometric study. Eye Contact Lens. 2011;37(1):2–5.
24. Alió JL, Peña-García P, Abdulla Guliyeva F, Soria FA, Zein G, Abu-Mustafa SK. MICS with toric intraocular lenses in keratoconus: outcomes and predictability analysis of postoperative refraction. Br J Ophthalmol. 2014;98(3):365–70.
25. Garzón N, Arriola-Villalobos P, Felipe G, Poyales F, García-Montero M. Intraocular lens power calculation in eyes with keratoconus. J Cataract Refract Surg. 2020;46(5):778–83.
26. Hashemi H, Heidarian S, Seyedian MA, Yekta A, Khabazkhoob M. Evaluation of the results of using Toric IOL in the cataract surgery of keratoconus patients. Eye Contact Lens. 2015;41(6):354–8.
27. Ghiasian L, Abolfathzadeh N, Manafi N, Hadavandkhani A. Intraocular lens power calculation in keratoconus; a review of literature. J Curr Ophthalmol. 2019;31(2):127–34.
28. Watson MP, Anand S, Bhogal M, Gore D, Moriyama A, Pullum K, Hau S, Tuft SJ. Cataract surgery outcome in eyes with keratoconus. Br J Ophthalmol. 2014;98(3):361–4.
29. Mol IE, Van Dooren BT. Toric intraocular lenses for correction of astigmatism in keratoconus and after corneal surgery. Clin Ophthalmol. 2016;10:1153–9.
30. Farideh D, Azad S, Feizollah N, Sana N, Cyrus A, Mohammad G, Alireza BR. Clinical outcomes of new toric trifocal diffractive intraocular lens in patients with cataract and stable keratoconus: six months follow-up. Medicine (Baltimore). 2017;96(12):e6340.
31. Sauder G, Jonas JB. Treatment of keratoconus by toric foldable intraocular lenses. Eur J Ophthalmol. 2003;13(6):577–9.
32. Navas A, Suárez R. One-year follow-up of toric intraocular lens implantation in forme fruste keratoconus. J Cataract Refract Surg. 2009;35(11):2024–7.
33. Visser N, Gast ST, Bauer NJ, Nuijts RM. Cataract surgery with toric intraocular lens implantation in keratoconus: a case report. Cornea. 2011;30(6):720–3.
34. Jaimes M, Xacur-García F, Alvarez-Melloni D, Graue-Hernández EO, Ramirez-Luquín T, Navas A. Refractive lens exchange with toric intraocular lenses in keratoconus. J Refract Surg. 2011;27(9):658–64.
35. Nanavaty MA, Lake DB, Daya SM. Outcomes of pseudophakic toric intraocular lens implantation in Keratoconic eyes with cataract. J Refract Surg. 2012;28(12):884–9.
36. Parikakis EA, Chatziralli IP, Peponis VG, David G, Chalkiadakis S, Mitropoulos PG. Toric intraocular lens implantation for correction of astigmatism in cataract patients with corneal ectasia. Case Rep Ophthalmol. 2013;4(3):219–28.
37. Yağcı R, Güler E, Kulak AE, Erdoğan BD, Balcı M, Hepşen İF. Repeatability and reproducibility of a new optical biometer in normal and keratoconic eyes. J Cataract Refract Surg. 2015;41(1):171–7.
38. Zhu X, He W, Zhang K, Lu Y. Factors influencing 1-year rotational stability of AcrySof Toric intraocular lenses. Br J Ophthalmol. 2016;100(2):263–8.

39. Montano M, López-Dorantes KP, Ramirez-Miranda A, Graue-Hernández EO, Navas A. Multifocal toric intraocular lens implantation for forme fruste and stable keratoconus. J Refract Surg. 2014;30(4):282–5.
40. Ouchi M, Kinoshita S. Implantation of refractive multifocal intraocular lens with a surface-embedded near section for cataract eyes complicated with a coexisting ocular pathology. Eye (Lond). 2015;29(5):649–55.
41. Moshirfar M, Walker BD, Birdsong OC. Cataract surgery in eyes with keratoconus: a review of the current literature. Curr Opin Ophthalmol. 2018;29(1):75–80.
42. Aiello F, Nasser QJ, Nucci C, Angunawela RI, Gatzioufas Z, Maurino V. Cataract surgery in patients with keratoconus: pearls and pitfalls. Open Ophthalmol J. 2017;11:194–200.
43. Bourges JL. Cataract surgery in keratoconus with irregular astigmatism. In: Goggin M, editor. Astigmatism: Optics, Physiology and Management. InTech; 2012. p. 93–102.
44. Jurkunas U, Azar DT. Potential complications of ocular surgery in patients with coexistent keratoconus and Fuchs' endothelial dystrophy. Ophthalmology. 2006;113(12):2187–97.
45. Labiris G, Panagiotopoulou EK, Ntonti P, Taliantzis S. Corneal ectasia following cataract extraction surgery in a patient with keratoconus: a case report. J Med Case Rep. 2019;13(1):296.
46. Oie Y, Kamei M, Matsumura N, Fujimoto H, Soma T, Koh S, Tsujikawa M, Maeda N, Nishida K. Rigid gas-permeable contact lens-assisted cataract surgery in patients with severe keratoconus. J Cataract Refract Surg. 2014;40(3):345–8.
47. Chanbour W, Harb F, Jarade E. A modified customized rigid gas permeable contact lens to improve visualization during phacoemulsification in Ectatic corneas. Med Hypothesis Discov Innov Ophthalmol. 2020;9(1):1–6.
48. Kanellopoulos AJ. Ten-year outcomes of progressive keratoconus management with the Athens protocol (topography-guided partial-refraction PRK combined with CXL). J Refract Surg. 2019;35(8):478–83.

Refractive Surgery in Management of Keratoconus

21

Jorge L. Alió, Ali Nowrouzi, and Jorge L. Alió del Barrio

21.1 Introduction

Keratoconus has always been considered a contraindication of refractive surgery since its early development. Refractive surgical procedures, simply speaking, were contraindicated and even the subject of negligence or wrong indication since early years. However, since the introduction of cross-linking and the improved knowledge of the progress of keratoconus, refractive surgical techniques have been applied successfully to keratoconus in selected cases. Intraocular refractive surgery with phakic intraocular lenses in stable keratoconus and selected customized corneal surface excimer laser treatments by total or corneal wavefront aberrometry have gained popularity as they improve the vision of these patients without the risk of inducing further problems.

Refractive surgery is frequently needed in keratoconus due to the aniseikonia and anisometropia generated by the evolution of the disease.

J. L. Alió (✉) · J. L. Alió del Barrio
Cornea, Cataract and Refractive Surgery Unit, Vissum (Miranza Group), Alicante, Spain

Department of Ophthalmology, Universidad Miguel Hernández de Elche, Alicante, Spain
e-mail: jlalio@vissum.com

A. Nowrouzi
Centro de Oftalmología Quirónsalud Marbella, Marbella, Spain

VISSUM Instituto Oftalmológico de Alicante, Alicante, Spain

This chapter brings together the most recent information about refractive surgical procedures in keratoconus, when they are indicated, how they are to be performed, and the results that have been reported so far by the evidence available.

Keratoconus provides a decrease in quality of life to the patients who suffer from it. The treatment used as well as the method to correct the refractive error of these patients may influence the impact of this disease. It is important to note the recent advances in collagen cross-linking for creating a stable corneal condition for the corneal refractive procedure, especially excimer laser surgery.

Corneal collagen cross-linking (CXL) is the treatment for progressive keratoconus, as it is the only available treatment option capable of halting the natural progression of the disease, achieving its stabilization in more than 90% of treated patients [1], and biomechanical studies have shown that CXL increases human corneal rigidity over three times [2]. Considering this increase in corneal stiffness, a cross-linked human cornea should be able to afford a limited tissue ablation without negatively impacting the stabilization of the corneal ectasia. Moreover, although CXL is capable of flattening the cone, this effect is usually limited (1-2D on average) and so the corrected distance visual acuity (CDVA) lines gain (1 line on average).

Excimer laser surgery can be used for refractive purposes in selected cases of stable keratoconus for lower refractive errors, but its use is

S. Das (ed.), *Keratoconus*, https://doi.org/10.1007/978-981-19-4262-4_21

controversial because of the association of a significant level of higher-order aberration in keratoconus corneas. This is why today excimer laser surgery is used as a therapeutic tool guided by aberrometry and looking for refractive therapeutic purposes and associated usually to collagen cross-link (CXL). This procedure aims to improve jointly the visual quality of the patient and the refraction of the treated eye.

Significant loss of CDVA lines (CDVA<0.8) may be potentially an indication of combined CXL-customized photorefractive keratectomy (PRK) treatment by corneal "reshaping" procedure, to increase regularity and recover part of the visual potential. By this therapeutic approach, contact lens dependence will be reduced, and the patient will be able to either wear spectacles again comfortably or remove the residual ametropia on an intraocular plane.

The first target on the visual rehabilitation of a keratoconic eye should be the regularization of the secondary irregular astigmatism and reducing higher-order aberrations (HOA), as the main problem of such patients is the dependence on rigid or scleral contact lenses due to the loss of lines of CDVA with spectacles. Corneal reshaping procedures aim to regularize the cornea by reducing HOA, and intracorneal ring segments (ICRS) are the paradigm of such procedures.

In recent years, several surface excimer laser ablation protocols combined with CXL treatment have been suggested as a therapeutic refractive procedure to "reshape" the keratoconic cornea (and so increase the visual potential at a spectacle plane) while halting the progression of the disease for cases of early or moderate keratoconus. This use of laser treatment as a combination with CXL is a new refractive therapeutic approach for keratoconus eyes.

21.2 Corneal Therapeutic Laser Refractive Surgery

The vast majority of evidence on using CXL simultaneous or before PRK to "reshape" the cornea applies to mild–moderate forms of keratoconus [3, 4]. Nevertheless, the idea is always to leave enough underlying stroma to be able to perform afterward a CXL procedure. This fact practically excludes more advanced cases with thinner corneas.

The major consideration when planning a combined procedure of PRK-CXL in a keratoconus patient is the expected post-ablation residual stromal thickness, as the safety of the subsequent CXL procedure must not be compromised. Combined PRK-CXL protocols have proven to be capable of halting the progression of the ectasia with similar efficacy to CXL alone [3, 4]. However, with better outcomes in CDVA, uncorrected distance visual acuity (UDVA), and spherical equivalent refraction, Kontadakis et al published the long-term outcomes of their protocol compared to CXL alone (mean follow-up of 3 years) [5].

Progressive keratoconus patients (with a mean age at operation of 28 years) were selected. The average ablation depth in the tPRK-CXL group was 33.9 μm. CDVA in the tPRK-CXL group improved from 0.26 to 0.09 (logMAR), while in the CXL alone group improved from 0.24 to 0.15 (differences among groups were significant postoperatively while not preoperatively). No patient lost more than 2 lines of visual acuity in any group, whereas 63% of eyes in the tPRK-CXL group gained 2 or more lines of CDVA, and only 27% of eyes in the CXL group did. In the same fashion, unaided distance visual acuity (UDVA) in the tPRK-CXL group improved from 0.83 to 0.27 (logMAR), while in the CXL alone group improved from 0.86 to 0.69 (differences among groups were significant postoperatively while not preoperatively). tPRK-CXL induced a significantly higher keratometric flattening than CXL alone. Spherical equivalent refraction in the tPRK-CXL group improved from −3.73 to −1.54D, while in the CXL alone group improved from −4.15 to −3.79D (differences among groups were significant postoperatively while not preoperatively). Depth of CXL treatment was also deeper in the tPRK-CXL group (299.7 vs 269.8 microns). No differences were found in endothelial cell density. Finally, 6.7% of eyes in both groups were suspicious of ectasia progression. 47% developed mild posterior stroma haze.

Different authors have reported equivalent outcomes with similar protocols [6].

It is an important issue that ablating corneal tissue in patients whose corneal biomechanics are already altered is a risk factor for ectasia becoming progressive, so PRK on its own without CXL should not be considered as the technique of choice in stable keratoconus due to doubts concerning long-term stability.

21.2.1 Combined Protocols: Efficacy and Safety

Nowadays, there is extensive evidence for combined PRK-CXL protocols regarding the safety of these procedures on halting the progression of the cone, while providing better visual outcomes than CXL alone, for cases of mild-to-moderate keratoconus [3, 4]. Different variety of protocols have been suggested, and they differ on the inclusion criteria, ablation depths, ablation patterns, CXL protocol (Dresden, accelerated or customized), use or not of MMC, and timing of the CXL (sequential or simultaneous to the PRK). We must remember that all these protocols use surface ablations (never LASIK or SMILE due to their impact on corneal biomechanics).

21.2.2 PRK + CXL: Simultaneous or Sequential?

CXL has a direct impact on corneal keratometry and aberrometry, so the manifest refraction changes are unavoidable. Because of this, some authors suggested performing the excimer ablation 6–12 months after the CXL, to have a more predictable and stable effect after the CXL effect on corneal topography [7]. However, we should remind that CXL effects on visual, topographic, and aberrometric parameters continue in the long term, even years after the CXL procedure, and do not become fully stable within the first postoperative year [8]. It is important to emphasize that further topographic changes can still happen even after 12 months in a sequential approach. CXL effect is proven to continue even years after the procedure (mainly in Dresden protocol), so overcorrections are possible and a specific refractive/visual target may not be achieved. The goal of such procedures is "therapeutic" and not "refractive," and the patient should be informed according to this idea.

Moreover, the sequential approach raises some other concerns: (a) The ablation rate of cross-linked corneas may vary from that of the untreated corneas, which may affect predictability; (b) corneal tissue already stiffened by CXL is removed during the PRK procedure, potentially diminishing the benefits of CXL; (c) the probability of post-PRK haze might differ since CXL induces apoptosis of anterior stromal keratocytes, which may lower the probability of postoperative haze formation if the excimer ablation is applied simultaneously. With a sequential approach, cross-linked stroma becomes repopulated by host keratocytes, which probably explains the higher risk of haze observed with this approach [9].

Kanellopoulos compared these techniques: The sequential group had topo-guided PRK 6 months after the CXL procedure (127 eyes); the simultaneous group had a CXL procedure immediately after topo-guided PRK with MMC (198 eyes) [10]. The latter demonstrated statistically superior results in CDVA, spherical equivalent (SE) reduction, keratometric flattening, and grade of corneal haze. Furthermore, it was not observed progression of ectasia in either group after a mean follow-up of 36 months, so they concluded that same-day simultaneous topography-guided PRK and CXL appear to be superior to sequential CXL with later PRK in the visual rehabilitation of progressing keratoconus [10].

Although a recent review reported that sequential CXL followed by surface ablation showed greater improvements in CDVA, SE, and refractive astigmatism compared to simultaneous PRK-CXL. These results might be biased since different protocols have been selected in the study [9] which needs further studies to confirm these results.

21.2.3 Transepithelial PTK + CXL with Better Results Compared to Manual Epithelial Debridement

Initially, Kymionis et al demonstrated that epithelial removal using 50 μm transPTK (tPTK) during CXL resulted in better visual and refractive outcomes in comparison with regular manual epithelial debridement [11]. It is important to take into consideration that 50 μm tPTK to remove the epithelium before CXL does not do the homogenized ablation even at the cone site. It will partially ablate some stroma at the apex of the cone (regularizing the cornea) considering that epithelial thickness gets thinner at this point and thicker around the cone [12]. Considering this finding, a properly customized ablation could enhance these results by a more controlled and personalized ablation of the cone stroma, and so topo-guided surface ablation protocols were developed.

Utilizing high-resolution OCT during transepithelial ablation might be a good solution to do highly double customized corneal ablation based on different epithelial layer thicknesses in keratoconus. Finally, the masking effect of the corneal epithelium is the greatest ally to regularize the abnormal keratoconic corneal stroma surface, so transPRK protocols have a higher rationale than regular PRK protocols with previous epithelial removal.

21.2.4 Wavefront-Guided PRK

Despite 50 μm maximum ablation criteria are commonly used, this limit has been established empirically and arbitrarily, and we shall remember that we are ablating tissue on a biomechanically altered cornea, and so the less ablation the better. Recently, new wavefront-guided protocols have been developed to minimize tissue removal by targeting only selected higher-order aberrations. By this approach, the target is to reduce irregular astigmatism. Nevertheless, by targeting some HOA only (with no compensatory additional tissue removal), a spherocylindrical shift still occurs, but corneal tissue removal depths are reduced to the minimum required to improve irregular astigmatism. After these, spectacles or phakic IOLs can be used at a later time to complete the visual rehabilitation (Fig. 21.1).

21.2.4.1 Surgical Technique

Ocular or corneal wavefront-guided transepithelial PRK with tissue-saving algorithm (targeting only the most relevant HOA, minimizing tissue removal, and not considering subjective refraction), with a limit of 325 μm of minimum residual stromal thickness after tPRK and before CXL is planned. Simultaneous pulsed accelerated CXL protocol (10 min riboflavin 0.1% soaking followed by 30 mW/cm [2] for 8 min; 7.2 J/cm [2]) is applied. No mitomycin C (MMC) is applied. Optical zone considered is 7.5 mm.

21.2.4.2 Outcomes

Gore et al published the long-term outcomes of their protocol (mean follow-up of 2 years) and compared the outcomes with a historical database of pulsed accelerated CXL only [13]. Progressive keratoconus patients (with a mean age at operation of 24 years) were selected. All treatments delivered were finally ocular wavefront-guided, as predicted tissue ablation depths in ocular wavefront-guided programming were significantly less than corresponding predicted tissue ablation depths for corneal wavefront-guided treatments (mean difference of 25 μm among both treatment plans). The average ablation depth in the tPRK-CXL group was 34 μm at the cone apex. CDVA in the tPRK-CXL group significantly improved from 0.28 to 0.15 logMAR, while in the CXL alone group improved from 0.22 to 0.17 (p = 0.06). Gains of CDVA lines were more common after tPRK–CXL (53% of eyes) than after CXL alone (29% of eyes). CDVA loss due to persistent anterior corneal haze occurred in 6% of tPRK–CXL cases and 13% of CXL alone cases. UDVA in the tPRK-CXL group improved from 0.72 to 0.52 logMAR, while in the CXL alone group remained stable (from 0.63 to 0.66). tPRK-CXL induced a significantly higher flattening of the maximum keratometry than CXL alone, while mean keratometry

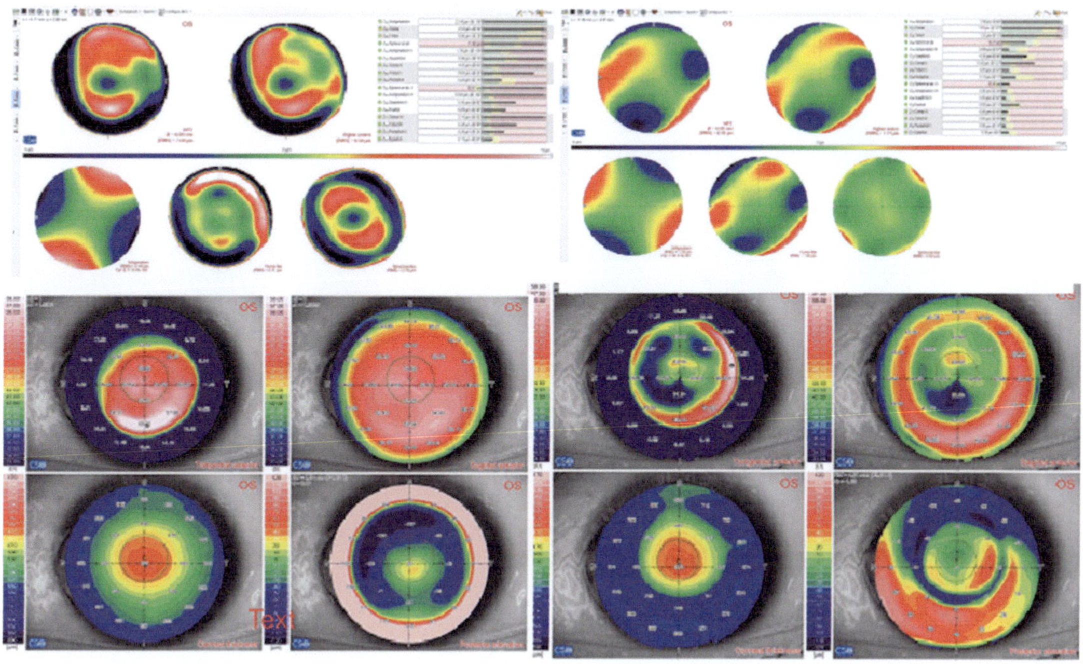

Fig. 21.1 Corneal anterior keratometry (down) and aberrometry (up) maps of a patient with moderate keratoconus (left) treated with a combined wavefront-guided transPRK with simultaneous Dresden protocol corneal collagen cross-linking (right). UDVA changed from 0.5 (decimal scale; preoperative) to 0.8 (6 months postoperative). CDVA changed from 0.6 (decimal scale; preoperative) to 0.9 (6 months postoperative)

remained stable in both groups. Manifest refraction in the tPRK-CXL group improved approximately 2D in the cylinder but showed 1D of myopic shift, while in the CXL alone group remained stable postoperatively. No differences were found in endothelial cell density; an increase in corneal densitometry (haze) was similar in both groups. Finally, 8% of eyes in both groups were suspicious of ectasia progression.

21.3 Therapeutic Refractive Surgery of Keratoconus with Phakic IOLs

In patients with contact lenses, intolerance implantation of pIOLs should be considered when the patient has stable refraction as ongoing keratoconus progression can affect the long-term outcomes. Phakic IOLs are also suitable for eyes without advanced keratoconus with acceptable best-corrected visual acuity or without highly irregular astigmatism. Recently, utilizing procedures such as reduction of irregular astigmatism and corneal regularization with ICRS and topography-guided transepithelial PRK (ttPRK) and wavefront-guided transepithelial PRK opens a great perspective of the possibility to exclusively correct higher-order aberrations (HOA) and improving CDVA to implant pIOL in these cases as a secondary approach [14].

It is obvious that pIOLs just can correct only spherical and cylindrical errors. Eyes with keratoconus are known to have significant HOAs, with high levels of vertical coma, primary coma, and coma-like aberrations, that could affect the visual quality [15].

These HOAs, which are uncorrected by pIOLs, could affect the final visual outcomes. For these cases with high HOAs, the wavefront-guided transepithelial PRK with CXL before implantation of pIOLs could be a good solution that permits obtaining better visual outcomes in such cases (Fig. 21.2) [16].

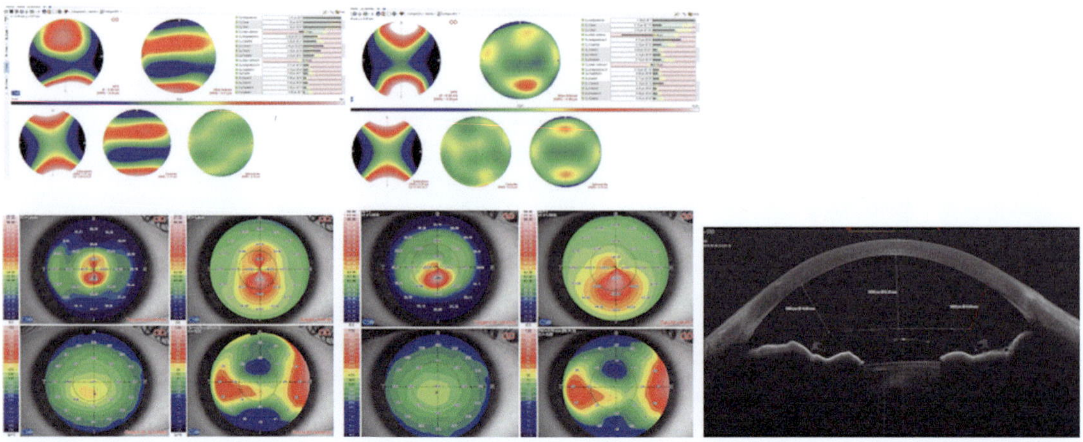

Fig. 21.2 Corneal anterior keratometry (down) and aberrometry (up) maps of a patient with moderate keratoconus (left) treated with a combined wavefront-guided transPRK with simultaneous Dresden protocol corneal collagen cross-linking (right). UDVA changed from 0.15 (decimal scale; preoperative) to 0.2 (6 months postoperative). CDVA changed from 0.3 (decimal scale; preoperative) to 0.5 (6 months postoperative). OCT (right) Phakic IOL toric Artiflex

21.3.1 Implantation Criteria

There are two major groups of implantation criteria for implantation of pIOLs in keratoconus patients. The first group is the minimum requirements for keratoconus eyes to define it as stable disease. The second group of implantation criteria is the essential anatomical requirement of the eye to be a good candidate for these kinds of implantation in general.

Correcting the refractive error in keratoconus using the pIOL is an off-label use of the lens. Particular care should be taken to ensure that the refractive error is stable or stabilized in these patients. Stable keratoconus may be defined as stable refraction in the eye with no surgical intervention for 2 years. Once the patient has attained stable refraction for 3 consecutive months, the keratoconus may be considered stable, although some authors believe in a longer period of six consecutive months to define it as stable. Indications for phakic IOL implantation in these cases should be BSCVA of 20/50 or better, clear central cornea, keratometric values ≤52.00D, stable refraction (cylinder ≤3.00D) for 2 years, refractive axes stability in 1 year, the optical power of steepest corneal meridian changes less than 1 diopter, and corneal thickness change less than 25 microns in 1 year [17].

Stabilized keratoconus is an essential requirement for implanting the pIOLs; if the keratoconus is not stable, the accepted approach will be stabilization of the disease at first utilizing other therapeutic options such as CXL, ICRs, and then after the stabilization confirmation planning to implant the pIOLs.

Some authors implanted toric pIOLS in mild-to-moderate progressive keratoconus after stabilizing the disease through CXL, ICRs, and confirmation of refractive and topographic stabilization before pIOLs implantation [18, 19].

Combined treatment planning for stabilization might be an essential approach in some cases before implanting pIOLs. For the safe implantation of these pIOLs, there are recommendations for each model that must be considered before the implantation.

As a general recommendation for all model minimal endothelial cell count, ECC should be at least 2400 with a coefficient of variation (CV) of more than 0.4 and hexagonality of more than 50% of all endothelial cells. Anterior chamber depth (ACD) should be more than 3 mm [20].

Another important consideration is the possibility of laser correction after pIOLs implantation to touch up residual undesirable refractive errors as well as possible causes of progression after pIOLs implantation which could be restabilized by CXL and correct possible new HOAs after such progressions.

Summarizing, if adequately selected, combined PRK-CXL procedures provide patients the benefit of stability offered by CXL but with the additional benefit of improved visual performance and quality of vision, which translates into a better quality of life with less dependence on contact lenses.

Financial Support This study has been supported in part by the Red Temática de Investigación Cooperativa en Salud (RETICS), reference number RD16/0008/0012, funded by Instituto de Salud Carlos III and co-funded by European Regional Development Fund (ERDF), "A way to make Europe."

References

1. O'Brart DPS. Corneal collagen crosslinking for corneal ectasias: a review. Eur J Ophthalmol. 2017;27(3):253–69.
2. Wollensak G. Crosslinking treatment of progressive keratoconus: new hope. Curr Opin Ophthalmol. 2006;17(4):356–60.
3. Al-Mohaimeed MM. Combined corneal CXL and photorefractive keratectomy for treatment of keratoconus: a review. Int J Ophthalmol. 2019;12(12):1929–38.
4. Zhu AY, Jun AS, Soiberman US. Combined protocols for corneal collagen cross-linking with photorefractive surgery for refractive Management of Keratoconus: Update on Techniques and Review of Literature. Ophthalmol Ther. 2019;8(Suppl-1):15–31.
5. Kontadakis GA, Kankariya VP, Tsoulnaras K, Pallikaris AI, Plaka A, Kymionis GD. Long-term comparison of simultaneous topography-guided photorefractive keratectomy followed by corneal cross-linking versus corneal cross-linking alone. Ophthalmology. 2016;123(5):974–83.
6. Alessio G, L'abbate M, Sborgia C, La Tegola MG. Photorefractive keratectomy followed by cross-linking versus cross-linking alone for management of progressive keratoconus: two-year follow-up. Am J Ophthalmol. 2013;155(1):54–65.e1.
7. Nattis AS, Rosenberg ED, Donnenfeld ED. One-year visual and astigmatic outcomes of keratoconus patients following sequential crosslinking and topography-guided surface ablation: the TOPOLINK study. J Cataract Refract Surg. 2020;46(4):507–16.
8. O'Brart DP, Patel P, Lascaratos G, Wagh VK, Tam C, Lee J, O'Brart NA. Corneal cross-linking to halt the progression of keratoconus and corneal ectasia: seven-year follow-up. Am J Ophthalmol. 2015;160(6):1154–63.
9. Bardan AS, Lee H, Nanavaty MA. Outcomes of simultaneous and sequential cross-linking with excimer laser surface ablation in keratoconus. J Refract Surg. 2018;34(10):690–6.
10. Kanellopoulos AJ. Comparison of sequential vs same-day simultaneous collagen cross-linking and topography-guided PRK for treatment of keratoconus. J Refract Surg. 2009;25(9):S812–8.
11. Kymionis GD, Grentzelos MA, Kounis GA, Diakonis VF, Limnopoulou AN, Panagopoulou SI. Combined transepithelial phototherapeutic keratectomy and corneal collagen cross-linking for progressive keratoconus. Ophthalmology. 2012;119(9):1777–84.
12. Reinstein DZ, Gobbe M, Archer TJ, Silverman RH, Coleman DJ. Epithelial, stromal, and total corneal thickness in keratoconus: three-dimensional display with Artemis very-high frequency digital ultrasound. J Refract Surg. 2010;26(4):259–71.
13. Gore DM, Leucci MT, Anand V, Fernandez-Vega Cueto L, Arba Mosquera S, Allan BD. Combined wavefront-guided transepithelial photorefractive keratectomy and corneal crosslinking for visual rehabilitation in moderate keratoconus. J Cataract Refract Surg. 2018;44(5):571–80.
14. Ferreira GA, Ghanem VC, Tavares RLP, Ghanem RC. Toric artisan after transepithelial topography-guided photorefractive keratectomy for higher-order aberrations following intrastromal corneal ring segments in keratoconus - Trioptics. Indian J Ophthalmol. 2020;68(11):2564–7.
15. Piñero DP, Alió JL, Alesón A, Escaf M, Miranda M. Pentacam posterior and anterior corneal aberrations in normal and keratoconic eyes. Clin Exp Optom. 2009;92(3):297–303.
16. Coskunseven E, Sharma DP, Grentzelos MA, Sahin O, Kymionis GD, Pallikaris I. Four-stage procedure for keratoconus: ICRS implantation, corneal cross-linking, Toric Phakic intraocular lens implantation, and topography-guided photorefractive keratectomy. J Refract Surg. 2017;33(10):683–9.
17. Espandar L, Meyer J. Keratoconus: overview and update on treatment. Middle East Afr J Ophthalmol. 2010;17(1):15–20.
18. Güell JL, Morral M, Malecaze F, Gris O, Elies D, Manero F. Collagen crosslinking and toric iris-claw phakic intraocular lens for myopic astigmatism in progressive mild to moderate keratoconus. J Cataract Refract Surg. 2012;38(3):475–84.
19. Alió JL, Peña-García P, Abdulla Guliyeva F, Soria FA, Zein G, Abu-Mustafa SK. MICS with toric intraocular lenses in keratoconus: outcomes and predictability analysis of postoperative refraction. Br J Ophthalmol. 2014;98(3):365–70.
20. Alió JL, Azar DT, editors. Management of complications in refractive surgery. 2nd ed. Springer; 2018.

22 Artificial Intelligence in the Diagnosis and Management of Keratoconus

Nicole Hallett, Chris Hodge, Jing Jing You, Yu Guang Wang, and Gerard Sutton

22.1 Introduction

Across all health paradigms, early disease diagnosis and the implementation of appropriate treatment protocols will optimize the potential short- and long-term outcomes for our patients. With the introduction of collagen cross-linking to halt the progression of keratoconus, early identification of both at-risk patients and those likely to progress is vital to maintaining best-corrected visual acuity. Often, both diagnosis and treatment decisions represent a nuanced combination of specialist experience and evidence-based outcomes. Diagnostic classifications and flow charts, which essentially aim to formalize the surgeon's approach, have been available for many years within the keratoconus literature; however, the increasing ability to generate significant clinical data combined with rapidly developing computational capabilities has provided corneal specialists an opportunity to be at the forefront of machine learning approaches [1]. Within this chapter, we aim to discuss the development of the algorithmic approach to the diagnosis and treatment of keratoconus with an emphasis on the recent incorporation of artificial intelligence within the clinical and surgical environment.

22.1.1 Machine Learning and Keratoconus

Machine learning techniques have been utilized across ophthalmic screening and analysis for a range of conditions including glaucoma, diabetic retinopathy, neovascular macular degeneration, uveitis, cataract surgery, and visual field interpretation [2–9].

N. Hallett · J. J. You
Faculty of Medicine and Health, Clinical Ophthalmology and Eye Health, Save Sight Institute, The University of Sydney, Sydney, NSW, Australia
e-mail: nhal6992@uni.sydney.edu.au; jing.you@sydney.edu.au

C. Hodge
Faculty of Medicine and Health, Clinical Ophthalmology and Eye Health, Save Sight Institute, The University of Sydney, Sydney, NSW, Australia

Vision Eye Institute, Chatswood, NSW, Australia

Graduate School of Health, The University of Technology, Sydney, NSW, Australia
e-mail: christopher.hodge@vei.com.au

Y. G. Wang
Institute of Natural Sciences, School of Mathematical Sciences, and Key Laboratory of Scientific and Engineering Computing of Ministry of Education (MOE-LSC), Shanghai Jiao Tong University, Shanghai, China
e-mail: yuguang.wang@sjtu.edu.cn

G. Sutton (✉)
Faculty of Medicine and Health, Clinical Ophthalmology and Eye Health, Save Sight Institute, The University of Sydney, Sydney, NSW, Australia

Vision Eye Institute, Chatswood, NSW, Australia
e-mail: gerard.sutton@vei.com.au

S. Das (ed.), *Keratoconus*, https://doi.org/10.1007/978-981-19-4262-4_22

To fully appreciate the potential role of machine learning within the keratoconus paradigm, it is necessary to have a basic understanding of artificial intelligence, in particular the general terminology and the relative advantages and disadvantages of the various existing approaches. In this section, we address the definitions commonly used within this environment and review the key technologies to provide a platform for the eventual assessment of current pathways researchers have taken to aid the diagnosis and treatment of keratoconus.

22.2 Introduction to Machine Learning and Artificial Intelligence

Rather than a specific approach, artificial intelligence (AI) itself represents a broad description for the collection of technologies utilized to perform tasks and solve problems without explicit human guidance [1]. This general-purpose technology can provide unique learning capabilities and the potential for wide-ranging improvements to the way we undertake medical research and assessment [2].

AI emerged as a simple theory as early as the 1950s, described as "giving computers the ability to learn without being programmed." [10] In medical imaging, a more appropriate definition of AI would be "a system's ability to correctly interpret external data, to learn from such data, and to use those learnings to achieve specific goals and tasks through flexible adaptation." [11] As evident through many recent advances in image recognition and pathology diagnosis, AI is ideally suited to medicine [12].

22.2.1 Machine Learning Terminology

Before considering the current and potential applications of AI to the field of ophthalmology and more specifically to keratoconus, it is important to define and explore key aspects of this field.

As the terminology often overlaps or is simply misused, some confusion exists around the relationships between AI, machine learning, and deep learning. As outlined in Fig. 22.1, artificial intelligence represents the overarching term, with machine learning and then deep learning being subsets within this broad area. Data mining and machine learning have the same goal of discovering the unknown properties within the data. Machine learning uses more modern statistical and mathematical methods, and the emerging deep learning technology facilitates models that can analyze data efficiently, powerfully, and on a much larger scale than traditional statistical analysis. The key distinction between statistics and machine learning is while statistics are used to provide inference based on a sample, machine

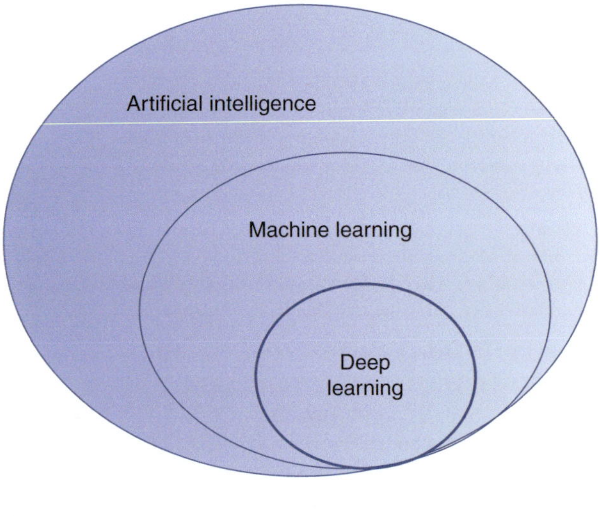

Fig. 22.1 Relationship between artificial intelligence, machine learning, and deep learning

learning seeks to result in repeatable predictions through the identification of patterns within the data.

Machine learning (ML) is the utilization of algorithms that are trained to improve through adapting to patterns in data by ongoing exposure and experience. Machine learning is classified as either supervised, semi-supervised, or unsupervised:

- Supervised learning identifies patterns to relate variables to measured outcomes, such as an automatically fitted regression model. Supervised learning, as the name suggests, is led by the researcher who provides the variables and/or research question.
- Semi-supervised learning utilizes labels provided by the researcher to infer classification or regression through the subsequent analysis.
- Unsupervised learning generally seeks to find patterns in unlabeled data and is external to researcher input.

It is important to note that within the management of big data, semi-supervised and unsupervised models are often utilized as data mining techniques to extend or generate a range of additional models. These can then be applied as precursors to supervised models, which will finally be employed to predict outcomes or undertake a rigorous statistical analysis [13, 14].

A node (or neuron) is the basic unit of a neural network. Similar to a biological neuron, these (neural) networks comprise significant numbers of nodes and layers (or perceptrons). Deep learning techniques typically rely on multiple layers for the eventual extraction and transformation of their features. The depth of the network may range from as few as three through to thousands of layers [15, 16]. Of note, the input for each successive layer is the output of the previous layer, meaning that multiple levels of representation correspond to different abstraction levels as they are learned through the model [17].

There are several characteristics that make deep learning both distinct and beneficial as a machine learning (ML) approach. One of the key differences between traditional machine learning methods and the modern deep learning (DL) method is that of feature engineering, which progressively extracts the most important features from the existing model prior to building the next iteration [18]. Traditional ML models learn mapping from input to output, and in classification problems, it learns to separate classes through a decision boundary often provided by the researcher (Fig. 22.2) [19]. They are therefore unable to learn decision boundaries for nonlinear data, nor is it capable of learning all the researcher required functions. These characteristics ultimately limit the problems that can be solved. Subsequently, DL has high generative and learning capacity; that is, the more data available, the

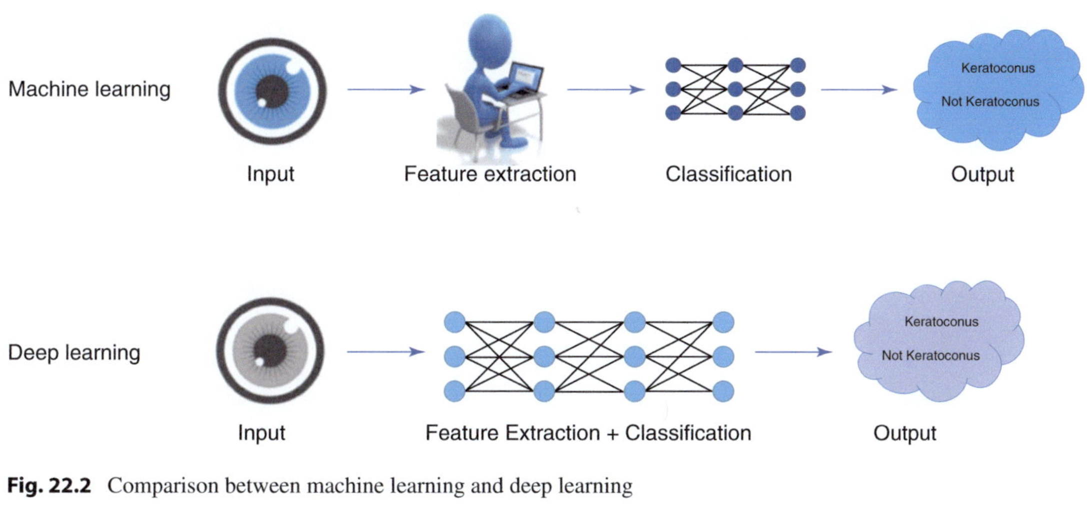

Fig. 22.2 Comparison between machine learning and deep learning

more inferences and relationships that can be developed from the data set. With the introduction of greater processing, deep neural networks (DNNs) can work on large amount of data leading to a better trained model with increased performance for prediction tasks. Deep learning also provides a significant platform for the ongoing transfer of knowledge. A model can be identified within a large data set and then transferred to a similar problem within a different dataset or population.

22.3 Neural Networks in Deep Learning

Within DL, there are numerous deep neural network models that facilitate the identification of patterns, characteristics, and features within the various classification relationships. Each neural network is comprised of a collection of neurons, which are appropriately linked. While the general network architecture is designed beforehand, the precise topological structure of DNNs is data-driven. Those most utilized, and relevant to ophthalmology, include multiperceptron, convolutional neural networks, and recurrent neural networks (Fig. 22.3) [20].

22.3.1 Multiperceptron (MLP) Neural Network

An MLP is a fully connected network where each node of the layer is connected to each node of the next layer. It is a feedforward neural network as inputs are processed in the forward direction [14]. The MLP maps and then applies weighting to various classifications. MLPs are utilized to solve problems, which involve image, tabular, or text data and subsequently have been used in determining positive diagnostic features for keratoconus inclusive of topographical maps and biomechanical data [21]. However, MLPs tend to lose the spatial features of an image impacting potential accuracy in identifying clinical features and do not have the ability to capture sequential information in the input data layer. This minimizes the ability to determine disease progression.

22.3.2 Convolutional Neural Networks (CNNs)

Convolutional neural networks that employ a sparse connection of nodes represent the most widely used DNN model, particularly within ophthalmology [6, 22–24]. Analogous to the function of the visual cortex, each node or neuron within the algorithm contains a weight that is multiplied through the input, which then "fires" at the determined threshold similar to a neuron firing in its own visual receptive field. This in turn contributes to the input at the next layer (convolution). Within the hidden layer of the CNN, a variety of additional layers including pooling, fully connected, and normalization layers work to extract and refine further relationships.

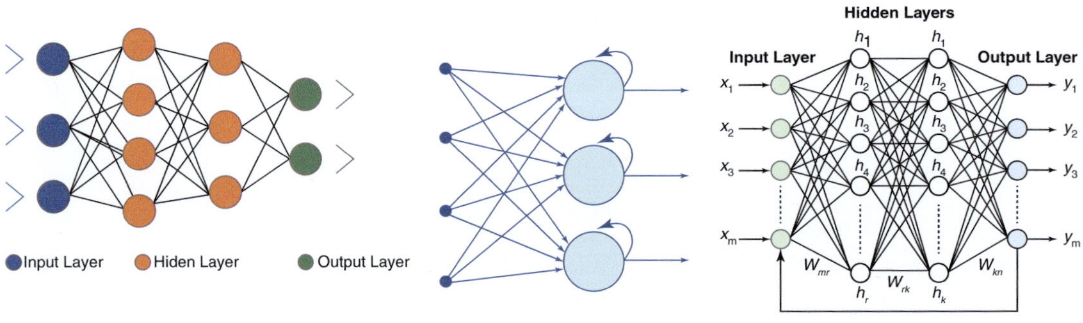

Fig. 22.3 From left to right, artificial neural network 7, recurrent neural network 7, convolutional neural network 8

The ability to extract additional features from input data suggests a greater capacity for learning without instruction representing a key potential advantage of CNNs. Further, they capture spatial features from an image, allowing accurate object identification, location, and relationship with other features. As would be expected within ophthalmology, CNNs have found a role in the diagnosis of conditions that utilize imaging, for example, diabetic retinopathy and glaucoma [25, 26].

22.3.3 Recurrent Neural Networks (RNNs)

Recurrent neural networks incorporate a looping or recurrent constraint within the hidden layer that enables the capture of sequential information at the prior input level. RNNs are specifically designed to identify patterns in sequences of data or images, therefore are commonly used with problems relating to audio or text information and, in particular, time-series data. The looping facility also provides an RNN with the ability to share parameters across different steps, which result in less parameters to train. This feature can further reduce computation time and costs. A disadvantage, albeit of any network that encapsulates feedback or looping mechanism, is the tendency to exaggerate increasing or decreasing gradient data. RNNs have recently been utilized to increase the identification of temporal features in fundus videos of glaucoma patients [27].

22.3.4 Limitations of Artificial Intelligence Programs

Similar to research based on standard data accumulation, the success of AI programs will be limited by access to information and the understanding of the condition investigated.

Basic training sets using homogenous data and populations limit the applicability and potential accuracy of output data [25, 28, 29]. For example, the use of retinal images from a single unit with restricted width of field or magnification may allow adequate interpretation using the diagnostic unit; however, the application would have reduced accuracy and therefore usability, across a range of devices. Similarly, the use of a single patient population will reduce the likelihood of incorporating phenotypes across a broad range. Keratoconus with its range of morphology and contributing factors represents a key example, and any AI-based application would benefit from including a wide range of data from multiple geographic and demographic cohorts. Rare diseases will be limited in the availability of large data albeit common disorders may paradoxically be impacted in a similar fashion due to the lack of routinely collected imaging. An example within ophthalmology would be biomicroscopic imaging of cataract, which is rarely done within busy ophthalmic practices [30].

Although one of the advantages of DL programs is the ability to extract a range of additional relationships from existing data, broader application to existing disease definitions or classifications is still essential. This is commonly described as the "ground truth" and ophthalmology contains several important examples including classification of keratoconus. The lack of a gold standard classification for keratoconus, for example, may inhibit how DL results can be interpreted. On a more theoretical level, the concept of the hidden layers used for calculation within DL requires a clinician to place their trust in a virtual "black box" of calculations. This may continue to limit widespread implementation of any programs until a clearer understanding is reached [31].

22.3.5 Open-Source Vs Purpose-Built?

Broadly, there are two key approaches to engaging with machine learning—open-source or purpose-built applications.

Open-source software facilitates easier implementation of machine learning by providing a platform, usually free to users, and then sample sections of code from each of the languages to undertake specific tasks. These libraries or frameworks provide many common algorithms, classification, and evaluation functions, which can then be utilized for interactive "workbench" applications, or embedded directly into the user's software and reused. The proliferation of free open-source software has made machine learning increasingly accessible to all users.

Purpose-built applications provide the user with a much deeper understanding of the algorithm and its functionality, increasing the potential complexity of the application and future optimization. However, this does require a range of specialty input, often from data scientists, and both platform and machine learning engineers, which may not be readily available to researchers [32, 33].

The decision to use open-source programs to refine existing code or derive a purpose-built application will be governed by the availability of existing programs that can be applied to the data and the ready access to data scientists.

22.3.6 Keratoconus and Artificial Intelligence

There is significant interest in applying AI to ophthalmology, in particular the challenge of keratoconus (KC), given the increasing development of broad ophthalmic data sets and expanding accessibility to machine learning algorithms. The focus of most current AI applications within this area has been the diagnosis and classification of the condition. More recently, understanding the contribution of risk factors, the likelihood of disease progression, and the optimization of key rehabilitative treatments such as intrastromal corneal rings have been investigated. A discussion of AI within KC is discussed below.

22.4 AI for Keratoconus Detection

Currently, topographic and tomographic mapping is the gold standard for keratoconus diagnosis. It is intuitive in that it represents the "ground truth" with which most subsequent algorithms have been compared [34]. Consequentially, the earliest attempts at machine learning were focused on diagnosis through the automation of topographical variables. In 1995, Maeda, Klyce, and Smolek described preliminary findings of a neural network trained on 11 parameters from the TMS-1 videokeratoscope that characterized corneal shape [35]. Despite a small training set, the network correctly classified 80% of the test maps against expert diagnosis with specificity greater than 90% for all parameters albeit with highly variable sensitivity (44–100%). Subsequent algorithms were instrumental in developing indices, which have been routinely incorporated into today's commercially available diagnostic topography units including, but not limited to Inferior–Superior Index (I-S Index), SRAX representing the degree of skewing of the steepest radial axes and therefore an expression of irregular astigmatism, and Keratoconus Percentage Index (KISA % Index), which is effectively a combination of these indexes [31, 36, 37]. The Belin–Ambrosio display has consolidated nine tomographical variables using regression analysis to identify corneas that differ significantly from normal. It is, however, designed to identify patients at risk of ectasia following refractive surgery rather than providing a diagnosis of keratoconus [38]. Using 55 indices measured with a dual Scheimpflug camera and decision tree classification algorithm, Smadja et al stated that the sensitivity and the specificity were 100% and 99.5%, respectively (Table 20.1) [54].

Stromal thinning is an integral feature in keratoconus, and the ability to measure corneal thickness provides specialists with the capacity to further increase the complexity of algorithms [61]. The Ambrosio relational thickness measure represented one of the first models adding corneal thickness to algorithms and has been shown to provide high specificity (85.5 to 100%) and sensitivity (88.9 to 99%) across multiple studies highlighting the benefits of incorporating pachymetry. Notably, these outcomes were enabled in moderate to severe cases of keratoconus and studies investigating differentiation of subclinical KC indicated considerable lower ranges of specificity (54–86.5%) and sensitivity (61–90.5%) [53, 62–64]. This is not uncommon in AI-based studies of sub-clinical KC where the

Table 20.1 Existing deep learning models for accuracy of keratoconus diagnosis (based on Kamiya et al. BMJ Open 2019; 9(9): e031313)

Author	Year	Sample size	Device	Machine learning	Input	Sensitivity	Specificity	Accuracy
Al-Timemy et al. [39]	2021	444 eyes	Pentacam	Ensemble of deep transfer learning	4 classifier maps	Avg. 90.8%	100%	Avg. 87.9%
Feng et al. [40]	2021	854 eyes	Pentacam HR	KerNet convolutional neural network	5 numerical matrices	NA	94.7%	Avg. 98%
Kato et al. [41]	2021	274 images	Pentacam HR	Convolutional neural network	Axial and pachymetry maps + age	77.8%	69.6%	81.4%
Langenbucher et al. [42]	2021	439 eyes	Corvis ST and Pentacam HR	24 different machine learning models	6 parameters	94.5%	NA	65.1%–95.2%
Bolarin et al. [43]	2020	169 eyes	Sirius	Multivariate logistic regression and ordinal logistic regression	17 variables	Avg. 64.6%	Avg. 93%	Avg. 78.7%
Isaarti et al. [44]	2020	812 eyes	Pentacam HR	Feedforward neural network	2 parameters	94%	99.9%	99.1%
Kuo et al. [31]	2020	354 images	Pentacam HR Corvis ST Tomey Videokeratoscope	3 convolutional neural network models compared	5 parameters	Avg. 93%	Avg. 95.8%	Avg. 94%
Shanthi et al. [45]	2020	205 eyes	Not specified	Support vector machine	31 parameters	94.2%	97.5%	91.8%
Shi et al. [46]	2020	121 eyes	Pentacam and a UHR-OCT prototype	Neural network classifier	49 parameters	98.5%	94.7%	93%
Zéboulon et al. [34]	2020	3000 images	Orbscan	Convolutional neural network	4 variables	100%	99%	99.3%
Dos Santos et al. [47]	2019	142	UHR-OCT	Custom neural network	72 images	NA	NA	99.56%
Issarti et al. [48]	2019	851	Pentacam	Feedforward neural network	19,881 matrices	97.78%	95.56%	96.56%
Kamiya et al. [49]	2019	543 eyes	Casia AS-OCT	Convolutional neural network	6 color-coded maps	100%	98.4%	99.1%
Yousefi et al. [50]	2018	3156 eyes	CASIA	Unsupervised machine learning	420 parameters	94.1%	97.7%	NA
Ruiz Hidalgo et al. [51]	2017	131	Pentacam	Support vector machine	25 parameters	NA	NA	92.6–98.0%
Ruiz Hidalgo et al. [52]	2016	860	Pentacam	Support vector machine	22 parameters	99.1%	98.4%	98.9%

(continued)

Table 20.1 (continued)

Author	Year	Sample size	Device	Machine learning	Input	Sensitivity	Specificity	Accuracy
Kovács et al. [53]	2016	135	Pentacam	Neural network	15 parameters	100%	95%	99% (AUROC)
Smadja et al. [54]	2013	372	Galilei	Decision tree	55 parameters	100%	99.5%	NA
Arbelaez et al. [55]	2012	3502	Sirius	Support vector machine	7 parameters	95.0%	99.3%	98.2%
Souza et al. [56]	2010	318	Orbscan	Neural network support vector machine and radial basis function neural network	11 parameters	NA	NA	71–99% (AUROC)
Twa et al. [57]	2005	244 eyes	Keratron topographer	Decision tree classifier	6912 points in polar coordinate grid	92%	93%	92%
Accardo & Pensiero [58]	2002	396	EyeSys	Neural network	9 parameters	94.1%	97.6%	NA
Smolek & Klyce [59]	1997	300	TMS-1	Neural network	10 parameters	100%	100%	100%
Maeda et al. [35]	1995	183	TMS-1	Neural network	11 parameters	44–100%	>90%	80%
Maeda et al. [60]	1994	200	TMS-1	Expert system	8 parameters	89%	99%	96%

NA Not applicable or not supplied; *UHR-OCT* Ultra-high-resolution optical coherence tomography; *AUROC* Area under receiver operating characteristic diagnosis of subclinical keratoconus is more complex and depends on numerous factors including subjective interpretation [60, 61]. Muftuoglu and coauthors used the D-index, a multimetric combination parameter composed of keratometric, pachymetric, pachymetric progression, and back elevation parameters to compare patients with KC in one eye and subclinical KC in the other against a control cohort of normal eyes. Although more sensitive than corresponding parameters, the algorithm still suggested diminished specificity in detecting subclinical KC [63]. Saad and Gatinel used a neural network to recognize specific classifications of corneal topography (Orbscan IIz, Bausch & Lomb, USA). The authors describe increased sensitivity (92.5%) and specificity (93%) when a combination of indices was used to detect subclinical KC [65]. A follow-up study using the same program in an Asian population, confirmed impressive specificity (98.1%) but lower sensitivity (70.8%) suggesting additional revision is required [66]. Arbelaez et al used curvature, thickness, and height data of both anterior and posterior corneal surface and pachymetry to train a support vector machine to aid classification of subclinical KC cases. The authors describe high sensitivity and specificity (93% and 98%, respectively) across a large cohort [55]. Although it remains difficult to compare these studies due to variable "ground truths," these outcomes reinforce that algorithms based on multiple metrics are significantly better than individual metrics alone in these at-risk cases [55]. This continues to represent one of the most pressing challenges for corneal specialists, particularly in reference to confirming patient suitability for laser refractive surgery.

Most models have concentrated on topography and tomography-based indices primarily due to machine availability. The incorporation of additional diagnostic variables such as corneal biomechanical properties and epithelial thickness has been explored more recently [21, 67–69].

Karimi et al employed a combination of clinical data, finite element method (FEM), and artificial neural network to establish a novel biomechanical-based diagnostic method based on contact and noncontact tonometry and topographic variables. Accuracy was 95.5% in the test cohort suggesting good, but not optimal outcomes [21]. A relative disadvantage of biomechanical tests such as the Corvis ST is the inability to visualize the distribution of the air puff over the corneal surface, which in KC patients is increasingly irregular, thereby leading to inaccurate, or at least variable outcomes. Rahmati and coauthors recently calculated the pressure distribution on the cornea's surface as a function of both the distance from the apex of the cornea and time, incorporating these new indices into a coupled, finite element (FE) optimization algorithm [69]. Further validation is required; however, these findings further increase our understanding of KC parameters and may provide additional benefits to future classification algorithms.

As discussed previously, CNNs perform comparatively well in pattern recognition and image classification tasks, likely making these algorithms an improved choice for the automated analysis of color-coded topographical and tomographical images [25, 70]. Abdelmotaal et al applied the CNN model to color-coded corneal maps of Scheimpflug images (Pentacam) to objectively classify eyes into normal, KC, and subclinical KC cohorts. The unsupervised model broke down data to the pixel level, thereby adding potentially greater spatial information [70]. This approach makes inherent sense in KC analysis where the changes across the cornea can be subtle, yet significant. The authors found substantial improvement in classification of all groups through the validation cohorts albeit additional incorporation of external datasets may further improve the model's broader applications [70]. In a similar fashion, Kamiya et al sought to evaluate the diagnostic accuracy of KC with machine learning and color-coded optical coherence tomography (OCT) maps. This study analyzed a cohort of mild-to-severe KC eyes against an age-matched control subset. The authors report an average accuracy of 87.4% in classifying KC albeit the cohort did not include eyes with subclinical KC, which represents a barrier to its use, at least in screening refractive surgery patients [49]. Lavric et al developed a CNN-based algorithm, KeratoDetect, utilizing pixel imagery from corneal topography, which is considered as the image preprocessing step [71]. To overcome the difficulties faced in collecting a large tomography dataset, the authors derived a stochastic model of the keratoconus eye using a baseline of 145 Scheimpflug tomographs, alongside biometry-related information. Although the algorithm demonstrated high KC detection accuracy, the platform of the derived tomography data suggested this as a supplementary tool only in the clinician disease diagnosis process [71].

Although not routinely available to clinical practices, the use of epithelial thickness in KC diagnostic assessment has been gaining validation across several studies. In a preliminary study undertaken by Silverman et al, the authors sought to develop and evaluate algorithms to differentiate normal and KC corneas through analysis of epithelial and stromal thickness data obtained through ultra-high-frequency ultrasound scans (Artemis) [68]. The study showed that epithelial remodeling in KC represents an independent means for differentiation of normal from advanced keratoconus corneas albeit the use of contact lens wearing patients in the test cohort may have represented a possible confounding factor. More recently, the same group developed a keratoconus classifier combining information from high-frequency ultrasound and topographical and pachymetry indices. The combined model had 97.3% sensitivity and 100% specificity in discriminating keratoconus from control patients. However, as per many studies, efficacy in subclinical KCs was yet to be determined [67]. Dos Santos and coauthors created a custom neural network (CorneaNet) trained on anterior segment ocular coherence images to segment healthy and keratoconic images based on epithelium, Bowman, and stromal layer thickness. The study found high accuracy in classifying keratoconus patients (validation accuracy: 99.56%). In contrast to previous approaches, the authors sought to minimize the potential parameters to increase the speed of the program, a practical endpoint for most busy practices. Of note, significantly diminishing the number of features of the convolutional layers, from over two million to 0.14 million, did not appear to impact validation accuracy, which decreased by only 0.1 points [47].

KC is considered primarily as a bilateral, albeit asymmetrical disease [72]. The creation of models using bilateral information, particularly in patients with one eye with frank KC and the other with minimal topographical or clinical changes is expected to introduce bias in any diagnostic algorithm. Although requiring consideration, it is notable that the use of automatic classifiers trained on bilateral data has been shown to be more effective than single parameters in discriminating fellow eyes of patients with preclinical signs of keratoconus from normal eyes [53].

Detection models for KC will continue to improve at a rapid pace; however, the incorporation of algorithms into clinical practice will remain a challenge for both logistical and theoretical reasons. Reinforcing existing diagnostic indices through AI-based models is likely key in engaging ophthalmologists. Kuo et al through a comparison of three pre-trained CNN models reported good accuracy of all models (>90% specificity and sensitivity); however, of particular note, they found that one of the models focused on the largest gradient difference in topographic maps, which corresponds well with diagnostic clues often used by ophthalmologists [31].

22.5 AI for Keratoconus Classification

Most studies have focused on the diagnosis of KC, which remains prudent. However, the classification of KC into stages may further assist detection of at-risk corneas and subsequent treatment planning for progressive and more advanced cases. Velázquez-Blázquez et al developed a predictive ordinal logistic regression model to classify KC patients through the analysis of optical, demographic, and geometric variables. Although overall accuracy was fair, the accuracy of early KC classification compared to subjective diagnosis provided the lowest outcome, which remains in line with current literature [73].

Shi et al developed an automated classification system with a focus on establishing grouping of clinically unaffected eyes in KC patients distinctly from a normal control population. Incorporating Scheimpflug imaging parameters and UHR-OCT, a neural network model was established as the classifier with an AUC for classifying normal from subclinical KC as 0.93. The authors found that OCT variables contributed more to the model than topographical imaging variables suggesting that subtle variations across groups may be more readily identified through corneal morphology. The combined approach, however, continued to provide the optimal outcomes [46].

Using topographic, tomographic, and thickness profiles, Yousefi et al undertook a stepwise process to developing an unsupervised model for patient clustering according to KC severity. In order to minimize potential prediction errors, the authors initially applied principal component analysis (PCA) to apply weighting to each parameter before final extraction as parameters most predictable of corneal status [50]. These components were then applied to a manifold learning model to group eyes with similar corneal characteristics together and/or to separate eyes with dissimilar characteristics as far away as possible. Overall sensitivity and specificity of 97.7% and 94.1%, respectively, demonstrating that an unsupervised model could cluster patients according to KC severity. The mean age of the sample was 69.7 years (± 16.2 years), which may represent a significant bias, at least with respect to using this as a model for estimating progression [50]. Zeboulon and coauthors have similarly used an unsupervised approach to classification with high accuracy (96.5%) albeit the model distinguished only between normal, KC, and patients with a history of refractive surgery [34].

22.6 AI for Keratoconus Progression

Although therapeutic treatments such as collagen cross-linking show an excellent safety profile, the decision to undertake surgery represents an important discussion with frank consideration of potential complications required [74]. Accurately identifying cases likely to progress either at or closely following the initial consultation would provide the surgeon with important information that could aid the patient's decision to undertake or delay surgery. Concurrently, proceeding earlier, with greater confidence of patient selection, would conceivably promote greater retention of corrected visual acuity. As of 2021, few existing AI models, however, have incorporated progression.

Kato et al [41] developed a CNN model to predict progression utilizing axial map, corneal thickness, and patient age in a retrospective cohort of KC patients [41]. Patient data were analyzed across 3 retrospective visits, and patients were allocated to CXL treatment groups or non-treatment, based on the application of a CNN (VGG-16) DL model with the highest accuracy at 81.4%. Our group conducted a study that developed a semi-supervised and unsupervised deep learning model to classify KC patients, before establishing a progression detection approach for the disease. Using a Bayesian deep neural network to classify KC patients and a Gaussian mixture model to cluster patients into 4 classes, the study utilized 29 variables retrospectively collected from topography, tomography, and clinical and demographic data. The study considered the Amsler–Krumeich (AK) classification as the ground truth. An average accuracy is 76% and 80% for supervised and unsupervised models, respectively [75]. Given these outcomes broadly match the findings of Kato et al, this suggests that these prediction models cannot currently be considered reliable enough for clinical utilization; however, they do demonstrate the emerging capabilities of DL for potential disease classification and thereby progression prediction [41].

22.7 Surgery Optimization

Variable corneal properties continue to impact the predictability of treatment outcomes in KC patients. Utilizing AI-based models may provide enabling specialists with a more optimal approach to interventions including intrastromal corneal ring segments (ICRS) [76, 77]. Valdes-Mas and coauthors first described a neural network to predict keratometry and corneal astigmatism changes following ISCR implantation. Error on the best models was under 1D (0.97D of corneal curvature and 0.93D of astigmatism) [76]. Later, Lyra and colleagues identified best mean absolute error value of 0.19 for corneal asphericity and 1.18D for mean keratometry values in an AI-based linear regression model in comparison with clinical data for ICRS (Ferrara segments) [77].

These outcomes are encouraging; however, they require additional revision prior to incorporation in the surgical decision-making process. Given the corresponding development of topographic guided collagen cross-linking, researchers may ultimately find greater benefits to creating models to optimize this more recent innovation.

22.8 Summary

Significant developments have been made to optimize AI-based applications to assist in the detection and classification of keratoconus. These innovations will continue to assist surgeons to identify patients either at risk of further progression or for sub-standard safety and efficacy outcomes following refractive-based procedures. Increasing availability and incorporation into existing diagnostic equipment will further enhance patient care. In developing these algorithms, consideration of the model and the comparative ground truth is essential in optimizing outcomes. This will continue to represent a key challenge in KC patients in subclinical cases. Researchers should strive to develop models based on heterogeneous populations and ideally a cross section of demographic, clinical, and tomographic parameters.

References

1. Gokul A, Patel DV, McGhee CN. Dr John Nottingham's 1854 landmark treatise on conical cornea considered in the context of the current knowledge of keratoconus. Cornea. 2016;35(5):673–8.
2. Wang P, Yuan M, He Y, Sun J. 3D augmented fundus images for identifying glaucoma via transferred convolutional neural networks. Int Ophthalmol. 2021;41(6):2065–72.
3. Wang XN, Dai L, Li ST, Kong HY, Sheng B, Wu Q. Automatic grading system for diabetic retinopathy diagnosis using deep learning artificial intelligence software. Curr Eye Res. 2020;45(12):1550–5.
4. Yellapragada B, Hornauer S, Snyder K, Yu S, Yiu G. Self-supervised feature learning and phenotyping for assessing age-related macular degeneration using retinal fundus images. Ophthalmol Retina. 2021;6(2):116–29.
5. Xu Z, Wang W, Yang J, Zhao J, Ding D, He F, Chen D, Yang Z, Li X, Yu W, Chen Y. Automated diagnoses of age-related macular degeneration and polypoidal choroidal vasculopathy using bi-modal deep convolutional neural networks. Br J Ophthalmol. 2021;105(4):561–6.
6. Zhang W, Chen Z, Zhang H, Su G, Chang R, Chen L, Zhu Y, Cao Q, Zhou C, Wang Y, Yang P. Detection of Fuchs' uveitis syndrome from slit-lamp images using deep convolutional neural networks in a Chinese population. Front Cell Dev Biol. 2021;9:684522.
7. Yu F, Silva Croso G, Kim TS, Song Z, Parker F, Hager GD, Reiter A, Vedula SS, Ali H, Sikder S. Assessment of automated identification of phases in videos of cataract surgery using machine learning and deep learning techniques. JAMA Netw Open. 2019;2(4):e191860.
8. Morita S, Tabuchi H, Masumoto H, Yamauchi T, Kamiura N. Real-time extraction of important surgical phases in cataract surgery videos. Sci Rep. 2019;9(1):16590.
9. Yousefi S, Kiwaki T, Zheng Y, Sugiura H, Asaoka R, Murata H, Lemij H, Yamanishi K. Detection of longitudinal visual field progression in glaucoma using machine learning. Am J Ophthalmol. 2018;193:71–9.
10. Lin SR, Ladas JG, Bahadur GG, Al-Hashimi S, Pineda R. A review of machine learning techniques for keratoconus detection and refractive surgery screening. Semin Ophthalmol. 2019;34(4):317–26.
11. Kaplan B, Farzanfar R, Friedman RH. Personal relationships with an intelligent interactive telephone health behavior advisor system: a multimethod study using surveys and ethnographic interviews. Int J Med Inform. 2003;71(1):33–41.
12. McGenity C, Treanor D. Guidelines for clinical trials using artificial intelligence - SPIRIT-AI and CONSORT-AI†. J Pathol. 2021;253(1):14–6.
13. Mooney SJ, Pejaver V. Big data in public health: terminology, machine learning, and privacy. Annu Rev Public Health. 2018;39:95–112.
14. LeCun Y, Bengio Y, Hinton G. Deep learning. Nature. 2015;521(7553):436–44.
15. Le WT, Maleki F, Romero FP, Forghani R, Kadoury S. Overview of machine learning: part 2: deep learning for medical image analysis. Neuroimaging Clin N Am. 2020;30(4):417–31.
16. Cui S, Tseng HH, Pakela J, Ten Haken RK, El Naqa I. Introduction to machine and deep learning for medical physicists. Med Phys. 2020;47(5):e127–47.

17. Pullen LC, Doctor AI, Am J. Transplantation. 2019;19(1):1–2.
18. Yang S, Zhu F, Ling X, Liu Q, Zhao P. Intelligent health care: applications of deep learning in computational medicine. Front Genet. 2021;12:607471.
19. Bouwmans T, Javed S, Sultana M, Jung SK. Deep neural network concepts for background subtraction: a systematic review and comparative evaluation. Neural Netw. 2019;117:8–66.
20. O'Byrne C, Abbas A, Korot E, Keane PA. Automated deep learning in ophthalmology: AI that can build AI. Curr Opin Ophthalmol. 2021;32(5):406–12.
21. Karimi A, Meimani N, Razaghi R, Rahmati SM, Jadidi K, Rostami M. Biomechanics of the healthy and Keratoconic corneas: a combination of the clinical data, finite element analysis, and artificial neural network. Curr Pharm Des. 2018;24(37):4474–83.
22. Grassmann F, Mengelkamp J, Brandl C, Harsch S, Zimmermann ME, Linkohr B, Peters A, Heid IM, Palm C, Weber BHF. A deep learning algorithm for prediction of age-related eye disease study severity scale for age-related macular degeneration from color fundus photography. Ophthalmology. 2018;125(9):1410–20.
23. Brown JM, Campbell JP, Beers A, Chang K, Ostmo S, Chan RVP, Dy J, Erdogmus D, Ioannidis S, Kalpathy-Cramer J, Chiang MF. Imaging and informatics in retinopathy of prematurity (i-ROP) research consortium. Automated diagnosis of plus disease in retinopathy of prematurity using deep convolutional neural networks. JAMA Ophthalmol. 2018;136(7):803–10.
24. Thompson AC, Jammal AA, Medeiros FA. A deep learning algorithm to quantify Neuroretinal rim loss from optic disc photographs. Am J Ophthalmol. 2019;201:9–18.
25. Ting DSJ, Foo VH, Yang LWY, Sia JT, Ang M, Lin H, Chodosh J, Mehta JS, Ting DSW. Artificial intelligence for anterior segment diseases: emerging applications in ophthalmology. Br J Ophthalmol. 2021;105(2):158–68.
26. Jeon H, Park KH, Kim H, Choi H. SD-OCT parameters and visual field defect in chiasmal compression and the diagnostic value of neural network model. Eur J Ophthalmol. 2020;31(5):2738–45.
27. Gheisari S, Shariflou S, Phu J, Kennedy PJ, Agar A, Kalloniatis M, Golzan SM. A combined convolutional and recurrent neural network for enhanced glaucoma detection. Sci Rep. 2021;11(1):1945.
28. Abràmoff MD, Garvin MK, Sonka M. Retinal imaging and image analysis. IEEE Rev Biomed Eng. 2010;3:169–208.
29. Gulshan V, Peng L, Coram M, Stumpe MC, Wu D, Narayanaswamy A, Venugopalan S, Widner K, Madams T, Cuadros J, Kim R, Raman R, Nelson PC, Mega JL, Webster DR. Development and validation of a deep learning algorithm for detection of diabetic retinopathy in retinal fundus photographs. JAMA. 2016;316(22):2402–10.
30. Ting DSW, Peng L, Varadarajan AV, Keane PA, Burlina PM, Chiang MF, Schmetterer L, Pasquale LR, Bressler NM, Webster DR, Abramoff M, Wong TY. Deep learning in ophthalmology: the technical and clinical considerations. Prog Retin Eye Res. 2019;72:100759.
31. Kuo BI, Chang WY, Liao TS, Liu FY, Liu HY, Chu HS, Chen WL, Hu FR, Yen JY, Wang IJ. Keratoconus screening based on deep learning approach of corneal topography. Transl Vis Sci Technol. 2020;9(2):53.
32. Oke I, VanderVeen D. Machine learning applications in pediatric ophthalmology. Semin Ophthalmol. 2021;36(4):210–7.
33. Alexeeff SE, Uong S, Liu L, Shorstein NH, Carolan J, Amsden LB, Herrinton LJ. Development and validation of machine learning models: electronic health record data to predict visual acuity after cataract surgery. Perm J. 2020;25:1.
34. Zéboulon P, Debellemanière G, Gatinel D. Unsupervised learning for large-scale corneal topography clustering. Sci Rep. 2020;10(1):16973.
35. Maeda N, Klyce SD, Smolek MK. Neural network classification of corneal topography. Preliminary demonstration. Invest Ophthalmol Vis Sci. 1995;36(7):1327–35.
36. Schwiegerling J, Greivenkamp JE. Keratoconus detection based on videokeratoscopic height data. Optom Vis Sci. 1996;73(12):721–8.
37. Steinberg J, Aubke-Schultz S, Frings A, Hülle J, Druchkiv V, Richard G, Katz T, Linke SJ. Correlation of the KISA% index and Scheimpflug tomography in 'normal', 'subclinical', 'keratoconus-suspect' and 'clinically manifest' keratoconus eyes. Acta Ophthalmol. 2015;93(3):e199–207.
38. Belin MW, Villavicencio OF, Ambrósio RR Jr. Tomographic parameters for the detection of keratoconus: suggestions for screening and treatment parameters. Eye Contact Lens. 2014;40(6):326–30.
39. Al-Timemy AH, Ghaeb NH, Mosa ZM, Escudero J. Deep transfer learning for improved detection of keratoconus using corneal topographic maps. Cogn Comput. 2021:1–6.
40. Feng R, Xu Z, Zheng X, Hu H, Jin X, Chen DZ, Yao K, Wu J. KerNet: a novel deep learning approach for keratoconus and sub-clinical keratoconus detection based on raw data of the pentacam system. IEEE J Biomed Health Inform. 2021;25(10):3898–910.
41. Kato N, Masumoto H, Tanabe M, Sakai C, Negishi K, Torii H, Tabuchi H, Tsubota K. Predicting keratoconus progression and need for corneal crosslinking using deep learning. J Clin Med. 2021;10(4):844.
42. Langenbucher A, Häfner L, Eppig T, Seitz B, Szentmáry N, Flockerzi E. Keratokonusdetektion und Ableitung des Ausprägungsgradesaus den Parametern des Corvis®ST : Eine Studie, basierend auf Algorithmen des Maschinenlernens [keratoconus detection and classification from parameters of the Corvis®ST : a study based on algorithms of machine learning]. Ophthalmologe. 2021;118(7):697–706.
43. Bolarín JM, Cavas F, Velázquez JS, Alió JL. A machine-learning model based on morphogeometric parameters for RETICS disease classification and GUI development. Appl Sci. 2020;10(5):1874.

44. Issarti I, Consejo A, Jiménez-García M, Kreps EO, Koppen C, Rozema JJ. Logistic index for keratoconus detection and severity scoring (Logik). Comput Biol Med. 2020;122:103809.
45. Shanthi S, Nirmaladevi K, Pyingkodi M, Dharanesh K, Gowthaman T, Harsavardan B. Machine learning approach for detection of keratoconus. In: IOP Conference Series: Materials Science and Engineering 2021, vol. 1055 (1). IOP Publishing. p. 012112.
46. Shi C, Wang M, Zhu T, Zhang Y, Ye Y, Jiang J, Chen S, Lu F, Shen M. Machine learning helps improve diagnostic ability of subclinical keratoconus using Scheimpflug and OCT imaging modalities. Eye Vis (Lond). 2020;7:48.
47. Dos Santos VA, Schmetterer L, Stegmann H, Pfister M, Messner A, Schmidinger G, Garhofer G, Werkmeister RM. CorneaNet: fast segmentation of cornea OCT scans of healthy and keratoconic eyes using deep learning. Biomed Opt Express. 2019;10(2):622–41.
48. Issarti I, Consejo A, Jiménez-García M, Hershko S, Koppen C, Rozema JJ. Computer aided diagnosis for suspect keratoconus detection. Comput Biol Med. 2019;109:33–42.
49. Kamiya K, Ayatsuka Y, Kato Y, Fujimura F, Takahashi M, Shoji N, Mori Y, Miyata K. Keratoconus detection using deep learning of colour-coded maps with anterior segment optical coherence tomography: a diagnostic accuracy study. BMJ Open. 2019;9(9):e031313.
50. Yousefi S, Yousefi E, Takahashi H, Hayashi T, Tampo H, Inoda S, Arai Y, Asbell P. Keratoconus severity identification using unsupervised machine learning. PLoS One. 2018;13(11):e0205998.
51. Ruiz Hidalgo I, Rozema JJ, Saad A, Gatinel D, Rodriguez P, Zakaria N, Koppen C. Validation of an objective keratoconus detection system implemented in a Scheimpflug Tomographer and comparison with other methods. Cornea. 2017;36(6):689–95.
52. Ruiz Hidalgo I, Rodriguez P, Rozema JJ, Ní Dhubhghaill S, Zakaria N, Tassignon MJ, Koppen C. Evaluation of a machine-learning classifier for keratoconus detection based on Scheimpflug tomography. Cornea. 2016;35(6):827–32.
53. Kovács I, Miháltz K, Kránitz K, Juhász É, Takács Á, Dienes L, Gergely R, Nagy ZZ. Accuracy of machine learning classifiers using bilateral data from a Scheimpflug camera for identifying eyes with preclinical signs of keratoconus. J Cataract Refract Surg. 2016;42(2):275–83.
54. Smadja D, Touboul D, Cohen A, Doveh E, Santhiago MR, Mello GR, Krueger RR, Colin J. Detection of subclinical keratoconus using an automated decision tree classification. Am J Ophthalmol. 2013;156(2):237–246.e1.
55. Arbelaez MC, Versaci F, Vestri G, Barboni P, Savini G. Use of a support vector machine for keratoconus and subclinical keratoconus detection by topographic and tomographic data. Ophthalmology. 2012;119(11):2231–8.
56. Souza MB, Medeiros FW, Souza DB, Garcia R, Alves MR. Evaluation of machine learning classifiers in keratoconus detection from orbscan II examinations. Clinics (Sao Paulo). 2010;65(12):1223–8.
57. Twa MD, Parthasarathy S, Roberts C, Mahmoud AM, Raasch TW, Bullimore MA. Automated decision tree classification of corneal shape. Optom Vis Sci. 2005;82(12):1038–46.
58. Accardo PA, Pensiero S. Neural network-based system for early keratoconus detection from corneal topography. J Biomed Inform. 2002;35(3):151–9.
59. Smolek MK, Klyce SD. Current keratoconus detection methods compared with a neural network approach. Invest Ophthalmol Vis Sci. 1997;38(11):2290–9.
60. Maeda N, Klyce SD, Smolek MK, Thompson HW. Automated keratoconus screening with corneal topography analysis. Invest Ophthalmol Vis Sci. 1994;35(6):2749–57.
61. Martínez-Abad A, Piñero DP. New perspectives on the detection and progression of keratoconus. J Cataract Refract Surg. 2017;43(9):1213–27.
62. Muftuoglu O, Ayar O, Ozulken K, Ozyol E, Akıncı A. Posterior corneal elevation and back difference corneal elevation in diagnosing forme fruste keratoconus in the fellow eyes of unilateral keratoconus patients. J Cataract Refract Surg. 2013;39(9):1348–57.
63. Muftuoglu O, Ayar O, Hurmeric V, Orucoglu F, Kılıc I. Comparison of multimetric D index with keratometric, pachymetric, and posterior elevation parameters in diagnosing subclinical keratoconus in fellow eyes of asymmetric keratoconus patients. J Cataract Refract Surg. 2015;41(3):557–65.
64. Ruiseñor Vázquez PR, Galletti JD, Minguez N, Delrivo M, Fuentes Bonthoux F, Pförtner T, Galletti JG. Pentacam Scheimpflug tomography findings in topographically normal patients and subclinical keratoconus cases. Am J Ophthalmol. 2014;158(1):32–40.e2.
65. Saad A, Gatinel D. Topographic and tomographic properties of forme fruste keratoconus corneas. Invest Ophthalmol Vis Sci. 2010;51(11):5546–55.
66. Xie Y, Zhao L, Yang X, Wu X, Yang Y, Huang X, Liu F, Xu J, Lin L, Lin H, Feng Q, Lin H, Liu Q. Screening candidates for refractive surgery with corneal tomographic-based deep learning. JAMA Ophthalmol. 2020;138(5):519–26.
67. Silverman RH, Urs R, RoyChoudhury A, Archer TJ, Gobbe M, Reinstein DZ. Combined tomography and epithelial thickness mapping for diagnosis of keratoconus. Eur J Ophthalmol. 2017;27(2):129–34.
68. Silverman RH, Urs R, Roychoudhury A, Archer TJ, Gobbe M, Reinstein DZ. Epithelial remodeling as basis for machine-based identification of keratoconus. Invest Ophthalmol Vis Sci. 2014;55(3):1580–7.
69. Rahmati SM, Razaghi R, Karimi A. Biomechanics of the keratoconic cornea: theory, segmentation, pressure distribution, and coupled FE-optimization algorithm. J Mech Behav Biomed Mater. 2021;113:104155.
70. Abdelmotaal H, Abdou AA, Omar AF, El-Sebaity DM, Abdelazeem K. Pix2pix conditional generative adversarial networks for Scheimpflug camera color-coded corneal tomography image generation. Transl Vis Sci Technol. 2021;10(7):21.

71. Lavric A, Valentin P. KeratoDetect: keratoconus detection algorithm using convolutional neural networks. Comput Intell Neurosci. 2019;2019:8162567.
72. Gomes JA, Rapuano CJ, Belin MW, Ambrósio R Jr. Group of Panelists for the global Delphi panel of keratoconus and Ectatic diseases. Global Consensus on Keratoconus Diagnosis. Cornea. 2015;34(12):e38–9.
73. Velázquez-Blázquez JS, Bolarín JM, Cavas-Martínez F, Alió JL. EMKLAS: a new automatic scoring system for early and mild keratoconus detection. Transl Vis Sci Technol. 2020;9(2):30.
74. Kobashi H, Tsubota K. Accelerated versus standard corneal cross-linking for progressive keratoconus: a meta-analysis of randomized controlled trials. Cornea. 2020;39(2):172–80.
75. Hallett N, Yi K, Dick J, Hodge C, Sutton G, Wang YG, You J. Deep learning based unsupervised and semi-supervised classification for keratoconus. In: 2020 International Joint Conference on Neural Networks (IJCNN); 2020. p. 1–7.
76. Valdés-Mas MA, Martín-Guerrero JD, Rupérez MJ, Pastor F, Dualde C, Monserrat C, Peris-Martínez C. A new approach based on machine learning for predicting corneal curvature (K1) and astigmatism in patients with keratoconus after intracorneal ring implantation. Comput Methods Prog Biomed. 2014;116(1):39–47.
77. Lyra D, Ribeiro G, Torquetti L, Ferrara P, Machado A, Lyra JM. Computational models for optimization of the intrastromal corneal ring choice in patients with keratoconus using corneal tomography data. J Refract Surg. 2018;34(8):547–50.

23 Changing Paradigm in the Diagnosis and Management of Keratoconus

Rashmi Sharad Deshmukh
and Pravin K. Vaddavalli

23.1 Introduction

Dr. Benedict Dudell first described keratoconus in 1736. However, the initial literature about the disease was unclear and confusing, with various names used to describe it, such as cornea conica, hyperkeratosis, prolapses corneae, sugar-loaf cornea, and staphyloma pellucidum. Around a century later, in 1844, Pickford described the conical cornea as a disease that is “intractable in nature and fatal to vision” and one in which “the pathology and treatment are so little understood.” While in the early years, literature and understanding of the disease depended on the authors’ insightful observations and clinical experiences, many of the observations published in that era are relevant even today. John Nottingham gave the first detailed description of keratoconus (KC) in 1854 in his landmark 270-page publication. Even more than 150 years later, keratoconus remains an enigmatic disease.

The advent of refractive surgeries called for a better understanding, early diagnosis, and effective management of patients with ectatic corneal disorders, including keratoconus. The past few decades have observed a rapid advancement in the understanding, diagnosis, and treatment of this condition.

R. S. Deshmukh · P. K. Vaddavalli (✉)
The Cornea Institute, L V Prasad Eye Institute, Hyderabad, Telangana, India
e-mail: rashmi.deshmukh@lvpei.org; pravin@lvpei.org

23.2 Epidemiology

Keratoconus was originally classified as a rare disease by the National Institute of Health, with an incidence lower than 1 per 2000 people [1]. However, it is now known that the occurrence of the disease is far more common than originally thought. The incidence and prevalence reported are inevitably subject to a bias for the methods used to diagnose keratoconus. Considering these limitations, the prevalence is highly variable, from 0.2/100,000 in Russia to as high as 3300/100,000 in Iran [2, 3]. A higher prevalence is reported in Asian and Middle Eastern population. A recent study from western India reported a prevalence of keratoconus as 1.61% in patients screened for refractive surgery [4]. A prevalence rate of 2.3% has been reported from rural central India in patients 30 years of age and older [5], while another population-based study from China reported a prevalence of 0.9% [6]. Studies from the Middle East have reported a prevalence rate of 3.3% in Lebanon [7], 2.34% in Israel [8], and 1.5% in Palestine [9]. In the United Kingdom, the reported prevalence ranged from 3.5 to 4.5/100,000. Studies from the United Kingdom have also reported a 5–9 times higher prevalence in the Asian population [1]. In the United States, the prevalence was about 54.5/100,000 population in 1986, which has increased to 1 per 375 in 2017 [10, 11]. Regardless of the potential bias that is induced due to the different diagnostic techniques, it is established that the reported

S. Das (ed.), *Keratoconus*, https://doi.org/10.1007/978-981-19-4262-4_23

prevalence of keratoconus has increased over the past three decades and is no more a rare disease.

Pediatric populations have a higher prevalence rate with the highest reported prevalence being 4790/100,000 in Saudi Arabia [12]. A study from New Zealand reported a prevalence of 520/100,000 in pediatric population overall, while that in Maori population was 2250/200,000 (4 times higher) [13].

Etiology of keratoconus is multifactorial and includes environmental and genetic factors. Atopy, eye rubbing, and ultraviolet light exposure are some of the established risk factors. Most cases are known to occur sporadically; however, familial aggregation, higher prevalence in certain ethnic groups, concordance in monozygotic twins, and associations with systemic syndromes such as Down's syndrome and Leber's congenital amaurosis indicate a genetic predisposition of keratoconus. In the Collaborative Longitudinal Evaluation of Keratoconus (CLEK) study, 13.5% of the patients reported a positive family history [14]. Other studies have reported 20–25% of patients have affected family members. The most common mode of inheritance described is autosomal dominant with incomplete penetrance and variable expression. However, a study based on a segregation analysis of 95 families suggested a possibility of autosomal recessive inheritance [15]. Additionally, a higher frequency observed in the children of consanguineous couples also suggests an autosomal recessive inheritance. A questionnaire-based study from Jerusalem reported that offspring of consanguineous couples had a four times higher risk of developing keratoconus than the ones with unrelated parents. Further, the authors reported that this association was stronger when the parents were first cousins, than second cousins [16]. Another study on Arab population reported a fivefold higher risk of keratoconus in children with related parents [17]. A strong effect of consanguinity could also explain a higher prevalence of keratoconus in certain ethnicities. There are several reports of keratoconus in twins with concordance in the topographic patterns. A study comparing monozygotic and dizygotic twins showed a higher prevalence in monozygotic twins suggesting a genetic association [18].

Several linkage and association studies have been performed to understand the genetic basis of the disease. Linkage loci have been identified on chromosomes 2, 5, 14, 15, and 16. Genome-wide association studies have suggested an association between central corneal pachymetry and sequence variants within or near several genes. These include ZNF469, FOXO1, FNDC3B, COL5A1, and COL8A2. Candidate genes have been studied in relation to the pathogenesis of keratoconus. The visual system homeobox 1 (VSX1) gene and superoxide dismutase 1 (SOD1) gene are two such genes being studied in patients with keratoconus [19].

23.3 Diagnosis

Traditional methods of diagnosing KC included clinical signs such as corneal thinning and steepening, Vogt's striae, Fleischer's ring, and scissoring reflex on retinoscopy. However, most of these signs appear after the keratoconus has caused significant corneal changes. A revolution in the armamentarium of diagnostic tools enabled diagnosing the disease at an earlier stage. Advancements in imaging technologies have allowed a detailed characterization of the corneal shape and anatomy.

23.4 Evolution in Topography

In the early part of the nineteenth century, Cuignet described the use of keratoscopes to study the shape of the cornea. The invention of a keratometer followed this to quantify the corneal curvature [20]. In 1880, Antonio Placido used a disk painted with black and white alternating concentric rings with a convex lens in the center for the examiner to visualize the cornea. The reflection of these rings from the anterior corneal surface would give a qualitative analysis of the corneal contour [21]. This disk came to be known as the "Placido disk." Images of the rings were photographed and compared to the reflections from spheres of known radius to obtain quantitative measurements of the corneal radius. In 1959, Reynolds and Kratt were the first to automate the Placido disk and develop a photo-electronic keratoscope [22]. A newer, more advanced version of the photo-electronic keratoscope was the corneascope, introduced in 1981 [23].

Placido-based topographers measure the anterior corneal surface, which helps identify minor changes in the anterior topography when the clinical examination is normal. One of the drawbacks, however, is that to measure the total corneal power, the device assumed a specific relationship between the anterior and posterior corneal surfaces. A good reflection from the anterior corneal surface needs a healthy tear film. Consequently, Placido-based topography is difficult in a patient with an unhealthy ocular surface.

Front surface corneal analysis evolved into a tomographic or 3-dimensional analysis, characterizing the posterior corneal topography and corneal thickness. Orbscan, incorporating the scanning-slit technology, became the first commercially available topographer to measure the posterior corneal surface. Several slit beams scanned the cornea, and a camera captured the cross sections illuminated by the slit beams to map the topographical features of the anterior and posterior corneal surface. Orbscan II took advantage of both the technologies and combined the slit-scanning system with the Placido disk topography [24]. The development of another technique, the Scheimpflug imaging, also enabled direct measurement of the posterior corneal surface. It is based on the Scheimpflug principle in which the depth of focus achieved is higher if the planes of the image, lens, and object are not parallel to each other [25]. Pentacam (OCULUS Inc.) and Galilei (Ziemer Group, Port, Switzerland) utilize this principle. The machine can then derive the topographic and power maps utilizing the thickness measurements. Very high-frequency ultrasound, employed by Artemis (ArcScan, Inc.), helped create three-dimensional images of the individual corneal layers in the posterior cornea. The increased resolution of the image, however, comes at the cost of decreased field of view [26].

The advances in topographical techniques were accompanied by the acquisition of a large amount of data. One of the challenges clinicians face is the interpretation of the vast information generated by these machines. Keeping this in mind, various classification systems and indices were developed to interpret these data and diagnose ectatic corneal diseases.

Marc Amsler was the first to give a classification system for keratoconus based on clinical signs in 1950. Central corneal radius, best-corrected visual acuity, pachymetry, and corneal transparency were used to classify keratoconus from stages 0–4. Muckenhirn, in 1984, added corneal eccentricity as an additional factor to be considered. Krumeich created a new classification using corneal radius, corneal thickness, induced myopia, and slit-lamp features.

Indices such as Rabinowitz and McDonnell were based on Placido disk topographers. Although lacking specificity, these indices were sensitive in detecting mild ectasias in patients with good visual acuity and an unremarkable slit-lamp examination [27]. However, it was soon evident that despite having a normal anterior corneal curvature, some cases progressed to have ectasias following refractive surgery [28]. Conversely, some cases remained stable post-refractive surgery despite having abnormalities in anterior keratometric data [29]. When Scheimpflug imaging became widely used, classifications and indices based on Scheimpflug topography came into being. These include the Keratoconus Index (KI), topographic keratoconus classification (TKC), and the recent ABCD classification that helps determine the progression of keratoconus.

Further advances and development of segmental tomography allowed characterization of individual corneal layers such as epithelium and Bowman's membrane. Studies have demonstrated epithelial thickness mapping to be a valuable tool in detecting early forms of keratoconus [30]. Using OCT, the authors have proposed Bowman's roughness index (BRI) that measures the irregularity of Bowman's membrane in mild forms of keratoconus. When combined with the epithelial thickness mapping, BRI had a good performance in detecting early keratoconus [31].

Beyond the analysis of corneal geometry, corneal biomechanical analysis has emerged as a valuable tool in enhancing the accuracy of detecting early forms of keratoconus and predicting the disease's tendency of progression [32]. It has been proposed that the changes in corneal pachymetry and keratometry observed in keratoconus are secondary to focal biomechanical weakening [33]. The first instrument introduced for in vivo biomechanical assessment was the Reichert ocular response analyzer (ORA). It was introduced as a noncontact tonometer (NCT) with a collimated air pulse deforming the central 5–6 mm of the cornea. The peak of the air pulse is adjusted according to the measured intraocular pressure (IOP), and the corneal deformation is measured by the apical reflex of an infrared light going toward the sensor through a pinhole system. The first-generation pressure-dependent parameters—corneal hysteresis (CH) and the corneal resistance factor (CRF)—had a statistically different distribution in keratoconus and normal cornea. However, there was a significant overlap found, which reduced its sensitivity and specificity. Higher accuracy was found using parameters derived from the waveform signal measuring deformation [34]. Accuracy was further improved when corneal biomechanical data were combined with tomographic data [35].

The Corvis ST (OCULUS Optikgeräte; Wetzlar, Germany) is the next generation NCT having a collimated air pulse, albeit with a fixed pressure pulse, combined with an ultra-high-speed Scheimpflug camera that monitors the corneal deformation response. Parameters derived from Corvis ST such as deformation amplitude, corneal velocities, the inverse concave radius of curvature, and corneal stiffness at first applanation improved the detection of corneal ectasias [36]. Although an overlap was evidenced between normal and keratoconus corneas, the use of artificial intelligence techniques has enabled improving accuracy in detecting mild forms of the disease [37]. Corvis corneal biomechanical index (CBI) was developed using linear regression analysis to combine corneal deformation parameters and horizontal thickness profile. The CBI is highly accurate in detecting clinical keratoconus [38]. The tomographic biomechanical index (TBI) was developed using artificial intelligence to combine the Scheimpflug-based tomography and biomechanical data. The ability of TBI to detect clinical ectasia is statistically higher than other tested parameters. In a study including 94 eyes of very asymmetric ectasia and fellow eye presenting with normal topography, TBI performed better than any other parameters tested in isolation [39].

Another promising technology emerging in analyzing corneal biomechanical properties is Brillouin microscopy. It is based on Brillouin scattering arising from the light rays incident on the medium of interest and the phonons in the same medium. It consists of a standard, inverted confocal microscope, and a double, virtually imaged phased array (VIPA) spectrometer [40]. Useful in measuring the corneal stiffness and mapping corneal modulus, this technique is not yet clinically available. In vivo and in vitro studies have shown focal mechanical weakening in the cone area compared to the rest of the cornea, corroborating with the concept of focal biomechanical weakening being the primary pathology leading to thinning and ectasia as secondary changes.

23.5 Treatment

Until the end of the last century, the treatment offered for keratoconus was limited to spectacles or rigid contact lenses for visual improvement and penetrating keratoplasties in more advanced cases, not benefiting from the former options [41]. The advent of collagen cross-linking (CXL) made it possible to prevent progression of the ectasia and reduce the need for keratoplasty. CXL was described by Wollensak and group in 2003 as a preventive approach to halt the progression of keratoconus [42]. The initial protocol known as the Dresden protocol involved epithelial debridement and soaking the cornea with riboflavin every 2 mins for 30 mins followed by ultraviolet

A (UVA) radiation exposure for 30 mins. A photochemical reaction between the riboflavin and UV-A radiation induces cross-links between the collagen fibrils in the corneal stroma. Although studies have demonstrated the Dresden protocol to be effective in arresting progression, this procedure posed specific challenges, including rapid oxygen depletion with higher fluence irradiances, limited riboflavin penetration through the epithelium, potential endothelial toxicity in thin corneas, and prolonged duration of the treatment. Advances and developments were made to overcome these challenges while maintaining the effect of CXL.

Based on the Bunsen–Roscoe law of reciprocity, accelerated protocols were conceptualized where the irradiances were increased, and treatment duration was reduced proportionately to deliver the same amount of surface dose. Consequently, protocols were introduced with an irradiance of 9 mW/cm [2] for 10 mins, 18 mW/cm [2] for 5 mins, and 30 mW/cm [2] for 3 mins, all delivering the same amount of surface dose as the conventional Dresden protocol (5.4 J/cm [2]). The shorter the duration of CXL, the lower is the efficacy of the procedure; however, they are safe and effective in halting the progression of keratoconus.

Higher irradiances, even though they help reduce the treatment duration, result in rapid oxygen depletion during the UV-A exposure. CXL is safer and more effective when it occurs in the presence of sufficient oxygen (type 2 reaction). On the other hand, when the process occurs in a low-oxygen environment (type 1 reaction), it not only results in fewer cross-links making the CXL less efficient but also generates hydrogen peroxide, which is a toxic by-product [43]. An effort to improve oxygen availability led to the introduction of pulsed therapy with on and off cycles. The "on" time (1–1.5 s) is when the UVA radiation exposure occurs, while the "off" time (1–1.5 s) is when the UVA is turned off, enabling replenishment of oxygen. Consequently, more oxygen is available with type 2 reaction taking place during the "on" time. It is vital to bear in mind that the oxygen replenishment occurs at a much slower pace than the consumption rendering short "on–off" cycles ineffective in complete restoration of oxygen. Studies have demonstrated the demarcation line to be deeper with pulsed protocols as compared to the continuous protocols [44]. However, whether the depth of the demarcation line can be used as an indicator for the success of cross-linking is still debatable.

Oxygen availability is also a challenge in transepithelial approaches where the epithelium consumes significantly higher oxygen than the stroma. The pulsed treatments would therefore have limited efficacy in epi-on treatments with higher irradiances [45]. Recent advances include using oxygen delivery goggles during accelerated transepithelial CXL and have reported improved visual acuity and keratometry values at 6 months of follow-up with no significant adverse effects [46].

Apart from oxygen consumption, intact epithelium acts as a barrier for effective penetration of riboflavin due to the molecule's hydrophilicity and large size. Also, the monophosphate molecules in the riboflavin increase the electronegativity of the solution, acting to repel the negatively charged proteoglycans present in the stroma. This further reduces the riboflavin penetration. Approaches to improve riboflavin delivery include using molecules like ethylenediaminetetraacetic acid, benzalkonium chloride, diluted ethanol, vitamin E, and trometamol, all agents to loosen the corneal epithelial tight junctions enabling riboflavin to penetrate through the intact epithelium. Iontophoresis is another method used to increase the transport of riboflavin through the stroma. Studies have shown the efficacy to be comparable to standard CXL [47]. Recently, Mazzotta et al described enhanced fluence pulsed light iontophoresis (EF I-CXL), where they combined pulsed light accelerated protocol with iontophoresis. The 3-year results of this technique showed the depth of demarcation line to be comparable to standard CXL [48]. Novel delivery systems using nanostructured lipid carriers have been designed, coupled with other molecules to enhance permeation (Transcutol P) or confer a positive charge on the molecule (Stearylamine)

[49]. A microemulsion system also has been developed and showed promising results in rabbit eyes [50].

Another potential problem to be addressed with conventional protocol is endothelial toxicity, especially in thin corneas. Customized epithelial debridement, hypotonic riboflavin solution, contact lens-assisted CXL, or lenticule-assisted CXL is some of the solutions postulated for CXL in such cases [51].

Advances have been made to provide refractive correction along with halting the keratoconus progression. Customized CXL is one such approach where maximum treatment is delivered at the cone's apex compared to the surrounding normal area. This allows for selective flattening in the cone area favoring limited normalization of the corneal shape. Other approaches include combining CXL with procedures like intracorneal ring segments (ICRS) or photorefractive keratectomy (PRK) in suitable candidates. These procedures, called "CXL plus," have an additional effect of refractive correction over halting keratoconus progression. ICRS with CXL reportedly helps in more irregular corneas with worse visual acuity. It can be performed as a combined procedure in the same sitting or as two separate staged procedures [52].

Tissue ablation in an ectatic cornea is likely to cause further biomechanical weakening. Protocols like Athens protocol (topography-guided PRK with CXL) and Cretan protocol (transepithelial PRK with CXL) have shown success in improving visual acuity and stabilizing keratoconus. It is crucial to maintain the corneal thickness of at least 400 microns when PRK and CXL are combined. Strategies have been developed to ablate minimal possible tissue with a satisfactory refractive outcome. One such strategy is the "minimized volume ablation," which has proven to be safe and effective in keratoconus grades I-III when combined with accelerated CXL [53]. "Central corneal regularization" (CCR) is another protocol that is effective in reducing higher-order aberrations and maximum keratometry values [54]. The Tel Aviv protocol involves 50 μ ablation for epithelium and anterior stroma combined with CXL. Around half of the manifest astigmatism is corrected, to which spherical ablation is added so that the total ablation is limited to 50 μ. It has reportedly been successful in halting progression and improving visual acuity without significantly thinning the cornea [55].

The last couple of decades have also seen a paradigm shift in keratoplasty procedures offered to keratoconus patients, shifting from full-thickness keratoplasties to a lamellar approach. Lamellar grafts improve the chances of graft survival and provide better visual outcomes by inducing lesser astigmatism. In 1877, a novel procedure of selectively transplanting the corneal stromal tissue without endothelial cells was described, which formed the basis of deep anterior lamellar keratoplasty (DALK), which is now widely performed for ectatic corneal diseases [56]. Earlier techniques of manual dissection further evolved into Descemet membrane baring techniques such as "big bubble" or "viscodissection" techniques that resulted in improved visual outcomes. Although the number of keratoplasty procedures has declined with the advent of CXL, lamellar keratoplasties still have a place in managing advanced cases not amenable to a conservative approach.

It is postulated that the fragmentation of Bowman's membrane plays an important role in the pathogenesis of keratoconus. Therefore, it has been theorized that the replacement of Bowman's layer might provide the essential biomechanical support and help maintain corneal shape. Bowman's layer transplant (BLT) has recently gained interest, particularly in corneas with low pachymetry or increased steepening, making them unsuitable for CXL plus procedures. BLT not only halts the progression of the ectasia but also causes corneal flattening and improved biomechanical strength [57]. Owing to the acellular nature of the Bowman's membrane, BLT is associated with prolonged survival rates, and there have not been any reports of rejection in the literature to date. The femtosecond laser has been used to create the stromal pockets to reduce the chances of micro-perforation. The use of intraoperative optical coherence tomography (OCT) helps improve the visualization of the dissection plane. In the classic technique, the graft is inserted at the mid-stromal level, but more recently, a modification has been described where the Bowman's layer is placed as an onlay subepithelial. Preliminary results of this technique are promising [58].

A newly developed femtosecond-assisted stromal pocket creation and insertion of the corneal lamella are termed "additive keratoplasty." This procedure helps increase the corneal thickness and biomechanical strength and cause flattening in the cone area. Studies have shown improved visual outcomes and biomechanical stability in both progressive and non-progressive keratoconus corneas [59, 60]. Recently, the results of the phase I trial of using decellularized stromal lenticule with or without autologous adipose tissue-driven stem cells have been published, showing a good safety profile [61].

23.6 Summary

It has been realized over time that keratoconus is not as rare a disease as was once thought. As with most conditions, it is evident that trends have changed from treating the disease to preventing the disease and diagnosing it at an early stage. Advances in the diagnosis and treatment of keratoconus are evolving rapidly due to the advent of refractive surgery, which necessitates screening patients for early signs of ectasia. Tissue engineering and regenerative therapies are being devised to target the disease at the cellular level. Efforts must be taken to educate the patients on the preventable causes of keratoconus and the newer techniques that offer opportunities to reduce the visual debilitation caused by the disease.

References

1. Ferrari G, Rama P. The keratoconus enigma: a review with emphasis on pathogenesis. Ocul Surf. 2020;18(3):363–73.
2. Gorskova EN, Sevost'ianov EN. Epidemiology of keratoconus in the Urals. Vestnik Oftalmologii. 1998;114(4):38–40.
3. Hashemi H, Khabazkhoob M, Fotouhi A. Topographic keratoconus is not rare in an Iranian population: the Tehran eye study. Ophthalmic Epidemiol. 2013;20(6):385–91.
4. Shilpy N, Shah Z, Singh S, Purohit D. Prevalence of keratoconus in refractive surgery cases in Western India. Middle East Afr J Ophthalmol. 2020;27(3):156–9.
5. Jonas JB, Nangia V, Matin A, Kulkarni M, Bhojwani K. Prevalence and associations of keratoconus in rural Maharashtra in Central India: the Central India eye and medical study. Am J Ophthalmol. 2009;148(5):760–5.
6. Xu L, Wang YX, Guo Y, You QS, Jonas JB, Beijing Eye Study Group. Prevalence and associations of steep cornea/keratoconus in Greater Beijing. The Beijing Eye Study. PLoS One. 2012;7(7):e39313.
7. Waked N, Fayad AM, Fadlallah A, El Rami H. Dépistage du kératocône dans une population universitaire au Liban [Keratoconus screening in a Lebanese students' population]. J Fr Ophtalmol. 2012;35(1):23–9.
8. Millodot M, Shneor E, Albou S, Atlani E, Gordon-Shaag A. Prevalence and associated factors of keratoconus in Jerusalem: a cross-sectional study. Ophthalmic Epidemiol. 2011;18(2):91–7.
9. Shehadeh MM, Diakonis VF, Jalil SA, Younis R, Qadoumi J, Al-Labadi L. Prevalence of keratoconus among a Palestinian tertiary student population. Open Ophthalmol J. 2015;9:172–6.
10. Godefrooij DA, de Wit GA, Uiterwaal CS, Imhof SM, Wisse RP. Age-specific incidence and prevalence of keratoconus: a Nationwide registration study. Am J Ophthalmol. 2017;175:169–72.
11. Kennedy RH, Bourne WM, Dyer JA. A 48-year clinical and epidemiologic study of keratoconus. Am J Ophthalmol. 1986;101(3):267–73.
12. Torres Netto EA, Al-Otaibi WM, Hafezi NL, Kling S, Al-Farhan HM, Randleman JB, Hafezi F. Prevalence of keratoconus in paediatric patients in Riyadh, Saudi Arabia. Br J Ophthalmol. 2018;102(10):1436–41.
13. Papali'i-Curtin AT, Cox R, Ma T, Woods L, Covello A, Hall RC. Keratoconus prevalence among high school students in New Zealand. Cornea. 2019;38(11):1382–9.
14. Zadnik K, Barr JT, Edrington TB, Everett DF, Jameson M, McMahon TT, Shin JA, Sterling JL, Wagner H, Gordon MO. Baseline findings in the collaborative longitudinal evaluation of keratoconus (CLEK) study. Invest Ophthalmol Vis Sci. 1998;39(13):2537–46.
15. Wang Y, Rabinowitz YS, Rotter JI, Yang H. Genetic epidemiological study of keratoconus: evidence for major gene determination. Am J Med Genet. 2000;93(5):403–9.
16. Gordon-Shaag A, Millodot M, Essa M, Garth J, Ghara M, Shneor E. Is consanguinity a risk factor for keratoconus? Optom Vis Sci. 2013;90(5):448–54.
17. Shneor E, Millodot M, Gordon-Shaag A, Essa M, Anton M, Barbara R, Barbara A. Prevalence of keratoconus among young Arab students in Israel. Int J Keratoconus Ectatic Corneal Dis. 2014;3(1):9–14.

18. Tuft SJ, Hassan H, George S, Frazer DG, Willoughby CE, Liskova P. Keratoconus in 18 pairs of twins. Acta Ophthalmol. 2012;90(6):e482–6.
19. Gordon-Shaag A, Millodot M, Shneor E, Liu Y. The genetic and environmental factors for keratoconus. Biomed Res Int. 2015;2015:795738.
20. Leahy A. Keratoscopy. Ind Med Gaz. 1884;19(7):184–6.
21. Placido A. Novo instrumento de exploração da córnea. Periodico d'Oftalmológica Practica. 1880;5:27–30.
22. Reynolds AE, Kratt HJ. The *photo-electronic keratoscope*. Contacto. 1959;3:53–9.
23. Rowsey JJ, Reynolds AE, Brown R. Corneal topography. Corneascope. Arch Ophthalmol. 1981;99(6):1093–100.
24. Cairns G, McGhee CN. Orbscan computerized topography: attributes, applications, and limitations. J Cataract Refract Surg. 2005;31(1):205–20.
25. Dubbelman M, Sicam VA, Van der Heijde GL. The shape of the anterior and posterior surface of the aging human cornea. Vis Res. 2006;46(6–7):993–1001.
26. Piñero DP, Plaza AB, Alió JL. Anterior segment biometry with 2 imaging technologies: very-high-frequency ultrasound scanning versus optical coherence tomography. J Cataract Refract Surg. 2008;34(1):95–102.
27. Maeda N, Klyce SD, Smolek MK, Thompson HW. Automated keratoconus screening with corneal topography analysis. Invest Ophthalmol Vis Sci. 1994;35(6):2749–57.
28. Ambrósio R Jr, Dawson DG, Salomão M, Guerra FP, Caiado AL, Belin MW. Corneal ectasia after LASIK despite low preoperative risk: tomographic and biomechanical findings in the unoperated, stable, fellow eye. J Refract Surg. 2010;26(11):906–11.
29. Reinstein DZ, Archer TJ, Gobbe M. Stability of LASIK in topographically suspect keratoconus confirmed non-keratoconic by Artemis VHF digital ultrasound epithelial thickness mapping: 1-year follow-up. J Refract Surg. 2009;25(7):569–77.
30. Li Y, Chamberlain W, Tan O, Brass R, Weiss JL, Huang D. Subclinical keratoconus detection by pattern analysis of corneal and epithelial thickness maps with optical coherence tomography. J Cataract Refract Surg. 2016;42(2):284–95.
31. Pahuja N, Shroff R, Pahanpate P, Francis M, Veeboy L, Shetty R, Nuijts RMMA, Sinha RA. Application of high resolution OCT to evaluate irregularity of Bowman's layer in asymmetric keratoconus. J Biophotonics. 2017;10(5):701–7.
32. Ambrósio R Jr, Nogueira LP, Caldas DL, Fontes BM, Luz A, Cazal JO, Alves MR, Belin MW. Evaluation of corneal shape and biomechanics before LASIK. Int Ophthalmol Clin. 2011;51(2):11–38.
33. Roberts CJ, Dupps WJ Jr. Biomechanics of corneal ectasia and biomechanical treatments. J Cataract Refract Surg. 2014;40(6):991–8.
34. Luz A, Lopes B, Hallahan KM, Valbon B, Fontes B, Schor P, Dupps WJ Jr, Ambrósio R Jr. Discriminant value of custom ocular response analyzer waveform derivatives in Forme Fruste keratoconus. Am J Ophthalmol. 2016;164:14–21.
35. Luz A, Lopes B, Hallahan KM, Valbon B, Ramos I, Faria-Correia F, Schor P, Dupps WJ Jr, Ambrósio R Jr. Enhanced combined tomography and biomechanics data for distinguishing Forme Fruste keratoconus. J Refract Surg. 2016;32(7):479–94.
36. Ambrósio R Jr, Lopes B, Faria-Correia F, Vinciguerra R, Vinciguerra P, Elsheikh A, Roberts CJ. Ectasia detection by the assessment of corneal biomechanics. Cornea. 2016;35(7):e18–20.
37. Salomão MQ, Hofling-Lima AL, Faria-Correia F, Lopes BT, Rodrigues-Barros S, Roberts CJ, Ambrósio R. Dynamic corneal deformation response and integrated corneal tomography. Indian J Ophthalmol. 2018;66(3):373–82.
38. Vinciguerra R, Ambrósio R Jr, Elsheikh A, Roberts CJ, Lopes B, Morenghi E, Azzolini C, Vinciguerra P. Detection of keratoconus with a new biomechanical index. J Refract Surg. 2016;32(12):803–10.
39. Ambrósio R Jr, Lopes BT, Faria-Correia F, Salomão MQ, Bühren J, Roberts CJ, Elsheikh A, Vinciguerra R, Vinciguerra P. Integration of Scheimpflug-based corneal tomography and biomechanical assessments for enhancing ectasia detection. J Refract Surg. 2017;33(7):434–43.
40. Scarcelli G, Besner S, Pineda R, Yun SH. Biomechanical characterization of keratoconus corneas ex vivo with Brillouin microscopy. Invest Ophthalmol Vis Sci. 2014;55(7):4490–5.
41. Seiler T. The paradigm change in keratoconus therapy. Indian J Ophthalmol. 2013;61(8):381.
42. Wollensak G, Spoerl E, Seiler T. Riboflavin/ultraviolet-a-induced collagen crosslinking for the treatment of keratoconus. Am J Ophthalmol. 2003;135(5):620–7.
43. Rubinfeld RS, Caruso C, Ostacolo C. Corneal cross-linking: the science beyond the myths and misconceptions. Cornea. 2019;38(6):780–90.
44. Mazzotta C, Traversi C, Caragiuli S, Rechichi M. Pulsed vs continuous light accelerated corneal collagen crosslinking: in vivo qualitative investigation by confocal microscopy and corneal OCT. Eye (Lond). 2014;28(10):1179–83.
45. Sun L, Li M, Zhang X, Tian M, Han T, Zhao J, Zhou X. Transepithelial accelerated corneal collagen cross-linking with higher oxygen availability for keratoconus: 1-year results. Int Ophthalmol. 2018;38(6):2509–17.
46. Mazzotta C, Sgheri A, Bagaglia SA, Rechichi M, Di Maggio A. Customized corneal crosslinking for treatment of progressive keratoconus: clinical and OCT outcomes using a transepithelial approach with supplemental oxygen. J Cataract Refract Surg. 2020;46(12):1582–7.
47. Vinciguerra P, Rosetta P, Legrottaglie EF, Morenghi E, Mazzotta C, Kaye SB, Vinciguerra R. Iontophoresis CXL with and without epithelial debridement versus standard CXL: 2-year clinical results of a prospective clinical study. J Refract Surg. 2019;35(3):184–90.

48. Mazzotta C, Bagaglia SA, Sgheri A, Di Maggio A, Fruschelli M, Romani A, Vinciguerra R, Vinciguerra P, Tosi GM. Iontophoresis corneal cross-linking with enhanced Fluence and pulsed UV-A light: 3-year clinical results. J Refract Surg. 2020;36(5):286–92.
49. Aytekin E, Öztürk N, Vural İ, Polat HK, Çakmak HB, Çalış S, Pehlivan SB. Design of ocular drug delivery platforms and in vitro - in vivo evaluation of riboflavin to the cornea by non-interventional (epi-on) technique for keratoconus treatment. J Control Release. 2020;324:238–49.
50. Lidich N, Garti-Levy S, Aserin A, Garti N. Potentiality of microemulsion systems in treatment of ophthalmic disorders: keratoconus and dry eye syndrome - in vivo study. Colloids Surf B Biointerfaces. 2019;173:226–32.
51. Deshmukh R, Hafezi F, Kymionis GD, Kling S, Shah R, Padmanabhan P, Sachdev MS. Current concepts in crosslinking thin corneas. Indian J Ophthalmol. 2019;67(1):8–15.
52. Hashemi H, Alvani A, Seyedian MA, Yaseri M, Khabazkhoob M, Esfandiari H. Appropriate sequence of combined Intracorneal ring implantation and corneal collagen cross-linking in keratoconus: a systematic review and meta-analysis. Cornea. 2018;37(12):1601–7.
53. Yang X, Liu Q, Feng Q, Lin H. Safety and efficacy of corneal minimized-volume ablation with accelerated cross-linking in improving visual function for keratoconus. Cornea. 2020;39(12):1485–92.
54. Iselin KC, Baenninger PB, Bachmann LM, Bochmann F, Thiel MA, Kaufmann C. Changes in higher order aberrations after central corneal regularization - a comparative two-year analysis of a semi-automated topography-guided photorefractive keratectomy combined with corneal cross-linking. Eye Vis (Lond). 2020;7:10.
55. Kaiserman I, Mimouni M, Rabina G. Epithelial photorefractive keratectomy and corneal cross-linking for keratoconus: the Tel-Aviv protocol. J Refract Surg. 2019;35(6):377–82.
56. Parker JS, van Dijk K, Melles GR. Treatment options for advanced keratoconus: a review. Surv Ophthalmol. 2015;60(5):459–80.
57. Tong CM, van Dijk K, Melles GRJ. Update on Bowman layer transplantation. Curr Opin Ophthalmol. 2019;30(4):249–55.
58. Dapena I, Parker JS, Melles GRJ. Potential benefits of modified corneal tissue grafts for keratoconus: Bowman layer 'inlay' and 'onlay' transplantation, and allogenic tissue ring segments. Curr Opin Ophthalmol. 2020;31(4):276–83.
59. Jin H, He M, Liu H, Zhong X, Wu J, Liu L, Ding H, Zhang C, Zhong X. Small-incision femtosecond laser-assisted Intracorneal concave Lenticule implantation in patients with keratoconus. Cornea. 2019;38(4):446–53.
60. Mastropasqua L, Nubile M, Salgari N, Mastropasqua R. Femtosecond laser-assisted stromal Lenticule addition Keratoplasty for the treatment of advanced keratoconus: a preliminary study. J Refract Surg. 2018;34(1):36–44.
61. Alió Del Barrio JL, El Zarif M, Azaar A, Makdissy N, Khalil C, Harb W, El Achkar I, Jawad ZA, de Miguel MP, Alió JL. Corneal stroma enhancement with Decellularized stromal laminas with or without stem cell Recellularization for advanced keratoconus. Am J Ophthalmol. 2018;186:47–58.

MIX
Papier aus verantwortungsvollen Quellen
Paper from responsible sources
FSC® C105338

If you have any concerns about our products,
you can contact us on
ProductSafety@springernature.com

In case Publisher is established outside the EU,
the EU authorized representative is:
Springer Nature Customer Service Center GmbH
Europaplatz 3, 69115 Heidelberg, Germany

Printed by Libri Plureos GmbH
in Hamburg, Germany